Microbial Biotechnology and Ecology

Volume-2

Microbial Biotechnology and Ecology

Volume-2

Deepak Vyas
G.S. Paliwal
P.K. Khare
R.K. Gupta

2024
Daya Publishing House®
A Division of
Astral International Pvt. Ltd.
New Delhi – 110 002

First Published, 2011

Reprinted, 2024

ISBN: 978-81-7035-694-3 (HB)

Published by : **Daya Publishing House®**
A Division of
Astral International Pvt. Ltd.
– ISO 9001:2015 Certified Company –
4736/23, Ansari Road, Darya Ganj,
New Delhi-110 002
Ph. 011-43549197, 23278134
E-mail: info@astralint.com
Website: www.astralint.com

Printed at : Replika Press Pvt. Ltd.

– Biography –

Late Prof. K.M. Vyas

Born on 19th September, 1942 in village Dharoan then in district Hamirpur and presently in district Mahoba (UP) in the family of Smt Radhika Rani and Sri Rooplal Vyas. Krishna Murari had his primary education in village and for the secondary education he moved to a Tehsil place in Charkhari. He obtained BSc from Maharaja College, Chhatarpur and MSc (Botany) degree from Sagour University, Sagar in 1963. Young Krishna Murari joined as a lecturer in the Botany Department then Sagour University, Sagour now Dr. H.S.G. V.V., Sagar (M.P.). Simultaneously joined PhD programme under the supervision of Prof SB Saksena (FNA), a renowned mycologist of that time. He did his PhD on "*Studies on the Ecology and Physiology of Soil Microorganisms in Relation to Soil Borne Plant Diseases*". For post doctoral work (1973-74), he went to Department of Biochemistry, University of Hull, England (UK). He worked on "*Production and Activity of Cell Wall Degrading Enzymes by Late Blight Fungus–Phytopthora infestens*" with Prof J Friend.

Foreign Visits

Visited and delivered lectures at various important Research Institutions and Universities of England, Scotland, Belgium and Holland, Imperial College of Science and Technology, London, Long Ashton Research Station, Bristol, University of Glasgow, International Agriculture Institute, Wageninghe, Phytopathologic Research Institute Baarn, Holland.

Outstanding Research Contributions

1. Successful control of *Phytophthora* diseases of pan by streptomycin and other antibiotics.
2. Antibiotics as a new group of plant growth regulators.
3. Control of mosquitoes by certain isolates of bacteria and fungi.
4. Fungal pathogenesis of plants with special reference of cell wall degrading enzymes and phenolics in fungal pathogenesis.

5. *Alectra parasitica*: a traditional drug for the treatment of leprosy and other skin diseases.
6. Fungal respiration with special reference to mycelial respiration of plant pathogenic fungi.
7. Rhizosphere, rhizoplane, phyllosphere and phylloplane microflora and their role in plant diseases.

Professor and Head

In August 1984 he became a professor and in the month of October he became Head of the Department. As soon as he assumed the duty of HOD he brought DRS programme from UGC to strengthen the teaching and research facilities. During the period of 17 years of headship he also brought DSA phase I and II, and laid a stone for Cosist (Assistant programme) under SAP programme of UGC.

Prof Vyas established a strong centre of research in Mycology and Microbiology at Sagar. Where he undertook and successfully completed various research projects funding by UGC, CSIR, ICMR etc. He has published his work in various journals of National and International repute. He has edited book "*Recent Advances in Microbiology*". More than 40 students have obtained PhD under his supervision. Many of his students are actively engaged in research work and are occupying prestigious position in country and abroad.

During his tenure department grow, and many learned people from country and abroad visited the department and deliver their talks. He organized many seminars/ symposia/ workshops and refresher courses. Beside his scientific tamper and aptitude he has got administrative skills and proved himself an administrator in various capacities.

Administrative Experiences

1. As Head of the Botany Department. Dr. H.S.G. V.V., Sagar: 17 years (November 1984 to October 2001).
2. As Dean Faculty of Life Science: 4 years (two terms: 1988-90 and 1996-98).
3. As University Proctor: 6 Years (1986-1982).
4. As Chairman Board of Studies in Botany: 6 years (two terms: 1984-87 and 1994-97).
5. As Chief Coordinator of University Examinations: (three terms: 1985-86, 1988-89, and 1994-1995).
6. As Coordinator UGC NET- Exam, December 1996, June 1997, December 1997 and June 1998.
7. As Member of Academic Council Dr. H.S. G. V.V., Sagar: 10 years.
8. As Member of Executive Council; As Dean Faculty of Life Science (1988-90) and as Senior Professor (1996-99).
9. As Member of Central Board of Studies in Botany, Bhopal (MP): 10 years.
10. As Vice Chancellor of Dr. H.S.G. V.V., Sagar on various occasions/ day (during short term leave vacancy).
11. As Programme Coordinator of DRS/ DSA phase I and II programme of UGC in Botany Dr. H.S.G. V.V., Sagar.
12. As Member, Board of Studies, RDC and Selection Committees of various Universities and Colleges: 14 years.
13. As Professor Incharge of Development, Dr. H.S.G. V.V., Sagar: 3 years.

14. As Chairman, Organizing Committee of various symposia and seminars.
15. As Coordinator of Refresher Course in Botany: (1995-1998).
16. As Director Development in Botany: 1 October 2001–30 April 2004.

He was retired on 30th April 2004. He was an amazing personality with strong will power. His fight against Hepatitis B was amazing. After obtaining superannuation from the university he joined as a Principal at Pt. Vasudev Prasad Tiwari Degree College, Jhansi. He worked for the welfare of humanity under the umbrella of Bundelkhand Janseva Samiti, Jhansi.

Prof. Vyas was a great source of inspiration for his students, family members. His untimely death created a vacuum not only in scientific community but also in the family. It is said that there is a woman behind every great man. In this case it is Mrs Urmila Vyas, since 1958 when she was married to Prof KM Vyas. She has sacrificed all her comforts and has taken over all the household responsibilities so that Prof KM Vyas could be free to devote all his time to academics. Any visitor to their home was deeply impressed by their modesty, simplicity and warmth of their hospitability.

The Vyas are a well knit family. They have well educated children. One son and three daughters. Son is Dr Deepak Vyas presently serving in the same Department (Botany), Dr. H.S.G. V.V., Sagar married with Mrs. Nisha Vyas who is lecturer in college and have two sons Siddhant and Vedant studying in school. Among the daughters, elder daughter is Dr Jyoti married with with Dr Sanjay Chaubey, having their own hospital at Jhansi and having two sons Rohan and Kartik, then Mrs Arti married with Sunil Sharma who is working as an area manager in private firm. Arti is lecturer in private college at Bhopal have two kids Shivani and Shreyansh. Younger daughter Mrs Bharti is married with Dr Anand Sharma. Who is working at Cambridge Hospital, London, England.

List of Publications

1. Vyas, A. D. Vyas and K.M. Vyas (2006). Microbial cellulases for Industrial application. Every man's Science XL (6) 411-416.
2. Sharma, C.D., A.N. Rai and K.M. Vyas (2006). An undescribed fungal genus of the forest flora of Madhya Pradesh J. Bot. Soc. Univ. Sagar, 41 : 94-98.
3. Vyas, A., A. Jain, D. Vyas and K. M. Vyas (2005). Production and partial characterization of cellulases by two *Aspergillus* spp. on pretreated low value ligno-cellulases. Proc. Natl. Acad. Sci. India, 75(B) p. 1-7.
4. Vyas, Ashish, D. Vyas and K.M. Vyas (2005). Biodiversity conservation through integrated participatory management J. Bot. Soc. Univ. Sagar, 40 : 178-189.
5. Dwivedi, O. P., R. K. Yadav, D. Vyas and K. M. Vyas (2004). Role of Potassium in the occurrence of VAM spores in the rhizosphre soils of Lantana species. In: Microbiology and Biotechnology for sustainable development. Ed. P.C. Jain, Pp. 248–253. CBS Publishers, New Delhi.
6. Yadav, R.K., O.P.Dwivedi, D. Vyas and K. M. Vyas (2004). Antifungal effect of *Microcystis* against Beetalvine *Phytophthora.* J. Basic and applied Myco. 3(1+2) : 105–107.
7. Vyas Ashish, Vyas Deepak and Vyas K.M. (2004). Production and optimization of cellulases on pretreated groundnut shell by *Aspergillus tenuis* AV49. Journal of Scientific and Industrial Research Vol. 64, Pp. 281-286.
8. Vyas, A., D. Vyas and K.M. Vyas (2004). Cellulolytic strains of *Aspergillu* and *Penicillium.* J. Bot.Soc.Univ. Sagar 39 66-71.

9. Yadav, R.K., O.P. Dwivedi, D. Vyas and K.M. Vyas (2003). Management of *Phytophthora* disease of betel vine by plant extracts J. Basic and Applied Mycol. 2 (1) : 79-82.
10. Agrawal, R., A.N. Rai and K.M. Vyas (2003). A new species of *Tretospora* from India. J. Basic and Applied Mycol. 2 (1) 48-49.
11. Soni, Anuradha, D. Vyas and K.M. Vyas (2003). Effect of VAM fungi on the growth and productivity of Soybean (*Glycine max.*) J. Basic and Applied Mycol. 2 (1) : 40-41.
12. Vyas, Ashish, D. Vyas and K.M. Vyas (2003). Screening of extra-cellular cellulase producing fungi from different lignocellulosic wastes. J. Basic and Applied Mycol. 2 (1) : 14-16.
13. Khare, N. and Vyas K.M. (2003). Effect of nitrogen sources on the production of pectolytic and cellulytic enzymes by *Rhizopus nodosus* and *Phytophthora nicotiana* J. Bot Soc. Univ. Sagar 36 : 87-94.
14. Dwivedi, O.P., R.K. Yadav, D. Vyas and K.M. Vyas (2002). Distribution of VAM fungi in the rhizosphere soils of Betel vine J. Phytopathol. 56 (2) : 228-229.
15. Dwivedi, O.P., Yadav, R.K., Vyas, D. and Vyas, K.M. (2002). Vesicular-Arbuscular Mycorrhizal Association with *Lantana* sp. In Sagar University Campus; in Different Disordered Systems INDIAS 2000. (eds) K. Fukawa, J.T. Watson, S.N. Saxena and S.K. Shrivastava, pp. 154-157. INDIAS Publication, Allahabad.
16. Vyas, D., O.P. Dwevedi, R.K. Yadav and K.M. Vyas (2002). Arbuscular Diversity of VAM Fungi. In frontiers of fungal diversity in India. (Eds.) G.P. Rao, C. Manoharachari, D.J. Bhat, R.C. Rajak and T.N. Lakhanpal pp. 873-889. International Book Distributing Company Lucknow, India.
17. Singh, N., Vyas, D., Gupta, U.S. and Vyas, K.M (1999). Physico-chemical properties of Sagar lake with special reference to *Microcystis* bloom in the proceeding of the New Millenium Conference on Retrospect of Indian Research on Environmental Pollution : Focus 21st Century, 38.
18. Sharma, C.D., Gadpandey, K.K., Firdousi, S.A., Rai, A.N. and Vyas, K.M. (1998). Three New species of *Cladosporium* from Madhya Pradesh, India. Indian Phytopath. 51 (2): 152-160.
19. Chaursia, J.P., Chaurasia, P. and Vyas, K.M. (1997). Effect of *Ocimum sanctum* leaf extract on betelvine *Phytophthora* disease; An ecofriendly new approach. Environment pollution in 21 Century (Ed). V.S. Bais. Narendra Publishing House, Delhi, p. 46-51.
20. Chaurasia, J.P. and Vyas, K.M (1997). *In vivo* evaluation of some homoeopathic drugs against betelvine *Phytophthora* disease, Indian Phytopath. 4:148-153.
21. Vyas, K.M., Chaurasia, J.P. and Mishra, A.S. (1996). Effect of hepar sulphate on betelvine *Phytopathora* disease. Madhya Bharti Journal, Dr HS Gour Vishwavidyalaya, Sagar, India 36A 40B: 65-71.
22. Vyas, K.M. and Firdousi, S.A. (1996). Leaf blight of *Terminalia tomentosa.* Indian Phytopathology (Accepted).
23. Vyas, K.M., Gadpandey, K.K., Sharma, C.D., Firdousi, S.A. and Rai, A.N. (1996). Two new Hyphomycetes from India. Mycological Research (Accepted).
24. Vyas, K.M., Sharma, C.D., Gadpandey, K.K., Rai, A.N. and Firdousi, S.A. (1996). Three new species of *Cladosporium* from Madhya Pradesh. Indian Phytopathological Society IARI, New Delhi (In press).

25. Vyas KM, Dubey MP and Sharma RS (1995). Low cost agronomic practice for soybean (*Glycine max*) cultivation in Madhya Pradesh. Indian Journal of Agriculture Sciences 65(10):743-745.

26. Vyas KM, Kumar R and Rai AN (1995). Two new *Alternaria* species from Uttar Pradesh. Acta Botanica Indica 23 (1): 151-153.

27. Vyas KM and Firdousi SA (1994). A new leaf spot disease of *Casearia tomentosa* caused by *Asteromella* species. Acta Botanica Indica 20: 120-121.

28. Vyas KM and Saxena AP (1993). Antimicrobial activity of *Alectra parasitica,* A rice var. *chitrakutensis* rau. Journal of Economic and Taxonomic Botany 17 (1) 55-59.

29. Vyas KM, Firdousi SA and Rai AN (1993). A new species of *Stenella* from India. Acta Botanica Indica 25: 131-132.

30. Vyas KM and Firdousi SA (1993). A new spot of *Miliusa tomentosa* Roxb. Acta Botanica Indica 21 (1): 124.

31. Vyas KM and Mehta A (1992). Degradation of plant tissues by fungal enzymes. In: Dubey NK and Sharma PD, Rastogi Publications, Meerut, India.

32. Vyas KM, Firdousi SA and Rai AN (1992). A new species of *Pseudocercospora* from India. Indian Phytopathology 45(4): 449-451.

33. Vyas KM, Firdousi SA and Rai AN (1992). A new species of *Pseudocercospora* from India. Acta Botanica Indica.

34. Vyas KM, Firdousi SA and Rai AN (1992). *Mycovellosiella adinae* Sp nov. from India. Indian Phytopathology 45(4): 451-452.

35. Vyas KM (1990). A new leaf spot disease of *Ficus begalensis* caused by *Coniothyrium olivaceum* from India. Acta Botanica Indica 1: 150.

36. Vyas KM, Firdousi SA and Rai NA (1990). *Pseudocercospora gymnosporinae* sp. nov. India. Mycological Research (UK in press).

37. Vyas KM, Firdousi SA and Rai NA (1990). A new host record of *Thielvia appendiculata* from India. Indian Phytopath 43(1): 124.

38. Vyas KM, Firdousi SA and Rai NA (1990). A new leaf spot disease of *Eleodendron glaucum* from India. Indian Phytopath 43(1): 122.

39. Vyas KM and Gupta DK (1989). Efficacy of *Bacillus subtilis* against Mosquito larvae (*Anophelis culicifacies*). Zeitschrift Fur Angewandte Zoologie (German Journal for Applied Zoology) 85-91.

40. Vyas KM and Chile SK (1989). Metabolism of ascorbic acid and *Piper betle* leaves under *Phytopathora* pathogenesis. Perspective in Mycological Research 1: 143-150.

41. Vyas KM and Tripathi HSS (1986). Production of toxin by *Xanthomaonas compestris* pv *betticola* causing leaf spot disease of *Piper betle* L. Acta Botanica Indica 14: 220-225.

42. Vyas KM and Saxena NK (1986). Microbial synthesis of 11-deoxy corticosteron from progesterone by a nutant of *Rhizophus nodosus* (Abst.) XIV International Congress of Microbiology: Menchester, England 7-13 September.

43. Vyas KM and Chile SK (1985). Electrolyte leakage from *Piper betle* leaves after infection with *Phytopathora parasitica* var *piperina*. Indian Phytopathology 38 (3): 529-530.

44. Vyas KM and Tripathi HSS (1985). Production of cellulolytic enzymes by *Xanthomonas compestris* pv *betticola*: *in vivo* and *in vitro*. Bull Bot. Soc. 33.

45. Vyas KM, Tripathi HSS, Saxena NK and Sadique Y (1985). Efficacy of hydroxyl stilbamidine isethionate USP against *Phytopathora parasitica* var *piperina*. Phytopathora Newsletters 13: 32-33.

46. Vyas KM, Saxena NK, Tripathi HSS and Sadique Y (1985). Complete control of *Phytopathora parasitica* var *piperina* by S-flurocytosine. Phytopathora News Letters 13: 30-31.

47. Vyas KM, Dubey GL and Dubey O (1985). Physico-chemical properties of linseed oil as affected by various seed borne fungi. Phytopath. z. 113: 66-70.

48. Vyas KM and Chile SK (1984). Efficacy of *Vinca rosea* extracts against protease from human pathogenic strain of *Trichophytom rubrum* sab. Hindustan Antibiotics Bull. 26: 114-116.

49. Vyas KM, Kher AK and Saxena SB (1984). Persistence of various fungicides in soil. Indian Phytopath 27(3): 574-576.

50. Vyas KM and Shrivastava A (1984). Effect of cholesterol on the toxicity of certain antibiotics against betelvine *Phytopathora*. Phytopathora News Letter 12 pp. 33.

51. Vyas KM, Soni, Saxena NK and Tripathi HSS (1984). Decline in the total reducing sugar content during the postharvest infection of *Lycopersicon lycopersicum* L. Karsgen fruits by *Bacillus fructodrestruens*. Bull Bot. Soc. 30-31: 69-71.

52. Vyas KM, Saxena NK and Tripathi HSS (1984). Cationic degradation of Streptomycine and Kanemycine by *Aspergillus niger* in broth cultures during fragmentation in shade flask. Hindustan Antibiotics Bulletin 26 (3 and 4) pp. 96-101.

53. Chile SK, Vyas KM and Singh R (1984). Induced resistance in *Piper betle* leaves in relation to *Phytopathora parasitica* var. *piperina*. Indian Phytopath. 37: 719-721.

54. Chile SK and Vyas KM (1984). Inhibitors of certain enzymes of *Botrydiplodia theobromae* in *Piper betle* leaf extract. Hindustan Antibiotics Bull. 26: 27-32.

55. Vyas KM and Chile SK (1984). Respiratory response of betlevine *Phytopathora* induced by various volatile oils. Jr Mycology Plant Path.

56. Vyas KM, Saxena NK and Tripathi HSS (1984). Accumulation of D.L. 3,4 dihydroxy-phenyalanine during the soft rot of *Lycopersicon esculentum* fruits caused by *Bacillus fructodestruens*. Abst. 36th Ann. Meeting Indian Phytopath (Hissar) 37: 401.

57. Vyas KM, Saxena NK and Tripathi HSS (1984). Postharvest accumulation of vitamin C induced by *Bacillus fructodestruens* in the *Lycopersicon esculentum* fruits. Abst. 36th Ann. Meeting Indian Phytopath, Hissar and paper published in Nat. Acad. Sci. Letters 7(4): 109-110.

58. Vyas KM and Shrivastava A (1984). Chemical control of betelvine *Phytopathora*. Abst. Symp. Chemical Control of Plant Disease. Indian Phytopath, Hissar.

59. Vyas KM and Singh R (1984). Nitrogen nutrition of *Phytopathora parasitica* var *piperina* (Dast) causing foot and leaf rot disease of *Piper betle* Linn. Proc. 71st Ind. Sci. Cong. Part III Abstract, 57: 26.

60. Vyas KM and Atri DC (1983). Pectolytic and cellulolytic activity during pathogenesis caused by *Botryodiplodia theobromae* Pat. In *Pyrus pyrifolia* Burm. fruits. Abst National Acad. Sci. (Biol.) Abst. No. 257 pp. 94.

61. Vyas KM and Chile SK (1983). Free amino acids in relation to *Phytopthora* leaf rot pathogenesis of Pan. Indian Phytopath 36(4): 626-628.

62. Vyas KM and Chile SK (1983). Dehydrogenase activity in *Piper betle* L. leaves infected with *Phytopathora parasitica* var. *piperina*. Indian Phytopath 36(4): 613-617.

63. Vyas KM and Sxena N (1983). Effect of antibiotics on certain cell wall degrading enzymes of *Rhizopus nodosus* and *Phytopathora nitotianae*. Hindustan Antibiotics Bulletin 25 (1 and 2) pp. 21-24.

64. Vyas KM and Shrivastava A (1983). In vitro efficacy of tetracycline against betelvine *Phytopathora*. Hindustan Antibiotics Bulletin 25 (1 and 2) pp. 15-17.

65. Vyas KM and Saxena AP (1983). Ethnobotany of Dhasan valley. Jr. of Econ. Tax. Bot., Jodhpur.

66. Vyas KM and Saxena AP (1983). Traditional treatment of leprosy and leucoderma by tribals from Bundelkhand UP. Bull. of Medico Ethn. Bot. Res. CCRAS, New Delhi.

67. Vyas KM and Thakur MS (1983). Production of plant growth regulators by some *Fusarium* species. Folia Microbial. 28: 124-129.

68. Vyas KM, Gupta DK and Shrivastava A (1983). In vitro antibacterial properties of some fixed oils. Proc 70th Ind. Sci Cong. Assoc 29.

69. Vyas, Chile SK and Shrivastava A (1982). Efficacy of some growth hormones on sporulation of betelvine *Phytopathora*. Bull. Bot. Soc. Univ. Saugar 29: 25-27.

70. Chile SK and Vyas KM (1982). Efficiency of carboxin in relation to *Phytopathora* leaf rot of *Piper betle*. Abstract 1st National Symposium of Synthetic Fungicides in Plant Disease Control in IARI, June 1982.

71. Chile SK, Vyas KM and Vyas RS (1982). Effect of culture filtrate of various fungi on sporulation of betelvine *Phytopathora*. Hind. Ant. Bull. 23: 25-26.

72. Chile SK and Vyas KM (1982). Effect of culture filtrate of various fungi on acidative enzymes of betelvine *Phytopathora*. Hind. Ant. Bull. 24: 26-28.

73. Vyas KM, Gupta DK and Chile SK (1982). A fruit rot disease of Momardiaca. Indian Phytopath 35(2): 351.

74. Vyas KM and Gupta DK (1982). Biological control of mosquito. IX Annual Conference of Indian Society of Human Genetics, Bhopal 58.

75. Vyas KM and Gupta DK (1982). Effect of *Aspergillus* mycotoxin on *Culex* larvae. Proc 69th Ind. Sci. Cong. Asso. Abstract 61.

76. Vyas KM and Thomas T (1982). On the abundance of *Trichoderma* species in the soil of Andaman and Nicobar Islands. Proc 69th Ind. Sci. Cong. Asso. Abstract 59.

77. Vyas KM and Saxena N (1982). Pectolytic enzymes of *Rhizopus nodosus* and *Phytopathora nictianae* in relation to electrolyte leakage and tissue maceration. Proc 69th Ind. Sci. Cong. Asso. Abstract 44.

78. Vyas KM and Saxena AP (1982). In vitro antimicrobial activity of some medicinal plants against human pathogens. Proc 69th Ind. Sci. Cong. Asso. Pt. III: 43-44.

79. Vyas KM, Singh R and Chile SK (1982). Nitrogen nutrition of *Phytopathora parasitica* var *piperina* (Dast) Causing foot rot and leaf rot diseases of *Piper betle* Linn. Jur. Biol. Res.

80. Vyas KM (1982). Peroxiodase and catalases in relation to betelvine. Phytopathora News Letters, USA 10: 8.

81. Vyas KM and Chile SK (1982). Breakdown of disease resistance in betelvine *Phytopathora* system by vitamin C. Phytopathora News Letters, USA 10: 6-7.
82. Vyas KM and Thakur MS (1982). Plant growth regulatory metabolites produced by fungi. Abstract Symp. Fermented Foods, Food Contaminants, Biofertlizers and Bioenergy pp. 54.
83. Vyas KM and Thoimas T (1982). *Gliocladium virens*- A new report from India. Geobios News reports 1: 45.
84. Vyas KM and Saxena AP (1981). *Martynia annua* Linn. A drug for Asthma, Itch and Eczema. Bull of Medico. Ethno Bot. Res. CCRAS, New Delhi II (3): 427- 429.
85. Vyas KM (1981). Problem and progress in *Phytopathora* diseases of Pan group discussion on improvement of betelvine cultivation. NBRI, Lucknow p 92-93.
86. Vyas KM, Thomas T and Gupta DK (1981). *Gilmaniella subornate*: A new report from India. Bull. Bot. Soc. Univ. of Saugar 28: 38.
87. Vyas KM, Thomas T and Gupta DK (1981). *Trichoderma pseudo-konningii* Rifai: A new report from India. Bull. Bot. Soc. Univ. of Saugar 28: 28.
88. Vyas KM (1981). Effect of culture filtrates of various fungi on sporulation of betelvine *Phytopathora*. Hind. Antibiot. Bot. 23: 25-26.
89. Vyas KM, Chourasia SC and Saxena SB (1981). Management of *Phytopathora* diseases of Pan (*Piper betle*). Abst. 3rd International Symposium on Plant Pathology (IPS) pp. 253.
90. Chile SK and Vyas KM (1981). Polyphenol oxidase in relation to betelvine *Phytopathora* pathogenesis of Pan. Phytopathora News Letters, USA 9: 40-41.
91. Vyas KM and Saxena AP (1981). Medicinal plants of Bundelkhand I.P preliminary ethnobotanical survey of Banda district UP. Proc. 68th Ind. Sci. Cong. Pt III (Abst): 147.
92. Vyas KM and Saxena AP (1981). Flora of Bundelkhand II. Hydrophytic tract of Ken-Baghain tract (Banda district UP). Ind. Soc. Weed. Sci. Abst: 40-41.
93. Vyas KM and Saxena AP (1981). Ethnobotanical records on infectious diseases from tribals of Banda district (UP). Ind. Soc. Weed. Sci. Abst: 40-41.
94. Vyas KM and Gupta DK (1981). Biological control of mosquitoes: I Effect of culture filtrate of certain *Aspergilli* on Anopheles larvae. Proc. 51 Session Nat. Acad. Sci.: 51.
95. Vyas KM and Chile SK (1981). Effect of the age of betel vine leaves on phenolics and *Phytopathora* rot. Ind. Sci. Cong.
96. Chile SK, Chourasia and Vyas KM (1981). Role of cuttings on the growth of the betel vine *Phytopathora*. Phytopathora News Letters, USA 8: 31.
97. Vyas KM and Chile SK (1980). Role of polyphenol oxidase in disease resistance with special reference to the betel vine *Phytopathora*. Symp. Plant Disease Problem at PAU, Ludhiana (Punjab) Abstract IIX.
98. Vyas KM, Chile SK and Saraf M (1980). Effect of some fungicides on sporulation of different isolates of betel vine *Phytopathora*. Bull. Bot. Univ. of Saugar, Sagar (MP) 27 pp. 16-18.
99. Vyas KM, Chourasia SC and Chile SK (1980). Role of infested soil and cuttings on the spread of betel vine *Phytopathora*. Phytopathora News Letters, USA 8: 28.
100. Vyas KM and Chile SK (1980). Role of infested soil and cuttings on the spread of betel vine *Phytopathora*. Symp. on Phytopathora Diseases of Tropical Plants (Calicut) pp. 22.

101. Vyas KM and Chile SK (1980). Varietal reaction of *Piper betle* leaves against different isolates of betel vine *Phytopathora*. Phytopathora News Letters, USA 8: 29.

102. Vyas KM, Chile SK and Vyas RS (1980). Two new diseases of cultivated plants. Indian Phytopath. 33(3): 493-495.

103. Vyas KM and Gupta M (1979). Studies on cell wall degrading enzymes in relation to banana fruit rot. Indian Phytopath. 32: 456- 457.

104. Vyas KM, Raghvan U and Saxena SB (1979). Studies on amino acid composition of mycelia of 14 of *Botryodiplodia theobromae* Pat. Bull. Bot. Soc. Univ. Saugar, 23-24: 21-25.

105. Vyas KM and Thakur MS (1979). Production of indole auxins by *Curvularia* spp. Abst. 66th Sess. Ind. Sci. Cong. p. 38.

106. Vyas KM and Dubey GL (1979). Physico-chemical properties of linseed oil as affected by various seed borne fungi. Abst. 66th Sess. Ind. Sci. Cong. p. 15.

107. Vyas KM and Saxena AP (1979). Flora of Bundelkhand I, A contribution to grasses of Banda and Hamirpur districts (UP). Bull. Bot. Soc. Univ. of Saugar, Sagar 25-26: 73-78.

108. Vyas KM and Chourasia SC (1979). Efficacy of certain antibiotics against betel vine *Phytopathora*. Phytopathora News Letters, USA 7: 28.

109. Vyas KM and Chourasia SC (1979). Leaf spot, a new disease of bakoli (*Mimusops elengi*) in Sagar, India 63: 806.

110. Vyas KM and Chourasia SC (1979). Oxidative metabolism under *Phytopathora* leaf rot pathogenesis of Pan. Phytopathora News Letters, USA 7: 27.

111. Vyas KM (1978). Effects of fungicides on the growth of *Phytopathora parasitica* var. *piperina* causing foot rot and leaf rot diseases of Pan. Proc. Nat. Acad. Sc. (Allahabad) 47 (B) III: 141-144.

112. Vyas KM and Chourasia SC (1978). Formation of cospores in vivo by *Phytopathora parasitica* var. *piperina*. Phytopathora News Letters USA, Feb. 1978, No. 6 pp. 42-43.

113. Vyas KM and Chourasia SC (1978). Leaf surface mycoflora in relation to *Phytopathora* leaf rot on Pan (*Piper betle*). Phytopathora News Letters USA, Feb. 1978, No. 6 pp. 40-41.

114. Vyas KM and Chourasia SC (1978). Host parasite interactions in betelvine *Phytopathora* varietal response to leaf rot pathogenesis. Phytopathora News Letters USA, Feb. 1978, No. 6 pp. 38-39.

115. Vyas KM (1978). Effect of fungal metabolites on the growth ot morphogenesis of crop plants. Abst. Ibid. pp. 43.

116. Vyas KM (1978). Studies on the molds and mycotoxins with special reference to mycoflora associated with the grains of jowar. Abst. All India Symposium on Physiology of Parasitism Jabalpur. pp. 20.

117. Vyas KM, Kazmi SM and Soni NK (1978). Studies on the antifungal properties of mamalian urine. Agriculture and Agro Industries Jur.

118. Chourasia SC, Vyas KM and Pathak RK (1977). In vitro inhibitory effects of certain fungicides in the growth of *Phytopathora parasitica* var. *piperina* causing foot rot and leaf rot diseases of Pan (*Piper betel* Linn.) Proc. Nat. Acad. Sci. Ind. 47(B) III: 141-144.

119. Vyas KM and Chourasia SC (1977). Effect of fungicides on the oxidative metabolism of *Phytopathora parasitica* var. *piperina* (Dast.) causing foot rot and leaf rot diseases of Pan (*Piper*

betel) in physiology of microorganism edited by KS Bilgrami Todays and Tomorrow Printers and Publishers, New Delhi 11-16.

120. Vyas KM and Jain SK (1977). Production of auxin like plant growth regulatory metabolites by soil fungi. In: physiology of microorganisms (Edited by KS Bilgrami), Todays and Tomorrow Printers and Publishers, New Delhi 331-340.

121. Vyas KM, Thind TS and Prakash V (1977). Effect of some antibiotics on the germination of coraınder seeds. Ind Jr. of Exp. Biol. Vol. 15, No. 3, March 77 pp. 247-248.

122. Vyas KM and Chourasia SC (1977). In vitro effect of some volatile oils against *Phytopathora parasitica* var. *piperina*. Jr. Res. Ind. Med. Yoga and Homoeo. 12:3. 139-142.

123. Vyas KM and Chourasia SC (1977). The influence of age and starvation on endogenous respiration of mycelium of *Phytopathora parasitica* var. *piperina*. Acta Botanica Indica 5: 54-57, 77.

124. Vyas KM (1976). Respiratory characterstics of plant pathogenic fungi, *Ibid*.

125. Vyas KM (1976). Production of cell wall degrading enzymes by *Botryodiplodia theobromae*, *Ibid*.

126. Vyas KM (1976). Microbial metabolites and plant growth promoting activity of some antifungal antibiotic compounds, *Ibid*.

127. Vyas KM (1976). Microbial metabolites and plant growth production of indole auxins by soil fungi, *Ibid*.

128. Vyas KM (1976). Effect of fungicides on the oxidative metabolism of *Phytopathora parasitica* var. *piperina* (Dast) causing foot rot and leaf rot of Pan (*Piper betle*). In: Physiology of Microorganisms (Edited by KS Bilgrami), Today and Tomorrow Publications pp. 11-16.

129. Vyas KM (1976). Interactions of soil microorganisms with *Phytopathora parasitica* var. *piperina*. Abst. Symp. on Physiology of Microorganisms held at Bhagalpur Feb. 1976.

130. Vyas KM and Chourasia SC (1976). Activity of some volatile oils against *Phytopathora parasitica* var. *piperina*. Indian Drugs Jan 9-15.

131. Vyas KM and Chourasia SC (1976). Influence of culture media on fungal respiration. Hind. Antibiot. Bull. Vol. 18: 3 and 4.

132. Vyas KM and Mehta P (1975). Effect of plat growth regulators on production and activity of cellulase. Ind. J. Exptl. Biol. Vol 14, 206-208.

133. Vyas KM and Chourasia SC (1975). Studies on leaf rot of Pan (*Piper betle*) varietal factors in relation to disease resistance. Symp. on Plant Pathlogical problems held at Udaipur 5(1): 10-11.

134. Vyas KM, Mehta P and Saxena SB (1975). Pathological studies of fruit rot diseases of tamato caused by *Alternaria solani* and *A. tenuis*. Indian Phytopath. Vol. XXVIII No 2, 247-252.

135. Vyas KM, Mehta P and Saxena SB (1975). Metabolic changes during pathogenesis of tomato fruit rot diseases. Indian Phytopath. Vol. XXVIII No 2, 253-255.

136. Vyas KM and Soni NK (1975). Effect of antibiotics and fungicides on the mycelial respiration and growth of *Rhizoctonia capsici*. Ind. Jr. Exptl. Biol. Vol. 13, pp. 216-218.

137. Vyas KM, Mehta P and Saxena SB (1975). Production of pectolytic enzymes by *Alternaria* sp. of various culture media. J. Ind. Bot. Soc. 200-206.

138. Vyas KM and Soni NK (1975). Responses of *Rhizotonia solani* Kuhn and *Colletotrichum capsici* (Syd.) Butler and Bisby to various chemical substances. Madhya Bharti Univ. Sagar, Vol. 22-23 pp. 43-48.

139. Vyas KM, Mehta P and Saxena SB (1975). Effect of native carbon sources and pH on the cellulolytic enzymes of *Alternaria solani* and *A. tenuis*. Science and Culture Vol. 41 pp. 400-402.

140. Vyas KM and Chourasia SC (1975). Effect of vitamins on the mycelial growth of *Phytopathora parasitica* var. *piperina*. Madhya Bharti, vol. 22 and 23 pp. 63-65.

141. Vyas KM and Soni NK (1975). Respiratory response of *Gleosporium papayae* induced by various substances. Proc. Ind. Sci. Acad. Vol. 41, Part B. No. 5 pp. 458-461.

142. Vyas KM, Saxena RK and Saxena SB (1974). Physiology of *Tectona grandis* leaves infected with *Uncinula ţectonae*. J. Indian Bot. Soc. 53: 256-270.

143. Vyas KM, Jain SK and Raghvan P (1974). Microbial metabolites and plant growth: Plant growth regulatory activity of culture filtrates of soil microorganisms and some antibiotic compounds. Abst. Symp. on Biology of Soil Microorganisms, Sagar pp. 35-36.

144. Vyas KM, Mehta P and Saxena SB (1974). Metabolic changes during pathogenesis of fruit rot diseases of tomato. MP Vigyan Acad. Bhopal Abst. pp. 7-8.

145. Vyas KM, Saxena SB and Soni NK (1974). Effect of antibiotics and fungicides on endogenous mycelial respiration and growth of *Rhizoctonia solani* Kuhn. and *Colletotrichum capsici* (Syd.) Butler and Bisby. MP Vigyan Acad. Bhopal Abst. pp. 5-6.

146. Vyas KM, Mehta P and Saxena SB (1974). Production of pectolytic and cellulolytic enzymes by *Alternaria* sp. during pathogenesis of tomato fruits. Hind. Antibiot. Bull. Vol. 16, No. 4 pp. 20-214.

147. Vyas KM, Mehta P and Saxena SB (1974). Effect of native carbon sources and pH on the pectolytic enzymes of *Alternaria* sp. during pathogenesis of tomato fruits. Hind. Antibiot. Bull. Vol. 40 Part B, No. 4 pp. 433-439.

148. Vyas KM, Pandey P and Soni NK (1974). Effect of antibiotics on endogenous mycelial respiration and growth of some plant pathogenic fungi. Hind. Antibiot. Bull. Vol. 16: 199-201.

149. Vyas KM and Soni NK (1973). Effect of the age of culture and starvation period on mycelial respiration. Bull. Bot. Soc., Univ. Saugar, Vol. 20 pp. 17-20.

150. Vyas KM and Saxena SB (1973). Studies on mycelial respiration of *Sclerotium rolfsii*. Proc. Ind. Nat. Acad. Vol. 39 Part B No. 5 569-575.

151. Vyas KM, Raghvan P and Jain SK (1973). Auxins like activity of the antibiotic aureofungin. Ḥind. Antibiot. Bull. Vol. 16 No 1 pp. 29-31.

152. Vyas KM and Jain SK (1973). Production of auxins by microorganisms. Hind. Antibiot. Bull. Vol. 11, pp 217-219.

153. Vyas KM and Soni NK (1973). Respiratory and growth responses of *Fusarium oxysporum* Sacc. induced by various substances. Ind J. Exptl. Biol. Vol. 11 pp. 217-219.

154. Vyas KM, Chourasia SC and Soni NK (1973). Efficiency of certain antibiotics against *Phytopathora parasitica* var. *piperina* causing leaf rot of Pan. Hind. Antibiot. Bull. Vol. 16 No. 1 pp. 4-8.

155. Vyas KM and Soni NK (1973). Effect of antifungal antibiotics on endogenous mycelial respiration of *Rhizoctonia solani*. Hind. Antibiot. Bull. Vol. 15, pp. 160-163.

156. Vyas KM, Raghavan P and Jain SK (1973). Synergistic interaction of cloremphenicol and IAA on the growth of *Avena* coleoptile sections. Hind. Antibiot. Bull. Vol. 15, pp. 81-83.

157. Vyas KM and Mishra AS (1972). Production of P-proline by soil microorganisms. Hind. Antibiot. Bull. Vol. 15 No 1 and 2 pp. 30-33.

158. Vyas KM, Soni NK and Saxena SB (1972). Effect of culture of various fungi on the mycelial respiration of *Fusarium oxysporum* Sacc. Hind. Antibiot. Bull. Vol. 14, pp. 179-180.

159. Vyas KM, Saxena SB and Jain BK (1972). Respiratory characteristics of some soil borne plant pathogenic fungi. J. Ind. Bot. Soc. 51: 92-96.

160. Vyas KM and Mehta P (1972). Control of fruit rot of tomatoes by phenolics and fungicides. Bull. Bot. Soc., Univ. Saugar, Vol. 19 pp. 35-37.

161. Vyas KM and Dubey GL (1972). Effect of plant growth regulators on the growth of *Sclerotium rolfsii*. Bull. Bot. Soc., Univ. Saugar, Vol. 19 pp. 35-37.

162. Vyas KM, Saxena SB and Soni SK (1972). Effect of plant growth regulators on oxygen uptake and growth of *Rhizoctonia solani* Kuhn and *Colletotrihum capsici* (Syd.) Butler and Bisby. Bull. Bot. Soc., Univ. Saugar, Vol. 19 pp. 24-27.

163. Vyas KM and Mehta P (1970-71). Production of cellulose and mycelial growth of *Alternaria solani* and *A. tenuis*. Bull. Bot. Soc., Univ. Saugar, Vol. 17 and 18 pp. 71-72.

164. Vyas KM and Soni NK (1970-71). Respiratory characteristics of mycelium of *Gleosporium papaya* P. Henn. Bull. Bot. Soc., Univ. Saugar, Vol. 17 and 18 pp. 48-50.

165. Vyas KM, Soni NK and Mishra AS (1970-71). Respiratory characteristics of *Gleosporium* infected papaya fruits in relation to disease development. Bull. Bot. Soc., Univ. Saugar, Vol. 17 and 18 pp. 48-50.

166. Vyas KM, Saxena SB and Atri DC (1970-71). Production of amino acids by soil fungi. Bull. Bot. Soc., Univ. Saugar, Vol. 17 and 18 pp. 31-34.

167. Vyas KM and Saxena SB (1962-64). The wood decaying fungi of Sagar. Madhya Bharti, Vol. 11-13 pp. 15-28.

List of Ph.D. Awarded Under the Supervision of Prof. K.M. Vyas

1. Mehta, Pradeep 1974. "Biochemical Investigations of Fruit-Rot Diseases of Tomatoes."
2. Jain, Satish Kumar 1975. "Studies on the Microbial Production of Auxins".
3. Chourasia, Shiv Charan 1976. "Studies on the Foot-Rot and Leaf-Rot Diseases of Pan (*Piper betle* L.) with Special Reference to Pathogenesis and Control Measures".
4. Raghavan (alias) Srinivasan, Parvati 1976. "Physiological Studies on the Effect of Antibiotics on Plants with Special Reference to their Growth Regulatory Effects"
5. Mishra, Jayendra Kumar 1979. Biochemical Studies on Some *Botryodiplodia* Rot with Special Reference to Cell-Wall Degrading Enzymes".
6. Arti, Dinesh Chandra 1980. "Study of Fruit-Rot Disease of *Pyrus pyrifolia* Caused by *Botryodiplodia theobromae*".
7. Dubey, Guljari Lal 1980."Fungal Succession in Relation to the Bio-deterioration of Linseed".

8. Thakur, Munna Singh 1981. "Studies on the Metabolities of Some Microorganisms and their Effects on Plant Growth".
9. Jain, Maya (nee) Singhai, Maya 1982. "Studies on Plant Growth Regulatory Activities of Certain Antibiotics".
10. Saxena, Neeraj 1982. "Studies on Cell Wall Degrading Enzymes in Relation to Fungal Pathogenesis".
11. Thomas, Thankamma 1982. "Studies on the Soil Fungi of the Andaman and Nicobar Islands".
12. Chiele, Satish Kumar 1983. "Studies on Host–Parasite Relationship with Special Reference to Betel–Vine *Phytopathora*".
13. Saxena, Anand Prakash 1983. "Studies on Some Medicinal Plants of Bundelkhand Region with Special Reference to their Antimicrobial Activity".
14. Gupta, Deepak Kumar 1984. "Studies on the Microbiological Control of Mosquito, Causing Malaria".
15. Shrivastava, Anjali 1985. "Studies on the Efficacy of Certain Antibiotics Against Betel-Vine *Phytopathora*".
16. Katare, Daya Shanker 1987. "Genetic Analysis of Metric and Quality Attributes in Tomato".
17. Saxena, Nitin Kumar 1987. "Microbial Transformation of Steroids".
18. Tripathi, Hari Har Sharran 1987. "Study on the Production and Activity of Toxic Metabolites by Certain Bacterial and Fungal Pathogens of *Piper betle* L".
19. Sadiq, Yasmin 1989. "Studies on the Role of Phenolic Compounds in Disease Resistance in Plants (with special reference to Betel-vine *Phytopathora*)".
20. Shrama, Pratap Bhanu 1991. "Study on the Effect of Cultural and Chemical Control Systems of Kharif Weeds in Tawa Command Area".
21. Firdousi, Shakeel Ahamad 1992. "Studies on the Fungal Disease of Some Important Forest Plant with Special Reference to the Foliage Diseases".
22. Sediq, Roohi 1992. "Studies on the Effect of Certain Factors on the Forest Vegetation of Sagar".
23. Tewari, Prem Narayan 1992. "Studies on Yield, Oil and Protein Content of Soybean as Affected by Fertility Levels, Different Stages of Sowing and Plant Density".
24. Malaiya, Ku. Seema 1992. "Antimicrobial Evaluation of Certain Medicinal Plants of Ethnobotanical-Importance".
25. Dubey, Mahadev Prasad 1993. "Effect of Soil Tilth Seed Inoculation and Sowing Methods on Growth and Yield of Soybean".
26. Goswami, Ravi Prakash 1994. "Studies on the Effect of Volatile Fungistatic Factors on Fungal Morphogenesis".
27. Dixit, Ashwini Kumar 1995. "Ethno-medicinal, Photochemical and Anti-microbial Studies of Some Medicinal Plants of Sagar District".
28. Chourasia, J.P. 1995. "Studies on the Management of Betalvine *Phytopathora* Diseases in Sagar".
29. Sharma, C.D. 1995. "Folicolus Fungal from the Forest Flora of M.P. with Special Reference to Deuteromycotina".

30. Goswami, Sita Ram 1995. "Response of Different Levels of Phosphetic Fertilizers and their Methods of Application on Growth Parameters Productivity and Quality of Soybean".
31. Malaiya, Manju 1998. "Studies on Antimicrobial Activity of Some Indian Traditional Remedies (Ethnomedicinal plants)".
32. Mishra, Avanish 1998. "Studies on the Biology of Some Ethno-medicinal Plants of Sagar Region".
33. Kaushal, A.K. 1998. "Role of Irrigation Schedule on Productivity of Sunflower".
34. Sthapak Smt. Madhu 2000. "Studies on the Fungal Diseases of Potato Under Storage Conditions at Sagar".
35. Nema Ku. Shushma 2000. "Studies on Some *Phytopathora* Species from Central India with Special Reference to their Reproduction".
36. Dwivedi, O.P 2003. 'Studies on Soil Microorganisms with Special Reference to Vesicular-Arbuscular Mycorrhizal (VAM) Fungal Association with Wheat Crop of Sagar Region".
37. Yadav, Rajesh 2003. "Studies on Integrated Management of Betelvine *Phytopathora*".
38. Agrawal, Roop Shikha 2004. "Studies on Fungal Diseases of Forest Plants of Mandla Region".
39. Jain, Ashish 2005. "Studies on Mushroom Cultivation with Special Reference to *Pleurotus* Species and their Marketing Potential in Sagar Region".
40. Vyas, Ashish 2005. "Studies on Microbial Biodiversity with Special Reference to their Cellulolytic Activity".
41. Soni Anuradha 2006. Studies on occurrence of VAM Fungi in leguminous crops of sagar.

Acknowledgements

A journey into unknown territory, this is how I felt at the onset of this task. The work undertaken has made me experience many ups and downs throughout the duration of compilation. Although I had been living with it days and nights but there are many people who have knowingly or unknowingly figured a major role in its completion. Although words are not sufficient to express my feelings but still I shall try to comprehend as far as I can and the feelings behind are really heartfelt.

This book is presented with obligation to the under mentioned with full acceptance of its limitations.

I thanks my Shredye Guru Ji Pt Omkar Dev Ji, whose wishes enabled me to reach this mile stone who showed me path to reach the destination and responsible for how to thank god.

I note down here with humility and pride that I am fortunate enough in having support of esteemed personalities like Prof. H.D. Kumar (FNA), BHU, Varanasi, Prof. D.P. Tiwari, Ex Head, Department of Botany, Govt. Science P.G. College, Jabalpur, Prof. C. Manoharachari (Emeritus Prof.), Department of Botany, Osmania University, Hyderabad, Prof. Anupam Dixit, Department of Botany, Allahabad University, Prof. S.P. Adhikari, Department of Biotechnology, Visva Bharti University, Shantiniketan (West Bengal), Prof K.L. Tiwari, Ex Head, Department of Biotechnology, Pt R.S. University, Raipur, Prof G.S. Paliwal (Emeritus Prof.) Senior Consultant National Afforestation and Eco-development Board, New Delhi, Prof H.K. Goswami, Ex Head, Department of Genetics, Barkatullah University, Bhopal and Prof. H.C. Lakshman, Head, Department of Botany, Karnataka University, Dharwad.

I am happy to remember my teachers who happened to be students of my father late Prof. K.M. Vyas, therefore I gratefully acknowledges Prof A.D. Adoni, Prof. T.R. Sahu, Prof. N.K. Soni, Prof. D.C. Atri, Prof. A.K. Kandya, Prof. P. Mehta, Prof. P.K. Khare, Prof. A.N. Rai, Prof. (Smt.) J. Dubey, Dr. A.S. Mishra, Dr. S.K. Yadav, Dr. N.P. Bhalla and my colleague Dr. A. Mehta, Dr. A. Biswas, Miss Poonam Dehariya and Dr. Ashok Shukla for their necessary help whenever I was in need.

I express sincere gratitude to all the authors who have contributed for this volume.

It gives me immense pleasure in acknowledging with sincere gratitude, the enthusiastic co-operation received from my students Dr. O.P. Dwivedi, Dr. Rajesh Yadav, Dr. Ashish Vyas, Dr. Anuradha Soni, Dr. Ashish Jain, Dr. Archana Dubey, Dr. Mahendra Mishra, Dr. Pradeep Singh, Dr. Prashant Soni, Dr. H.C. Gena, Pramod Richhariya, Meenakshi Mishra, Anjuli Chaubey, Javed Ahmad Wagay and Mrs. Anuradha Shukla.

I express a deep valuation to all the non-teaching staff especially Dr. Pradeep Tiwari, K.K. Dixit, J.P. Chaubey, P. Gujre and Shailesh Katare of the department for their time to time help and co-operations.

It is beyond the capacity of all the words to express my respect and profound affection for my mother Mrs. Urmila Vyas. Today whatever I am that is only by virtue of her love, care, affection and blessings. At this juncture I can not forget my wife Mrs. Nisha and children Sidhhant and Vedant and pain taken and sacrifices made by them can not be summed up. They remained as a source of constant inspiration; I bow down before their love and affection towards me. The love and affection extended by my sisters Dr. Jyoti, Arti and Bharti, and their family is memorable.

Last, but certainly not the least, I must thanks to Mr. Nafees of Perfect Computers for designing this cover page in a careful and elegant manner, which is miraculous. I also thank Mr. Anil Mittal of Daya Publishing House for publishing the volume a scientific tribute to my father.

Deepak Vyas

H.D. Kumar

Ph.D. (London). FASc. FNASc, FNA

Formerly Professor of Botany,
Dean, Faculty of Science, and Coordinator,
Biotechnology Programme
Banaras Hindu University

Phone (Res.): (0542) 2315180

**214, Saketnagar, Naria,
VARANASi – 221 005**

Foreword

Microbes, the real masters of life on Earth, are both a boon and bane for the planet. Our microbial friends live within our body, protecting us from disease, aiding digestion, and preserving immunity. On the other side, some of the deadliest diseases are caused by viruses and pathogenic bacteria. Whereas beneficial fungi are an asset to the industrialist and the environment, pathogenic fungi cause havoc and can devastate cereal crops and fruit trees.

The present volume is a Festschrift in honour of my long-term friend, late Prof. K.M. Vyas, a reputed mycologist with strong interest in microbiology. This volume includes some 50 chapters including 23 on microbiology, 13 on biotechnology and 14 on ecology. These chapters are authored by senior professors and younger scientists. The editors are practising researchers and I have pleasure in commending this Festschrift to all those interested in the exciting fields of mycology, microbiology and general biology.

H.D. Kumar

Preface

With the advent of new technologies, the knowledge of science is expanding in new dimensions every day. The frequent review of the state of our knowledge not only to keep ourselves up to date but also to provide over the various strategies ought to be adopted for further revolution of science in all its sphere.

As one know that presently existing life form are evolve from the microorganisms during the course of evolution. These microorganisms can adapt to virtually any physio-chemical environment and are found everywhere.

Despite their huge importance, the fact is that much of what we know about and microbial processes is based on the work done on only a harmful of species-weed like species which can be readily grown in laboratory culture. The vast majority of microorganisms found in nature (Perhaps over 95 per cent) have not so far been cultured but earnest attempts are under ways to grow as many of them as possible in culture.

One most striking property of many microorganisms is the highly promiscuous mode of gene transfer among unrelated or remotely related taxa. Such horizontal (lateral) gene transfers have been the subject of intense research activity in the past few years, in view their strong bearing on the applicability of the biological species concept and the Linnaean system of binominal nomenclature to prokaryotes.

Technological advancement has revolutionized and transform microbiology with biotechnology and created exciting opportunities for agriculture, medicine, industry and environment remediation the organism involved in these mechanisms mostly belongs to bacteria, fungi, cyanobacteria etc.

To keep pace with the growing knowledge in every field of science, our agenda for the coming few years should be to identify the key organizational and genetic principles underlying various morphogenetic processes in both prokaryotes and eukaryotes, while also pursuing the laborious elucidation of the molecular network that control the organizational of living matter.

Considering the importance of microorganism and their biotechnological processes are the major contents of the monograph. Beside microbiology and biotechnology few chapters on ecology are included.

Editors

Contents

Biography: Late Prof. K.M. Vyas vii

Acknowledgements xxi

Foreword xxiii

Preface xxv

List of Editors & Contributors xxxiii

— Volume 1 —

— MICROBIOLOGY —

1. *Rhizobium* Biofertilizer: Retrospect and Prospects 3
S.K. Sethi and S.P. Adhikary

2. Microbial Diversity: Its Role in Ecosystem Maintenance 29
Jamaluddin

3. Thermophilic Cyanobacteria: The Wonder Organisms 34
Vidhi Verma and Meenakshi Banerjee

4. Cyanobacteria: Phenotypic to the Genotypic Diversity 41
A. Srivastava, P. Singh, A. Singh, S.S. Singh and A.K. Mishra

5. Hydrogen Production by Cyanobacteria 60
Deepak Vyas and Rajan Kumar Gupta

6. **Cyanobacterial Toxins** 94
U.S. Gupta, Deepak Vyas and Rajan Kumar Gupta

7. **The Toxins of Cyanobacteria** 150
Mukesh Kumar

8. **Antibacterial Potential of Diazotrophic Cyanobacteria: A Natural Strategy to Maintain Nitrogen Budget in Tropical Lowlands** 162
Usha Pandey

9. **Histochemical Studies on Some Petro-Plants Infected with AM Fungus (*Glomus fasciculatum*)** 168
H.C. Lakshman

10. **Biodiversity of VAM Fungi Associated with Some Common Medicinal Plants of Bihar** 189
A.K. Roy and A.N. Singh

11. **Association of Vesicular Arbuscular Mycorrhizal Fungi with Ornamental Plants** 201
Bhaskar Chaurasia and P.K. Khare

12. **Perspective of AM Fungi in Agroforestry Systems** 209
Ashok Shukla, A. Kumar, D. Vyas, A. Jha, M. Kamalvanshi and N. Chakravarty

13. **Arbuscular Mycorrhizal Fungi: The Hidden Heroes of the Soil** 225
Deepak Vyas, Meenakshi Mishra, Pradeep Singh, Ashok Shukla and R.K. Gupta

14. **Cumulative Effect of VAM Fungi** 256
O.P. Dwivedi, Meenakshi Mishra, Pradeep K. Singh, Pramod Kumar Richhariya, Prashant Soni and Deepak Vyas

15. **Some Additions to the Foliicolous Fungi from the Forest Flora of Madhya Pradesh, India** 268
P. Chauksay, A.N. Rai and Naveen Verma

16. **Current Status of Sesame and Niger Diseases and Their Management** 275
Sushma Nema, T.S. Rajpurohit and M.N. Khare

17. **Integrated Disease Management of *Piper betle*** 293
Deepak Vyas and Rajesh Yadav

18. **Thermophilic Fungi: Occurrence, Characteristics and Enzymatic Potential** 303
Naveen Kango

19. **Biodiversity and Conservation of Mushroom in Chhattisgarh Region** 320
M.P. Thakur, C.S. Shukla and V.K. Yadav

20. **Mushrooms: A Nutritive Food for Human Beings** 344
Poonam Dehariya, Anjuli Chaubey and Deepak Vyas

21. Mushroom: The Beneficial Fungi **353**
Anjuli Choubey, Deepak Vyas, Poonam Dehariya, A.K. Pandey and D.C. Atri

22. *Trichoderma* Species: The History and Evolution of Current Concepts of Biological Control **377**
Pradeep Kumar Singh and Deepak Vyas

— Volume 2 —

— BIOTECHNOLOGY —

23. Fungitoxic Potential of Essential oil and Extracts from Higher Plants in the Management of Postharvest Deterioration: A Review **393**
Anupam Dikshit, Ravindra Kumar Pandey, Rohit Kumar Mishra, Piyush Mishra and Ahsan Kamran

24. Carbonic Anhydrase: An Ancient Enzyme with Multidimensional Roles **439**
Anjana Sharma, Rajesh Pujari and Abhishek Bhattacharya

25. Pharmacological Potential of Mushrooms **452**
Alka Karwa and Mahendra Rai

26. Significance of GM Crops in Modern Agriculture **472**
Shweta J. Sabannavar, H.C. Lakshman, Mahesh B. Byatanal and C. Maya

27. Plant DNA Banking for Biodiversity Assessment and Conservation Research **484**
D. Thangadurai, M.A.A. Pinheirho De Car Valho, D.P. Biradar, Hemanth K.N. Vasathaiah, B. Suresh and Ganesh R. Hegde

28. Progress in Biotechnology of Guava (*Psidium guajava* L.) **501**
Nasim Akhtar

29. Hepatoprotective Medicinal Plants: A Review **520**
Siddhartha Singh, A. Mehta and P. Mehta

30. Cyanobacterial Exploitation in Biotechnology **525**
B.D. Kaushik

31. Effect of Herbicides on Mitosis, Nucleic Acids and Protein Contents in *Corchorus* and Soybean Plants **544**
A.K.S. Chouhan and S.K. Yadav

32. Biotechnological Potential of Cyanobacteria **553**
Surendra Singh

33. Plants and Rhizobium Techniques **571**
Pooja Agrawal

34. **Quest for a Novel Tuberculosis Vaccine: A Global Endeavor** 577
Umesh Dutta Gupta, Vijender Singh and Pushpa Gupta

35. **Silver Nanoparticles: A New Generation of Antimicrobial Agents** 591
Mukesh K. Upadhyay, Devendra Jain, Abhijeet Singh, Sushma Rishi and Narayan Rishi

36. **Phenolic Quantification and Anti-Aging Activity of *Morchella esculenta*** 606
Javed Ahmad Wagay , Ashok Shukla, Anjuli Choubey, Poonam Dehairya and Deepak Vyas

37. **Antibacterial Potential of *Morchella esculenta* Against Some Human Pathogenic Bacteria** 616
Javed Ahmad Wagay, Poonam Dehariya, Anjali C. and Deepak Vyas

38. **Production and Partial Characterization of Fungal and Bacterial Cellulases on CMC and Cellulose Powder** 624
Deepak Vyas and Ashish Vyas

— ECOLOGY —

39. **Lichen Bioindicator Communities in Achanakmar: Amarkantak Biosphere Reserve, Madhya Pradesh and Chhattisgarh** 669
Satya and D.K. Upreti

40. **Silvipastoral Systems: The Solution for the Sustainable Production in Semi Arid Tropics** 683
R.K. Bhatt, A.K. Mishra and H.S. Tiwari

41. **Agroforestry: Conservation of Natural Resources, Biomass Production and Climate Moderations** 708
Ashok Shukla and V.D. Tripathi

42. **Soil Mycoflora of Forest Field at Jagdalpur Region** 724
K.L. Tiwari, S.K. Jadhav and S. Kunjam

43. **Study of Life-Forms and Biological Spectrum of Forest of Sagar District, Madhya Pradesh** 729
A.S. Thakur and P.K. Khare

44. **Environmental Impact of Fly Ash on Soil Health, Yield and Nutrient Uptake by Rice** 741
T. Thomas, Ram Bharose, Arun A. David, H. Thomas and R.K. Tamphasana

45. **Eutrophication: Causes, Consequences and Control Measures** 766
Ashu and Mukesh Kumar

46. **Aquatic Biodiversity Assessment should Trigger Freshwater Body Monitoring and Conservation** 773
S.D. Guru and H.K. Goswami

47. **Eco-Physiological Effects of Red Mud Waste of an Aluminium Industry on the Seed Biology of a Crop Plant** 780

Alka Sahu, Anita R. Patnaik, R.K. Behera and A.K. Panigrahi

48. **Effect of Pollution in Groundwater Quality and Soil Health of Naini Area at Allahabad City** 827

Saurabh Upadhyay, Arun A. David, T. Thomas, H. Thomas, R.K. Tamphasana and Ram Bharose

49. **Modifying Influence of Woody Perennials on Atmospheric Deposition of Nutrient Ions in a Dry Tropical Region of India** 837

J. Pandey

50. **Trends and Determinants of Health Practices Profile Among the Baigas** 846

Arun K. Jain and A.N. Sharma

Author Index 859

Subject Index 861

List of Editors & Contributors

Editors

Dr. Deepak Vyas
Assistant Professor, Department of Botany, Dr. H.S.G. University, Sagar – 470 003, M.P.

Prof. G.S. Paliwal
Senior Consultant, Regional Centre of the National Afforestation and Eco-development Board, Ministry of Environment and Forests, Government of India, New Delhi

P.K. Khare
Professor, Department of Botany, Dr. H.S.G. University, Sagar – 470 003, M.P.

Dr. R. K Gupta
Assistant Professor, Department of Botany, Govt. P.G. College, Rhishikesh

Associate Editors

Prof. A.K. Pandey
Chairman, M.P. Govt. Private University Commission, Bhopal, M.P.

Dr. Jamaludin
Emeritus Prof. Department of Biological Sciences, R.D. University Jabalpur, M.P.

Dr. Neeraj Khare
Department of Botany, Dr. H.S.G. University, Sagar – 470 003, M.P.

Contributors

Adhikary, S.P.
Department of Biotechnology, Vishwa-Bharti University, Shantiniketan, West Bengal

Agrawal, Pooja
Department of Applied Microbiology and Biotechnology, Dr. H.S.G. University, Sagar – 470 003, M.P.

Akhtar, Nasim
Department of Biotechnology, GITAM University, Gandhi Nagar Campus, Rushikonda, Vishakapatnam – 530 045

Ashu
Department of Botany, Sahu Jain PG College, Najibabad – 246 763, U.P.

Atri, D.C.
Department of Botany, Dr. H.S.G. University, Sagar – 470 003, M.P.

Banerjee, Meenakshi
Laboratory of Algal Biotechnology, Department of Bioscience, Barkatullah University, Bhopal, M.P.

Behera, R.K.
Department of Botany, Berhampur University, Berhampur – 760 007, Orissa

Bharose, Ram
School of Forestry and Environment, SHIATS-Deemed University, Allahabad

Bhatt, R.K.
Indian Grassland and Fodder Research Institute, Jhansi – 284 003, U.P.

Bhattacharya, Abhishek
Bacteriology Lab, Department of Biological Sciences, Rani Durgavati University, Jabalpur, M.P.

Biradar, D.P.
Department of Agronomy, UAS, Dharwad – 580 005

Byatanal, Mahesh B.
Post Graduate Department and Research in Botany (Microbiology Lab), Karnataka University, Dharwad – 580 003

Chakravarty, Neha
National Research Centre for Agroforestry, Jhansi – 284 003, U.P.

Chaubey, Anjuli
Lab of Microbial Technology and Plant Pathology, Department of Botany, Dr. H.S.G. University, Sagar – 470 003, M.P.

Chauksay, P.
Department of Botany, Dr. H.S.G. University, Sagar – 470 003, M.P.

Chaurasia, Bhaskar
Department of Botany, Dr. H.S.G. University, Sagar – 470 003, M.P.

Chouhan, A.K.S.
Department of Botany, Dr. H.S.G. University, Sagar – 470 003, M.P.

David, Arun A.
School of Forestry and Environment, SHIATS-Deemed University, Allahabad

Dehariya, Poonam
Lab of Microbial Technology and Plant Pathology, Department of Botany, Dr. H.S.G. University, Sagar – 470 003, M.P.

Dikshit, Anupam
Biological Product Laboratory, Department of Botany, University of Allahabad, Allahabad –211 002

Diwedi, O.P.
Lab of Microbial Technology and Plant Pathology, Department of Botany, Dr. H.S.G. University, Sagar – 470 003, M.P.

Goswami, H.K.
24, Kaushalnagar, PO Misrod, Bhopal – 462 047, M.P.

Gupta, Pushpa
National JALMA Institute for Leprosy and Other Mycobacterial Diseases, Agra – 282 001

Gupta, Rajan Kumar
Department of Botany, Govt. P.G. College, Rishikesh, Uttarakhand

Gupta, U.S.
Department of Zoology, Dr. H.S.G. University, Sagar – 470 003, M.P.

Gupta, Umesh Dutta
National JALMA Institute for Leprosy and Other Mycobacterial Diseases, Agra – 282 001

Guru, S.D.
Department of Botany, Ranchi Women's College, Ranchi, Jharkhand

Hegde, Ganesh R.
Department of Botany, Sri Krishnadevaraya University, Anantapur – 515 0003

Jadhav, S.K.
School of Studies in Biotechnology, Pt. Ravishankar Shukla University, Raipur – 492 010,

Jain, Arun K.
Department of Anthropology and Tribal Development, GG University, Bilaspur, C.G.

Jain, Devendra
School of Life Sciences, Jaipur National University, Jaipur – 302 025, Rajasthan

Jamaluddin
Ex Group Coordinator and Director, Tropical Forest Research Institute, Jabalpur, M.P.

Jha, Anuradha
National Research Centre for Agroforestry, Jhansi – 284 003, U.P.

Kamalvanshi, Madhavi
National Research Centre for Agroforestry, Jhansi – 284 003, U.P.

Kamran, A.
Biological Product Laboratory, Department of Botany, University of Allahabad, Allahabad –211 002

Kango, Naveen
Department of Applied Microbiology and Biotechnology, Dr. H.S.G. University, Sagar – 470 003, M.P.

Karwa, Alka
Department of Biotechnology, S.G.B. Amravati University, Amravati – 444 602

Kaushik, B.D.
Division of Biotechnology, Netaji Subash Institute of Technology, Sector 3, Dwarka, New Delhi – 110 078

Khare, M.N.
Agricultural Research Station, Mandor, Jodhpur, Rajasthan (Ex. Dean and Professor Emeritus, Plant Pathology)

Khare, P.K.
Department of Botany, Dr. H.S.G. University, Sagar – 470 003, M.P.

Kumar, Anil
Principal Scientist (Plant Pathologist), National Research Centre for Agroforestry, Jhansi – 284 003, U.P.

Kumar, Mukesh
Department of Botany, Sahu Jain PG College, Najibabad – 246 763, U.P.

Kunjam, S.
School of Studies in Biotechnology, Pt. Ravishankar Shukla University, Raipur – 492 010,

Lakshman, H.C.
Department of Botany, Microbiology Laboratory, Karnataka University, Dharwad -- 580 003, Karnataka

Maya, C.
Department of Botany, Bangalore University, J.B. Campus, Bangalore – 560 056

Mehta, A.
Department of Botany, Dr. H.S.G. University, Sagar – 470 003, M.P.

Mehta, P.
Department of Botany, Dr. H.S.G. University, Sagar – 470 003, M.P.

Mishra, A.K.
Indian Grassland and Fodder Research Institute, Jhansi – 284 003, U.P.

Mishra, P.
Biological Product Laboratory, Department of Botany, University of Allahabad, Allahabad –211 002

Mishra, Arun Kumar
Laboratory of Microbial Genetics, Department of Botany, Banaras Hindu University, Varanasi – 221 005

Mishra, R.K.
Biological Product Laboratory, Department of Botany, University of Allahabad, Allahabad –211 002

Nema, Sushma
Senior Scientist, Plant Pathology, AICRP (S&N) J.N.K.V.V., Jabalpur

Pandey, A.K.
Chairman, M.P. Council Pvt University Ltd., Bhopal

Pandey, J.
Department of Botany, Banaras Hindu University, Varanasi – 221 005, U.P.

Pandey, R.K.
Biological Product Laboratory, Department of Botany, University of Allahabad, Allahabad – 211 002

Pandey, Usha
Faculty of Science and Technology, MG Kashividya Pith, Varanasi – 221 005, U.P.

Panigrahi, A.K.
Department of Botany, Berhampur University, Berhampur – 760 007, Orissa

Pataik, Anita R.
Department of Botany, Berhampur University, Berhampur – 760 007, Orissa

Pujari, Rajesh
Bacteriology Lab, Department of Biological Sciences, Rani Durgavati University, Jabalpur, M.P.

Rai, A.N.
Department of Botany, Dr. H.S.G. University, Sagar – 470 003, M.P.

Rai, Mahendra
Department of Biotechnology, S.G.B. Amravati University, Amravati – 444 602

Rajpurohit, T.S.
Pathologist, Oilseeds (Rajasthan Agricultural University)

Richhariya, Pramod K.
Lab of Microbial Technology and Plant Pathology, Department of Botany, Dr. H.S.G. University, Sagar – 470 003, M.P.

Rishi, Narayan
School of Virology, Amity University, Noida, U.P.

Rishi, Sushma
School of Virology, Amity University, Noida, U.P.

Roy, A.K.
Department of Botany, T.M. Bhagalpur University, Bhagalpur – 812 007

Sabannavar, Shweta J.
Post Graduate Department and Research in Botany (Microbiology Lab), Karnataka University, Dharwad – 580 003

Sahu, Alka
Department of Botany, Berhampur University, Berhampur – 760 007, Orissa

Satya
Lichenology Laboratory, National Botanical Research Institute (CSIR), Rana Pratap Marg, Lucknow – 226 001, U.P.

Sethi, S.K.
PG Department of Biotechnology, Utkal University, Bhubaneswar – 751 004, Orissa

Sharma, A.N.
Department of Anthropology, Dr. H.S.G. University, Sagar – 470 003, M.P.

Sharma, Anjana
Bacteriology Lab, Department of Biological Sciences, Rani Durgavati University, Jabalpur, M.P.

Shukla, Ashok
Lab of Microbial Technology and Plant Pathology, Department of Botany, Dr. H.S.G. University, Sagar – 470 003, M.P.

Shukla, C.S.
Department of Plant Pathology, Indira Gandhi Agricultural University, Raipur – 492 006, Chhattisgarh

Singh, A.
Laboratory of Microbial Genetics, Department of Botany, Banaras Hindu University, Varanasi – 221 005

Singh, A.N.
Department of Botany, T.M. Bhagalpur University, Bhagalpur – 812 007

Singh, Abhijeet
School of Life Sciences, Jaipur National University, Jaipur – 302 025, Rajasthan

Singh, P.
Laboratory of Microbial Genetics, Department of Botany, Banaras Hindu University, Varanasi – 221 005

Singh, P.K.
Department of Botany, Dr. H.S.G. University, Sagar – 470 003, M.P.

Singh, Siddhartha
Department of Botany, Dr. H.S.G. University, Sagar – 470 003, M.P.

Singh, Surendra
Centre of Advanced Study in Botany, Banaras Hindu University, Varanasi – 221 005, U.P.

Singh, Vijendra
Institute of Microbial Technology, Chandigrah – 160 036

Singh. S.S.
Laboratory of Microbial Genetics, Department of Botany, Banaras Hindu University, Varanasi – 221 005

Soni, Prashant
Department of Botany, Dr. H.S.G. University, Sagar – 470 003, M.P.

Srivastava, A.
Laboratory of Microbial Genetics, Department of Botany, Banaras Hindu University, Varanasi – 221 005

Suresh, B.
Department of Applied Genetics, Karnatak University, Dharwad – 580 003

Tamphasana, R.K.
Department of Applied Geology, Dr. H.S.G. University, Sagar – 470 003, M.P.

Thakur, A.S.
Department of Botany, Govt College, Khurai, Sagar – 470 117, M.P.

Thakur, M.P.
Department of Plant Pathology, Indira Gandhi Agricultural University, Raipur – 492 006, Chhattisgarh

Thangadurai, D.
Department of Botany, Karnatak University, Dharwad – 580 003

Thomas, H.
Department of Applied Geology, Dr. H.S.G. University, Sagar – 470 003, M.P.

Thomas, T.
School of Forestry and Environment, SHIATS-Deemed University, Allahabad

Tiwari, H.S.
Indian Grassland and Fodder Research Institute, Jhansi – 284 003, U.P.

Tiwari, K.L.
School of Studies in Biotechnology, Pt. Ravishankar Shukla University, Raipur – 492 010, C.G.

Tripathi, V.D.
National Research Centre for Agroforestry, Jhansi – 284 003, U.P.

Upadhyay, Mukesh K.
School of Life Sciences, Jaipur National University, Jaipur – 302 025, Rajasthan

Upadhyay, Saurabh
School of Forestry and Environment, SHIATS-Deemed University, Allahabad

Upreti, D.K.
Lichenology Laboratory, National Botanical Research Institute (CSIR), Rana Pratap Marg, Lucknow – 226 001, U.P.

Valho, MAA Pinheirho De Car
ISO Plexis Germplasm Bank, Department of Biology, University of Madeira, Funchal 9000-390, Portugal

Vasathaiah, Hemanth K.N.
Center for Viticulture and Small Fruit Research, Florida A and M University, 6505 Mahan Drive, Tallahassee, Florida 32317, USA

Verma, Naveen
Department of Botany, Dr. H.S.G. University, Sagar – 470 003, M.P.

Verma, Vidhi
Laboratory of Algal Biotechnology, Department of Bioscience, Barkatullah University, Bhopal, M.P.

Vyas, Ashish
Division of Biotechnology, Lovely Professional University, Ludhiana (Punjab)

Vyas, Deepak
Lab of Microbial Technology and Plant Pathology, Department of Botany, Dr. H.S.G. University, Sagar – 470 003, M.P.

Wagay, Javed Ahmad
Lab of Microbial Technology and Plant Pathology, Department of Botany, Dr. H.S.G. University, Sagar – 470 003, M.P.

Yadav, Rajesh
ABR PG College, Anpra, Sonbadhra, U.P.

Yadav, S.K.
Department of Botany, Dr. H.S.G. University, Sagar – 470 003, M.P.

Yadav, V.K.
Department of Plant Pathology, Indira Gandhi Agricultural University, Raipur – 492 006, Chhattisgarh

Biotechnology

Microbial Biotechnology and Ecology (2011) *Pages* **393–438**
Editors: **Deepak Vyas, G.S. Paliwal, P.K.Khare and R.K Gupta**
Published by: **DAYA PUBLISHING HOUSE, NEW DELHI**

Chapter 23

Fungitoxic Potential of Essential Oil and Extracts from Higher Plants in the Management of Postharvest Deterioration: A Review

☆ ***Anupam Dikshit*, Ravindra Kumar Pandey, Rohit Kumar Mishra, Piyush Mishra and Ahsan Kamran***

Biological Product Laboratory, Department of Botany, University of Allahabad, Allahabad – 211 002

ABSTRACT

Postharvest losses of stored products are enormous due to fungal deteriorations. Although, there are number of synthetic fungicides available in the market for checking these deteriorations, they have several side effects such as high toxicity, long degradation periods, their concentration in food chain, chronic poisoning through the continuous intake of small quantities, development of new races of pathogens, non-biodegradable nature and exhaustible source. The history of pesticide development has been instructive to us in term of benefits derived as well as the hazard, which accompany the indiscriminate use of these poisonous chemicals. Therefore, we must search the new sources of pesticides, which in addition to their efficiency must be safe and selective to target pests or pathogen. Plants are very rich sources of bioactive chemicals such as phenolics, polyphenols, quinones, flavones, flavonoids, flavonols, tannins, cumarins, terpenoids, lectins and polypeptides. The essential oil fraction of botanicals is often the most inhibitory chemical to growth and survival

* E-mail: anupambplau@rediffmail.com

of microorganisms. They are highly enriched with terpenoids. Further they are volatile, biodegradable, and environmentally safe and are easily available in local environment. Therefore, present communication reviews the work done in investigating the fungitoxic potential of essential oils and extracts from higher plants in fungal deterioration of stored products.

Keywrds: *Myotoxins, Fungitoxic, Biodeterioration.*

Introduction

It is estimated that between 60 to 80 per cent of all grains produced in the tropics are stored by farmers. For small farmers, the main purpose of storing grains is to ensure household food supplies. It also provides a form of saving to cover future cash needs through sale or for barter or gift exchange. Small quantities of grains are also stored for seed. Farmers who produce surplus may also store grain for sale later to take advantage of seasonal price rise. A traditional farm storage system provides maximum protection against deterioration of commodity by inclement weather and pests. Farm storage system have evolved over a long periods to satisfy these requirements. Most are well adapted to their environment and losses are generally low, often below 5 per cent of grain weight over a storage season (Tyler and Boxall, 1984). However, for resource poor farmers, even losses of this magnitude have important implications for food security. In addition to storage of food grains at farmer's level, the governments of different countries also procure and store them for reasons of food security for its growing population. There was spiral increase in populations of several countries including India. In case of India, it has crossed one billion marks in 2000 A.D. and it will give India the dubious distinction of being the most populated country in the world by 2025 A.D. Therefore, the challenge of feeding ever-growing population of human being shall be very difficult task. We can not meet such a challenge with the increase in food production alone but their protection from deterioration caused by fungi and other pests during storage have to be given due emphasis (Shukla, 1997).

In developing countries, fungal pests cause the greatest losses during storage to cereals and other durable commodities. Deteriorations due to fungi are due to unhygienic conditions of storage and this in turn is associated with initial high moisture content of the stored products or absorption of moisture during storage due to defects in the storage system (Stinson *et al.*, 1980). There are several storage fungal pests that cause deteriorations in stored commodities. The most common among them are– *Aspergillus flavus, A. niger, A. clavatus, A. terreus, A. versicolor, A. candidus, Alternaria alternata, Curvularia lunata, Cladosporium cladosporoides, C. herbarum, Epicoccum nigrum, Emericella nidulans, Emericella rugulosa, Fusarium acuminatum, F. moniliforme, Mucor hiemalis, Penicillium citrinum, P. chrysogenum, P. expansum, P. funiculosum, P. italicum, Rhizopus arrhizus, Rhizopus nigricans, Syncephalastrum racemosum* etc. Several of these fungal pests such as species of *Aspergillus, Penicillium, Fusarium, Alternaria* and *Cladosporium* etc. not only bring about deterioration in the quality and quantity of agricultural produce in storage and transit but also create health hazards in animals and human beings, by producing toxic metabolites in the form of mycotoxins in the stored commodities. These organisms are capable of growing under a diversity of conditions of moisture, pH and temperature. If the mould growth occurs, there is always the concomitant possibility of mycotoxin production (Zohri and Abdel-Gawad, 1993).

Mycotoxins are dangerous chemical that cause several complications in the body. They are carcinogenic, hepatoxic, nephrotoxic and teratogenic. Extreme toxicity of mycotoxins lies in the fact that they are extremely stable and dangerous in minute quantities. Further, once formed they cannot be removed from the commodity concerned by processing or removal of visible mould growth. They are heat stable, so they cannot be destroyed by cooking. Since mycotoxins are extremely toxic, regulatory and industry guidelines limit are set at very low levels. In developing countries often the good quality products are exported while substandard produce unacceptable to foreign buyers (because they exceed regulatory limits for mycotoxin content) is sold to the domestic market (Dawson, 1991). Therefore, the mycotoxin contamination of food and feeds is not a particular problem to the developed world, although heavy economic costs are incurred in ensuring low concentrations of mycotoxins (Mannon and Johanson, 1985). In poorer developing countries, such contamination has more serious consequences, affecting agricultural economies, reducing annual production and good quality exports and seriously affecting the health of the population.

To control fungal deterioration of agricultural produce, many organic and inorganic fungicides have been developed and are being used. The use of many of these has, however, been restricted due to their undesirable side effects such as a high and acute toxicity, the long degradation periods, their concentration in food chain, the suspected dangers of chronic poisoning through the continuous intake of small quantities. Besides, due to development of new races of pathogens, many of these fungicides are gradually becoming out of date (Dikshit, 1980). Furthermore, the sources of these synthetic fungicides are largely petrochemicals, which are exhaustible. Therefore, hunt for inexhaustible sources of such chemotherapeutants is highly desirable. According to Brandes (1967) much of our efforts are being wasted in routine testing of the standard fungicides, when there is a pressing need to investigate new sources of effective fungicides.

Fungitoxic Potential of Higher Plants

Green plants appear to be the reservoir of effective chemotherapeutants and can provide reversible source of useful pesticides (Swaminathan, 1978). Tropical floras, in contrast to their temperate zone counterparts, have developed a more efficient and varied defence mechanism because of the far severe conditions for survival. They, thus provide a rich and intriguing source for isolating natural secondary plant metabolites, which exhibit interesting antimicrobial properties. Although only some 15,000 secondary plant metabolites have been chemically identified, their total number may exceed 4,000,000 (Saxena, 1993). They are vast cornucopia of defense chemicals. Recent reports on the possibility of use of higher plants and their constituents have indicated their usefulness in providing fungicides which are largely non-phytotoxic, more systemic and easily biodegradable (Fawcett and Spencer, 1969; Beye, 1978). They are sustainable, can be continuously propagated year after year and do not have any negative impact on the environment as long as care is taken to avoid the propagation of plants from foreign ecosystems which might, therefore, become established as weeds.

Farmers use plants as storage protectants since long times. Further, where plants are used as storage protectants, they are almost always applied to control insect pests. This is reflected in volumes of research directed to identifying insecticidal or insect repellent plants and plant extracts. Nevertheless, some work has been undertaken to determine whether plants can control storage fungi. Most workers have investigated the properties of spices as inhibiting agents of mycelial growth of *Aspergillus* species and of its toxin production. *Syzygium aromaticum* (cloves) have been found to be particularly effective, often completely inhibiting both fungal growth and toxin production (Hitokoto *et al.*, 1980; Mabrouk and El-Shayeb, 1980). Many commercially available spices and herbs, turmeric, basil, marjoram, anise, cumin and coriander are able to completely inhibit toxin production, but only partially inhibit fungal mycelial growth (Hitokoto *et al.*, 1980). Aqueous extracts of weeds and medicinal plants have also been found to inhibit toxin production by *Aspergillus flavus*. These include *Ricinus communis, Arnebia nobilis* and *Nicotiana plumbaginifolia*. (Bilgrami *et al.*, 1980). Other fungi, *Fusarium solani, F. phaseoli* and *Verticillium albo-atrum*, have been shown to be susceptsible to tannins extracted from bark of various trees, including chestnut and wattle (Lewis *et al.*, 1967). In addition to above several other fungi, have been shown to be susceptible to essential oils extracted from higher plants (angiosperms and gymnosperms). A recent compilation of work on fungitoxicity of higher plants against dominant storage fungi and a few other fungi have been made as under:

Abutilon indicum (Malvaceae)

Jain *et al.* (1979) reported the toxicity of oil isolated from leaves against *Alternaria robi, Aspergillus flavus, A. fumigatus, A. nidulans, A. niger, Cladosporium hebarum, Fusarium moniliforme, Helminthosporium* sp. *Penicillium digitatum, P. italicum, Rhizopus nigricans* and *Trichothecium roseum.*

Acorus calamus (Araceae)

Samuel (1993) isolated the oil from the rhizome and reported its toxicity against *Fusarium moniliforme* and *Helminthosporium oryzae* at a minimum dose of 500 ppm. The oil possessed fungistatic activity at MIC but turned fungicidal at 4000-ppm conc. The active principle isolated from the oil was recognized as Aṣarone. The volatile oil at its MIC was reported to possess toxicity against *Aspergillus flavus, A. nidulans, Cladosporium herbarurn, Drechslera sativa, Fusarium oxysporum, Macrophomina phaseolina, Rhizoctonia solani* and *Sclerotium rolfsii.* It did not show any phytotoxicity on seed germination and seedling growth of *Oryza sativa* and *Hordeum vulgare.* Siddiqui *et al.* (2003) reported the fungitoxicity of the essential oil against *Helminthosporium oryzae* and *Fusarium moniliforme* at a minimum dose of 500 ppm (0.5×10^3ml/l), and it was fungistatic in nature.

Adenocalymma allicea (Bignoniaceae)

Chaturvedi (1979) reported 0.3 per cent yield of water-soluble essential oil containing 10 major and 35 minor components. The oil inhibited the mycelial growth of *Alternaria raphani, A. solani, Cephalosporium sacchari, Cladosporium cladosporioides, Colletotrichum lindemutheanum, C. truncatum, Fusarium moniliforme, F. solani, Paecilomyces* sp. *Rhizoctonia bataticola, R. solani* and *Talaromyces* sp. at 500 ppm (0.5×10^3ml/l). The oil killed *Helminthosporium oryzae* within 30 minutes (by contact). The antifungal factor was thermostable and retained its toxicity up to 21 days of storage. The oil controlled leaf spot disease in paddy without showing any adverse side effects on the host plant (Chaturvedi *et al.*, 1987).

Aegle mormelos (Rutaceae)

Rao and Joseph (1971) found that the oil was toxic to *Curvularia lunata, Fusarium moniliforme, Helminthosporium sacchari, Physalospora tucumanensis* and *Sclerotium rolfsii.* The leaves yielded 0.4 per cent oil, which killed 40 mycelial discs (5 mm. in diameter) of the test fungus *Rhizoctonia solani* within 2 hours (by contact) and completely inhibited the mycelial growth of *Helminthosporium corbonum* at 0.3 per cent (3.0×10^3 ml/l) dose (Srivastava, 1981). The thermostable fungitoxic factor of the oil retained its toxicity upto 105 days in storage at room temperature and was non phytotoxic to seed germination of *Vigna mungo* (Renu *et al.*, 1986).

Ageratum conyzoides (Asteraceae)

Rao (1976a) reported that the leaf oil was toxic to *Colletotrichum capsici, Helminthosporium oryzae, H. turcicum, Penicillium chrysogenum, P. javanicum* and *Pyricularia setariae.* It was also found to be toxic against *Alternaria helianthi, Fusarium moniliforme, F. solani, Pyricularia oryzae, Pythium vexans, Rhizoctonia bataticola* and *R. solani* (Sharma *et al.*, 1978). Chandra and Dikshit (1981) recorded fungistatic nature of the oil at 0.2 per cent (2.0×10^3 ml/l) concentration against *Absidia ramosa, Alternaria alternata, A. citri,*

A. raphani, Aspergillus flavipes, A. fumigatus, A. oryzae, A. quadrilineatus, A. ruber, A sydowi, A. tamarii, A. terreus, Botryodiplodia theobromae, B. palmicolum, Botrytis cinarea, Cladosporium cladosporioides, Colletotrichum falcatum, C. gloeosporioides, Cunninghamella elegans, Curvularia lunata, Fusarium oxysporum, Geotrichum candidum, Gloeosporium fructigenum, Penicillium funiculosum, P. expansum, Rhizopus arrhizus and *Tricothecium roseum*. Chandra (1984) reported that the oil controlled the blue mould rot during storage of oranges, caused by *Penicillium italicum* at 0.1 per cent (1.0×10^3 ml/l) concentration. Singh *et al.* (1986a) reported that the mycelial disc of *Epidermophyton floccosum, Microsporum canis* and *Trichophyton mentagrophytes* were completely killed when dipped in 4000-ppm (4.0×10^3ml/l) dose of the oil. The isolated de-methoxy ageratochromene, the antifungal principle of the oil, which was found toxic at 1000 ppm (1.0×10^3ml/l) against the dermatophytes tested.

Ageratum haustonianum (Asteraceae)

The leaf oil was found toxic at 100-ppm (0.1×10^3 ml/l) concentration, possessing fungistatic nature against *Blastomyces dermatitides, Epidermophyton floccosum, Histoplasma capsulatum, Trichophyton mentagrophytes, T. simii, T. terrestre, T. tonsurans, T. verrucosum* and *T. violaceum*. However, it killed *Microsporum gypseum* with in one second at 300-ppm (0.3×10^3 ml/l) dose by contact (Pandey *et al.*, 1983a). Pandey *et al.* (1983b) reported that the fungitoxic factor of the oil was thermostable and fungistatic against *Fusarium lateritium* at 0.05 per cent (0.5×10^3ml/l) concentration.

Aglaja odorata (Meliaceae)

Kakrani and Nair (1982) reported that the seed oil possessed toxicity against *Rhizopus oryzae*.

Allium sativum (Liliaceae)

Skinner (1955) reviewed in detail the antimicrobial spectrum of the volatile as well as non-volatile component of the plant and its active principle, allicin. Further publication of the Maruzzella and Liquroi (1958), Maruzzella and Baiter (1959), Maruzella *et al.* (1960), Thind and Dahiya (1977), Petricic *et al.* (1978), Singh and Singh (1981), and Singh and Deshmukhi (1984) revealed that the oil possessed toxicity against a wide range of fungi including *Absidia spinosa, Alternaria alternata, A. tenuis, Aspergillus flavus, A. fumigatus, A. japonicus, A. nanus, A. nidulans, A. sydowi, Candida albicans, C. monosa, Cephalosporium sacchari, Claviceps purpurea, Curvularia lunata, Erysiphe polygoni, Fusarium nivale, F. solani, Helminthosporium gramineum, Lentinus lepideus; Lenzites trabea, Polyporus versicolor, Trichoderma viride, Microsporum gypseum* and *Verticillium terrestrae.*

Allium cepa (Liliaceae)

The oil has been reported fungitoxic against many fungi *viz. Alternaria alternata, Aspergillus niger, Botrytis allii, Claviceps purpurea Chrysosporium tropicum, Keratinophyton terreum, Malbranchea pulchela, Microsporum gypseum, Phytophthora infestans* and *Verticillium tenuipes* (Meruzzella and Baiter, 1959; Korableva and Patapova, 1966; Jain and Agarwal, 1978; Singh and Deshmukhi, 1984).

Alpinia galanga (Zingiberaceae)

The oil extracted from rhizome was toxic at 4000 ppm (4.0×10^3ml/l) concentration to *Absidia ramose, Alternaria alternata, A. raphani, A. solani, Aspergillus fumigatus, A. versicolor, Cephalosporium sacchari, Colletotrichum capsici, C. gloeosporioides, C. tinosporae, Epicoccum roseum, Fusarium moniliforme, F. oxysporium, F. solani, Helminthosporium carbonum, H. gramineum, H. maydis, H. turcicum, H. oryzae, Pestalotia versicolor, Pyricularia oryzae, Talaromyces* sp. and *Trichoderma viride* (Tripathi, 1980). The active principle of the oil was thermolabile and it got destroyed during autoclaving but remained unaffected by temperature upto 100°C and by storage upto 91 days at room temperature. Tripathi *et al.* (1983) during preliminary *in-vivo* trials observed that the oil prevented the appearance of symptoms of leaf spot disease in paddy without affecting the germination and seedling growth of host plant. Janseen and Scheffer (1985) isolated acetoxychavicol, the active principle of the oil and reported its fungitoxicity at 250 mg/ml doses against *Aspergillus niger, Candida albicans, Epidermophyton floccosum, Penicillium expansum, Trichophyton mentagrophytes, T. rubrum* and *T. concentricum.*

Alseodaphne keanamia (Lauraceae)

The leaves and bark extracts of plant were screened for antifungal activities. Various pathogens were used *viz. Aspergillus niger, A. flavus, Trichoderma* sp. and *Cladosporium* sp. (Versha Parcha *et al.*, 2003).

Ammoides pusilla (Apiaceae)

Oil from aerial parts showed antimicrobial activity against eight strains of bacteria, several fungi and yeast such as *Aspergillus niger* and *Candida albicans.* GC and GC/MS of oil showed 46 constituents among which thymol (44.5 per cent), γ-terpinene (32.9 per cent) and p- cymene (13.5 per cent) were the chief. (Laouer *et al.*, 2003)

Amomum subulatum (Zingiberaceae)

Kumar (1992) reported that the volatile oil was toxic to *Aspergillus flavus, A. ochraceus, Fusarium oxysporum* and *Penicillium citrinum* at a conc. of 1000 ppm. The nature of fungotoxicity was static at MIC but turned fungicidal at a conc. of 8000 ppm.

Anaphalis controrta (Asteraceae)

Saxena *et al.* (1984) found that the leaf oil was toxic to *Aspergillus niger, Microsporum gypseum* and *Penicillium notatum.*

Anethum graveolens (Apiaceae)

Rao and Joseph (1971) reported that seed oil was toxic to *Candida albicans, Epidermophyton floccosum, Trichophyton mentagrophytes* and *T. rubrum.* Later, it was reported toxic to species of *Aspergillus, Curvularia* and *Penicillium* (Chaursia and Kher 1978a, b); *Alternaria* sp., *Aspergillus candidus, A. flavus, A. fumigatus, A. nidulans, A. niger, Cladosporium herbarium, Cunninghamella echinulata, Fusarium monilliforme, F. oxysporum, Helminthosporium sacchari, Microsporum cocci, M. gypseum, Mucor mucedo, Penicillium digitatum, Rhizopus* sp., *Trichophyton mentagrophytes, T. rubrum* and *Trichothecium roseum* (Sharma and Singh, 1979b) and *Alternaria tenuis, A. fumigatus, Candida albicans, C. tropicallis, Diplodia natalensis, Keratinomyces ajelloi, Microsporum gypseum, Penicillium digitatum, P. italicum, Trichophyton equinum* and *T. rubrum* (Narsimha Rao and Subba Rao, 1982; Arora and Pandey, 1984 a.b; Saksena, 1984). The oil showed fungistatic nature at 1000 ppm (1.0×10^3 ml/l) dose, against *Alternaria alternata, Aspergillus flavus, A. awamori, A. niger, A. ochraceus, A. parasiticus, A. sydowi, A. terreus, Candida tropicalis, Cladosporium herbarum, Epidermophyton floccosum, Fusarium moniliforme, F. oxysporum, Microsporum gypseum, Nigrospora oryzae, Penicillium chrysogenum, P. citrinum, Rhizopus nigricans* and *Trichophyton mentagrophytes* (Dubey, 1986). The toxic principle of the oil *i.e.* Anethol, proved non phytotoxic to seed germination and seedling growth of *Pisum sativum* and was not affected by temperature as well as by long storage duration at room temperature (Dubey, 1986).

Angelica archenglica (Apiaceae)

Korta and Starzyk (1963) reported toxicity of the oil against *Candida albicans, C. krusci, C. parakrusei, C. pelliculosa, C. silosis, C. stellatoidea* and *C. tropicalis*. Later, its toxicity was reported against *Nannizzia fulva, N. gypsea* and *N. incurvata* (Gautam *et al.*, 1980).

Apium graveolens (Apiaceae)

Rao and Joseph (1971), Sharma and Singh (1979 b) and Narsimha Rao ànd Subba Rao (1982) reported that the oil from seeds produced marked inhibitory zones in cultures seeded with spores of *Candida albicans, Epicoccum floccosum, Epidermotophyton floccosum, Trichophyton mentagrophytes. T. rubrum, Alternaria* sp., *Aspergillus candidus, A. flavus, A. fumigatus, A. nidulans, A. niger, Cladosporium herbarum, Cunninghamella echinulata, Fusarium moniliforme, F. oxysporum, Helminthosporium sacchari, Microsporum cocci, M. gypseum, Mucor mucedo, Penicillium digitatum, Rhizopus* sp. and *Trichothecium roseum.*

Arnica latifolia (Asteraceae)

Singh (1976) reported the toxicity of the oil against *Candida albicans, Cephalosporium sacchari, Ceratocystis paradoxa, Curvularia lunata, Fusarium moniliforme, Helminthosporium sacchari, Physalospora tucumanensis, Trichophyton rubrum* and *Sclerotium rolfsii.*

Artemisia absinthium (Asteraceae)

Kaul *et al.* (1976) reported the toxicity of oil at 1:1000 (1.0×10^3 ml/l) dilution against *Candida albicans, C. utilis* and *Aspergillus niger.*

Artemisia capillaris (Asteraceae)

Ikenaka *et al.* (1956) reported that the oil was toxic to *Alternaria kikuchiana, Aspergillus awamori, A. niger, A. oryzae, Gibberella fujikuroi, G. bataticola, G. sanbinetii, Colletotrichum miyabeanus, Penicillium chrysogenum, Pyricularia oryzae* and *Rhizopus javanicus.* Imai *et al.* (1956) isolated Capillin the antifungal factor of the oil.

Artemisia cina (Asteraceae)

Vichkanova *et al.* (1972) reported the toxicity of the oil against *Candida albicans, Microsporum lanceoletum* and *M. gypseum.*

Artemisia martima (Asteraceae)

Dikshit and Husain (1984) reported the toxicity of the oil against *Microsporum gypseum, Trichophyton equinum* and *T. rubrum.*

Artemisia vestita (Asteraceae)

The toxicity of the oil at 1:1000 (1.0×10^3 ml/l) dilutions against several dermatophytes was reported by Kaul *et al.* (1976). Gautam *et al.* (1980) reported the toxicity of this oil against *Nannizzia fulva, N. gypsia* and *N. incurvata.*

Azadirachta indica (Meliaceae)

Kher and Chaurasia (1977), Thind and Dahiya (1977) and Jain and Agrawal (1978) reported the toxicity of the oil against some kerationophylic fungi *viz. Verticillium tenuipes, Keratinophyton terreum, Malbrachea pulchella* and *Chrysosporium tropicum.* Later, Singh and Singh (1981) and Dwivedi and Dubey (1986) reported the complete inhibition of the conidial and sclerotial germination of *Erysiphe polygoni* and *Macrophomina phaseoli* by the volatile vapour of the oil.

Blumea membranacea (Asteraceae)

Zutshi and Mehta (1977) and Sharma *et al.* (1978) reported the toxicity of the oil against *Alternaria helianthi, Fusarium moniliforme, Helminthosporium oryzae, H. turcicum, Pyricularia setariae* and *Rhizoctonia solani*. Later, its toxicity was reported against *Aspergillus luchuensis, A. sydowi* and *Cladosporium cladosporioides.*

Bothriocloa perrtusa (Poaceae)

Jain *et al.* (1979) reported that the oil was inhibitory to *Alternaria robi, Aspergillus flavus, A. fumigatus, A. niger, A. nidulans, Cladosporium herbarum, Rhizopus nigricans* and *Trichothecium roseum.*

Boswellia serrata (Burseraceae)

Garg (1974) reported that the oil possessed toxicity against *Curvularia geniculata, C. pallescens, Fusarium culmorum, F. oxysporum* and *Pythium aphanidermatum*. Girgune *et al.* (1978) reported its inhibitory activity against *Alternaria helianthi, Fusarium solani, Helminthosporium oryzae, H. turcicum* and *Rhizoctonia solani* and found that the oil contains α-thuzene, α-pinene and α-phellendrene.

Caesulia axillaris (Asteraceae)

The antimicrobial activity of the oil was first reported by Zutshi *et al.* (1975) and later confirmed by Geda *et al.* (1978). The oil was fungicidal to *Helminthosporium oryzae* at 0.5 per cent (5.0×10^3ml/l) concentration and it controlled leaf spot disease of paddy at 0.025 per cent (0.25×10^3 ml/l) concentration with no side effects on the host plant (Pandey *et al.*, 1982a). The antifungal factor of the oil was thermostable, durable up to 180 days of storage and could bear increased inoculum density (Pandey *et al.*, 1982).

Caesalpinia sappan (Caesalpiniaceae)

The toxicity of the oil against *Aspergillus nidulans* was reported by Yadav *et al.* (1978).

Calamus sp. (Arecaceae)

Arora and Pandey (1984a) reported toxicity of the oil against *Alternaria tenuis, Diplodia natalensis, Penicillium digitatum* and *P. italicum.* The oil was used as preservative to prevent fungal deterioration of fruits of *Citrus reticulata* during storage (Arora and Pandey 1984b).

Calamintha nepeta (Lamiaceae)

In-vitro microbicidal properties of the essential oil of *Calamintha nepeta* were studied on *Aspergillus niger, A. parasiticus, Rhizopus oryzae, Rhizoctonia oryzae-sativae, Candida albicans* and *Colletotrichum musae.* The essential oil showed the highest activity against *R. oryzae-sativae* and *C. albicans.* (Tajo *et al.*, 1999).

Callistemon lanceolatus (Myrtaceae)

Dwivedi *et al.* (1990) tested the oil against *Macrophomina phaseolina* and found to be toxic at 500, 1000 and 2000 ppm (0.5×10^3 ml/l, 1.0×10^3 ml/l, 2.0×10^3 ml/l doses.

Capsicum annuum (Solanaceae)

The toxicity of the oil was tested against *Aspergillus niger* by Capek (1955).

Carum balbocastanum (Apiaceae)

The toxicity of the oil against *Aspergillus fumigatus, Curvularia lunata* and *Trichoderma viride* was reported by Nigam and Rao (1977).

Carum carvi (Apiaceae)

Slavenas (1963) reported that the oil from fruits possessed toxicity against *Aspergillus niger*. Do Vgich (1971) recorded the toxic nature of the oil against *Aspergillus oryzae, Alternaria tenuis* and *Penicillium chrysogenum*. The oil was later reported to possess toxicity against *Aspergillus flavus, A. fumigatus, A. versicolor, Fusarium* sp., *Trichoderma viride* and *Curvularia* sp. (Nigam and Rao, 1977). *Aspergillus candidus, A. nidulans, Cladosporium herbarum, Cunninghmella echinulata, Fusarium moniliforme, F. oxysporum, Helminthosporium sacchari, Microsporum cocci, M. gypseum, Mucor mucedo, Penicillium digitatum, Rhizopus* sp., *Trichophyton mentagrophytes, T. rubrum* and *Trichothecium roseum* (Sharma and Singh, 1979b) as well as *Candida tropicalis* and *Rhizopus oryzae* (Narayanan *et al.*, 1980a).

Carum roxburghianum (Apiaceae)

Nigam and Rao (1977) observed that the oil produced marked inhibitory zone in cultures seeded with spores of *Aspergillus flavus, A. fumigatus, A. oryzae, Alternaria tenuis, Curvularia* sp. and *Trichoderma viride*.

Cassia sp. (Caesalpiniaceae)

Maruzzela and Liquori (1958) and Maruzzella *et al.* (1960) reported the toxicity of the oil against *Lentinus lepideus, Lenzites trabea* and *Polyporus versicolor*.

Cedrus deodara (Pinaceae)

Dikshit *et al.* (1979) isolated 2.72 per cent oil from root wood and reported that the oil was toxic to *Helminthosporium oryzae* at 3000 ppm (3.0×10^3 ml/l) concentration. Dikshit (1980) reported that the thermostable fungitoxic factor of the oil retained its toxicity during storage up to 600 days and sustained heavy inoculum density but got destroyed by autoclaving when kept at 20 lbs per square inch pressure for 20 minutes. The oil at 3000 ppm (3.0×10^3 ml/l) dose inhibited the growth of *Absidia romosa, Alternaria brasicae, A. raphani, A. solani, Aspergillus carneus, A. flavipes, A. fumigatus, A. niger, A. versicolor, Cephalosporium sacchari, Cladosporiun* sp., *Colletotrichum falcaturn, C. lindemuthianum, C. tinosporae, Cornespora casicola, Fusarium moniliforme, F. solani, Pacilomyces* sp., *Pyricularia oryzae, Talaromyces* sp. and *Trichoderma viride*. The oil killed the test fungus *H. oryzae* in 3 hr. by contact at 3.0×10^3 ml/l concentration in 90 min at 5×10^3 ml/l, while the contact of pure oil killed the fungus in seconds. Dikshit and Dixit (1982) demonstrated that the oil successfully prevented the appearance of symptoms of leaf spot disease in paddy without any adverse effect on seed germination and general growth of the host plant (Dikshit *et al.*, 1982). Dikshit *et al.* (1983) reported that the oil at 5.0×10^3 ml/l dose controlled the fungal deterioration of fruits of *Foeniculum vulgare* and *Coriandrum sativum* during storage.

Centella asiatica (Apiaceae)

Minija and Thoppil (2003) studied the antimicrobial activity of oil on six fungi *viz. Aspergillus niger, A. parasiticus, Rhizopus oryzae, Candida albicans, Fusarium solani* and *Colletotrichum musae*. The essential oil showed remarkable activity against *A. niger, R. oryzae, F. solani* and *C. albicans*.

Cestrum diurnum (Solanaceae)

Renu *et al.* (1980) reported that the leaves yielded 0.22 per cent water soluble oil which exhibited toxicity against *Absidia ramosa, Alternaria alternata, A. brassicae, A. raphani, A. solani, Aspergillus flavipes,*

A. flavus, A. fumigatus, A. terreus, C. cladosporioides, Colletotrichum capsici, C. falcatum. C. gloeosporioides, C. tinosporae, Curvularia lunata, Epiccoccum sp., *Fusarium moniliforme, F. oxysporum, F. solani, Helminthosporium carbonum, H. gramineum, H. maydis, H. oryzae, H. turcicum, Pacilomyces* sp., *Pyricularia oryzae, Penicillium decumbens, Pestalotia versicolor, Phoma* sp., *Rhizoctonia batalicola, Talaromyces* sp., *Trichoderma viride* and *Trichothecium roseum* at 0.7 per cent (7.0×10^3ml/l) concentration and killed the test fungus, *Rhizoctonia solani* in 12 hrs by contact. The fungitoxic factor of the oil sustained heavy inoculum density and remained unaffected by temperature treatment and storage upto 400 days. The seeds of *Vigna mungo* when soaked in 0.7 per cent (7.0×10^3 ml/l) dilution of the oil for 12 hrs. did not show any adverse effect on their germination and seedling growth (Srivastava, 1981).

Chenopodium ambrosioides (Chenopodiaceae)

Kumar, *et, al.* (2007). extracted essential oil from the leaves of *Chenopodium ambrosioides* Linn. (Chenopodiaceae) and tested against the aflatoxigenic strain of test fungus *Aspergillus flavus* Link. The oil completely inhibited the mycelial growth at100 µg/ml. The oil exhibited broad fungitoxic spectrum against *Aspergillus niger, Aspergillus fumigatus, Botryodiplodia theobromae, Fusarium oxysporum, Sclerotium rolfsii, Macrophomina phaseolina, Cladosporium cladosporioides, Helminthosporium oryzae* and *Pythium debaryanum* at 100 µg/ml. Kishore *et al.* (1982b) reported that the oil from inflorescence was fungicidal to *Absidia romosa, Alternaria alternata, Aspergillus flavus, A. fumigatus, A. nidulans, A. niger, A. versicolor, Cladospoium cladosporioides, Chaetomium globosum, Colletotrichum capsici, C. falcutum, C. gloeosporioides, Curvularia lunata, Fusarium moniliforme, F. oxysporum, Helminthosporium maydis, Pacilomyces* sp., *Penicillium italicum* and, *Rhizopus arrhizus* at 1000 ppm (1.0×10^3 ml/l) concentration.

Chloroxylon swietenia (Rutaceae)

Garg and Oswal (1982) reported the toxicity of the oil at 1 : 50 (20×10^3 ml/l) dilution against *Aspergillus oryzae, A. terreus* and *Candida albicans.*

Cicer arietinum (Leguminosae)

Rao and Joseph (1971) reported that the oil from the seed husk was toxic to *Cephalosporium sacchari, Ceratocystis paradoxa, Curvularia lunata, Fusarium moniliformae, Helminthosporium sacchari, Physalospora tucumanesis, Rhizopus arrhizus* and *Sclerotium rolfsii.*

Cinnamomum sp. (Lauraceae)

The bark oil was reported to be toxic against *Aspergillus niger* by Capek (1955). Later Mukherjee (1974) reported that oil completely prevented the sporulation in *Alternaria solani, Curvularia lunata, Fusarium solani* and *Helminthosporium oryzae.*

Cinnamomum camphora (Lauraceae)

Suri and Thind (1979) reported the toxicity of the oil against *Aspergillus fumigatus* and *Penicillium notatum*. Tiwari *et al.* (1988) found that the oil at 1.0×10^3ml/l effectively reduced the decay due to *Aspergillus niger* of onion during storage. Dwivedi *et al.* (1990) tested the oil against *Macrophomina phaseolina* and found to be toxic at 0.5×10^3 ml/l, 1.0×10^3 ml/l and 2.0×10^3 ml/l doses. This fungus causes root rot disease of crops.

Cinnamomum tamala (Lauraceae)

Girgune *et al.* (1978) reported that the bark oil which contained α-phellendrene was toxic to *Alternaria helianthi, Fusarium moniliforme, F. solani, Helminthosporium oryzae, Pythium vexans, Rhizoctonia bataticoia* and *R. solani.*

Cinnamomum zeylanicum (Lauraceae)

Chaurasia and Kher (1978a, b) reported that the bark oil possess fungitoxicily. Jain and Agrawal (1978) reported toxicity against *Chrysosporium tropicum, Keratinophyton terreum, Malbranchea pulchella* and *Verticillium tenuipes*. Suri and Thind (1979) reported toxicity against pathogen *viz. Keratinophyton terreum, Malbranchea pulchella* and *Trichophyton mentogrephytes*. Narayan *et al.* (1980 b) reported that the oil at 1:64 dilution inhibited the mycelial growth of *Aspergillus fumigatus, A. niger, Candida troipicalis, Fusarium* sp. and *Rhizopus oryzae* whereas Saxena (1989) reported the toxicity of the bark oil against *Candida albicans, Keratinomyces ajelloi, Microsporum gypseum, Trichophyton equinum* and *T. rubrum*. Mishra *et al.* (1989) isolated the essential oil from leaves and reported its toxicity against *Aspergillus flavus* at 2.0×10^3 ml/l dose. Tiwari *et al.* (1994) reported that the vapour emitted by bark completely inhibited the mycelial growth of *A. flavus* and *A. niger*. Tiwari *et al.* (1998) found that the bark oil of *Cinnamomum zeylanicum* having the insect repellent activity against the pulse bettle, *Callosobrachus chinensis* L. by olfactometer. The minimum doses of repellency and LC 50 were found to be 0.002 per cent and 0.004 per cent respectively. Besides, the insect repellent potency of the oil was found to be thermostable and posses long shelf life at its absolute repellency concentration (0.004 per cent). Thus the oil of *Cinnamomum* demonstrated its activity as potent insecticides which may prove its usefulness as biodegradable, indigenous and herbal preservatives for safe storage of gram meant for human consumption.

Citrus aurantifolia (Rutaceae)

Gupta and Singh (1982) reported the toxicity of leaf oil against many fungi *viz. Aspergillus fumigatus, A. nidulans, A. niger, Cunninghamella echinulata, Cladosporium herbarum, Fusarium moniliforme, F. oxysporum* and *Rhizopus* sp. Narsimha Rao and Subba Rao (1982) reported the toxicity of the oil against human pathogenic fungi *viz. Candida albicans, Epidermophyton floccosum, Trichophyton mentagrophytes* and *T. rubrum*.

Citrus aurantifolium (Rutaceae)

Rao and Joseph (1971) reported that the oil was toxic to *Candida albicans, Cephalosporium sacchari, Ceratocystis paradoxa, Curvularia lunata, Epidermophyton floccosum, Fusarium moniliforme, Helminthosporium sacchari, Physalospora tucumanesis, Sclerotium rolfsii, Trichophyton mentagrophytes* and *T. rubrum*.

Cinnamomum bergamia (Rutaceae)

Ceruti *et al.* (1982) reported the toxicity of the oil against *Aspergillus flavus, A. fumigatus, Fusarium oxysporum, Penicillium digitatum* and *Trichophyton mentagrophytes*.

Citrus sinensis (Rutaceae)

The oil from epicarp exhibited strong fungitoxicity at 0.5 per cent concentration against *A. flavus, P. italicum* and *Alternaria alternata* as a contact toxicant. The oil at the same concentration inhibited heavy doses of inocula and exhibited quick killing action. The pesticidal action of the oil was thermostable upto 80°C and lasted even upto 24 months. The oil was broad spectrum (Shukla *et al.*, 2000).

Citrus lemon (Rutaceae)

de Souza *et al.* (2005) noted that oil and the phytochemicals citral, eugenol and mircene showed significant antimould activity. Among the products that evidenced the antimould activity citral and eugenol showed the lowest minimum inhibitory concentration, which was 1 per cent and 4 per cent respectively. The mould strains assayed are *Fusarium* sp. *Rhizopus* sp. *Aspergillus flavus, A. niger* and *Penicillium* sp.

Citrus medica (Rutaceae)

Essien, *et al.* (2008) evaluated the in vitro antifungal effect of the essential oil of *Citrus medica* L. on storage fungi of *Arachis hypogea* L. stored for 6 months using the disc diffusion agar method. The oil exhibited a wide spectrum of fungitoxicity, inhibiting all 14 fungus species tested. Thus, the oil can be exploited as a fumigant against storage fungi for the preservation of stored legume seeds due to its wide range of activity, non-phytotoxicity, and long-term persistence of fungitoxicity. Dubey (1981) isolated 0.5 per cent oil from the leaves and found it to be a mixture of 3 major and 10 minor components. The oil was fungistatic at 2000 ppm (2.0×10^3 ml/l) concentration against the test fungi, *Aspergillus flavus* and *A. versicolor.* The fungitoxic factor of the oil was susceptible to temperature treatment beyond 80°C but retained its toxicity up to 380 days during storage at room temperature. Dubey *et al.* (1982 a, b) reported that the oil at 2000 ppm (2.0×10^3 ml/l) dose, inhibited the mycelial growth of the *Acrophialospora fusispora, A. racemosa, Acremonium* sp., *Alternaria alternata, A. solani, Aspergillus nidulans, A. niger, A. flavipes, A. fumigatus, A. rubber, Chaetomium* sp., *Cladosporium cladosporioides, Colletotrichum capsici, Curvularia lunata, Paecilomyces varioti, Penicillium pinophilum, Rhizopus* sp. and *Trichoderma viride.* The vapour of the oil also controlled fungal deteriorations of the seeds of *Coriandrum sativum* and *Foeniculum vulgare* at 4000-ppm (4.0×10^3 ml/l) concentration up to 120 days in storage, without showing any adverse effect on their germination and seedling growth. Mishra *et al.* (1989) isolated the essential oil from leaves and reported its toxicity against *Aspergillus flavus* at 2000-ppm (2.0×10^3 ml/l) dose.

Citrus reticulata (Rutaceae)

The germicidal property of the leaf oil was first reported by Murdoch and Allen (1960). They reported that the oil was toxic to species of *Aspergillus* and *Torula.* Baiter (1971) reported that the fungitoxicity of the oil against *Candida albicans* and *Trichoderma lignorum* was due to its adverse effect on respiration. Devis and Smooth (1972) reported that the oil from fruits peels inhibited the spore germination of *P. digitatum.* Alderman and Marth (1976) reported that the oil inhibited the growth as well as aflatoxin production in *Aspergillus parasiticus.*

Citrus sinensis (Rutaceae)

Singh *et al.* (1978b) reported toxicity of the oil against *Nannizzia incurvata* (+), *N. incurvata* (–), *Botryotrichum kerotinophyllum* and *Malbranchea aurantica.*

Clerodendrum inerme (Verbinaceae)

Singh *et al.* (1979b) reported the toxicity of the oil against *Alternaria* sp., *Aspergillus candidus, A. flavus, A. fumigatus, A. nidulans, A. niger, Cladosporium herbarum, Cunninghamella echinulata, Fusarium moniliforme, F. oxysporum, Helminthosporium sachhari, Microsporum cocci, M. gypseum, Mucor mucedo, Penicillium digitatum, Rhizopus* sp., *Trichophyton mentagrophytes, T. rubrum* and *Trichothecium roseum.*

Coleus ambonicus (Lamiaceae)

Srivastava (1990) reported its toxicity against *Aspergillus flavus,* and *A. niger* at 1.0×10^3 ml/l concentration. The nature of toxicity was fungistatic at MIC but turned fungicidal at 0.3×10^3 ml/l concentration. Besides, the essential oil also inhibited the mycelial growth of 33 fungal species at its MIC.

Coriandrum sativum (Apiaceae)

Capek (1955) and Slavenas (1963) reported that the oil was toxic to *Aspergillus niger*. Inhibitory effect of the oil against *Alternaria tenuis, Aspergillus oryzae* and *Penicillium chrysogenum* was demonstrated by Do Vgich (1971). Sharma and Singh (1979b) reported that the oil was toxic to *Alternaria* sp., *Aspergillus candidus, A. flavus, A. fumigatus, A. nidulans, Cladosporium herbarum, Cunninghamella echinulata, Fusarium moniliforme, F. oxysporum, Helminthosporium sachhari, Microsporum cocci, M. gypseum, Mucor mucedo, Penicillium digitatum, Rhizopus* sp., *Trichophyton mentagrophytes, T. rubrum* and *Trichothecium roseum*. The oil was studied by Garg and Siddiqui (1992) *in vitro* for its antifungal activity against 18 fungal organisms using "Filter Paper Disc Agar Diffusion Technique". The strong antifungal activity against *Alternaria alternata, Curvularia lunata, Pestalotia psidi, Phytopthora parasitica, Trichoderma viride* and *Collectotrichum capsici* can be exploited.

Cuminum cyminum (Apiaceae)

Nigam and Rao (1977) reported that the oil produced inhibitory zone in culture seeded with *Aspergillus fumigatus, Fusarium tenuis*, and *Trichoderma viride* but was ineffective against *Aspergillus flavus, A. versicolor, A. oryzae, Curvularia* sp., *Penicillium javanicum* and *P. funiculosum*. Sharma and Singh (1979b) using filter paper disc technique reported that *Alternaria* sp., *Aspergillus candidus, A. flavus, A. nidulans, A. niger, Cladosporium herbarum, Cunninghamella echinulata, Fusarium moniliforme, F. oxysporum, Helminthosporium sacchari, Microsporum cocci, M. gypseum, Mucor mucedo, Penicillium digitatum, Rhizopus* sp. *Trichophyton mentagrophytes. T. rubrum* and *Trichothecium roseum* were susceptible to the oil. Saksena (1984) reported that the fungitoxic efficacy of the oil against *Aspergillus fumigatus, Candida albicans, C. tropicalis, Keratinomyces ajelloi, Microsporum gypseum, Trichophyton equinum* and *T. rubrum* was superior to griseofulvin. Singh and Upadhyay (1991) also reported that the oil was strongly fungitoxic against *Aspergillus flavus* and *A. niger*. Oil from seeds of *Cuminum cyminum* contained more than 60 compound principal among them were cumin aldehyde (36 per cent), β-pinene (19.3 per cent), p-cymine (18.4 per cent) and γ-terpinene (15.3 per cent). Antimicrobial testing showed high activity against *Aspergillus niger* and yeast *Saccharomyces cereviceae* and *Candida albicans*. (Jirovetz *et al.*, 2005)

Curcuma amada (Zingiberaceae)

Rao and Joseph (1971) reported that rhizome oil was toxic to *Cephalosporium sacchari, Ceratocystis paradoxa, Curvularia lunata, Fusarium moniliforme, Helminthosporium sacchari, Physalospora tucumanensis* and *Sclerotium rolfsii*. Banerjee and Nigam (1978a) and Mahajan *et al.* (1978) reported antifungal activity of the oil against *Aspergillus niger, A. flavus, Curvularia oryzae, Helminthosporium oryzae, Microsporum gypseum, Penicillium javanicum, P. liliacinum, Pestalotia lapagericola, Trichoderma viride* and *Trichophyton mentagrophytes*.

Curcuma angustifolia (Zingiberaceae)

Banerjee and Nigam (1977) reported that 0.1 ml of 1 : 1000 dilution of the oil produced significant inhibitory zone in cultures of *Aspergillus flavus, A. niger, Curvularia* sp., *P. lilacinum, Pestalotia lapagericola, Trichoderma viride* and *Trichophyton mentagrophytes*.

Curcuma cassia (Zingiberaceae)

Garg and Jain (1998) reported the toxicity of the rhizome oil against *A. niger* and *A. fumigatus*.

Curcuma aromatica (Zingiberaceae)

Toxicity of the rhizome oil was reported against *Aspergillus flavus, A. niger, Curvularia oryzae, Helminthosporium oryzae, Microsporum gypseum, Penicillium javanicum, P. lilacinum, Pestalotia lapagericola, Trichoderma viride* and *Trichophyton mentagrophytes*. (Rao, 1976b and Banerjee *et al*., 1978b).

Curcuma longa (Zingiberaceae)

The rhizome oil was reported to possess toxicity against *Aspergillus flauvs, A. niger, Curvularia oryzae, Helminthosporium oryzae, Microsporum gypseum, Penicillium javanicum, P. lilacinum, Pestalotia lapagericola, Trichoderma viride* and *Trichophyton mentagrophytes* (Banerjee and Nigam, 1978a, b). Chandi *et al*. (1999) reported that the turmeric leaf and rhizome oils were fungicidal against *Candida albicans* MTCC-183. Leaf oil showed better activities in comparison to rhizome oil. Leaf oil killed the test pathogen with in 1-15 minute. The activities were well compared with standard antifungal drugs. The essential oil from the rhizomes of *Curcuma longa* has been studied for antifungal activity against five fungi *viz. Aspergillus niger, A. fumigatus, Curvularia lunata, Fusarium psidi* and *Rhizopus oryzae* (Garg and Jain, 2003). Gurdip Singh *et al*. (2003) reported that the rhizome oil was toxic to several bacteria and is better antifungal as compared to synthetic fungicides. The oil has no adverse effect on seed germination and seedling growth of some common agricultural crops. The fungitoxic spectrum shows that oil has strong fungitoxic activity (100 per cent mycelial inhibition) against *Colletotrichum falcatum, Fusarium moniliforme*, and *Helminthosporium oryzae* at 1000-ppm concentration and against *Aspergillus niger, Curvularia pallescens, Fusarium oxysporum* and *Periconia atropurpurea* at 2000 ppm concentration. Mycelial growth of *A. flavus, Curvularia lunata* and *Rhizoctonia solani* was completely inhibited at 3000-ppm concentration.

Curcuma zedoaria (Zingiberaceae)

Rao and Joseph (1971) reported the toxicity of the oil against *Cephalosporium sacchari, Ceratocystis paradoxa, Curvularia lunata, Fusarium moniliforme, Helminthosporium sacchari, Physalospora tucumanensis* and *Sclerotium rolfsii*. Mishra and Dixit (1978), Banerjee and Nigam (1978b) and Banerjee *et al*. (1978b) reported toxicity of the oil against *Alternaria tenuis, Aspergillus flavus, A. niger, Curvularia oryzae, Fusarium nivale, Helminthosporium oryzae, Microsporum gypseum, Penicillium lilacinum, P. javanicum, Pestalotia lapagericola, Trichoderma viride* and *Trichophyton mentagrophytes*. Narsimha Rao and Subba Rao (1982) further reported the antifungal spectrum of the oil against many pathogenic fungi including *Candida albicans, Epidermophyton floccosum* and *Trichophyton rubrum*.

Cydonia oblonga (Rosaceae)

Shikhaliev (1974) reported that the oil from fruits was toxic to *Fusarium avenaceum*.

Cymbopogon citratus (Poaceae)

The toxicity of the oil against *Microsporum gypseum* and *Penicillium notatum* was reported by Sawhney *et al*. (1977). Arora and Pandey (1977) reported that the oil was not only toxic to *Penicillium italicum* but also controlled blue mould decay of citrus fruits during storage. Handique and Singh (1990) extracted essential oil from a mutant strain M-81 of lemon grass and tested against *Rhizoctonia solani, Sclerotium rolfsii* and *Sclerotinia sclerotiorum* at 100 ppm (0.1×10^3 ml/l). The growth of *Rhizoctonia solani* and *Sclerotinia sclerotiorum* was decreased by 67 per cent and 40 per cent respectively whereas it was ineffective against *Sclerotium rolfsii*. Dwivedi *et al*. (1990) tested the oil against *Macrophomina phaseolina* and found to be toxic at 500, 1000 and 2000 ppm (0.5×10^3 ml/l, 1.0×10^3 ml/l and 2.0×10^3 ml/l) doses. Oil and leaf powder of *Cymbopogon citratus* (lemon grass) at 0.1 and 0.25 per cent (v/w) and ground leaves at 10 per cent (w/w) significantly reduced deterioration and aflatoxin production in shelled melon seeds inoculated with toxigenic *Aspergillus flavus, A. niger, A. tamarii* and *Penicillium citrinum* (Bankole and Joda, 2003).

Cymbopogon flexuosus (Poaceae)

Saksena (1984) reported the toxicity of the oil agaisnt *Aspergillus fumigatus, Candida albicans, C. tropicalis, Keratinomyces ajelloi, Microsporum gypseum, Trichophyton equinum* and *T. rubrum*. The oil from leaves was strongly toxic against following storage fungal pests *viz. Aspergillus flavus, Penicillium italicum* and *Alternaria alternata*. The oil showed broad spectrum, inhibited heavy doses of inocula, thermostable and toxicity persisted for at least 12 months (Shukla *et al.*, 2000). The minimum bioactive concentration with fungicidal action of the oil was found to be 0.2 µl/ml for *Alternaria alternata*, 0.4 µl/ml for *A. flavus, A. fumigatus, A. parasiticus, Cladosporium cladosporioides, P. italicum, P. digitatum* and a number of other fungi, and 0.5 µl/ml for *Botrytis cyneria* and *Helminthosporium oryzae*. The bioactivity of oil was broad spectrum, thermostable and lasted upto 48 months. The oil was used for *in vivo* controlling postharvest spoilage of *Malus pumilo* (Shahi *et al.*, 2002). de Souza *et al.* (2005) noted that oil from *Cymbopogon citratus* and the phytochemicals citral, eugenol and mircene showed significant antimould activity. Among the products that evidenced the antimould activity citral and eugenol showed the lowest minimum inhibitory concentration, which was 1 per cent and 4 per cent respectively. The mould strains assayed are *Fusarium* sp. *Rhizopus* sp. *Aspergillus flavus, A. niger* and *Penicillium* sp.

Cymbopogon martinii (Poaceae)

Kala *et al.* (1984) reported that the oil from shoots completely prevented the growth and production of hepatocarcinogenic aflatoxin by *Aspergillus parasiticus*. Jeyalakshmi *et al.* (1997) evaluated the oil against chili fruit rot caused by *Colletotrichum capsici* (syd) Butler and Bisby at different concentration *viz.* 0.1, 0.075, 0.05, 0.025, 0.01 and 0.005 percent *in-vitro* following poisoned food technique and spore germination assay. It exerted cent percent inhibition on mycelial growth and spore germination even at 0.025 per cent concentration. Because of its strong fungitoxic activity it may be exploited for the management of chili fruit rot disease. Babu *et al.* (2000) to test the antifungal properties of palma rosa [*Cymbopogan martinii* (Roxb.) Watson] oil used it against *Alternaria solani*, the tomato leaf blight pathogen. Palma rosa oil inhibited the mycelial growth and spore germination of *A. solani* at 0.3 per cent concentration. Mycelial growth and spore germination were observed at very low concentration of the oil (below 0.2 per cent).

Cymbopogon nardus (Poaceae)

The growth and production of hepatocarcinogenic aflatoxin by *Aspergillus parasiticus* was reduced when cultures were supplemented with graded concentration of the oil (Kala *et al.*, 1984).

Cymbopogon winteriunus (Poaceae)

Sawhney *et al.* (1977) reported that the oil possessed toxicity against *Microsporum gypseum* and *Penicillium notatum*.

Cyperus scariosus (Cyperaceae)

Lahariya and Rao (1979) reported that the oil was toxic to *Aspergillus fumigatus, A. niger, Chrysosporium tropicum, Malbranchea pulchella, Microsporum gypseum* and *Penicillium lilacinum*. Dikshit and Hussain (1984) reported inhibitory effect of the oil against *Trichsophyton equinum* and *T. rubrum*.

Dalbergia sissoo (Fabaceae)

Jain *et al.* (1979) reported toxicity of the oil against *Alternaria solani, Aspergillus flavus, A. fumigatus, A. nidulans, A. niger, Cladosporium herbarum, Cunninghamella* sp., *Fusarium moniliforme, Helminthosporium* sp., *Penicillium digitatum, P. italicum, Rhizopus nigricans* and *Trichothecium roseum.*

Daucus carota (Apiaceae)

Chaurasia and Kher (1978a, b) and Grover and Rao (1978a) reported that the oil was toxic to species of *Aspergillus, Curvularia* and *Penicillium.*

Dinnetia tripetala (pepperfruit)

Essential oil and phenolic extracts inhibited growth of several food borne microorganisms including sp. of *Penicillium* and *Aspergillus* (Ejechi and Akpomedaye, 2004).

Dysoxylum malabaricum (Meliaceae)

Parcha *et al.* (2003) tested for antimicrobial activity of essential oil from the leaves of *Dysoxylum malabaricum* against *Aspergillus niger, A. flavus, Penicillium* sp. and *Candida albicans.* The oil was found effective in inhibiting the growth of all the organisms. Maximum inhibition was found in case of *C. albicans.*

Eucalyptus sp. (Myrtaceae)

The effectiveness of *Eucalyptus* oil to control the black mould of onion bulbs was observed by Tiwari *et al.* (1988) and it was found that the oil at 1.0×10^3 ml/l concentration effectively reduced the decay as well as the sprouting of stored onions. Oil showed inhibitory effect on the mycelial growth of three soil borne plant pathogen *viz., Sclerotium rolfsii, Rhizoctonia solani* and *Sclerotinia rolfsii* (Handique and Singh, 1989). Suri and Thind (1979) reported that the *Eucalyptus camaldulensis* oil was toxic to *Aspergillus fumigatus, Penicillium notation* and some human pathogens. Kaul and Nigam (1977) and Sampurna and Nigam (1979) reported that the *E. citriodora* oil was toxic to *Aspergillus niger, Candida albicans, C. utilis, Keratinophyton terreus, Malbranchea pulchella* and *Trichophyton mentagrophytes.* Suri *et al.* (1979) recorded that the pure oil of *E. citriodora* controlled fruit rot of apple caused by *Clathridium corticola* and 1: 1000 dilution of the same oil completely checked the growth of *A. niger, C. corticola* and *Microsporum gypseum.* The toxicity of the *E. citriodora* oil against *Aspergillus flavus, A. fumigatus, Fusarium oxysporum* and *Penicillium digitatum* was also reported by Ceruti *et al.* (1982). Haerdtl (1962) reported the fungitoxicity of the volatile constituent from *E. gennii* against *Aspergillus niger.* Egawa *et al.* (1977) isolated gallic acid and unidentified isomers of benzene from the volatile constituent of the same plant and reported that the compounds were inhibitory to conidial germination of *Cochliobolus benaus.* However, Arora and Pandey (1984a, b) recorded the toxicity of the oil against *Alternaria tenuis, Diplodia metalensis* and *Penicillium digitatum.* Ceruti *et al.* (1982) reported the toxicity of the *E. globulus* oil against *Aspergillus flavus, A. fumigatus, Fusarium oxysporum, Penicillium digitatum* and *Trichophyton mentagrophytes.* Benjinali *et al.* (1984) reported that the oil possessed broad antifungal spectrum and Dwivedi and Dubey (1986) observed that the oil was inhibitory to sclerotial germination of *Macrophomina phaseoli.* Ceruti *et al.* (1982) recorded the toxicity of the *E. piperita* oil against *Aspergillus flavus, A. fumigatus, Fusarium oxysporum,* and *Penicillium digitatum* and *Tichophyton mentagrophytes.* Shahi *et al.* (1997) noted that essential oils from *Eucalyptus citriodora, E. dalarympleana, E. laveopinea, E. pauciflora* at 1000 ppm showed complete inhibition of the storage spoilage test fungus *Penicillium italicum.* The oil of *E. dalarympleana* and *E. laveopinea* showed fungistatic toxicity against the test fungus at 3000-ppm but the oil of *E. laveopinea* showed partial inhibition at 3000 ppm. The oil of *E. citriodora* at 1000-ppm exhibited fungicidal nature and withstood heavy inoculum. Shahi *et al.* (2002) noted that essential oil extracted from leaves of *Eucalyptus pauciflora* showed toxicity against fungal pests *viz.*, sp. of *Alternaria, Aspergillus, Penicillium,* and *Rhizopus.* The effective pesticidal concentration (EPC) of the oil was found to be 0.3×10^3, 0.4×10^3, 0.5×10^3 and 0.6×10^3ml/l respectively inhibiting the mycelial growth of the tested pests completely.

Eugenia bracteata (Myrtaceae)

Rao and Joseph (1971) recorded that the oil was toxic to *Cephalosporium sachhari, Ceratocystis paradoxa, Curvularia lunata, Fusarium moniliforme, Helminthosporium sacchari, Physalospora tucumanensis* and *Sclerotium rolfsii.*

Eugenia caryophylata (Myrtaceae)

Clove oleoresin at 0.2 to 0.8 per cent (v/v) was studied against the test microorganisms such as *Candida albicans, Pencillium citrinum, Aspergillus niger* and *Trichophyton mentagrophytes.* It was highly effective against *T. mentagrophytes* and *Candida albicans. P. citrinum* and *A. niger* were relatively more resistant. Clove oleoresin was first dispersed in sugar solution and then used for antifungal testing (Nunez *et al.*, 2001)

Eugenia heyneana (Myrtaceae)

Rao and Joseph (1971) recorded the toxicity of the oil against *Ceratocystis paradoxa, Curvularia lunata, Helminthosporium sacchari* and *Physalospora tucumanensis.* Garg (1974) while testing the range of antifungal activity reported that the oil was toxic to *Curvularia geniculata, C. cappescens, Fusarium culmorum, F. oxysporum, Helminthosporium* sp. and *Pythium aphanidermatum.* Narsimha Rao and Subba Rao (1982) recorded toxicity of the oil against *Candida albicans, Epidermophyton floccosum, Trichophyton mentagrophytes* and *T. rubrum.*

Eupatorium ayapana (Asteraceae)

Chaurasia and Kher (1978a, b) reported toxicity of the oil against species of *Aspergillus, Curvularia and Penicillium.* Sharma and Singh (1979b) recorded toxicity of the oil against *Alternaria* sp., *Aspergillus candidus, A. flavus, A. fumigatus, A. nidulans, A. niger, Cladosporium herbarum, Cunninghamella echinulata, Fusarium moniliforme, F. oxysporum, Helminthosporium sacchari, Microsporum cocci, M. gypseum, Mucor mucedo, Penicillium digitatum, Rhizopus* sp., *Trichophyton mentagrophytes, T. rubrum* and *Trichothecium roseum.*

Eupatorium cannabinum (Asteraceae)

Dubey, *et al.* (2007) extracted essential oil of *Eupatorium cannabinum,* it was found to be fungitoxic in nature against *Botryodiplodia theobromae* and *Colletotrichum gloeosporioides* causing stem end rot disease and anthracnose disease in mango respectively. Dwivedi *et al.* (1990) tested the oil against *Macrophomina phaseolina* and found to be toxic at 500, 1000 and 2000 ppm (0.5×10^3 ml/l, 1.0×10^3 ml/l and 2.0×10^3 ml/l) doses.

Eupatorium capillifolium (Asteraceae)

Chandra *et al.* (1982c) reported that the leaves yielded 1 per cent of the oil which was fungitoxic to *Absidia ramose, Alternaria raphani, Aspergillus awamori, A. sydowi, Colletotrichum capsici, C. gloeosporioides, Curvularia lunata, Helminthosporium oryzae* and *Rhizoctonia solani* at 1.0×10^3 ml/l dose. They further reported that the fungitoxicity of the oil was enhanced at pH 7 and pH 9.

Eupatorium triplinerve (Asteraceae)

Garg (1974) reported that the leaf oil was toxic to *Aspergillus candidus, A. fumigatus, A. nidulans, A. terreus, Curvularia geniculata, C. pallescens, Fusarium culmorum, F. oxysporum, Paecilomyces* sp., *Penicillium chrysogenum, Helminthosporium* sp., *Pythium aphanidermatum, Trichoderma viride* and *Trichurus* sp.

Feronia elephantum (Rutaceae)

Sharma *et al.* (1978) reported that the oil, which contained estragol, was toxic to *Alternaria helianthi, Colletotrichum capsici, Fusarium moniliforme, F. solani, Helminthosporium oryzae, H. turcicum, Pythium vexans, Pyricularia setariae, Rhizoctonia bataticola* and. *R. solani.* Zutshi *et al.* (1975), Zutshi and Mehta (1977) and Gupta and Singh (1982) reported that the oil possessed toxicity against *Aspergillus fumigatus, A. niger, A. nidulans, Cladosporium herbarum, Cunninghamella echinulata, Fusarium moniliforme, F. oxysporum* and *Rhizopus* sp. Dubey (1993) reported the toxicity of the oil against *Aspergillus flavus* and *A. niger* at 1.0×10^3 ml/l doses and was fungicidal.

Ferula jaeschkeana (Apiaceae)

Gautam *et al.* (1990) reported that the oil was toxic to *Nannizzia fulva, N. gypsea* and *N. incurvata.*

Foeniculum vulgare (Apiaceae)

Ozcan *et al.* (2006) examined the chemical composition of the flower and unripe and ripe fruits from fennel (bitter) (*Foeniculum vulgare* ssp. *piperitum*) by gas chromatography and gas chromatography-mass spectrometry. The main identified components of the flower and unripe and ripe fruit oils were estragole (53.08 per cent, 56.11 per cent, and 61.08 per cent), fenchone (13.53 per cent, 19.18 per cent, and 23.46 per cent), and α-phellandrene (5.77 per cent, 3.30 per cent, and 0.72 per cent), respectively. The oils exerted varying levels of antifungal effects on the experimental mycelial growth of *Alternaria alternata, Fusarium oxysporum,* and *Rhizoctonia solani.* The 40 ppm concentrations of fennel oils showed inhibitory effect against mycelial growth of *A. alternata,* whereas 10 ppm levels were ineffective. Capek (1956) reported toxicity of the oil against *Aspergillus flavus.* Later Do Vgich (1971) reported the toxicity against *Alternaria tenuis, Aspergillus oryzae* and *Penicillium chrysogenum.* Sharma and Singh (1979b) reported the toxicity against *Alternaria* sp., *Aspergillus candidus, A. flavus, A. fumigatus, A. nidulans, A. niger, Cladosporium herbarum, Caninghamella echinulata, Fusarium moniliforme, F. oxysporum, Helminthosporium sacchari, Microsporum cocci, M. gypseum, Mucor mucedo, Penicillium digitatum, Rhizopus* sp., *Trichophyton mentagrophytes, T. rubrum, Trichothecium roseum.* However, Narayan *et al.* (1980a) reported the toxicity of the oil against *A. fumigatus, A. niger, Candida tropicalis* and *Rhizopus oryzae.* Shukla (1987) reported that the fungitoxic factor of the oil was thermostable and remained active during storage upto 365 days. The antifungal efficacy of the oil was not affected when the inoculum density of *Penicillium italicum* was increased. Shukla and Tripathi (1987a) reported that the oil at 1.5×10^3 ml/l completely inhibited the mycelial growth of *Alternaria alternata, A. tenuissima, Aspergillus awamori, A. ochraceus, A. parasiticus, A. sydowi, A. tamarii, A. terreus, Botryodiplodia theobromae, Colletotrichum capsici, Curvularia lunata, C. pallascens, Drechslera hawaiiensis, D. oryzae, Epicoccum nigrum, Fusarium acuminatum, F. equiseti, F. semitectum, F. udum, Macrophomina phaseolina, Mwemnoniella echinata, Nigrospora oryzae, Penicillium chrysogenum, P. citrinum* and *Rhizopus nigricans* and enhanced the seed germination *of Arachis hypogea.*

Geranium sp. (Geraniaceae)

Sampurna and Nigam (1979) and Saksena (1984) reported that the oil was toxic to *Aspergillus fumigatus, Candida albicans, C. tropicalis, Keratinophyton terreum, Keratinomyces ajelloi, Microsporum gypseum, Trichophyton rubrum* and *T. equinum.*

Glossocardia bosvallia (Asteraceae)

Pathak and Dixit (1984) reported toxicity of the oil against *Aspergillus niger, Botryodiplodia theobromae, Botryotrichum keratinophyllum, Chrysosporium tropicum, Microsporum gypseum, Malbranchea pulchella, Phytophthora parasitica* var. *piperina* and *Rhizopus nodosus.*

Hedychium spicatum (Zingiberaceae)

Samuel and Tripathi (1994) reported that the essential oil extracted from the rhizome completely inhibited the mycelial growth of *Helminthosporium oryzae* and *Fusarium moniliforme* at a minimum dose of 1000 ppm. The nature of toxicity against the test fungi at this concentration was fungistatic but turned fungicidal at 5000 ppm dose. Temperature treatment upto 120°C and storage up to 365 days (at 28 + 2°C) did not alter the fungistatic efficacy of the oil. The oil exhibited broad fungitoxic spectrum and proved non-phytotoxic to seed germination and seedling growth of *Oryza sativa* and *Hordeum vulgare.*

Helichrysum italicum (Asteraceae)

Chirkina and Osipova (1974) reported that the oil obtained from flowers showed the presence of eugenol, furfural, geroniol, neusol and pinene and inhibited the growth of *Candida albicans.*

Hypericum patulum (Hyperaceae)

Kumar (1992) reported the toxicity of the oil against *Aspergillus flavus, A. ochraceus,* and *Fusarium oxysporum* at 1.2×10^3ml/l. The oil was fungistatic at its MIC and remained static even upto 10×10^3 ml/l conc. of the oil.

Hyptis suaveolens (Lamiaceae)

Pandey *et al.* (1982c) recovered 0.22 per cent oil from the leaves and reported its toxicity at 4.0×10^3 ml/l concentration against *Aspergillus flavus, A. rubrum, A. versicolor, Chaetomium globosum, Cladosporium cladosporioides, Fusarium oxysporum, Helminthosporium oryzae, Microsporum gypseum, Monilia sitophila, Pyricularia oryzae, Rizopus arrhizus, Trichophyton equinum, T. mentagrophytes* and *T. rubrum.* They further reported that the thermostable antifungal factor of the oil was most effective at pH 9 and remained unaffected by autoclaving and storage upto 180 days. They also observed that the oil successfully prevented the leaf spot disease of paddy without showing any toxicity to the host plant. However, Singh *et al.* (1983a) reported that the oil at 1.0×10^3 ml/l concentration completely inhibited the mycelial growth of *Epidermophyton floccosum, Microsporum canis* and *Trichophyton mentagrophytes.*

Hyssopus officinalis (Lamiaceae)

Do Vgich (1971) reported the toxicity of the oil against *Alternaria tenuis, Aspergillus oryzae* and *Penicillium chrysogenum.*

Inula cuspidata (Asteraceae)

Chauhan and Saxena (1985) reported that the oil was toxic to *Aspergillus flavus, A. fumigatus, A. glaucus, A. nidulans* and *A. terreus.*

Inula racemosa (Asteraceae)

Mishra and Dixit (1978) reported that the oil possessed toxicity against *Colletotrichum capsici* and *Fusarium moniliforme.* Later Mishra *et al.* (1979a) recorded toxicity of the oil against *Alternaria helianthi, Fusarium solani, Helminthosporium turcicum, H. oryzae, Pyricularia setariae, Pythium vexans, Rhizoctonia bataticola* and *R. solani.*

Juniperus communis (Pinaceae)

The toxicity of the oil against *Aspergillus niger* was reported by Slavenas and Razinskaite (1962) and Slavenas (1963). Dwivedi *et al.* (1990) tested the oil against *Macrophomina phaseolina* and found to be toxic at 500, 1000 and 2000 ppm (0.5×10^3 ml/l, 1.0×10^3 ml/l, 2.0×10^3ml/l). This fungus causes root rot disease of crops.

Juniperus macropoda (Pinaceae)

Singh *et al.* (1978b) and Mishra and Chauhan (1984) reported that the oil possessed toxicity against *Botryotrichum keratinophyllum, Epidermophyton floccosum, Malbranchea aurantica, Nannizzia incurvata* (+), *N. incurvata* (–) and *Trichophyton rubrum.*

Juniperus verginiana (Pinaceae)

Mall *et al.* (1985) reported that the wood oil was fungistatic to *Candida pseudotropicalis, Epidermophyton floccosum, Microsporum gypseum, Sporothrix schenekii* and *Trichophyton rubrum* at 1.0×10^3 ml/l dose but became fungicidal at 6.0×10^3 ml/l.

Lantana camara (Verbinaceae)

Avadhoot and Verma (1978) reported that the seed oil was toxic to *Candida albicans, Curvularia lunata* and *Fusarium oxysporum.* Sharma and Singh (1979b) reported the toxicity of the oil against *Alternaria* sp., *Aspergillus candidus, A. flavus, A. fumigatus, A. nidulans, A. niger, Cladosporium herbarum, Cunninghamella echinulata, Fusarium moniliforme, Helminthosporium sacchari, Microsporum cocci, M. gypseum, Mucor mucedo, Penicillium digitatum, Rhizopus* sp., *Trichophyton mentagrophytes, T. rubrum* and *Trichothecium roseum.*

Lantana indica (Verbinaceae)

Rao and Joseph (1971) and Narsimha Rao and Subba Rao (1982) reported that the oil was toxic to *Candida albicans, Epidermophyton floccosum, Trichophyton mentagrophytes* and *T. rubrum.*

Laurus nobilis (Lauraceae)

The toxicity of the oil against *Aspergillus niger* was reported by Capek (1955).

Lepidogathis hyalina (Acanthaceae)

The essential oil of *L. hyalina* inhibited the mycelial growth of *Aspergillus flavus, A. niger* and some bacteria (Yadava, 1986).

Lapidium ruderale (Brassicaceae)

Singh *et al.* (1984) reported that the oil from growing tips was toxic to *Aspergillus flavus* at 1.0×10^3 ml/l dose.

Leucus aspera (Lamiaceae)

Rao and Joseph (1971) and Narsimha Rao and Subba Rao (1982) reported the toxicity of the oil against *Candida albicans, Epidermophyton floccosum, Trichophyton mentagrophytes* and *T. rubrum.*

Lippia alba (Verbinaceae)

Dwivedi *et al.* (1990) tested the oil against *Macrophomina phaseolina* and found to be toxic at 500, 1000 and 2000 ppm. This fungus causes root rot of crops. de Souza *et al.* (2005) noted that oil from

Lippia alba, Lippia microphylla and the phytochemicals citral, eugenol and mircene showed significant antimould activity. Among the products that evidenced the antimould activity citral and eugenol showed the lowest minimum inhibitory concentration, which was 1 per cent and 4 per cent respectively. The mould strains assayed are *Fusarium* sp., *Rhizopus* sp., *Aspergillus flavus, A. niger* and *Penicillium* sp.

Lippia javanica (Verbinaceae)

Leaves of Bangladeshi *Lippia javanica* gave essential oil content of 0.15 per cent. Thirty-three compounds comprising 99.3 per cent of the oil were identified by GC/MS. The major constituents were geraniol (29 per cent), neral (19.3 per cent), isopropenyl acetophenone (15.9 per cent) and linalool (10.6 per cent). The oil was tested for fungitoxic properties against six pathogens. The minimum concentration for absolute inhibition of the *Alternaria alternata, Fusarium equiseti. Curvularia lunata, Colletotrichum corchori* was found to be 250 ppm and *Macrophomina phaseolina, Botrydiplodia theobromae* were found to be 750 ppm and 1000 ppm respectively (Chowdhury *et al.*, 2003).

Majorana hortensis (Lamiaceae)

Yadav and Saini (1991) reported its antimicrobial activity against *Aspergillus fumigatus* and *A. niger.*

Melaleuca leucadendron (Myrtaceae)

Dubey *et al.* (1983 b) reported that the leaf oil was fungistatic to *Colletotrichum capsici, Curvularia lunata, Helminthosporium oryzae, Pyricularia oryzae, Pythium aphanidermatum, P. debaryanum, Rhizoctonia solani* and *Syncephalastrum* sp. at 0.05×10^3 ml/l but at 0.5×10^3 ml/l it turned fungicidal. However, at 0.5×10^3 ml/l the oil was proved to have no adverse effect on seed germination and seedling growth of *Phaseolus aureus*. Mishra *et al.* (1989) isolated the essential oil from leaves and reported its toxicity against *Aspergillus flavus* at 2.0×10^3ml/l dose.

Melissa officinalis (Lamiaceae)

Dikshit and Hussain (1984) reported the toxicity of the oil against *Microsporum gypseum, Trichophyton equinum* and *T. rubrum.*

Melissa parviflora (Lamiaceae)

The toxicity of the oil against *Colletotrichum* sp. was reported by Lakshmi and Rao (1978).

Mentha arvensis (Lamiaceae)

Kumar, *et al.* (2007) extracted essential oils from *Mentha arvensis*, it was found to be effective against strains of *A. flavus* and completely stopped the radial mycelial growth of *A. flavus* at 0.10 mg mL^{-1}. It was found to be superior over the synthetic fungicides tested and showed a broad fungitoxic spectrum against *A. niger, A. fumigatus, Botryodiplodia theobromae, Cladosporium cladosporioides, Fusarium oxysporum, Helminthosporium oryzae, Macrophomina phaseolina* and *Sclerotium rolfsii* at 0.10 mg mL^{-1}. Sanyal and Verma (1969) reported that the oil was fungitoxic. Later Arora and Pandey (1977, 1984a,b) reported the toxicity of the oil against *Alternaria tenuis, Diplodia metalensis, Penicillium digitatum* and *P. italicum.* Chaurasia and Kher (1978a, b) and Dikshit *et al.* (1979) noted the toxicity of oil against *Aspergillus* sp., *Curvularia lunata,* and *Helminthosporium oryzae.* While Gautam *et al.* (1980) noted the toxicity of oil against dermatophytes *viz. Nannizia fulva, N. gypsea, N. incurvata.* Ceruti *et al.* (1982) reported the toxicity of the oil against *Aspergillus flavus, A. fumigatus, Fusarium oxysporum* and *Trichophyton mentagrophytes.* Singh *et al.* (1983a) recorded that the oil at 2.0×10^3 ml/l was fungicidal to *Absidia ramose, Alternaria brassicae, A. raphani, A. solani, Aspergillus niger, A. lindemuthianum, C. tinosporae, Fusarium monoliforme, F. solani, Paecilomyces fusisporus, Talaromyces* sp. and *Trichoderma viride.* Kala *et al.* (1984) reported that the oil significantly reduced aflatoxin production in *Aspergillus parasiticus.* Arora and Pandey (1984 b) reported that the oil can be successfully exploited for control of blue mould decay in citrus fruits during storage.

Mentha citrata (Lamiaceae)

Sawhney *et al.* (1977) noted the toxicity of the oil against *Microsporum gypseum* and *Penicillium notatum.*

Mentha lavanduliodora (Lamiaceae)

Ceruti *et al.* (1982) reported the oil was toxic to *Aspergillus flavus, A. fumigatus, Fusarium oxysporum, Penicillium digitatum* and *Trichophyton mentagrophytes.*

Mentha piperita (Lamiaceae)

The fungitoxicity of the oil against *Fusarium moniliforme* and *Penicillium luteum* was reported by Makorova (1961) and Kovacs (1964). Gautam *et al.* (1980) reported toxicity of the oil against some dermetaphytes *viz., Nannizzia fulva, N. gypseum* and *N. incurvata.*

Murraya exotica (Rutaceae)

The toxicity of the leaf oil against *Alternaria alternaria, A. solani, Aspergillus flavus, A. fumigatus, A. nidulans, A. niger, Cladosoporium herbarum, Cunninghamella* sp., *Fusarium moniliforme, Helminthosporium* sp., *Penicillium digitatum, P. italicum, Rhizopus nigricans* and *Trichothecium roseum* was first reported by Jain *et al.* (1979). Later Gupta and Singh (1982) reported the toxicity against *Cunninghamella echinulata, Fusarium moniliforme, F. oxysporum* and *Rhizopus* sp.

Murraya paniculata (Rutaceae)

Garg (1974) reported that the oil was inhibitory to *Curvularia geniculata, C. pallescens, Fusarium culmorum, F. oxysporum, Helminthosporium* sp. and *Pythium aphanidermatum.*

Myristica fragrans (Myristicaceae)

Srivastava (1990) reported that the essential oil of *M. fragrans* was toxic to *Aspergillus flavus* and *A. niger* at 2.0×10^3ml/l and 1.0×10^3ml/l doses respectively. The nature of fungitoxicity was found to be fungistatic even at a higher concentration of 15×10^3 ml/l. However, the oil also proved fungitoxic to 33 fungal species.

Nardostachys jatamansi (Valerianaceae)

Girgune *et al.* (1978) reported toxicity of the oil against *Alternaria helianthi, Colletotrichum capsici, Fusarium solani, Helminthosporium oryzae, H. turcicum, Pyricularia setariae, Pythium vexans, Rhizoctonia bataticola* and *R. solani.* Mishra *et al.* (1995) reported that the oil at 1.0×10^3 ml/l conc. inhibited the growth of *Aspergillus flavus, A. niger* and *Fusarium oxysporum.* The oil also proved effective against six other fungi at the same conc. and did not adversely affect seed germination and seedling growth of *C. arietinum* and *Cajanus cajan.*

Nepeta cataria (Lamiaceae)

Makorova (1961) reported the toxicity of the seed oil against *Aspergillus flavus, A. versicolor, Fusarium tenuis* and *Trichoderma viride.* Rao and Nigam (1978) isolated d-limonene, p-cymene, citronellyl acetate, carvone and d-citroneual from oil and reported that each component possessed fungitoxicity. Agarwal *et al.* (1979) reported that the oil besides being anti-helminthic also possessed toxicity against *Aspergillus flavus, A. niger, Curvularia lunata, C. oryzae, Microsporum gypseum, Penicillium chrysogenum, P. javanicum* and *Trichoderma viride* either at 1:10 or at 1:1000 dilutions. Rathee *et al.* (1982) reported that carvone was antifungal factor of the oil and was toxic to *Alternaria helianthi, Colletotrichum capsici, Fusarium moniliforme, F. solani, Helminthosporium oryzae, H. turcicum, Pyricularia setariae, Pythium vexans, Rhizoctonia bataticola* and *R. solani.*

Ocimum adscendens (Lamiaceae)

Asthana and Singh (1981) isolated oil from leaves and reported its fungicidal toxicity against *Aspergillus flavus* and *A. niger* at 4.0×10^3 ml/l and 0.2×10^3 ml/l concentration respectively. Asthana *et al.* (1982) reported the toxicity against *Helminthosporium oryzae* and reported that the oil controlled fungal deterioration of *Vigna radiata* during storage without affecting its seed germination and seedling growth. Asthana (1984) recorded that the oil at 0.4×10^3 ml/l conc. completely inhibited the growth of *Alternaria alternata, A. citri, Aspergillus awamori, A. flavipes, A. fumigatus, A. nidulans, A. ochraceus, A. sydowi, A. terreus, Chaetomium globosum, Cladosporium cladosporioides, Colletotrichum capsici, C. gloeosporioides, Gleosporium fructigenum* and *Trichothecium roseum* and its fungitoxic factor was not affected by temperature treatment up to 100°C and storage up to 360 days.

Ocimum basilicum (Lamiaceae)

Herath and Abeywickrama (2008) isolated essential oil of *Ocimum basilicum* most effective chemical component is eugenol inhibiting conidial germination of *Colletotrichum musae* and *Fusarium proliferatum in vitro.* Do Vgich (1971) reported toxicity of the oil against *Alternaria tenuis, Aspergillus oryzae* and *Penicillium chrysogenum.* Kaul and Nigam (1977) and Sawhney *et al.* (1977) recorded the toxicity against *Aspergillus niger, Candida albicans, C. utilis, Microsporum gypseum* and *Penicillium notatum.* Lahariya and Rao (1979) reported that the oil was toxic to *Aspergillus fumigatus, A. niger, Chrysosporium tropicum, Malbranchea pulchella, Microsporum gypseum* and *Penicillium lilacinum* while inhibition of *Diplodia metalensis, Penicillium digitatum* and *P. italicum* was reported by Arora and Pandey (1984a, b). Reuveni *et al.* (1984) reported that cineole, linalool, methyl chavicol and eugenol were probably the active constituents of the oil which completely inhibited the growth of *D. metalensis* and *Fusarium oxysporum.* Dube *et al.* (1989) reported that the essential oil completely inhibited the mycelial growth of 22 species of fungi including mycotoxin producing strains of *Aspergillus flavus* and *A. parasiticus* at 1.5×10^3 ml/l concentration. It also exhibited significant insect repellent activity against *Allacophora foveicollis.*

Ocimum canum (Lamiaceae)

Rao and Joseph (1971) reported that the leaf oil was toxic to *Candida albicans, Cephalosporium sacchari, Ceratocystis paradoxa, Curvularia lunata, Epidermophyton floccosum, Fusarium moniliforme, Helminthosporium sacchari, Physalospora tucumanensis, Sclerotium rolfsii, Trichophyton mentagrophytes* and *T. rubrum.* Jain and Agarwal (1978) observed presence of methyl heptone, eugenol and geraniol in the oil, which was toxic to *Chrysosporium tropicum, Keratinophyton tenuipes, Malbranchea pulchella* and *Verticillium tenuipes.* Bhargava *et al.* (1979) isolated 1.4 per cent of the oil from leaves and recorded its toxicity against *Aspergillus flavus* and *A. versicolor* at 3.0×10^3 ml/l. Bhargava *et al.* (1981) reported fungistatic nature of the oil at 3.0×10^3 ml/l which become fungicidal at 6.0×10^3 ml/l concentration. Dubey (1981) noted the toxicity of the thermostable fungitoxic factor, which remained active during storage up to 390 days. Narsimha Rao and Subba Rao (1982) reported that the oil inhibited the growth of *E. floccosum.* Dubey *et al.* (1983 a) reported that the oil successfully prevented fungal deterioration of

Foeniculum vulgare and *Coriandrum sativum* during storage without showing any phytotoxic effect on the treated commodities. Mishra *et al.* (1989) isolated the essential oil from leaves and reported its toxicity against *Aspergillus flavus* at 2000 ppm (2.0×10^3 ml/l). Thakur *et al.* (1989) isolated linalool from the *Ocinum canum* oil and tested against *Rhizoctonia solani* and *Fusarium solani*. It was found to be strongly fungitoxic to the test fungi.

Ocimum citriodora (Lamiaceae)

Sawhney *et al.* (1977) reported the toxicity of the oil against *Microsporum gypseum* and *Penicillium notatum*.

Ocimum gratissimum (Lamiaceae)

The toxicity of the oil against *Microsporum gypseum* and *Penicillium notatum* was reported by Sawhney *et al.* (1977) and Grover and Rao (1977). Singh *et al.* (1983a) reported that the oil at 1.0×10^3 ml/l completely inhibited the growth of *Epidermophyton floccosum, Microsporum canis* and *Trichophyton mentagrophytes*. Tripathi *et al.* (1985) reported the toxicity against *Alternaria alternata, Colletotrichum capsici* and *Sclerotium rolfsii* at 0.25×10^3 ml/l, 0.5×10^3 ml/l conc. respectively. They further reported that the oil possessed fungistatic nature at lower doses but became fungicidal at higher doses and when chemically analyzed yielded myrcene, b-pinene, p-cymene, linalyl acetate, terpineol, terpinyl acetate, linalool, geranial, citroneollol and eugenol each exhibiting toxicity against *A. alternata, C. capsici* and *S. rolfsii* at different doses. Dixit (1986) isolated eugenol from the oil and reported that the oil as well as eugenol can be used to prevent bakery bread from fungal deterioration during storage. Mishra *et al.* (1989) isolated the essential oil from leaves and reported its toxicity against *Aspergillus flavus* at 2000 ppm. Thakur *et al.* (1989) isolated the main constituent eugenol from the *Ocimum* oil. 0.1 per cent of eugenol inhibited the radial growth of *Sclerotium rolfsii, Rhizoctonia* sp. and *Alternaria alternata*. *O. gratissimum* was found to exhibit absolute toxicity against the tested fungi *A. flavus* and *A. niger* (Sharma, 2000).

Ocimum killimandscharicum (Lamiaceae)

Suri and Thind (1979) reported the toxicity of the oil against *Aspergillus fumigatus* and *Penicillium notatum*.

Ocimum sanctum (Lamiaceae)

Oil from leaves showed absolute toxicity against *Aspergillus flavus* but was moderately active against *A. niger* (Sharma, 2000).

Ocimum thesiforum (Lamiaceae)

Rao and Joseph (1971) reported the toxicity of the oil against *Cephalosporium sacchari, Ceratocystis paradoxa, Curvularia lunata, Fusarium moniliforme, Helminthosporium sacchari, Physalospora tucumanensis* and *Sclerotium rolfsii*.

Ocimum viridae (Lamiaceae)

Thakur *et al.* (1989) isolated thymol from the oil. 0.1 per cent of thymol inhibited the growth of *Rhizoctonia solani* and *Sclerotium rolfsii*.

Oenanthe javanica (Apiaceae)

Sharma and Singh (1979 a) reported the toxicity of the oil against *Alternaria* sp., *Aspergillus candidus, A. flavus, A. fumigatus, A. niger, Cladosporium herbarum, Cunninghamella echinulata, Fusarium moniliforme,*

F. oxysporum, Helminthosporium sacchari, Microsporum cocci, M. gypseum, Mucor mucedo, Penicillium digitatum, Rhizpus sp., *Trichophyton mentagrophytes, T. rubrum* and *Trichothecium roseum.*

Oenanthe marjorana (Apiaceae)

Capek (1955) recorded toxicity of the oil against *Aspergillus niger*. Maruzzella and Liguroi (1958) and Maruzzella *et al.* (1960) noted that the oil was inhibitory to *Lentinus lepideus, Lenzites trabea* and *Polyporus versicolor.*

Oenanthe vulgaris (Apiaceae)

Korta and Staryzk (1963) recorded mycostatic action of the oil against *Candida albicans, C. tropicalis, C. parakrusei, C. krusei, C. pelliculose, C. stellatoidea* and *C. silosis.*

Parthenium hysterophorus (Asteraceae)

Sharma and Singh (1979) reported that the oil completely inhibited the growth of *Alternaria* sp., *Aspergillus candidus, A. flavus, A. fumigatus, A. nidulans, A. niger, Cladosporium herbarum, Cunninghamella echinulata, Fusarium moniliforme, F. oxysporum, Helminthosporium sacchari, Microsporum cocci, M. gypseum, Mucor mucedo, Penicillium digitatum, Rhizopus* sp., *Trichophyton mentagrophytes, T. rubrum* and *Trichothecium roseum.*

Pastinaca sativa (Apiaceae)

Do Vgich (1971) reported toxicity of the oil against *Alternaria tenuis, Aspergillus oryzae* and *Penicillium chrysogenum.*

Piperomia pellucida (Piperaceae)

Singh *et al.* (1980) reported that the leaf oil completely inhibited the mycelial growth of *Absidia ramosa, Aspergillus fumigatus, A. niger, A. versicolor, Cephalosporium sacchari, Chaetomium globosum, Cladosporium cladosporioides, Colletotrichum falcatum, C. gloeosporioides, Curvularia lunata, Helminthosporium carbonum, H. gramineum, H. maydis, H. oryzae, H. sturcicum, Trichoderma viride* and *Trichothecium roseum* at 2.0×10^3 ml/l and the fungitoxic factor of the oil was thermostable as well as durable during storage up to 150 days. Later, Singh *et al.* (1983b) noted that the oil sustained heavy inoculum density and killed the test fungus, *H. oryzae* within 15 minutes (by contacts). They further observed that the oil successfully prevented the leaf spot disease in paddy without affecting the germination, seedling growth and morphology of the host plant.

Petroselinum crispum (Apiaceae)

Crisan and Hodisan (1975) reported the toxicity of the oil against *Alternaria alternata.*

Peucedanum oreoselnum (Apiaceae)

Crisan and Hodisan (1975) reported the toxicity of the oil against *Alternaria alternata.*

Phytolacca americana (Phytolaccaceae)

Vichkanova *et al.* (1972) reported the toxicity of the oil against *Candida albicans, Microsporum gypseum* and *M. lanantum.*

Pimpinella anisum (Apiaceae)

Capek (1956) reported the toxicity of the oil against *Aspergillus niger*. Shukla and Tripathi (1987b) recorded that the oil at 1.0×10^3 ml/l completely inhibited the mycelial growth of *Aspergillus flavus* and

Penicillium italicum and antifungal factor of the oil remained unaffected by temperature treatment up to 100°C and storage up to 365 days. They isolated anethole as antifungal principle of the oil and reported its fungistatic nature of toxicity at 0.6×10^3 ml/l against *Alternaria alternata, A. tenuis, Aspergillus awamori, A. fumigatus, A. parasiticus, A. sydowi, A. tamarii, A. terreus, Colletotrichum capsici, Curvularia lunata, C. pallascens, Epicoccum nigrum, Fusarium acuminatum, F. equiseti, F. moniliforme, F. oxysporum, F. semitectum, F. udum, Macrophomina phaseolina, Nigrospora oryzae, Penicillium chrysogenum, P. citrinum* and *Rhizopus nigricans*. Seed dressing with anethole at 5.0×10^3 ml/l completely prevented the fungal deterioration of groundnut during storage without affecting its germination and seedling growth (Shukla, 1987).

Pinus pondorosa (Pinaceae)

Cobb *et al.* (1968) detected the presence of comphene, carvene, limonene, myrcene, oleoresin, phellendrene and pinene in the oil which possessed toxicity against *Ceratocystis annosus, C. minor, C. pilifera, C. schrenkiana* and *Fames annosus*.

Pinus sylvestris (Pinaceae)

Melvin and Krupa (1971) and Krupa and Nylund (1972) reported that the oil contained some volatile organic constituents, which were toxic to *Fomes annosus* and *Phytophthora cinnamoni* and also to the mycorrhizal fungi of the plant from which the oil was isolated.

Piper betel (Piperaceae)

Dubey (1986) reported fungistatic nature of the oil against *Aspergillus flavus* at 0.5×10^3 ml/l dose, which remained unaffected by autoclaving, temperature treatment, storage and heavy inoculum density. He further reported that the oil showed no adverse effect on seed germination and seedling growth of *Pisum sativum*. Dubey and Tripathi (1987) isolated eugenol as antifungal principle of the oil and reported its fungistatic nature at 0.2×10^3 ml/l dose against *Alternaria alternata, Aspergillus awamori, A. fumigatus, A. parasiticus, A. sydowi, A. terreus, Botrydiplodia theobromae, Curvularia lunata, Nigrospora oryzae, Penicillium citrinum* and *Rhizopus nigricans*.

Piper nigrum (Piperaceae)

Chaurasia and Kher (1978 a, b) reported that the oil possessed toxicity against *Curvularia lunata* and species of *Aspergillus, Penicillium* and *Rhizopus*.

Pogostemon plectranthoides (Lamiaceae)

Kaul and Nigam (1977) recovered 0.5 per cent oil from leaves and reported its toxicity against *Aspergillus niger, Candida albicans* and *C. utilis* at 1:1000 dilution.

Polyalthia longifolia (Annonaceae)

Narsimha Rao and Subba Rao (1982) recorded toxicity of the oil against *Candida albicans, Epidermophyton floccosum, Trichophyton mentagrophytes* and *T. rubrum*.

Premna tomentosa (Verbinaceae)

Rao and Joseph (1971) reported the toxicity of the oil against *Cephalosporium sacchari, Ceratocystis paradoxa, Curvularia lunata, Fusarium moniliforme, Helminthosporium sacchari, Physalospora tucumanensis* and *Sclerotium rolfsii*.

Prunus amygdalus (Rosaceae)

Singh (1976) reported the toxicity of the oil against *Colletotrichum falcatum, Helminthosporium oryzae* and *Pyricularia oryzae.*

Psidium guajava (Myrtaceae)

Nigam and Rao (1977) reported the toxicity of the oil against *Aspergillus flavus, A. fumigatus, A. oryzae, A. versicolor, Curvularia* sp., *Fusarium tenuis, Penicillium funiculosum, P. javanicum* and *Trichoderma viride.* Kamran (2008) tested the oil against *Aspergillus fumigatus, A. niger, A. ochraceous, Penicillium expansum* and *Alternaria alternata.*

Psoralea corylifolia (Leguminosae)

Grovers and Rao (1979) and Sharma and Singh (1979 b) noted toxicity of the oil against *Alternaria* sp., *Aspergillus candidus, A. flavus, A. fumigatus, A. nidulans, A. niger, Cladosporium herbarum, Cunninghamella echinulata, Fusarium moniliforme, F. oxysporum, Helminthosporium sacchari, Microsporum cocci, M. gypseum, Mucor mucedo, Penicillium digitatum, Rhizopus stolonifer, Trichophyton mentagrophytes, T. rubrum* and *Trichothecium roseum.*

Putranjiva roxburghii (Euphorbiaceae)

Tripathi and Kumar (2007) collected samples of peanut seeds from stores in eastern Uttar Pradesh, India and examined for their associated mycoflora and insects. The oil of *Putranjiva roxburghii* exhibited the greatest toxicity. The oil was found to be fungicidal and thermostable at its minimum inhibitory concentration (MIC) of 400 ppm evaluated against the dominant fungi, *Aspergillus flavus* and *Aspergillus niger*, as well as *Trogoderma granarium.* Kumar and Tripathi (2003) reported the fungitoxic properties of the oil against *Aspergillus flavus* and *A. niger* and insect *Trogoderma granarium* causing heavy deterioration in fresh seeds of ground nut during storage.

Raphanus sativus (Brassicaceae)

The seed oil was reported to possess toxicity at 1:1000000 dilutions against *Alternaria brassicae, Fusarium avenaceum* and *Phoma* sp. (Nehrash, 1961). Sehgal (1961) reported that the fungitoxic property of members of Brassicaceae was due to presence of isocyanates.

Randia dumentorium (Rubiaceae)

Mishra *et al.* (1979 b) reported the toxicity of the oil against *Colletotrichum capsici* and *Fusarium solani.*

Rosa indica (Rosaceae)

Maruzzella (1963) reported that the oil used in perfumery was toxic to *Claviceps graminicola, C. purpurea, Colletotrichum graminicola, Gibberella fujikuroi, G. zeae* and *Helminthosporium turcicum.*

Salvia officinalis (Lamiaceae)

Brieskorm (1950) and Crisan and Hodisan (1975) reported that the oil was toxic to *Mucor mucedo* and *Penicillium glaucum.*

Santalum album (Santalaceae)

Singh (1976) reported the toxicity of the oil against *Colletotrichum falcatum, Helminthosporium oryzae,* and *Pyricularia oryzae.* Dikshit and Hussain (1984) recorded toxicity against *Microsporum gypseum, Trichophyton equinum* and *T. rubrum.*

Satureja delmatica (Lamiaceae)

Korta and Staryzk (1963) reported that the oil possessed toxicity against *Candida albicans*, *C. krusei*, *C. parakrusei*, *C. pelliculosa*, *C. silosis*, *C. stellatoidea* and *C. tropicalis*.

Satureja hortensis (Lamiaceae)

The oil possessed toxicity against *Candida albicans*, *C. krusei*, *C. parakrusei*, *C. pelliculosa*, *C. stellatoidea*, *C. tropicalis* (Korta and Staryzk, 1963), and *Aspergillus oryzae*, *Alternaria tenuis* and *Penicillium chrysogenum* (Do Vgich, 1971).

Selinum tenufolium (Apiaceae)

Murari and Mathela (1978) and Mathela and Sinha (1978) reported the toxicity of the oil against many fungi.

Sequoia sempervirens (Taxodjaceae)

Hital *et al*. (1977) reported the toxicity of the oil against different species of *Aspergillus*.

Seseli indicum (Apiaceae)

Dwivedi *et al*. (1990) tested the oil against *Macrophomina phaseolina* and found to be toxic at 0.5×10^3 ml/l, 1.0×10^3 ml/l and 2.0×10^3 ml/l doses. This fungus causes root rot disease of crops. Chaturvedi and Tripathi (1989) reported the toxicity of the oil against *Aspergillus niger*, *A. flavus* and *Fusarium oxysporum* at 8.0×10^3 ml/l concentration.

Sassafras officinalis (Lauraceae)

Singh *et al*. (1978b) reported toxicity of the oil against *Botryotrichum keratinophyllum*, *Malbranchea aurantica*, *Nannizzia incurvata* (+) and *N. incurvata* (–).

Skimmia laureda (Rutaceae)

Sampurna and Nigam (1979) reported that the oil possessed toxicity against *Keratinophyton terreum*, *Malbranchea pulchella* and *Trichophyton mentagrophytes*.

Sphaeranthus indicus (Asteraceae)

Rao and Joseph (1971) reported that the oil was toxic to *Cephalosporium sacchari*, *Ceratocystis paradoxa*, *Curvularia lunata*, *Fusarium moniliforme*, *Helminthosporium sacchari*, *Physalospora tucumanensis* and *Sclerotium rolfsii*.

Syzygium aromaticum (Myrtaceae)

Capek (1955) reported the toxicity of the oil against *Aspergillus niger*. However, the oil was also inhibitory to 8 species of keratinophilic fungi (Thind and Dahiya, 1977). Khan *et al*. (1994) found that the flower bud extract of *Syzygium aromaticum* exhibited absolute toxicity against *Aspergillus niger* and *Curvularia ovoidea*, inhibiting the mycelial growth completely.

Syzygium caryophyllata (Myrtaceae)

Singh (1976) reported the toxicity of the oil against *Colletotrichum falcatum*, *Helminthosporium oryzae* and *Pyricularia oryzae*.

Syzygium cumini (Myrtaceae)

The oil possessed toxicity against *Cephalosporium sacchari, Ceratocystis paradoxa, Curvularia lunata, Fusarium moniliforme, Helminthosporium sacchari, Physalospora tucumanensis* and *Sclerotium rclfsii* (Rao and Joseph, 1971 and Grover and Rao, 1978b).

Thuja orientalis (Cupressaceae)

Nigam and Rao (1977) reported that the oil was toxic to *Aspergills flavus, A. fumigatus, A. oryzae, A. versicolor, Curvularia* sp., *Fusarium tenuis, Penicillium funiculosum, P. javanicum* and *Trichophyton viride.*

Thujopsis dalabrata (Cupressaceae)

Uchida (1928) reported toxicity of the oil against *Merulius lacrymans* and *Polyporus lacrymans.* Later, Okazaki and Homma (1953) observed that the fungitoxicity of the oil against *Achorion* sp. and species of *Epidermophyton* and *Trichophyton* was due to the presence of kinokitiol, 1-rhodinic acid and thujopsol.

Thymus vulgaris (Lamiaceae)

The toxicity of the oil against *Aspergillus niger* was first reported by Capek (1955). Later Do Vgich (1971) reported toxicity against *Alternaria tenuis, Aspergillus oryzae* and *Penicillium chrysogenum,* and Ceruti *et al.* (1982) against *Aspergillus flavus, A. fumigatus, Fusarium oxysporum, Penicillium digitatum* and *Trichophyton mentagrophytes.*

Thymus serpyllum (Lamiaceae)

Oil extracted from dried, crushed flowering plants showed antifungal properties against *A. flavus, A. awamori, A. niger, A. foetidus* and *A. oryzae.* It also inhibited all the three stages of asexual reproduction *i.e.* spore germination, mycelial growth and spore formation (Rahman *et al.*, 2003)

Trachyspermum ammi (Apiaceae)

Nigam and Rao (1977) reported that the oil was toxic to *Fusarium tenuis.* Sharma and Singh (1979b) and Narayan *et al.* (1980a) recorded that the oil was inhibitory to *Alternaria* sp., *Aspergillus candidus, A. flavus, A. fumigatus, A. nidulans, A. niger, Candida tropicalis, Cladosporium herbarum, Cunninghamella echinulata, Fusarium moniliforme, F. oxysporum, Helminthosporium sacchari, Microsporum canis, M. gypseum, Mucor mucedo, Penicillium digitatum, Rhizopus oryzae, Trichophyton mentagrophytes, T. rubrum* and *Trichothecium roseum.* Singh *et al.* (1986b) reported toxicity of the dethymolysed oil against *Alternaria brassicae, A. solani, Cephalosporium sacchari, Cladosporium cladosporioides, Colletotrichum falcatum, C. lindemuthianum, C. tinosporae, Cornespora casicola, Fusarium solani, Helminthosporium oryzae, Paecilomyces* sp., *Talaromyces* sp. and *Trichoderma viride.* Dikshit and Hussain (1984) reported toxicity against *Microsporum gypseum, Trichophyton equinum* and *T. rubrum,* and Saksena (1984) against *Candida albicans, C. tropicalis* and *Keratinomyces ajelloi.* Singh *et al.* (1986b) reported that the oil at 900 ppm (0.9×10^3 ml/l) dilution killed *Epidermophyton floccosum, Microsporum canis* and *Trichophyton mentagrophytes* within 20 seconds (by contact). Tripathi *et al.* (1986) reported fungicidal nature of the oil against *Alternaria alternata, A. solani, Aspergillus flavipes, A. flavus, A. niger, A. ochraceus, A. sydowi, A. tamarii, A. terreus, A. versicolor, Botrytis cinerea, Colletotrichum capsici, C. falcatum, Curvularia lunata, C. pallescens, Chaetomium globosum, Fusarium semitectum, Monilia pruinosa* and *Penicillium funiculosum* at 800 ppm (0.8×10^3 ml/l). They further added that the fungitoxic factor remained unaffected by temperature treatment up to 100°C and storage at room temperature up to 365 days. The seeds of

Arachis hypogea when dressed at 5000 ppm (5.0×10^3 ml/l) of the oil and stored for 12 months showed no fungal contamination indicating the grain protection efficacy of the oil. Thymol and p-cymene were isolated as antifungal principles of the oil and reported to possess toxicity against *Aspergillus flavus* and *A. niger* at 1.0×10^3ml/l concentration (Tripathi *et al.*, 1986).

Valeriana wallichii (Valerianaceae)

Suri and Thind (1979) reported the toxicity of the oil against *Aspergillus fumigatus* and *Penicillium notatum.*

Vitex negundo (Verbenaceae)

Uppalpati and Rao (1979) reported the toxicity of the oil against species of *Colletotrichum, Fusarium, Helminthosporium* and *Trichoderma.* Dwivedi *et al.* (1990) tested the oil against *Macrophomina phaseolina* and found to be toxic at 500, 1000 and 2000 ppm (0.5×10^3 ml/l, 1.0×10^3 ml/l, 2.0×10^3 ml/l). This fungus causes root rot of crops.

Vitiveria zizanoides (Poaceae)

Singh *et al.* (1978b) reported the fungitoxicity of the oil against *Botryotrichum keratinophyllum, Malbranchea aurantica, Nannizzia incurvata* (+) and *N. incurvata* (–). Dikshit and Hussain (1984) reported toxicity against *Microsporum gypseum, Trichophyton equinum* and *T. rubrum.*

Zanthoxylum alatum (Rutaceae)

The essential oil recovered from the fruits, at 2.0×10^3 ml/l dose was fungistatic to 24 fungi, including the aflatoxin producing strains of *Aspergillus flavus* and *A. parasiticus.* (Dubey *et al.*, 1990).

Zanthoxylum avicennae (Rutaceae)

Chen *et al.* (1990) extracted essential oil by steam distillation. Separation of essential oil yielded 27 compounds, out of which 22 were identified using Gas Chromatography. Citral, 1-octanol, 4-methyl-1-6 acetohexanol and linalool showed anti-mildew activity.

Zingiber officinale (Zingiberaceae)

Sharma and Singh (1979b) reported toxicity of the oil against *Alternaria* sp., *Aspergillus candidus, A. flavus, A. fumigatus, A. nidulans, A. niger, Cladosporium herbarum, Cunninghamella echinulata, Fusarium moniliforme, F. oxysporum, Helminthosporium sacchari, Microsporum cocci, M. gypseum, Mucor mucedo, Penicillium digitatum, Rhizopus* sp., *Trichophyton mentagrophytes, T. rubrum* and *Trichothecium roseum.* Singh and Singh (1981) recorded complete inhibition of conidial germination of *Erysiphe polygoni.* Singh *et al.* (1983b) isolated citral (3, 7 dimethyl 1-2, 6-octadieneal) as antifungal principle of the oil and reported its toxicity against *Fusarium nivale.* Singh *et al.* (1999) studied the activity of the aqueous extract of Zingiber *officinalis* on *Sclerotinia sclerotiorum* which causes stem rot of gram and reported that growth and sclerotium formation were completely inhibited at 80,000 ppm and above.

Efficacy and Applications

Several hundred-research papers are published each year on the antimicrobial activity or other functional activity of botanicals from higher plants, and a complete review of all of them is beyond the scope of this article. The most excellent ones are given above. A brief discussion on efficacy and application of antimicrobial botanicals from higher plants is crucial. The antimicrobial botanicals, which have the potential to be used as storage protectants, can be divided into several useful categories, including phenolics, polyphenols, quinones, flavones, flavonoids, flavonols, tannins, cumarins, terpenoids, lectins and polypeptides (Cowan, 1999). Many herbs, such as thyme, contain multiple active compounds, which represent different chemical families. The essential oil fraction of botanicals is often the most inhibitory chemical fraction to growth and survival of microorganisms. Essential oils are highly enriched with terpenoids. Examples of herbs and spices containing terpenoids which have been shown to have antimicrobial activity include allspice, basil, bay, burdock, cinnamon, paprika, chilli pepper, clove, eucalyptus, dill, gotu kola, grape fruit seed extract, horseradish, lemon verbena, oregano, paod' arco, papaya, peppermint, rosemary, savory, sweet flag, tansy, tarragon, thyme, turmeric, valerian and willow (Duke, 1985; Cate, 2000). The other major chemical group found in plants, which has been frequently reported to have antimicrobial and antifungal activity, is the sulfoxide/ isothiocyanate family, which includes onion, garlic, mustard and members of the *Brassica* family. Approximately 30 per cent of essential oils, which have been examined, are inhibitory to bacteria, and more than 60 per cent of essential oil derivatives have been shown to be inhibitory to fungi (Chaurasia and Vyas, 1977; Cowan, 1999).

The mechanism of action for the antimicrobial activity of botanical storage protectants is not fully understood. However, terpenoids and phenolics are thought to exert inhibitory action against microorganisms by membrane disruption (Cichewick and Thorpe, 1996; Lambert *et al.*, 2001; Schultes, 1978). Simple phenols and flavonoids appear to inhibit growth by binding to biochemicals essential for metabolism (Peres *et al.*, 1997). Both coumarins and alkaloids are thought to inhibit growth of microorganisms at the genetic level (Hoult *et al.*, 1996; Rahman and Chaudhary, 1995).

Although numerous studies have been done *in vivo* to evaluate the antimicrobial activity of botanicals, only a few studies have been done with stored products for preventing or controlling mould growth. Inhibition of fungal growth on coriander and fennel seeds dressed with 0.5 per cent concentration of *Cedrus* oil has been reported (Dikshit 1980). Seeds of coriander showed good result when fumigated with essential oil from *Citrus media* and *Ocimum canum* at their MIC (Dubey *et al.*, 1983). *In vivo*, application *Cymbopogon citratus* oil showed that growth of *Aspergillus flavus* was greatly checked (Mishra *et al.*, 1994). Seeds of wheat and groundnut fumigated with oil from *Eucalyptus citriodora* showed excellent result (Shukla, 1997). Oil and leaf powder of *Cymbopogon citratus* significantly reduced deterioration and aflatoxin production in shelled melon seeds inoculated with toxigenic *Aspergillus flavus, A. niger, A. tamarii* and *Penicillium citrinum* (Bankole and Joda, 2003). Use of *Trachyspermum ammi* oil inhibits growth of dominant storage fungi such as species of *Aspergillus, Penicillium,* and *Alternaria* etc. *in-vivo* condition.

These studies show that some botanicals have the potential to be effective storage protectant although product development to optimize functionality and flavour will be challenging. More studies are needed on applications of botanicals from higher plants in storage protection to fully understand how best to optimize their use.

Safety

Use of many plants in storage protection is commonly regarded as safe but some plants contain noxious compounds, which may render them unsafe for both animals and humans to consume. Toxicology axiom."The dose makes the poison" also apply in some cases. It means that a substance that is safely consumed in the diet at low levels may be unsafe if consumed at a higher level in the diet. Therefore, the data demonstrating that the botanical is safe when consumed at the higher level is needed. And it is virtually difficult to find typical toxicological data such as Acceptable Daily Intake and No Effect Level. Further, there may be unusual sensitivities of some parts of the population to specific herbal compounds or strong aromatic ingredients. Therefore, while using botanicals in storage protection these points should be duly emphasized to avoid negative nutritional or health consequences.

A Sure Future for Botanical Storage Protectants

We are currently limited to a rather small number of antimicrobial agents, which have been used for many years with little expansion, and there is a real need to expand the list of storage protectants, which can be used to ensure safety and quality of stored products. These systems may have synergistic or additive uses with one another or may also be used with conventional antimicrobial compounds. The future of naturally occuring antimicrobial system seems sure, as new storage protection systems are being rapidly developed and used in a variety of storage products.

Acknowledgements

The authors are thankful to the Head, Department of Botany, University of Allahabad, Allahabad for providing the facilities and to the Council of Scientific and Industrial Research, New Delhi for providing financial assistance.

References

Agarwal, R., Kharya, M.D. and Srivastava, R. (1979). Antimicrobial and antihelmintic activities of essential oil of *Nigella sativa* L. Family Ranunculaceae (Kalajira). *Indian J. Expl. Biol.* 17(11): 1264-1265.

Alderman, G.G. and Morth. E.H. (1976). Inhibition of growth and aflatoxin production of *Aspergillus parasiticus* by *Citrus* oils. *Z. Lebensm. Unters, Forsch.* 160: 353-358.

Arora, R. and Pandey, G.N. (1977). The application of essential oils and their isolates for blue mould decay control in *Citrus reticulata. J. Food Sci. Technol.* 14: 15-16.

Arora, R. and Pandey, G.N. (1984). Effect of essential oils on *Citrus* decay pathogens. *Biol. Mem.* 9(1): 69-72.

Arora, R. and Pandey, G.N. (1984). Application of essential oil and their isolates as preservative of *Citrus reticulata. Biol. Mem.* 9(1): 98-104.

Asthana, A. (1984). Studies on volatile activity of some higher plants against fungal deterioration of *Vigna radiata* (L.) Wilczak during storage. *Ph.D. Thesis*, University of Gorakhpur, Gorakhpur, India.

Asthana, A. and Singh, A.K. (1981). Fungitoxic properties of essential of *Ocimum adscendens. J. Indian Bot. Soc.* (Suppl.). 60:13.

Asthana, A., Chandra, H., Dikshit, A. and Dixit S.N. (1982). Volatile fungitoxicants from leaves of some higher plants against *Helminthosporium oryzae. Z. Pflanzen Krankheiter Pflanzens Chutz.* 89:475-479.

Avadhoot, Y. and Verma, K.C. (1978). Antimicrobial activity of essential oil of seeds of *Lantana camara* var. *aculeata* Linn. *Indian Drugs Pharm.* 13: 41-42.

Babu, S., Seetharaman, K., Nandakumar, R. and Johnson. I. (2000). *In vitro* antifungal activity of Palmarosa (*Cymbopogon martinii* (Roxb.) Watson) oil against *Alternaria solani. Indian Perfumer* 44 (4): 275-277.

Baiter, J. (1971). Effect of *Citrus* oil on respiration of *Trichoderma lignorum*. *Z. Labensm. Unters-Forsch* 169: 22-25.

Banerjee, A. and Nigam, S.S. (1977). Antifungal activity of the essential oil of *Curcumu angustifolia. Indian J. Pharm.* 39: 143.

Banerjee, A. and Nigam, S.S. (1978). Antimicrobial efficacy of the essential oil of *Curcuma longa*. *Indian J. Med. Res.* 68: 864-866.

Banerjee, A. and Nigam, S.S. (1978). Antifungal efficiency of the essential oils derived from the various species of the genus *Curcuma* Linn. *J. Res. Indian Med. Yoga Homeo.* 13: 63-70.

Bankole, S.A. and Joda, A.O. (2003). Effect of lemon grass oil (*Cymbopogon citratus* Stapf.) powder and essential oil on mould deterioration and aflatoxin contamination of melon seeds (*Colocynthis citrullus* L.). *E-mail: sabankole@juno.com*

Benjinali, B., Tanaqui–Elaraki, A., Ayadi, A. and Ihlal, M. (1984). Method to study antimicrobial effects of essential oils. Application to the antifungal activity of six morocean essences. *Journal Food Protection.* 47(10): 748-752.

Beye, F. (1978). Insecticides from Vegetable Kingdom. *Plant Research and Development* 7: 13-31.

Bhargava, K.S., Dixit, S.N., Dubey, N.K. and Tripathi, R.D. (1979). Fungitoxic properties of *Ocimum canum. J. Indian Bot. Soc. (Suppl.)* 58: 20.

Bhargava, K.S., Dixit, S.N., Dubey N.K. and Tripathi R.D. (1981). Fungitoxic properties *of Ocimum canum. J. Indian Bot. Soc.* 60: 24-27.

Bigrami, S.K., Misra, R.S., Sinha, K.K and Singh, P. (1980). Effect of some wild and medicinal plant extracts on aflatoxin production and growth of *Aspergillus flavus* in liquid culture. *Indian Botanical Society* 59: 123-126.

Bishop, C.D. and Thornton, I.B. (1997). Evaluation of antifungal activities of essential oils of *Monarda citriodora* var. *citriodora* and *Melaleuca alternifolia* on postharvest pathogens. *J. Essential Oil Research*, USA. 9 (1): 77-82.

Brandies, G.A. (1967). Commercial development of fungicides (Discussion): 246-247. In Holten *et al.* (eds.) Plant Pathology problems and progress, 1908-1958. *Indian University Press*, Allahabad, India.

Brieskorm, C.M. (1950). Active ingradients of *Salvia offinalis* VI. Bactericidal activity of oil. *Dage Arch. Pharma.* 283: 33-35.

Capek, A. (1955). Phytoncides of species. *Prumsyl Potranin* 6: 433-435.

Capek, A. (1956). Phytoncides of anise and fennel. *Prumsyl Potranin* 7: 260-262.

Cate, M. (2000). Antimicrobial and Toxicological characteristics of commercial herbal extracts and the antimicrobial efficacy of herbs in marinated chicken. *M.S. thesis* directed by F. A. Draughon, May, Univ. of Tennessee, Knoxville.

Ceruti, A., Sacco, T. and Vinai. A. (1982). Action of some essential oils on fungal growth, *Allionia* 25: 5-8.

Chandi, C.R., Dash, S.K., Mishra, R.K. and Charyulu, J.K. (1999). *In-vitro* evaluation of antimycotic activity of turmeric (*Curcuma longa* L.) essential oils against *Candida albicans* and *Cryptococcus neoformans. Indian Perfumer* 43(4): 172-178.

Chandra, H. (1984). Evaluation of some higher plants for their volatile activity against blue mould rots of orange. *Ph.D. thesis*, University of Gorakhpur, Gorakhpur, India.

Chandra, H. and Dikshit, A. (1981). Volatile Fungitoxicant from the leaves of *Ageratum conyzoides* against *Colletotrichum capsici* and *Penicillium italicum*. *J. Indian Bot. Soc.* (*Suppl.*) 60:13.

Chandra, H., Asthana, A., Tripathi, R.D. and Dixit S.N. (1980). Fungitoxicity in the vapours from the fruits of *Cinnamomum cecidodaphne*. *Jour. Ind. Bot. Soc.* (*suppl.*) 59:19.

Chandra, H., Pandey, D.K., Tripathi, N.N. and Dixit, S.N. (1982). Toxicity of the essential oil of *Eupatorium capillifolium* against *Helminthosporium oryzae*. *Indian Perfumer* 26 (3-4): 231-236.

Chaturvedi, R. (1979). Evaluation of higher plants for their fungitoxicity against *Helminthosporium oryzae*. *Ph.D. Thesis*, University of Gorakhpur, Gorakhpur, India.

Chaturvedi, R., Dikshit, A and Dixit, S.N. (1987). *Adenocalyma allicea*. A new source of natural fungitoxicant. *Tropical Agriculture* 64(4): 318-322.

Chaturvedi, R.V. and Tripathi, S.C. (1989). Fungitoxic, physiochemical and phytotoxic properties of essential oil of *Seseli indicum*. *W and A Journal of Phytopathology* 124 (1-4): 316-322.

Chaurasia, S.C. and Vyas, K.K. (1977). *In vitro* effect of some volatile oil against *Phytophthora parasitica* var. *piperina*. *J. Res. Indian Med. Yoga Homeoath*. 24-26.

Chaurasia, S.C. and Kher, A. (1978). Inhibitory effects of essential oils of three medicinal plants against various fungi. *Indian Drugs Pharm*. 13: 7-9.

Chaurasia, S.C. and Kher, A. (1978). Activity of essential oils of three medicinal plants against various pathogenic and non-pathogenic fungi. *Indian J. Hosp. Pharm*.15: 139-141.

Chawdhary, J.U., Yusuf. M., Jaripa Begum, Sultana, S.A. and Husain, M.M. (2003). Composition and Fungitoxic properties of the essential oil of *Lippia javanica* leaves. *Indian perfumer* 47(4): 385-388.

Chen. S.F., Zhu, L.P., Lu, B.Y., Yu, K.K., Lin, Z.S. (1990). Studies on essential oil from *Zanthoxylem avicennae* (Lam.) D.C. and its antimildew activity. *Acta Botanica Sinica* 31(1): 49-53.

Cichewick, R.H. and Thorpe, P.A. (1996). The antimicrobial properties of chile pepper (*Capsicum* species) and their use in Mayan medicine. *J. Ethanopharmacol*. 52: 61-70.

Chirkina, N.N. and Osipova, E.A. (1974). Antimicrobial properties of essential oil from everlasting flower *Helichrysum italicum* cultivated in Crimea. *Biol. Nauki* 17: 86-89.

Cobb Jr. F.W., Kristie, M., Zavarin, E. and Barber Jr. H.W. (1968). Inhibitory effects of volatile olioresin component on *Fomes annosus* and four *Ceratocystis* sp. *Phytopath*. 58: 1327-1335.

Cowan, M.M. (1999). Plant products as antimicrobial agents. *Clin. Microbiol. Rev*. 12: 564-582.

Crisan, A. and Hodisan, V. (1975). Investigations on fungistatic and flungicidal action of some extracts and volatile oils from medicinal plants. *Contributii Botanica* 171-179.

Davis, P.L. and Smoot, J.L. (1972). Germination of *Penicillium digitatum* spores as affected by solutions of volatile components of *Citrus* fruits. *Phytopath*. 62: 488-489.

Dawson, R.J. (1991). A global view of the mycotoxin problem. In: Champ B.R., Higley E., Hocking, A.D., Pitt, J.I. (eds.) *Fungi and mycotoxin in stored products*. Canberra: ACIAR Proc.36: 22-28.

de Souza, E.L., de Oliveira Lima, E., de Luna, K.R., de Sousa, F. and de Sousa, C.P. (2005). Inhibitory action of some essential oils and phytochemicals on the growth of various mould isolated from foods. *Brazilian Arch. Biology and Technology* 48(2): 245-250.

Dikshit, A. (1980). Fungitoxic evaluation of some plants and active product (Cedrus oil). *Ph.D. Thesis*, University of Gorakhpur, Gorakhpur, India.

Dikshit, A., Dubey, N.K., Tripathi, N.N., Tripathi, R.D. and Dixit, S.N. (1982). Control of fungal deterioration by some species during storage by the essential oil of *Cedrus deodara, A supplement to Annals of Applied Biology* 100: 56-57.

Dikshit, A. Singh, A.K., Tripathi, R.D. and Dixit, S.N. (1978). The volatile fungitoxic activity of *Cedrus deodara. Proc. Symp. Plant Disease Problems*, Jaipur, 47.

Dikshit, A., Naqvi, A.A. and Hussain, A. (1986). *Schinus molle*: A new source of fungitoxicant. *Appl. Environ. Microbiol.* 15: 1085-1088.

Dikshit, A., Singh, A.K., Tripathi, R.D. and Dixit, S.N. (1979). Fungitoxic and phytotoxic properties of some essential oils. *Bio. Bull. Indian* 1: 45-51.

Dikshit, A. and Hussain, A. (1984). Antifungal action of some essential oils against animal pathogens. *Fitoterapia* 55 (3): 171-176.

Dikshit, A., Dubey, N.K., Tripathi, N.N., Dixit, S.N. (1983). *Cedrus* oil- A promising storage fungitoxicant. *J. Stored Prod. Res.* 19(4): 159-162.

Dixit, K. (1986). Evaluation of some higher plants and their products for preservation of some food stuffs against fungal deterioration during storage. *Ph. D. Thesis*. University of Gorakhpur, Gorakhpur, India.

Dovgich, N.A. (1971). Antimicrobial effect of essential oils. *Microbiol. Zh.* 33: 253-259.

Dube, P. and Tripathi, S.C. (1987). Studies on antifungal, physico-chemical and phytotoxic properties of essential oil of *Piper betel. Pflan. Und. Pflanzen. Shutz.* 94: 235-242.

Dubey, R.K., Kumar, R. and Dubey, N.K. (2007). Evaluation of *Eupatorium cannabinum* Linn. oil in enhancement of shelf life of mango fruits from fungal rotting. *World J Microbiol Biotechnol.* 23:467–473.

Dube, S., Kumar, A. and Tripathi, S.C. (1990). Antifungal and insect repellant activity of essential oil of *Zanthoxylum alatum. Annals of Botany* 65:75-76.

Dube, S., Upadhyay, P.D. and Tripathi, S.C. (1989). Antifungal, physicochemical and insect repellant activity of essential oil of *Ocimum basilicum. Canadian J. Bot.*67: 2085-2087.

Dubey, N.K. (1981). Studies on volatile activity of some higher plants against fungi causing seed deterioration in storage. *Ph.D. Thesis*, Univ. of Gorakhpur, Gorakhpur, India.

Dubey, N.K., Bhargava, K.S. and Dixit, S.N. (1983). Protection of some stored food commodities from fungi by essential oils *of Ocimum canum* and *Citrus medica. Indian J. Tropical Plant Disease* 1: 177-179.

Dubey, N.K., Kishore, N. and Singh, S.K. (1983). Antifungal properties of the volatile fraction of *Melaleuca leucadendron. Trop. Agric.* (Trinidad) 60 (3): 227-228.

Dubey, N.K., Kishore, N., Tripathi, N.N., Tripathi R.D. and Dixit S.N. (1982). Fungitoxicity of the essential oil of *Citrus medica* against storage fungi. *Suppl. Ann. Appl. Biol.* 100: 58-59.

Dubey, N.K., Dixit, S.N. and Bhargava, K.S. (1982). Evaluation of leaf extracts of higher plants against some storage fungi. *J. Indian Bot. Soc.* 5: 20-22.

Dubey, N.K., Kishore, N., Tripathi, N.N., Tripathi, R.D. and Dixit, S.N. (1981). Fungitoxicity of the essential oils of *Ocimum canum* against *Aspergillus flavus* and *A. vesicolor*. *Indian Perfumer* 25 (2): 1-5.

Dubey, P. (1986). Studies on antifungal activity of some essential oils. *Ph.D. Thesis*. University of Gorakhpur, Gorakhpur, India.

Duke, P.J. (1985). "Hand book of Medicinal Herbs." *CRC Press, Inc.* Boca Raton, Fla.

Dwivedi, R.S. (1993). Biopesticidal plant protection for substainable crop productivity. Presidential address. *Botany section, 80th Indian Science Congress Association*. Goa 1-35.

Dwivedi, R.S. and Dubey, R.C. (1986). Effect of volatile fractions of two medicinal plants on germination of *Macrophomina phaseolina* Sclerotia. *Trans. Brit. Mycol. Soc.* 87(2): 326-328.

Dwivedi, S.K., Kishore, N., Dwivedi, S.K. (1990). Fungitoxicity of some essential oils against *Macrophomina phaseolina*. *Indian Perfumer* 34(1): 20-21.

Dwivedi, S.N. and Shukla T.N. (1990). Mycoflora of gram seeds in different agroclimatic regions and their pathology. *Indian Phytopathology* 43: 98-99

Egawa, A., Tsulsui, D., Talsuyama, R. and Halta, T. (1977). Antifungal substances found in leaves of *Eucalyptus* sp. *Experientia* 33: 889–890.

Ejechi, B.O. and Akpomedaye, D.E. (2005). Activity of essential oil and phenolic acid extracts of Pepperfruits (*Dennetia tripetala* G. Baker, Anonaceae) against some food-borne microorganisms. *African J. Biotechnology* 4 (3): 258-261.

Essien, P.E., Essien, J.P., Basil, N. and Ebong, G.A. (2008). Physicochemical Properties and Fungitoxicity of the Essential Oil of *Citrus medica* L. against Groundnut Storage Fungi. *Turk J Bot.* 32, 161-164.

Fawcett, C.H. and Spencer, D.M. (1969). Natural antifungal compounds: 637-669. In Torgeson, D.C. (eds.) Fungicides an Advance Treatise Vol. II. *Academic Press*, New York and London.

Garg, S.C. (1974). Antifungal activity of some essential oils. *Indian J. Pharm.* 36: 46-47.

Garg, S.C. and Jain, R.K. (1998). Antimicrobial efficacy of essential oil from *Curcuma cassia*. *Indian J. Microbiology* 38: 169-170.

Garg, S.C. and Jain, R.K. (2003). Antimcrobial activity of the essential oil of *Curcuma longa*, *Ind. Perfumer* 47(2): 199-202.

Garg, S.C. and Oswal, V.B. (1982). *In-vitro* antifungal activity of the essential oil of *Chloroxylon swietenia* Roxb. Coram. *Indian Drugs* 19(5): 189-190.

Garg, S.C., Siddiqui IV. (1992). *In-vitro* antifungal activity of the essential oil of *Coriandrum sativum* Linn. *J. Research and Education In: Indian medicine* 11(3): 11-13.

Gautam, M.P., Jain, P.C. and Singh, K.V. (1980). Activity of some essential oils against dermatophytes. *Indian Drugs* 17(9): 269-270.

Geda, A. and Bokadia, M.M. (1979). Antifungal activity of the essential oil of *Blumea membranacea*. *Ind. Drugs Pharma.* 14: 21-22.

Geda, A., Saxena, S.P. and Bokadia, M.M. (1978). *In-vitro* antimicrobial efficiency of essential oil against human pathogenic bacteria and phytopathogenic fungi. *Indian Drugs* 15: 253-255.

Girgune, J.B., Jain, N.K. and Garg, B.D. (1978). Antifungal activity of some essential oils. *Indian Drugs* 16: 24-26.

Girgune, J.B., Jain, N.K. and Garg, B.D. (1978). Antimicrobial activity of the essential oil from *Leucas cilliata* (Labiatae). *Indian Drugs Pharm. Ind.* 13: 39-40.

Grover, G.S. and Rao, J.T. (1977). Investigation on the anti-microbial efficiency of essential oils of *Ocimum sanctum* and *O. gratissimum* L. *Perfumer U. Kosmet* 58: 326-328.

Grover, G.S. and Rao, J.T. (1978). *In-vitro* antimicrobial studies of essential oil of *Eugenia jambolana. Indian Drugs* 15: 143-144.

Grover, G.S. and Rao, J.T. (1979). *In-vitro* antimicrobial studies of the essential oil of *Psoralea corylifolia. Indian Perfumer* 23: 135-137.

Grover, G.S., Rao, J.T. (1978). *In-vitro* antimicrobial studies of essential oil of *Daucus carota. Indian Drugs Pharm.* India 13: 39-40.

Gupta, C. and Singh, V.P. (1982). *In-vitro* antifungal effect of the essential oils of some medicinal plants. *Science and culture* 48(2): 441-443.

Haerdtl, H. (1962). Fungicidal properties of oils and solid filters. *Deuts. and pothek,* Ztd. 102: 447-448.

Handique, A.K. and Singh, H.B. (1990). Antifungal action of Lemon grass oil on some soil-borne plant pathogens. *Indian Perfumer* 34(3): 232-234.

Handique, A.K. and Singh, H.B. (1989). Antifungal activity of *Eucalyptus* oil on some soil-borne plant pathogens. *Ind. Drugs* 26(6): 274-276.

Herath, H. and Abeywickrama, K. (2008). *In-vitro* application of selected essential oils and their major components in controlling fungal pathogens of crown rot in Embul banana (*Musa acuminate*-AAB) *International Journal of Food Science and Technology*. 43, 440–447.

Hital, S.H., Zedan, H.H., Haggag, M.Y. and Saliman, P.M. (1977). Volatile of *Sequoia semipervirens* Engl. *Egypt. J. Pharm. Sci.*18: 85-91.

Hitokoto, H., Morozumi, S., Wauke, T., Sakai, S. and Kurata, H. (1980). Inhibitory effects of spices on growth and toxin production of toxigenic fungi. *Applied and Environmental Microbiology* 39: 818-822.

Hoult, J.R.S. and Paya. M. (1996). Pharmacological and biochemical action of simple coumarins: Natural products with therapeutic potential. *Gen. Pharmacol.* 27: 713-722.

Ikenaka, T., Ikeda, N., Taneka, K. and Sugawara, S. (1956). Studies on the essential oil of *Artemisia capillaris* Thumb. I. Antifungal activity of essential oil (4). *Bayer Synp.* 5: 325-343.

Imai, K., Ikeda, N., Tanaka, K. and Sugawara, S. (1956). Studies on the essential oil *of Artemisia capillaris* Thumb. I. Antifungal activity of the essential oil (2) Isolation of the antifungal principle. *J. Pharm. Soc. Jap.*76: 400-406.

Jain, P.C. and Agarwal, S.C. (1978). Notes on the activity of some odoriferous organic compounds against some keratinophillic fungi. *Trans. Mycol. Soc. Jap.* 19: 197-200.

Jain, P.K., Charia, A.K., Sharma, S.K. and Bokadia, M.M. (1979). Study of some essential oils for their antifungal activities. *Indian Drugs* 16: 122-123.

Janseen, A.M. and Scheffer, J.J.C. (1985). Acetoxychavicol acetate an antifungal component of *Alpinia galanga. Plant Medica* 6: 507-511.

Jeyalakshmi, C. and Seetharaman, K. (1997). Antifungal properties of palmarosa oil against *Colletotrichum capsici* causing fruit rot of chilli. *Indian Perfumer* 41(3): 106-108.

Jham, G.N., Dhingra, O.D., Jardim, C.M. and Valente, V.M.M. (2005). Identification of the major fungitoxic component of cinnamon bark oil. *Fitopatol. Bras.* 30 (4) July/Aug. 2005.

Jirovetz, L., Buchbauer, G., Stoyanova, A.S., Georgiev, E.V., and Damianova S.T. (2005). Composition, quality control and antimicrobial activity of the essential of cumin (*Cuminum cyminum*) seeds from Bulgaria that had been stored for up to 26 years. *J. Food Science and Technology* 40(3): 305.

Kakrani, H.K. and Nair, G.V. (1982). Antibacterial and antifungal activity of volatile oil from the seeds of *Aglaca odoratissima. Fitoterapia* 53(4): 107-109.

Kala, P.K., Tripathi, R.K., Gupta, K.C. and Singh, A.K. (1984). Effect of some essential oil on growth and aflatoxin production by *Aspergillus parasiticus* in stored grains. *Pesticides* 18: 43-46.

Kamran, A. (2008). Studies on antifungal action of some biochemotherapeutants. *Ph.D. Thesis,* University of Allahabad, Allahabad, India.

Kaul, V.K., and Nigam, S.S. (1977). Antibacterial and antifungal studies of some essential oils. *J. Res. Indian Med. Yoga Homeo* 12: 132-135.

Kaul, V.K., Nigam, S.S. and Dhar, K.L. (1976). Antimicrobiol activities of essential oils of *Artemisia absinthium* Linn., *A. vestita* Wall and *A. vulgaris* Linn. *Indian J. Pharm.* 38: 21.

Khan, S.A. and Tripathi, N.N. (1994). Volatile antifungal activity of some higher plants against storage fungi. *Neo Botanica* 2: 111-119.

Kher, A. and Chaurasia, S.C. (1977). Antifungal activity of essential oils of three medicinal plants, *Indian Drugs* 15: 41-42.

Kishore, N., Srivastava, O.P., Dubey N.K. and Dixit, S.N. (1982). Evaluation of the essential oils from the inflorescence of *Chenopodium ambrosioides* L. against *Rhizoctonia solani. Indian Perfumer* 26(2): 228-230.

Korableva, N.P. and Patapora, L.M. (1966). Role of essential oil in resistance of onion to microorganism. *Biokhim Osn. Zashch. Rost. Acad. Nauk. S.S.R.* Inst. Biochem. 79-88.

Korta, J. and Starzyk, J. (1963). Investigation on antibiotic properties of essential oils of certain species of Umbelliferae. *Acta Botanica Cracoviensia* 6: 149-160.

Kovacs, G. (1964). Studies on antibiotic substances from higher plants with special reference to their plant pathological importance. *K. Vet. Hjsk. Arsskr.* 47-92.

Krupa, S. and Nylund, *I.E.* (1971). Ectomycorrhizae of Pine III. Growth inhibition of two root pathogenic fungi by volatile organic constituents of ectomycorrhizal root systems of *Pinus sylvestris. Eur. J. For. Path.* 2: 88-94.

Kumar, A. (1992). Evaluation of some essential oils against mycotoxin producing fungi deteriorating pulses during storage. *Ph.D. Thesis,* University of Gorakhpur, Gorakhpur, India.

Kumar, N. and Tripathi, N.N. (2003). *Putranjiva* oil an ecofriendly herbal bio-pesticide. *Indian Phytopath.* 56 (3): 352.

Kumar, R., Dubey, N.K., Tiwari, O.P., Tripathi, Y.B. and Sinha, K.K. (2007). Evaluation of some essential oils as botanical fungitoxicants for the protection of stored food commodities from fungal infestation. *Journal of the Science of Food and Agriculture.* 87(9) p 1734-1743.

Kumar, R., Mishra, A.K., Dubey, N.K. and Tripathi, Y.B. (2007). Evaluation of *Chenopodium ambrosioides* oil as a potential source of antifungal, antiaflatoxigenic and antioxidant activity. *Int. J. Food Microbiol.* 115(2):159-64.

Lahariya, A.K. and Rao, J.T. (1979). *In-vitro* antimicrobial studies of the essential oil of *Cyperus scariosus* and *Ocimum basilicum*. *Indian Drugs* 16(7): 150-152.

Lakshmi, U.S. and Rao, J.T. (1978). Antimicrobial efficacy of the essential oil of *Melissa parviflora*. *Indian Drugs* 16(3): 69.

Lambert, R.J.W., Skandamis, P.N., Coote, P.J. and Nychas, G.J.E. (2001). A study of the minimum inhibitory concentration and mode of action of oregano essential oil, thymol and carvacrol, *J. Appl. Microbiol.* 91: 453-562.

Laouer, H., Zerrouq, M.M., Sahli, F., and Chaker, A.N. (March/April 2003). Composition and antimicrobial activity of *Ammodes pusilla* (Brot.) Breistr. essential oil. *J. Essential Oil Research*.

Lewis, J.A. and Papavizas, G.C. (1967). Effects of tannins on spore germination and growth of *Fusarium solani* f. *phaseoli* and *Verticillium albo-atrum*. *Canadian J. Microbiology* 13: 1655-1661.

Mabrouk, S.S. and El-Shayeb, N.M.A. (1980). Inhibition of aflatoxin formation by some spices. *Lebensm. Unters. Forsch* 171: 344-347.

Mahajan, V., Omray, A.K. and Verma, K.C. (1978). Antimicrobial activity of essential oil from rhizome of *Curcuma* sp. *Indian Perfumer* 22(4): 293-295.

Mall, H.V., Asthana, A., Dubey, N.K. and Dixit, S.N. (1985). Toxicily of Cedar wood oil against some dermatophytes. *Indian Drugs* 22: 296- 298.

Mannon, J., Johanson, E. (1985). Fungi down on the farm. *New Scient* 28:12-16.

Marruzzella, J.C. (1963). The effect of perfume oils on the growth of phytopathogenic fungi. *Plant Dis. Rep.* 47: 756-757.

Maruzzela, J.C., Baiter, J. and Katz, A. (1959). Further studies on the action of perfume oil vapours on microorganism. *Perfume Essent. Oil Res.* 50: 955-957.

Maruzzella, J.C. and Baiter, J. (1959). The action of essential oils on phytopathogenic fungi. *Plant Dis. Rep.* 43 (11): 1143-1147.

Maruzzella, J.C. and Liguroi, L. (1958). The *In-vitro* antifingal activity of essential oils. *J. Amer. Pharm. Ass. Sci. Ed.* 47: 250-254.

Maruzzella, J.C., Sorandis, D.A., Sorandis, J.B. and Grabon, G. (1960). Action of odoriferous organic chemicals and essential oil on wood destroying fungi. *Plant Dis. Rep.* 44: 789-792.

Mathela, C.S. and Sinha, G.K. (1978). Antibacterial and antifungal study of some indigenous essential oils. *J. Res. Indian Med. Yoga Homeo.* 13(3): 122-124.

Melvin, E. and Krupa, S. (1971). Studies on ectomycorrhizae of Pine III. Growth inhibition of mycorrhizal fungi by volatile organic constituents *of Pinns sylvestris* (Scots Pine) roots. *Physiol. Plant* 25: 337-340.

Miniza, J. and Thoppil. *I.E.* (2003). Antimicrobial activity of *Centella asiatica* (L.) Urb. essential oil. *Indian Perfumer* 47(2): 179-181.

Mishra, A. (1993). Evaluation of some essential oils for the control of fungi producing aflatoxin in pulses during storage. *Ph.D. Thesis,* Awadh University, Faizabad, India.

Mishra, A.K. and Dubey, N.K (1990). Fungitoxic properties of *Prunus persica* oil. *Hindustan Antibiot. Bull.* 32(3-4): 91-93.

Mishra, A.K. and Dubey, N.K. (1994). Evaluation of some essential oils for their toxicity against fungi causing deterioration of stored food commodities. *Applied and Environmental Microbiology* 60: 1101-1105.

Misra, D., Mishra, M. and Tiwari, S.N. (1997). Toxic effect of volatiles from *Callistemon lanceolatus* on six fungal pathogens of rice. *Indian Phytopath.* 50 (1): 103-105.

Mishra, A.K., Dwivedi, S.K. and Kishore, N. (1989). Antifungal activity of some essential oil. In *Nat. Aca. Sci. Letters* 12(10): 33-36.

Mishra, D., Chaturvedi, R.V. and Tripathi, S.C. (1995). The fungitoxic effect of the essential oil of the herb *Nardostachys jatamansi* D.C. *Tropical Agri.* 72(1): 48-52.

Mishra, P. and Chauhan, C.S. (1984). Antimicrobial studies of the essential oil of the berries of *Juniperus macropoda* Boiss. *Hindustan Antibio. Bull.* 25(182): 38-40.

Mishra, S.B. and Dixit, S.N. (1978). Antifungal properties of leaf extract of *Ranunculus scleratus* L. *Experientia* 34: 1442.

Mishra, S.H., Chaturvedi, S.C. and Dixit, V.K. (1979). Antimicrobial activity of essential oil of *Inula racemosa*. *Indian Drugs* 16(7): 141-143.

Mishra. S.H., Chaturvedi, S.C. and Dixit, V.K. (1979). Anti-microbial activity of essential oil of *Randia dumentorium* Lank. *Indian Perfumer* 23(1): 59-60.

Misra, S.B. and Dixit, S.N. (1978). Fungitoxic activity of volatile fraction of three plants. *Indian Perfumer* 22: 61-62.

Mokurova, V.A. (1961). The action of antimicrobial substances from higher plants on the causal agents of maize disease. *Nauk. Dokl. Vysk. Shkol. Biol. Sci.* 4: 152-154.

Mukherjee, N. (1974). Antifungal activities of some oils and detergents. I. Action on spore germination, growth and sporulation of some plant pathogenic fungi. *Z. pflazenkrank, Pflanzen Schutz.* 81: 468-471.

Murari, N.D. and Mathela, C.S. (1978). Antifungal studies of some indigenous essential oils. *Indian Perfumer* 22(4): 291-292.

Murdoch, D.I. and Allen, W.E. (1960). Germicidal effect of orange peel oil and d-limonene in water and orange juice. I. Fungicidal properties against yeast. *Food Techol.* 14: 441-445.

Narayan, V., Rao, K.K. and Giridhar, R. (1980). Antimicrobial activity of essential oil of *Cinnamomum zeylanicum* Bl. *Indian Drugs* 17(11): 360-362.

Narayan, V., Rao, K.K. and Giridhar, R. (1980). The *in vitro* efficiency of essential oils of some umbelliferous plants. *Indian Drugs* 17(12): 394-396.

Narsimha Rao, B.G.V. and Subba Rao, P. (1982). The efficacy of some essential oils on pathogenic fungi. *Flavour Industry* 3: 368.

Nehrash, A.K. (1961). The antimicrobial properties of cultivated radish I. The antimicrobial activity of extracts and essential oil from cultivated and wild radish. *J. Microbiol.* Kiew, 23: 32-37.

Nigam, S.S. and Rao, T.S.S. (1977). Antimicrobial efficacy of some Indian essential oils. In Kapoor, L.D. and Ramkrishanan, 1977 (eds.) *Advances in essential oil industry*. Today and Tomorrow's Printers and Publishers, New Delhi, India. 177-180.

Nunez, L., Aquino, M.D. and Chirife, J. (Apr./Jun. 2001). Antifungal properties of Clove oil (*Eugenia caryophylata*) in sugar solution. *Braz. J. Microbiol.* 32(2).

Okazaki, K. and Homma, A. (1953) Antibacterial activity of higher plants XXVI. Antimicrobial effect of essential oil, I. Oil of *Thujopsis dolabrata* and its components. *J. Pharm. Soc.* Japan, 74: 174-176.

Ozcan, M.M., Chalchat, J.C., Arslan, D., Ates, A. and Unver, A. (2006). Comparative essential oil composition and antifungal effect of bitter fennel (*Foeniculum vulgare* ssp. *piperitum*) fruit oils obtained during different vegetation. *J Med Food* 9 (4) 552–561.

Palanisami, A., Manickam, A. and Neelakantan, S. (1990). Fungal flora and aflatoxin production in relation to postharvest practices in groundnut. *Madras Agricultural Journal* 77(1): 26-31.

Pandey, D.K. Chandra, H., Tripathi, N.N. and Dixit, S.N. (1983). Mycotoxicity in leaves of some higher plants with special reference to that of *Ageratum houstonianum. Mil. Mykosen.* 26(11): 565-573.

Pandey, D.K., Chandra, H. and Tripathi, N.N. (1982). Volatile Fungitoxic activity in higher plants with special reference to that of *Callistemon lanceolatus* D.C. *Phytopath. Z.* 105: 175-182.

Pandey, D.K., Chandra, H., Tripathi, N.N., and Dixit, S.N. (1983). Toxicity of the essential oil of *Ageratum houstonianum* against *Fusarium lateritium. Beitr. Biol. Pflanz.* 58(1): 115-122.

Pandey, D.K., Tripathi, N.N., Tripathi, R.D. and Dixit S.N. (1982). Fungitoxic and phytotoxic properties of the essential oil of *Caesulia axillaris* Roxb. (Campositae) *Angew. Botanik* 56: 259-267.

Pandey, D.K., Tripathi, N.N., Tripathi, R.D. and Dixit, S.N. (1982). Fungitoxic and phytotoxic properties of the essential oil of *Hyptis suaveolens. J. Plant Disease and Protection* 89(6): 344-349.

Parcha, V., Gahlot, M., Kumar, P. and Bishwas, S.A.S. (2003). Antimicrobial activity of *Alseodaphne keanamia* extracts. *Ind. Perfumer* 47(1): 87-90.

Parcha, V., Gahlot, M. and Bajaj, B.K. (2003). Antimicrobial activity of essential oil of *Dysoxylum malabaricum. Indian Perfumer* 47 (2): 183-187.

Pathak, A.K. and Dixit, V.K. (1984). Antifungal and antibacterial studies on essential oil of *Glossocardia bosvallia. Indian Perfumer* 28(2): 91-94.

Peres, M.T., Monache, F.D., Cruz; A.B., Pizzolatti, M.G. and Yunes, R.A. (1997). Chemical composition and antimicrobial activity of *Croton urucurana* Baillon (Euphorbiaceae). *J. Ethnopharmacol.* 56: 223-226.

Petricic, J., Kupinic, M. and Lulie, B. (1978). Garlic (*Allium sativum* Linn.) Antifungal effects of some component of volatile oil. *Acta. Pharm. Jugosal.* 28: 41-43.

Rahman, M.U., Gul, S. (May-June 2003). Mycotoxic effect of *Thymus serpyllum* oil on the asexual reproduction of *Aspergillus* species. *J. Essential Oil Research.*

Rahman, A. and Chaudhary, M.I. (1995). Diterpinoid and steroidal alkaloids. *Nat. Prod. Rep.* 12: 361-379.

Rao, B.G.V.N. and Joseph, P.L. (1971). Activity of some essential oils towards phytopathogenic fungi. *Riechest Aromas Koir* 21: 405-410.

Rao J.T. (1976). The *in vitro* antimicrobial effects of the essential oil of *Ageratum conyzoides. Riecht. Aromen. Koerperf* 26: 50.

Rao, J.T. (1976). Antifungal activity of some essential oil of *Curcuma aromatica. Ind. J. Pharma.*38: 53-54.

Rao, T.S.S. and Nigam, S.S. (1978). Chemical and antimicrobial examination of the essential oil from the seeds of *Nigella sativa* var. *aromatica*. Abstracts of papers presented at the seminar on "*Advances in Aromatic plants and Aroma chemicals*" by Essential oil Association of India held at Bombay, 8-9th April, Session-I, ab-18.

Rathee, P.S., Mishra, S.M. and Kousal, R. (1982). Antimicrobial activity of essential oil, fixed oil and unsapioniafiable matter of *Nigella saliva* L. *Indian J. Pharm. Sci.* 44(1): 8-10.

Renu, Mall, H.V., Dubey, N.K. and Dixit, S.N. (1986). Mycotoxic properties of the essential oil of *Aegle mermelos* Corr. *Beitr. Biol. Pflanzen Go.* 325-331.

Renu, Tripathi, R.D. and Dixit, S.N. (1980). Fungitoxic properties of *Cestrum diurnum. Naturwiss* 67: 150.

Renuveni, R., Fleischer, A. and Putieysky, E. (1984). Fungistatic activity of essential oil from *Ocimum basillicum* Chemotypes. *Phytopath. Z.* 110(1): 20-22.

Saksena, N.K. (1984). Comparative evaluation of some essential oils for their antifungal action some dermatophytes. *Indian Perfumer* 28(1): 35-37.

Sampurna, T. and Nigam, S.S. (1979). Efficacy of some Indian oils against *Trichophyton mentagrophytes, Malbranchea pulchella* and *Keratinophyton terreum*, at different conc. *Indian Drugs Pharm.* India 14(4): 20-30.

Samuel, C.O. (1993). Evaluation of essential oils for their toxicity against some seed-borne pathogen. *Ph.D. Thesis*, University of Gorakhpur, Gorakhpur, India.

Samuel, C.O. and Tripathi, S.C. (1994). Fungitoxic properties of essential oil of *Hedychium spicatum. Indian Perfumer* 38(4): 105-111.

Sanyal, A. and Verma, K.C. (1969). *In-vitro* antibacterial and antifungal activity of *Mentha arvensis* var. *piperescenes* oil obtained from different sources. *Indian J. Microbiol.* 9: 23-24.

Sawhney, S.S., Suri, A.K. and Thind, T.S. (1977). Antimicrobial efficacy of some essential oil *in vitro. Indian Drugs* 15: 30-32.

Saxena, A.R. (1980). Evaluation of higher plants for their fungitoxic properties, *Ph.D. Thesis*, University of Gorakhpur, Gorakhpur, India.

Saxena, V.K., Sahai, A. and Sandhya, G. (1984). Studies on antimicrobial efficacy of essential oil of the leaves of *Anaphalis centorta. India Perfumer* 28 (3-4): 177-178.

Saxena, R.C. (1993). Neem as a source of natural insecticides: An Update-*Proc. Symp. on Botanical Pesticides* at Central Tobacco Research Institute, Rajamundry.

Schultes, R.E. (1978). The kingdom of plants. In "Medicines from the Earth," ed. W.A.R.Thompson. 208. McGraw-Hill Book Co., New York.

Sehgal, J.M. (1961). Antimicrobial substances from flowering plants. I. Antifungal substances. *Hindustan Antibiotics. Bull.* 4: 3-29.

Shahi, S., Shukla, A.C., Dikshit, S. and Dikshit, A. (1997). Modified spore germination inhibition technique for evaluation of candidate fungitoxicant (*Eucalyptus* sp.) H. W. Dehne *et al.* eds. *Proc.* 4th *Int. Symp. Diagnosis and Identification of Plant Pathogens*, Kluwer Academic Publishers, Netherlands, 253-263.

Shahi, S.K., Shukla A.C., Patra, M. and Dikshit, A. (2002). Use of essential oil as botanical-pesticide against postharvest spoilage in fruits, *Malus pumilo*. *J. BioControl*, Kluwer Academic Publishers. 00: 1-10.

Shahi, S.K., Shukla A.C. and Dikshit, A. (2002). *Eucalyptus pauciflora*: A potential source of ecofriendly pesticide, PROTECTON. *Proc. National Seminar on Plant Biotechnology for Sustainable Hill Agriculture.* (eds.) Kumar, N., Negi, P.S. and Singh, N.K. 149-152.

Sharma, N. (2001). Preservation of dried fruits and nuts from biodeterioration by natural plant volatiles. Donahaye, E. J. *et al.*, eds. (2001) *Proc. Int. Conf. CAF in stored Products*, Executive Printing Services, Clovis California, USA, 195-208.

Sharma, G.P., Jain, N.K. and Garg, B.D. (1978). Antifungal activity of some essential oils, *Indian Drugs* 16: 21-23.

Sharma, S.K. and Singh, V.P. (1979). Antifungal activity of the essential oil of *Oenanthe javanica*. *Indian Drugs* 17: 289-291.

Sharma, S.K. and Singh, V.P. (1979). Antifungal activity of some essential oils. *Indian Drugs and Pharm. Ind.* 14: 3-6.

Sharma, A. and Gautam, M.P. (1977). Investigation on the antifungal activity of volatile oil derived from *Nepeta hindostana* (Roth) Hains. *Indian Drugs Pharm. Ind.*12: 33-34.

Sharma, G.P., Jain, N.K. and Garg, B.D. (1978). Antifungal activity of some essential oils. *Indian Drugs* 16: 21-23.

Shukla, A.C. (1997). Fungitoxic studies of some aromatic plants against storage fungi, *Ph D Theis*, University of Allahabad, Allahabad, India.

Shukla, A.C., Shahi, S.K. and Dikshit, A. (1997). Fungicidal toxicity of the essential oil of *Cymbopogon flexuosus* against some storage fungi. *Proc. 49th Annual meeting and National Symposium on emerging issues in Plant Pathology*, Jabalpur. (abs.) 20.

Shukla, A.C., Shahi, S.K. and Dikshit, A. (2000). Epicarp of *Citrus sinensis*: A Potential source of natural pesticide, *Indian Phytopathology* 53(3): 318-322.

Shukla, H.S. (1987). Studies on some volatile fungitoxic constituents of some higher plants. *Ph.D. Thesis*, University of Gorakhpur, Gorakhpur.

Siddiqui, N., Samuel, C.O. and Tripathi, S.C. (2003). Fungitoxic properties of essential oil of *Acorus calamus*. *Indian Phytopath.* 56(3): 355.

Singh, A.K. (1980). Antifungal activity of volatile fractions of some higher plants. *Ph. D. Thesis*, University of Gorakhpur, Gorakhpur, India.

Singh, A.K., Dikshit, A., Sharma, M.L. and Dixit, S.N. (1980). Fungitoxic activity of some essential oils. *Eco. Bot.* 34(2): 186-190.

Singh, A.K., Dikshit, A. and Dixit, S.N. (1983). Fungitoxic properties of essential oil of *Mentha arvensis* var. *piperascens*. *Perfumer and Flavorist* 8: 55-58.

.Singh, A.K., Dikshit, A. and Dixit, S.N. (1983). Antifungal studies of *Peperomia pellucida*. *Beitr. Biol. Pflanzen* 58:.357-368.

Singh, A.K., Tripathi, S.C. and Dixit, S.N. (1978). Fungitoxicity of volatile fraction of some angiospermic plants. *Proc. Symp. Environ. Sci. and Human welfare*, Ujjain, India, 13.

Singh, G., Singh, B.S. and Kumar, B.V.A. (1978). Antimicrobial activity of the essential oil of four medicinal plants against some keratinophilic fungi. *Indian Drugs* 16: 44-45.

Singh, G., Upadhyay, R.K. (1991). Fungitoxic activity of cumaldehyde main constituents of the *Cuminum cyminum* oil. *Fitoterapia* 62(1): 87.

Singh, G., Upadhyaya, R.K., Narayanan, C.S., Padmkumar, K.P. and Rao, G.P. (1993). Chemical and fungitoxic investigations on the essential oil of *Citrus sinensis* (L) Pers, *Zeitschriftfuer Pflanzenkrankheiten-und-Pflanzenschutz*, Germany. 100 (1): 69-74.

Singh, H.B. and Singh, U.P. (1981). Effect of volatile of some plant extracts and their oil on conidia of *Erysiphae polygoni*. DC. *Aust. Plant. Path.*10 (4): 66-67.

Singh, J. and Tripathi, N.N. (1999). Inhibition of storage fungi of blackgram. (*Vigna mungo* L.) by some essential oils. *Flavour Fragr. J.* 14 (1-4).

Singh, K.V. and Deshmukhi, S.K. (1984). Volatile constituents from members of Liliaceae and spore germination of *Microsporum gypseum* Comples. *Fitoterpia* 55(5): 297.

Singh, L. (1976). Effect of some oil on *in vitro* growth of three phytopathogenic fungi. *J. Indian Bot. Soc.* 55: 186-189.

Singh, R.B., Singh, J. and Singh, H.B. (1999). Effect of ginger (*Zingiber officinale* Roscoe) extracts on growth and sclerotium (Lib) de Bary. *Indian Perfumer* 43(2): 60-63.

Singh, S.K., Dubey, N.K., Tripathi, S.C. and Singh, S.K. (1984). Fungitoxicity of some essential oils against *Aspergillus flavus*. *Indian Perfumer* 28(3-4): 164-166.

Singh, S.P., Dubey, P. and Tripathi, S.C. (1986). Antifungal properties of essential oil of *Ageratum conyzoides L. Nat. Acad. Sci. Lett.* 9(4): 97-99.

Singh, S.P., Dubey, P. and Tripathi, S.C. (1986). Fungitoxic properties of the essential oil of *Trachyspermum ammi. Sprague–Mykosen* 29(1): 37-40.

Singh, Y., Tripathi, R.D., Tripathi, N.N. and Dixit, S.N. (1983). The isolation and properties of fungitoxic principle from *Zingiber officinale. India J. Pl. Pathol.*1: 89-96.

Skinner. F.A. (1955). Antibiotics, In: *Modern method of plant Analysis Vol. VII*, Peach. K. and Tracey, M.N. (eds.) Springer I Verlag, Berlin, 626-726.

Slavenas, J. (1963). Physiological role of essential oils. *Obschch Zakonomer Rosta. Razu. Rast. Dokl. Nauk. Konz. Vilnyus* 313-338.

Slavenas. J. and Razinskaite. D. (1962). Some studies of phytoncidal substances and *Juniperus* oil from common Juniper Leit. *T.S.R. Moks. Akad. Darbai, Er. C.* 4(2): 63-74.

Srivastava, L. (1990). Fungitoxic evaluation of volatile constituents of some higher plants against fungi infesting dry fruits during storage, *Ph.D. Thesis*, Gorakhpur University, Gorakhpur.

Srivastava, R. (1981). Evaluation of higher plants for their fungitoxicity against *Rhizoctonia solani* Kuhn. *Ph.D. Thesis*, University of Gorakhpur, Gorakhpur, India.

Stinson, E.E., Billis, D.D., Osman, S.F., Sciliano, J., Ceponis, M.J., Heisler, *E.G.* (1980). Mycotoxin production by *Alternaria* species grown on apples, tomatoes and blueberries. *Agric. Food Chem.* 28: 960-963.

Suri, R.K. and Thind, T.S. (1979). *In-vitro* antifungal efficacy of some essential oils. *East Pharm.* 22(257): 109-110.

Suri, R.K., Nigam, S.S. and Thind, T.A. (1979). *In-vitro* antimicrobial efficacy of essential oil of *Eucalyptus citriodora*. *Indian Drugs* 14(3): 35-37.

Swaminathan, M.S. (1978). Inaugural Address *First Bot. Conference*, Meerut, India: 1-31.

Thind, T.S. and Dahiya, M.S. (1976). Inhibitory effect of essential oils of some medicinal plants against soil inhabiting dermatophytes. *Indian Drugs* 14: 17-20.

Thind, T.S. and Dahiya, M.S. (1977). Inhibitory effect of essential oil of four medicinal plants against some keratinophillic fungi. *East Pharm* 20: 147-148.

Thakur, R.N., Singh, P. and Khosla, M.K. (1989). *In-vitro* studies on antifungal activity of some aromatic oils. *Indian Perfumer* 33(4): 257- 260.

Tiwari, R., Dixit, K. and Dixit, S.N. (1994). Studies on fungitoxic properties of essential oil of *Cinnamomum zeylanicum* Breyn. *Indian Perfumer* 38 (3): 98-104.

Tiwari, R., Dixit, V. and Behal, K. (1998). Insect repellent activity of the essential oil of *Cinnamomum zeylanicum* Breyn. bark. *Indian Perfumer* 42(2): 68-72.

Tiwari, R., Mishra, D.N. and Upadhyay, P.S. (1988). Efficacy of some plant volatiles for the control of black mold of onion caused by *Aspergillus niger* Van Tiegh. during storage. *L. Nat. Acad. Sci.* 2(11): 345-347.

Tripathi, N.N. (1980). Fungitoxicity in some higher plants. *Ph. D. Thesis*, University of Gorakhpur, Gorakhpur, India.

Tripathi, N.N., Dubey, N.K., Dikshit, A., Tripathi, R.D. and Dixit, S.N. (1983). Fungitoxic properties of *Alpinia galanga* oil. *Trop. Sci. Res.* 1(1): 49-52.

Tripathi, R.D., Banerji, R., Sharma, M.L., Balasubramanyam, V.R. and Nigam, S.K. (1985). Toxicity of essential oil from the new strain of *Ocimum gratissimum* (Clocimum) against Betilvine Pathogenic Fungi. *Agric. Biol. Chem.* 49(8): 2277-2282.

Tripathi, S.C., Singh, S.P. and Dube, S. (1986). Studies on antifungal properties of *Trachyspermum ammi* (L.) Sprague. *Phytopath. Z.* 116: 113-120.

Tripathi, N.N. and Kumar, N. (2007). *Putranjiva roxburghii* oil-A potential herbal preservative for peanuts during storage. *Journal of Stored Product Research.* 43(4) p 435-442.

Tyler, P.S. and Boxall, R.A. (1984). Postharvest loss reduction Programmes: A decade of activities:- What consequences? *Tropical Stored Products Information* 23: 13-28.

Uchida, S. (1928). In essential oils of leaves of "Hibs" wood and its relation to the resistance of the wood to destruction by fungi. *J. Soci. Chem.* India, 31: 501-508.

Uppalpati, L. and Rao, J.T. (1979). Antimicrobial properties of the essential oil of *Vitex negundo* Linn. *Indian Drugs Pharm.* 14: 31-33.

Vichkanova, S.A., Adeqina, V.V. and Izosimova, S.B. (1972). Essential oil as a source of new antifungal preparations. *Fintontsidy mater–Soveshch*, Naukova Dumka, Kiev.123-126.

Yadava, R.N. (1986). *In-vitro* antimicrobial studies on the essential oil of *Lepidagathis hylina* Nees. *Indian Perfumer* 30(4): 481-482.

Yadava, R.N., Saxena, V.K. and Nigam, S.S. (1978). Antimicrobial activity of the essential oil of *Caesalpinia Sappan* L. *Indian Perfumer* 22: 73- 75.

Zohri, A.A., Abdel-Gawad, K.M. (1993). Survey of mycoflora and mycotoxins of some dry fruit in Egypt. *Basic Microbiol.* 33: 279-288.

Zutshi, S.K. and Mehta, S.C. (1977). Screening of some essential oils for antifungal properties. *Indian Drugs and Pharma.* 12: 13-14.

Zutshi, S.K., Joshi, S.K. and Bokadia, M.M. (1975). Antimicrobial activity of some Indian essential oils. *Indian J. Pharm.* 37: 129–130.

Microbial Biotechnology and Ecology (2011) *Pages* **439–451**
Editors: **Deepak Vyas, G.S. Paliwal, P.K.Khare and R.K Gupta**
Published by: **DAYA PUBLISHING HOUSE, NEW DELHI**

Chapter 24

Carbonic Anhydrase: An Ancient Enzyme with Multidimensional Roles

☆ *Anjana Sharma, Rajesh Pujari and Abhishek Bhattacharya*

Bacteriology Lab, Department of Biological Sciences, Rani Durgavati University, Jabalpur, M.P.

ABSTRACT

Carbonic anhydrases catalyze the reversible hydration of CO_2 and are ubiquitous in highly evolved eukaryotes and in single cell prokaryotes. The existence of the enzyme in five classes and its identification in thermophillic species from the Archaea domain indicates the systematic evolution along with metabolic and phylogenetic diversity of the enzyme. The enzyme plays an important role in the maintaining the ionic concentration and pH; interconversion of CO_2 and HCO_3^-; homeostasis; photosynthesis and inorganic ion transport. Recently new roles related to gluconeogenesis and pathogenesis has also been assigned to this multifaceted enzyme. Thus in nut shell the enzyme has been envisaged to provide an enroute into the Biochemistry, Physiology and Pathology of individual organism.

Introduction

Carbonic anhydrases (CA) (Carbonate hydrolases; E. C. 4.2.1.1.) has long been one of the most well characterized zinc metalloenzymes that fall into three distinct evolutionary and structural classes *i.e.* α- (alpha), β- (beta) and γ- (gamma) however, recently another two classes has been investigated *i.e.* δ- (delta) and ε- (epsilon) class CA. Although α-class enzymes, particularly mammalian CA II have been the subject of extensive structural studies but for the β-class, consisting of a wide variety of prokaryotic and plant chloroplast CAs, the structural data is quite limited.

Physiologists predicted the existence of CA almost 70 years ago that plays a lead role in catalyzing as well as overcoming the slow-rate conversion between carbon dioxide and bicarbonate. Thereafter, for the first time carbonic anhydrase was purified from erythrocytes (Meldrum and Roughton, 1933; Stadie and O' Brien, 1933) and was further identified, belonging to α-class containing a zinc ion (Keilin and Mann, 1940). The first report of bacterial CA was presented in 1963 by Veitch and Blankenship. A large number of α-CA isoenzymes, primarily from mammalian species have subsequently been identified and characterized revealing different aspects of their molecular structures (Supuran, 2008). The reaction catalyzed, $CO_2 + H_2O \longleftrightarrow HCO_3^- + H^+$, the interconversion of carbon dioxide and bicarbonate, is of fundamental physiological and biochemical importance, relating in various *in vivo* context to pH or ionic balance and metabolic flux (Henry, 1996). Besides these, innumerable number of function makes the enzyme highly significant either in the perspectives of physiology or pathology and therapeutic concerns. Therefore, present review discusses and unravels the enigmatic roles of CA in lieu of different type of functions and existence in different forms in various living sources.

Carbonic Anhydrase: Ubiquitous Nature of the Enzyme

The ubiquitously expressed zinc metalloenzymes, present in prokaryotes and eukaryotes being encoded by three distinct, evolutionarily unrelated gene families: α-CAs (prevalent in vertebrates, bacteria, algae and cytoplasm of green plants), the β-CAs (predominant in bacteria, algae and chloroplasts of both mono as well as dicotyledons), the γ-CAs (mainly in archaea and some bacteria) and another class, the δ-CA was found to be present in marine diatoms, respectively (Supuran, 2008). The comparison of sequences and crystal structures of mammalian and plant CAs demonstrates that they evolved independently and therefore designated as α- and β-class respectively however an additional independently evolved γ-class was reported by Alber and Ferry (1994) for which the phylogenetic analyses predict an ancient origin (Smith *et al.*, 1999).

The α-class is the best characterized class with 16 isozymes identified in mammals with different catalytic activity, subcellular localization and tissue distribution (Supuran, 2008) (Table 24.1). Several isozymes were implicated in various disease states for which treatment frequently involves the application of sulfonamides that inhibit CA activity (Supuran *et al.*, 2008). Prokaryotic α-class enzymes have been compared with other two classes.

Though less study has been made for β-class CA but the first crystal structure for any β-class CA was reported by Mitsuhashi *et al.* (2000). β-class CA, as presumed earlier belonged to higher plants only but were later isolated from a variety of algae (Yagawa *et al.*, 1987; Hiltonen *et al.*, 1995; Eriksson *et al.*, 1996) and found to be widely distributed in bacteria and archaea domain (Smith *et al.*, 1999). The characterization of enzymes from the β-class revealed sharp differences from the other three classes. The α–class and γ–class enzymes are strictly monomers and trimers, respectively however, members of the β-class are dimers, tetramers, hexamers and octamers which suggested a dimer as the basic building block (Kimber and Pai, 2000). Phylogenetic analyses indicated that the β-class is more diverse than the other two classes (Smith *et al.*, 1999). Sequence alignment indicated that only 5 residues (three zinc ligand, one aspartate and one arginine residue) were completely conserved (Smith *et al.*, 2000). Plant sequences were found to form two monophyletic clades representing dicot and monocot plants (Smith *et al.*, 1999). Carbonic anhydrase obtained from *Pisum sativum* was found to be a dimer of homodimers whereas CA obtained from algae was a homodimer in which the monomer was found to be composed of two internally repeated structures each with an active site (Tripp *et al.*, 2001).

Gamma-class CA was thought to have evolved between 3.0 and 4.5 billion years ago (Smith *et al.*, 1999) and therefore preceded evolution of the α-class at 200-300 million years ago (Hewett-Emmett and Tashian, 1996; Jiang and Gupta, 1999). The only γ-class enzyme characterized was "Cam" from the archaeon *Methanosarcina thermophila* (Alber and Ferry, 1994). Cam was found to be a homodimer that adopts a left-handed parallel β-helical fold (Kisker *et al.*, 1996) and heterologously produced in *E. coli* at high levels to yield a zinc enzyme (Alber and Ferry, 1996). However, iron and cobalt-substituted forms exhibit greater CO_2 hydration rates than the zinc enzyme (Alber *et al.*, 1999) and it was thought that possibly Cam functions in *M. thermophila* using a different transition metal than zinc (Tripp *et al.*, 2001).

Table 24.1: Distribution of Various Human CA Isoforms with Different Catalytic Activities

Isozyme	*Kcal/Km* (M^{-1} s^{-1})	*Subcellular Localization*	*Tissue/Organ localization*
hCAI	5.0 x 10^7	Cytosol	Erythrocytes, GI tract
hCAII	1.5 x 10^8	Cytosol	Erythrocytes, GI tract, eye, bone osteoclasts, kidney, lung, testis, brain
hCAIII	3.0 x 10^5	Cytosol	Skeletal muscle, adipocytes
hCAIV	5.1 x 10^7	Membrane-bound	Kidney, lung, pancreas, brain, capillaries, colon, heart muscle
hCAVA	2.9 x 10^7	Mitochondria	Liver
hCAVB	9.8 x 10^7	Mitochondria	Heart and skeletal muscle, pancreas, kidney, spinal cord, GI tract
hCAVI	4.9 x 10^7	Secreted (saliva, milk)	Salivary and mammary glands
hCAVII	8.3 x 10^7	Cytosol	CNS
hCAVIII	–	Cytosol	CNS
hCAIX	5.5 x 10^7	Transmembrane	Tumours, GI mucosa
hCAX	–	Cytosol	CNS
hCAXI	–	Cytosol	CNS
hCAXII	3.5 x 10^7	Transmembrane	Renal, intestinal, reproductive epithelia, eye, tumours
hCAXIII	4.3 x 10^7	Cytosol	Kidney, brain, lung, gut, reproductive tract
hCAXIV	3.9 x 10^7	Transmembrane	Kidney, brain, liver
hCAXV	9.6 x 10^7	Membrane-bound	Kidney

Francois Morel and co-workers have reported the purification of a 27-kDa monomeric CA called TWCA1, from marine diatom *Thalassiosira weissflogii* (Roberts *et al.*, 1997) that was classified under a separate class called δ-class. The catalytic zinc ion was shown by X-ray absorption spectroscopy to be coordinated by three histidines and a water molecule, similar to the active sites of α-class and γ-class CAs and the near-edge spectra revealed that the active site geometry is similar to that of α-class enzymes (Cox *et al.*, 2000). The existence of a water molecule as a fourth ligand suggested that δ-class CA also follows the zinc hydroxide mechanism of the other three classes (Tripp *et al.*, 2001).

Although TWCA1 has biochemical properties similar to the three known classes of CA however the deduced sequence of the gene encoding TWCA1 revealed no significant identity to the three classes. Therefore TWCA1 is the prototype for a fourth class of CA that has been designated as the δ–class (Tripp *et al.*, 2001). During the conditions in which the level of TWCA1 was found low in *T. weissflogii*, in that case a 43-kDa cadmium-specific CA has been expressed (Lane and Morel, 2000). The sequence of the gene encoding δ–CA has not yet been reported (Tripp *et al.*, 2001).

Carbonic anydrases are widespread enzymes, present in mammals in 16 different isoforms (Supuran, 2008). Some of these ioszymes are cytosolic (CA I, II, III, VII and XIII) others are membrane-bound (CA IV, IX, XII, and XIV), CA V is mitochondrial by origin and CA VI is secreted in the saliva and milk. Three cytosolic a catalytic forms of CA *i.e.* CA related proteins (CARP) are also known (CARPVIII, CARPX and CARPXI). The catalytically isoforms, which play important physiological and pathological functions are strongly inhibited by aromatic and heterocyclic sulfonamides.

Under the name of CA, Meldrum and Roughton (1933) were the first to describe a new enzyme present in R.B.Cs. They purified the enzyme further and gave a detailed account of it's properties and the kinetics of the enzyme. Isoenzymes of CA later isolated not only from mammalian blood but also from other tissues of dog like kidney (Byvoet and Gotti, 1967), prostrate, uterus (McIntosh, 1969; 1970), stomach, colon, caecum (Carter and Parsons, 1970a; 1970b; 1971) and rumen epithelial tissue (Carter, 1971). Later different forms of the enzyme have been isolated from erythrocytes of man, green monkey, baboon, horse, pig, guinea pig, rat, blue-white dolphin and yellowfin tuna (Lindskog *et al.*, 1971; Anderson *et al.*, 1972; Laurentt-Tabusse *et al.*, 1972). CA has also been isolated from erythrocytes of sheep (Tanis *et al.*, 1970). The major form of CA from dog erythrocytes has been isolated and characterized by Soliman and Klub (1974). CA XII is a membrane glycoprotein with an active extracellular CA domain that overexpressed on cell surfaces of certain renal cell cancers (Ulmasov *et al.*, 2000). The last mammalian α-CA isoform (CAXV) has now been isolated, purified and characterized along with representatives of the α-, β-, γ-, and δ-classes from various pathogenic organisms from across the phylogeny.

During the past few decades, considerable efforts have been made on investigations of the properties and function of the enzyme carbonic anhydrase from microbial sources. Progress reviewed by Lindskog *et al.* (1971) and Maren (1967) paved the way to achieve knowledge of the kinetic behaviour of the enzyme as well as structural features. The presence of CA activity in bacteria was firstly reported by Veitch and Blankenship (1963) who measured significant activities in strains of several species of the genus *Neisseria* and in a strain of *Streptococcus salivaria*. The highest activity found was in *Nesseria sicca*, strain 6021. Gill *et al.* (1984) observed an intracellular CA but not periplasmic in *Rhodospirillum rubrum* however, the biological function of this enzyme has not yet been investigated. Guilloton *et al.* (1992) established the existence of CA in *E. coli* and identified that the enzyme is being encoded by *cyn operon*. Later Alber and Ferry (1994), purified and characterized CA from *Methanosarcina thermophila* grown in acetate and was the first report on CA from the archaeal domain. The enzyme represented a prototype of the γ-class of CAs. Methanogenic anaerobes have been the largest group within archaea, a domain which has been phylogenetically closer to the eukarya than to the bacteria (Woese *et al.*, 1990).

Later Braus-Stromeyer *et al.* (1997) detected the prevalence of CA activity in *Acetobacterium woodii, Acetohalobium arabaticum, Clostridium formicoaceticum, Sporomusa silvacetica, Moorella thermoautotrophica, Moorella thermoacetica subsp. "pratumsolum", Sporomusatermitida* and *Thermoanaerobacter kivui. A. woodii* was found to exhibit highest CA specific activity (approximately 14 U mg of protein^{-1}) of all the microbes represented till date. In 1999, Smith and Ferry reported a plant type β-class CA in the thermophilic methanoarchaeon *Methanobacterium thermoautotrophicum* reflecting no esterase activity however the enzyme had a KCal value of 1.7×10^4 S^{-1}. The results revealed that the β-class CA extends not only into the archaea domain but also into the thermophilic prokaryotes. *Rhodopseudomonas palustris*, a purple non-sulfur bacterium behaved surprisingly as it was observed that the organism exhibited CA activity when grown anaerobically but not aerobically (Puskas *et al.*, 2000).

Enigmatic Role of Carbonic Anhydrase

CAs were shown to be present in a multitude of prokaryotes, where it plays many important functions such as respiration, transport of CO_2 and photosynthesis (Supuran, 2008). Therefore, CA is widely distributed in nature and participates in various functions which includes facilitated diffusion of CO_2, interconversion of CO_2 and HCO_3^- during photosynthesis and biosynthetic processes, pH homeostasis and ion transport (Tashian, 1990; Coleman, 1991). Methanogenic anaerobes exhibit CA activity whereby they obtain energy for growth by producing methane from the reduction of CO_2 with H_2 or by the conversion of methyl groups of acetate, methanol or methanolamines to methane (Boone *et al.*, 1993) and also has been proposed that CA is required for an CH_3CO^{2-}/HCO_3^- antiport system.

In addition to the physiological reactions CAs catalyze a variety of other reactions (Figure 24.1) such as: hydration of cyanate to carbamic acid or of cyanamide to urea; aldehyde hydration to gem-diols; hydrolysis of carboxylic or sulfonic esters as well as other hydrolytic processes (Brig *et al.*, 1999; Guerri *et al.*, 2000; Supuran and Scozzafava, 2000; Supuran *et al.*, 2003).

The Carbonic anhydrase role was also found to be involved in many other biochemical and pathological processes which includes electrolyte secretion in various tissues and organs, biosynthetic reactions such as gluconeogenesis, lipogenesis and ureagenesis, bone resorption, calcification and tumorigenicity (Supuran and Scozzafava, 2000; 2002). Being involved in pathological basis for a number of diseases, the enzyme has been an important therapeutic targets with the potential to be inhibited to treat a range of disorders including oedema, glaucoma, obesity, cancer, epilepsy and osteoporosis (Supuran, 2008). There are atleast 25 clinically used drugs have been reported to possess significant CA inhibitory properties to treat several diseases *viz.* acetazolamide, methazolamide,

$$O=C=O + H_2O \longleftrightarrow HCO_3^- + H^+$$

$$O=C=NH + H_2O \longleftrightarrow H_2NCOOH$$

$$HN=C=NH + H_2O \longleftrightarrow H_2NCONH_2$$

$$RCHO + H_2O \longleftrightarrow RCH(OH_2)^{\bullet}$$

$$RCOOAr + H_2O \longleftrightarrow RCOOH + ArOH$$

$$RSO_3Ar + H_2O \longleftrightarrow RSO_3H + ArOH$$

$$ArF + H_2O \longleftrightarrow HF + ArOH \quad (Ar = 2,4\text{-dinitrophenyl})$$

$$PhCH_2OCOCl + H_2O \longleftrightarrow PhCH_2OH + CO_2 + HCl$$

$$RSO_2Cl + H_2O \longleftrightarrow RSO_3H + HCl \quad (R = Me; Ph)$$

Figure 24.1: Reactions Catalyzed by α-Class Carbonic Anhydrases

ethoxzolamide, sulthiame, dichlorophenamide, dorzolamide, brinzolamide, indisulam, topiramate, zonisamide, sulpiride, COUMATE, EMATE, celecoxib, valdecoxib and saccharin (Table 24.2).

Table 24.2: Biomedical Applications of Inhibitors of Carbonic Anhydrase Isoforms

Sl.No.	Compound	CA Isoforms (as therapeutic targets)	Application
1.	Acetazolamide	CAII, VA,VB, VII, VI, IX, XII, XIII and XIV	Nor-mercurial diuretic and glaucoma treatment
2.	Methazolamide	-do-	Qedema treatment and glaucoma treatment
3.	Ethoxzolamide	-do-	-do-
4.	Sulthiame	-do-	Glaucoma treatment
5.	Dichlorophenamide	-do-	Qedema treatment
6.	Dorzolamide	-do-	Glaucoma treatment
7.	Brinzolamide	-do-	-do-
8.	Indisulam	-do-	Treatment of cancer (antitumoric)
9.	Topiramate	CAII, VII, VA, VB, VI, XII and XIII	Antiepileptic
10.	Zonisamide[a]	CAII, VA, VB, IX	Antiepileptic, treatment for neuropathic pain, bipolar disorder, migraine, obesity, eating disorders, parkinsons disease
11.	Sulpiride[a]	CAVI, XII	Antipsychotic
12.	COUMATE	CAIX and XII*	Anticancer
13.	EMATE	CAIX and XII*	-do-
14.	Celecoxib	CAII	Antinflammatory
15.	Valdecoxib	CAXII and CAII	
16.	Saccharin	CA VII[a]	
17.	Fluorescent sulphonamide derivative	CAIX	Anticancer
18.	Pyridinium derivative	-do-	-do-
19.	Chlorothiazide and Hydrochlorothiazide	CAII, IV, XII and XIV	Diuretics
20.	Quinethazone	CAII, CAIV, XII and CAXIV	-do-
21.	Metolazone	-do-	-do-
22.	Chlorthalidone	-do-	-do-
23.	Indapamide	-do-	-do-
24.	Furosemide	-do-	-do-
25.	Bumetamide	-do-	-do-

a: Low affinity to other isoforms.

Furthermore, evidences have been laid down that various forms of organisms such as protozoa, fungi and bacteria were found to exhibit virulence and growth as a parasite due to carbonic anhydrase activity and therefore the aspect has emerged as a new and recent directive for research. *Plasmodium falciparum* (Krungkrai *et al.*, 2005), *Helicobacter pylori* (Nishimori *et al.*, 2006; 2007), *Mycobacterium tuberculosis* (Suarez Covarrubias *et al.*, 2005), *Candida albicans* (Klengel, 2005) and *Cryptococcus neoformans* (Morgensen *et al.*, 2006; Bahn *et al.*, 2005) are some of the organisms that have been well characterized in terms of their pathogenicity due to CA activity. Later it has been proved that the class of CA prevalent in the organism is critical for the growth or virulence of these pathogens and infact for their different degrees of resistance to the currently available drugs. An α-class CA (pfCA) is prevalent in *P. falciparum*. Possess catalytic properties that are distinct to that of the human host enzymes CA I and CA II and plays a major role in causing malaria. On the other hand *H. pylori*, organism responsible for different gastric mucosal lesions, including gastritis, stomach ulcers and gastric cancer (Nishimori *et al.*, 2006; 2007) exhibits both α- and β-class CAs called hpαCA and hpβCA, respectively. Both the classes of CAs are essential for the survival of the pathogen and plays crucial role in acid acclimatization of the pathogen within the human stomach (Supuran, 2008). Concrete evidence was put forth when it was revealed that inhibition of the two enzymes leads to the death of the bacteria and a possible eradication of *H. pylori* from the stomach thereby making the enzyme, a druggable target (Nishimori *et al.*, 2006; 2007). Another remarkable aspect was revealed by Suarez Covarrubias *et al.* (2005) when it was established that *M. tuberculosis Rv3588c* gene required for *in vivo* growth of the pathogen and the gene encodes for a β-class CA with an activity that is highly dependent on pH, being active at pH 8.4 but not at pH 7.5. As identified by Muhlschlegel's and Heitman's groups (2005), the signaling role of CAs in *C. albicans* and *C. neoformans* was evident proving that CA is important for the virulence of these two fungal pathogens.

Valdivia and Falkow (1999), investigated the inevitable role of *mig-5*, a gene encoding a putative β-class CA in facultative intracellular pathogen *Salmonella typhimurium* and was found that the gene get induced 24-fold upon infection in host macrophages and it was necessary for bacterial survival within the host. Sharma *et al.* (2008) investigated the prevalence of Carbonic anhydrase in diversified genera that includes *Enterobacter, Aeromonas, Shigella* and *Klebsiella* and observed that all the organisms exhibited CA activity irrespective of their magnitude of production, low or high. Noticeably, it was observed that high level of CA activity was more predominant in the organisms, those which were urease positive and are opportunistic pathogen thereby indicating that CA might play a role in their pathogenesis or microbial virulence, results in accordance to the earlier reports of Smith *et al.* (1999).

Multidimensional Properties of the Enzyme

Enzymes, the regulatory bodies within an organism has been represented by their known specificity towards substrate and their typified allotted function within a biological system and in nature all enzyme do follow the natural rule however, Carbonic anhydrase rules as an exception that deviates from the nature's rule in the sense that it has multiple functions to carry out and that which are not at all correlated with each other and the enzyme is meant for several diverse metabolic pathways as mentioned earlier and hence known for its multidimensional properties. It performs different functions under different physiological conditions. The same enigmatic behaviour is also evident from the reports of Liljas and Laurberg (2000). The enzyme belongs to different classes that evolved independently and have no sequence homology. The amino acid sequences are strikingly different however inspite of the differences in sequence, all forms of CA have an essential zinc ion in the active site.

The active sites show essential features of remarkable similarity though structurally there exists a wide variations. All of the CAs are completely different from one another at the level of their tertiary and quarternary structures (Figure 24.2). Gamma-class CA exhibits a primitive β-helix structure where short repeated amino acid sequence produces the main part of the protein fold whereas the α- and β-CAs have folds that are constructed by different arrangements of α-helices and β-strands.

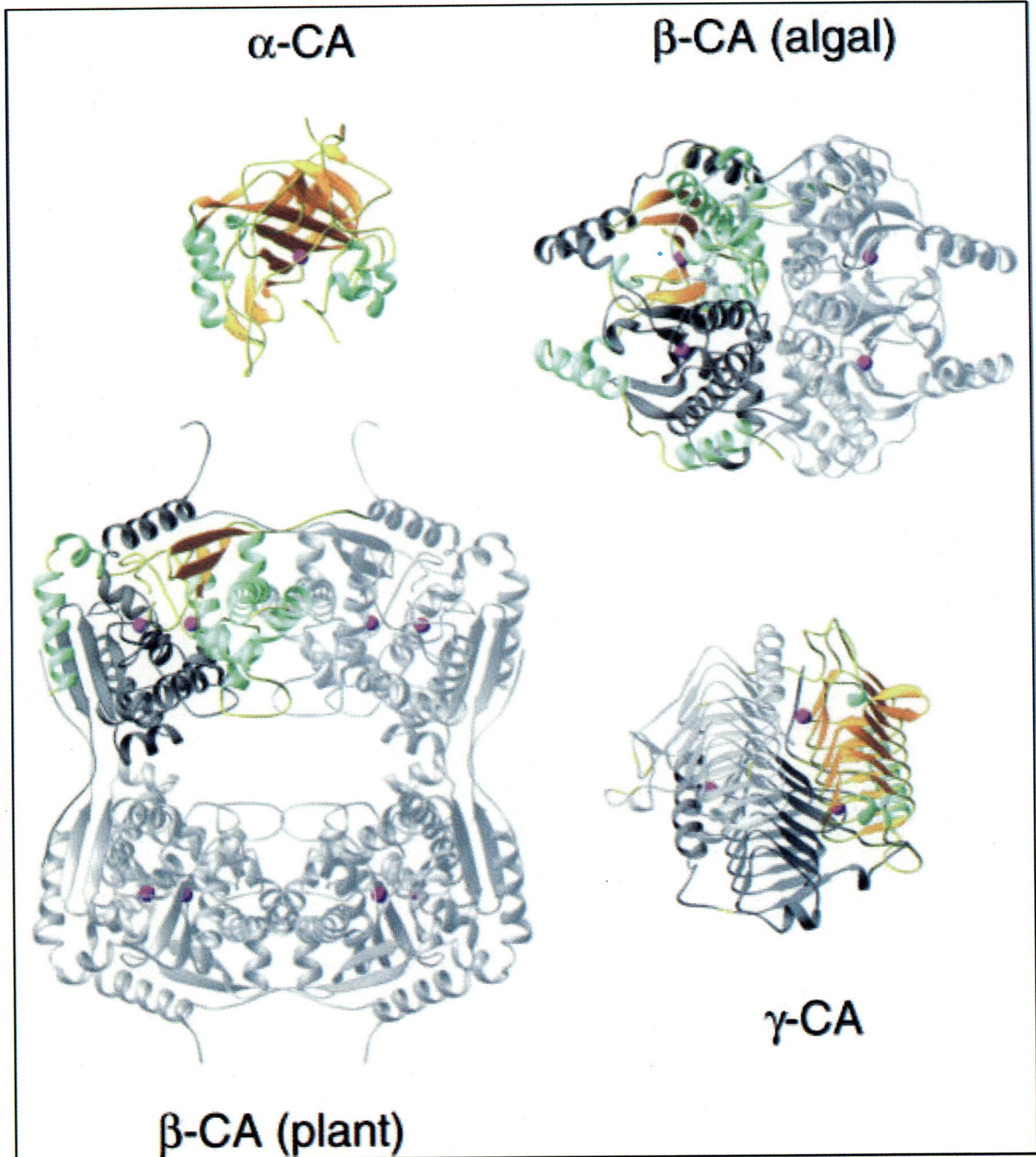

Figure 24.2: The Tertiary Structures of the Three Forms of Carbonic Anhydrase

Differences in quarternary structure exist even within the class of β-CA (Figure-2) where algal β-CA is a dimer with internal repeat and on the same hand, plant β-CA is an octamer which does not based on 4-fold but on repeated 2-fold symmetry.

Therefore, within the same class remarkable dissimilarity exist though the enzyme is same and performing the same function. The active site retains a zinc ion in common however, the zinc ion ligands are completely different and hence the essential residues of the active sites differ as well (Figure 24.3). More striking difference is that β-CAs from plant has an acetate ion bound to the zinc while the acetate ion is being replaced by aspartate in the algal β-CA.

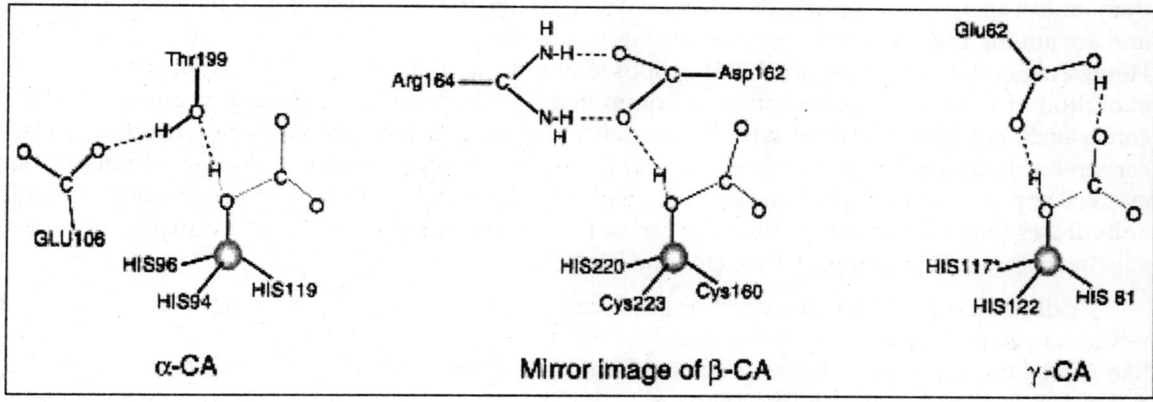

Figure 24.3: Schematic Representations of the Active Sites of the Three Forms of Carbonic Anhydrase

Inspite of the differences, these enzymes catalyzes reaction in common where the zinc ion activates a water molecule that reacts with CO_2 or destabilizes bicarbonate in the reverse reaction. Therefore, CA illustrates a detail enigmatic account that being the same enzyme it strongly holds a versatile nature.

Highlighting the genomics account and expression of the enzyme, Fukuzawa *et al.* (1990) investigated that *Chlamydomonas reinhardtii*, an alga encodes two different CAs within the same genome as gene *CAH1* and *CAH2* and are being expressed and regulated under different physiological conditions. The 5′ upstream gene *CAH1* encodes a major periplasmic CA and its level of expression is rapidly induced under low CO_2 level in the presence of light while the 3′ downstream gene *CAH2* encodes another periplasmic isozyme induced at high CO_2 level *i.e.* 1-5 per cent CO_2.

In regards to the cellular localization the enzyme exhibit a great diversity as the enzyme have different destination in different model systems such as either extracellular or intracellular. When intracellular it could be cytosolic, periplasmic, membrane bound and transmembranal and secreted outside a cell when extracellular by nature.

Carbonic anhydrase enzyme has been a strong example and representative of convergent evolution and hence though differ distinctly still has its unique features to correlate. It has been of significant interest to denote that the enzyme has evolved three times completely in an independent way (Liljas and Laurberg, 2000) thereby generating enzymes in several different isoforms that appears to be different superficially but are actually posssess great underlying similarities.

Ferry *et al.* (1999) detected the prevalence of β-class and γ-class carbonic anhydrases in methanoarachaea and established that carbonic anhydrases are widely distributed in prokaryotes and that the β-class and γ-class carbonic anhydrases are predominant. They also documented that these two classes of enzymes are of ancient origin. On the other hand presence of both β-class and γ-class carbonic anhydrases in thermophilic chemolithoautotrophs has been established suggesting that ancient carbon dioxide fixation pathways are dependent on carbonic anhydrase for efficient Carbondioxide fixation. However, Alber and Ferry (1996) purified the carbonic anhydrase enzyme from the archaeon methanosarcina thermophila which was noticeably found to be distinct from the α- and β- class, and is the prototype of a different class *i.e.* γ-class.

Ferry *et al.* (1999) found that β-class carbonic anhydrases occur not only in species of archaea domain, but also in thermophilic prokaryotes with an obligate chemilithoautotrophic mode of growth, and are among the species that represent some of the deepest branches of the universal tree of life. Hewwett-Emmett and Tashain (1996) proposed about the α-class carbonic anhydrase so that the evolution of this class has been from a common ancestral gene 0.5-0.6 billion years ago and the consistency has been followed with the evidence that few prokaryotic genomes encoding α-class carbonic anhydrases. However, Ferry *et al.* (1999) claimed that the γ-class carbonic anhydrases has evolved approximately 4.2 billion years ago, with the major cluster of bacterial and archaeal carbonic anhydrases thereby supporting that the carbonic anhydrases must be extremely ancient enzymes, existing before the divergence of archaea and bacteria domains.

Additional support for an ancient origin of carbonic anhydrase is the presence of the β-class and γ-classes in thermophiles representing deep branches of the universal tree of life that includes organisms like *C. hydrogenoformans, M. thermoautotrophicum, Methanococcus janaaschii, Sulfolobus solfataricus, P. furiosus, Pyrococcus horikoshii* etc. (Ferry *et al.*, 1999).

Evidence against prevalence of carbonic anhydrase was obtained from freshwater, marine, mesophilic, thermophilic, aerobic, anaerobic, pathogenic, symbiotic, methylotrophic, acetotrophic, methanogenic, acetogenic, autotrophic, heterotrophic and photosynthetic species (Ferry *et al.*, 1999). Prokaryotic carbonic anhydrases also have medical significance as are represented by several pathogenic species, suggesting the possibility that carbonic anhydrase exhibit some role and is required for microbial virulence. Evidence in support of this has been documented by Valdivia and Falkow (1997) for a gram-negative, facultative intracellular pathogen *S. typhimurium*. Expression of mig-5, a gene encoding a putative β-class carbonic anhydrase has been induced upto 24 fold upon infection in host macrophages and it is necessary for bacterial survival within the host.

Eriksson *et al.*, 1996 reported the prevalence of carbonic anhydrase in the green unicellular alga, *Chlamydomonas reinhardtii* when grown under Carbondioxide–limiting conditions and further the enzyme was characterized as 22-kDa polypeptide in *C. reinhardtii*, one more additional feature to the molecular nature of carbonic anhydrase with respect to the usual molecular weight of carbonic anhydrase that ranges between 29kDa–35kDa. Localization study of the enzyme in *C. reinhardtii* revealed that the enzyme was localized and induced within the mitochondria by a lowering of the partial pressure of Carbondioxide in the growth medium. The study brought-in a significant role of carbonic anhydrase in adaptation of the alga to low Carbondioxide conditions and thus provides the basis for experimental studies of mitochondrial carbonic anhydrases, which has been a rarely localized enzyme in living systems other than mammalian isoforms hCA VA and hCAVB.

Soltes-Rak *et al.*, 1997 identified and characterized Carbonic anhydrase from two disparate cyanobacteria, *Anabaena* sp. strain PCC 7120 and *Synechococcus* sp. strain PCC 7942 and was found out that the enzyme resembled to be of vertebrate-type. Carbonic anhydrase and that they revealed significant sequence similarity to human CA I and CA II as well as of *Chlamydomonas reinhardtii*. In addition, the similarity of the active-site structure of the cyanobacterial Carbonic anhydrase indicated that it could be an important tool for structural studies on amino acid substitutions resulting in the evolution of the highly efficient vertebrate CA II isoforms.

Marine diatom, *Phaeodactylum tricornutum* exhibited a single intracellular Carbonic anhydrase under different conditions *viz.* air-grown, and at reduced levels, in high Carbondioxide grown cells of the alga as per the study made by Satoh *et al.*, 2001. However, no external Carbonic anhydrase activity was detected irrespective of growth under cardondioxide conditions. Acetazolamide (2mM), a strong and specific inhibitor of Carbonic anhydrases had little effect on the affinity for dissolved inorganic carbon, thereby suggesting that internal Carbonic anhydrase was crucial for the operation of a carbon concentrating mechanism in *P. tricornutum*. Their study concluded that intracellular Carbonic anhydrase appeared to play a major role in acquiring and supplying substrate for photosynthesis in marine diatoms. Later *P. tricornutum* Carbonic anhydrase was described during the study to be the first β-class Carbonic anhydrase in a diatom species.

The other diatom Carbonic anhydrase isolated from *T. weissflogii* (TWCA1), showed no homology to the known algal Carbonic anhydrases and therefore a fundamental difference of carbon acquisition among algal phyla was proposed by Roberts *et al.* (1997).

Xia and Gao (2005) detected the prevalence of Carbonic anhydrase and it's activity from fresh green algae *Chlorella pyrenoidosa* chick and *C. reinhardtii* Dang cells when grown under different Carbondioxide concentrations within a range of 3-186 µmol/L. They observed the prevalence of both intracellualar and extracellular Carbonic anhydrase through activity and furthermore they concluded that the extracellular Carbonic anhydrase can be induced by a change in environmental Carbondioxide concentration and it was presumed to play an important role in photosynthesis by maintaining the inorganic carbon species equilibrium at the site of transport or diffusion into cells however with the increased Carbondioxide concentration in the medium both intracellular and extracellular Carbonic anhydrase activity exhibited a significant decline but to varying extents. And thus it implied that the susceptibility of Carbonic anhydrase activity to Carbondioxide enrichment was species dependent.

Intracellular Carbonic anhydrase in *Chlorella* species and *C. reinhardtii* was found to be of two types: (*i*) a soluble Carbonic anhydrase localized within the Cytosol as reported by Xia and Gao (2005) and (*ii*) an insoluble membrane-bound Carbonic anhydrase associated with the chloroplast however in contrast to this Sultemeyer (1998) earlier reported an intracellular Carbonic anhydrase in mitochondria during acclimation to low Carbondioxide concentrations in *C. reinhardtii*.

Concluding Remarks

Literature reviewed in this report is with an intention to putforth the uncommon role (with respect to nature, structure, function, expression level and evolution) of a common enzyme (being ubiquitous) in nature. A single biological derivative encompassing a number of functionality has reached a new height exceptionally in the field of biochemistry, physiology and pathology. The same molecule has gained a great foot hold now in terms of applied biotechnology either in regards to the approach of medical diagnosis on one hand and carbondioxide sequestration on the other hand whereby researchers foresee an ultimate alternative towards disease cure and eradicating the problem of global warming through exploitation of its CO_2 hydration activity, respectively. These facets let us assume the multidimensionality in total for the enzyme Carbonic anhydrase.

The enzyme seeks due importance and recognition being a novel entity and lays down path to unravel several other biological hurdles for researchers in the time to come. Further detail understanding is deemed necessary and the authors are paving the way for deep interaction of the molecule in biochemical and physiological perspectives to shape-up the dynamicity of the molecule.

References

Alber BE and Ferry JG. (1994). *Proc Natl Acad Sci USA* 91: 6909–6913.

Anderson B Nyman PO and Strid L. (1972). *Biochem Biophysics Res Commun* 48: 670-677.

Boone DR Whitman WB and Rouveiere P. (1993). in *Methanogenesis*, ed. Ferry JG (Chapman and Hall, London) pg 35-80.

Braus-Stromeyer S, Schnappauf G, Braus GH, Gobner A and Drake HL. (1997). *J Bacteriol* 179: 7197–7200.

Brigarti F Manganin S Scozzafava Vernaglione G and Supuran CT. (1999). *J Biol Inorg Chem* 4: 528-536.

Byvoet P and Gotti A. (1967). *Mol Pharm* 3: 142-152.

Carter MJ. (1971). *Biochem Biophysics Acta* 235: 222-236.

Carter MJ and Parsons DS. (1970 a). *Biochem biophysics Acta* 206: 190-192.

Carter MJ and Parsons DS. (1971). *J Physiol* 215: 71-94.

Carter MJ and Parsons DS. (1970 b). *J Biol Chem* 120: 797-808.

Coleman JR. (1991). 14: 861-867.

Cronk JD, Endrizzi JA, Cronk M and Zhang KYJ. (2001). *Protein Science* 10 : 911-922.

Errikson M Karlsson J Ramazanov Z Gardershrom P and Sameulsson G. (1996). *Proct Natl Acad Sci.* 93: 12031-12034.

Gill SR, Fedorka PJ, Tweten RK and Sleeper BP. (1984). *Arch Microbiol* 138: 113–118.

Henry RP. (1996). *Annu Rev Physiol* 58 : 523-538.

Hewett-Emmett D and Tashian RE. (1996). *J Bacteriol* 178: 3270-3274.

Hiltonen T Karlsson J Clarke AK and Sameulesson G. (1995). *Planta* 195 : 345-351.

Kimber MS and Pai EF. (2000). *EMBO* 19: 1407-1418.

Laurent-Tabuse G Giraud N and Limozin n. (1972). *Biochem Biophysics Res Commun* 54: 809-821.

Lindskog S Hederson LE Kaman KK Lijlas A Nyman PO and Strandberg B. (1971). *The Enzymes*, vol V (Boyer PO). 3rd edn pp. 587-665 Academic Press, New York.

Maren TH (1967). *Physiol Rev* 47: 595.

McIntosh JEA. (1969). *J Biol Chem* 114: 463-476.

McIntosh JEA. (1970). *J Biol Chem* 120: 299-310.

Meldrum NO and Roughton FJW. (1933). *J Physiol* 80 : 113-141.

Mitsuhashi S Mizurhima T yamashita E Yamato m and Trukihara T. (2000). *J Biol Chem* 275 : 5521-5526.

Pushkas LG, Inui M, Zahan K and Yukawa H. (2000). *Microbiology* 146: 2957–2966.

Roberts SB lane TW Morel FMM. (1997). *J Phycol* 33: 845-850.

Satoh D Hiraoka Y Colman B and Matsuda Y. (2001). *Plant Physiol* 126: 1459-1470.

Smith KS Zakubzick C, Whittam TS and Ferry JG. (1999). *Proc Natl Acad Sci USA* 96: 15184–15189.

Soltes-Rak E mulligan ME and Coleman JR. (1997). *J Bacteriol* 179: 769-774.

Stadie WC and O' Brien H. (1933). *J Biol Chem* 103 : 521-529.

Sultemeyer D. (1998). *Can J Biol* 76: 962-972.

Supuran CT. (2008). *Current Pharmaceutical Design* 14 : 603-614.

Supuran CT and Scozzofava A. (2000). *Exp Opin Ther* 10: 575-600.

Supuran CT Scozzofava A Vernaglione G and Supuran CT. (1999). *J Biol Inorg Chem* 4: 528-536.

Tashian RE. (1990). *Biossays* 10: 186-192.

Tripp BC Smith K and Ferry JG. (2001). 276: 46615-48618.

Ulmasov B Waheed A Shah GN Grubb HJ Sly WS and Silverman DN. (2000). 97: 14212-14217.

Valdivia RH and Falkow S. (1997). *Science* 277: 2007–2011.

Veitch FP and Blakenship LC. (1963). Carbonic anhydrase in bacteria. *Nature* 197: 76-77.

Woere CR Kandler O and Wheelis ML. (1990). Towards a natural system of organisms: proposals for the domains Archea, Bacteria and Eukarya. *Proc Natl Acad Sci USA* 87: 4576-4579.

Xia J and Gao K. (2005). Impacts of elevated CO_2 concentration on biochemical composition, carbonic anhydrase and nitrate reductase activity of freshwater green algae. *J Integrative Plant Biology* 47(6): 668-675.

Yagawa Y, Shiraiwa Y and Miyachi S. (1984). Carbonic anhydrase from the blue green algae (cyanobacterium). *Anabaena variabilis*. *Plant Cell Physiol* 25: 775–783.

Microbial Biotechnology and Ecology (2011) Pages 452–471
Editors: Deepak Vyas, G.S. Paliwal, P.K.Khare and R.K Gupta
Published by: DAYA PUBLISHING HOUSE, NEW DELHI

Chapter 25

Pharmacological Potential of Mushrooms

☆ *Alka Karwa and Mahendra Rai*

Department of Biotechnology, S.G.B Amravati University, Amravati – 444 602

ABSTRACT

Biodiversity of mushrooms in India reveals a wide spectrum of culinary and pharmacologically important species that shows a wide spectrum of bioactivity. These are traditionally being utilized and modern techniques of molecular biology are continuously being worked for the same. Certain activities of mushrooms like immunomodulator, antitumor and anti HIV effects are being exploited increasingly. Mushrooms after all are now no longer mysterious: they may inspire excitement, fascination and even wonder. Nature's oldest art, the food of the Gods, the mushroom promise to be the next marvel after the green revolution.

Introduction

Mushrooms have always been mysterious. Their extraordinary biology, history, appearance, flavors, folklore, cuisine, gathering and more, adds to the mystery. Mushrooms are the invaluable link in the energy chain whose enzymes break the tough lignin of the wood and scavenge the organic material found in the forest floor. Their role is as nature's trash burners. There are thousands of regularly harvested edible fungi in the world, in addition to literally hundreds of thousands of other edible species. Some species are highly priced because they cannot be cultivated and are often harvested from natural settings.

There is an enormous development in the food industry and mushroom production in particular in the past few decades. Mushrooms comprise an unlimited source of neutraceutical and pharmacological products with immunomodulator potential. Medicinal mycology is largely practiced in China, Japan, and to some extent in India and some Eastern countries since time immemorial. The power of mushrooms is considered divine. The multifaceted uses of mushrooms as food, medicine, feed, dyes and anti aging device besides ecological balance are continuously being exploited in different parts of the globe (Rai and Tidke, 2005). Most of the identified mushrooms have important salutary effects on health and in treating diseases.

Increasingly, many varieties of mushroom are becoming popular, and these offer a wider range of tastes and textures. Many are cultivated versions of wild mushrooms, now called specialty mushrooms, while others are varieties that haven't yet been domesticated and so must be picked in the wild and, therefore, tend to be rather expensive. Many specialty mushrooms are available in dried form; some are canned or jarred, as well as fresh.

The first reference of occurrence of basidiomycetes was recorded by Montagne in 1842 (Sathe, 1979). Manjula, (1983) later on compiled 'A revised list of agaricoid and boletoid basidiomycetes from India and Nepal'. Biodiversity and occurrence of basidiomycetes in India was studied by various workers (Sathe and Deshpande, 1979, Natrajan and Raman, 1983, Purkayastha and Chandra, 1985, Verma *et al.*, 1987, Lakhanpal 1995, Pradeep *et al.*, 1998, Vrinda *et al.*, 1999 and Atri *et al.*, 2000).

Culinary Awareness and Acceptance

Mushroom is frequently mentioned as an alternative resource for food. The modern mushroom culture produces more proteins per unit area of land than by any other form of agriculture. Its use as food is probably as old as cultivation itself. But the nutritive value of mushroom was recognized only in recent times. Not usually thought of as a particularly good source of nutrients, mushrooms actually rank rather high in nutritive value. They contain a substantial amount of B vitamins, selenium, copper, and some other trace minerals. Mushrooms are low in calories (a cup of raw mushrooms has about 20 calories). Moreover, researchers have discovered antibacterial and other medicinal components, including anti-tumor compounds called triterpenoids in many mushrooms.

A large population of India is vegetarian. With human population billowing as rapidly as it is, conventional agriculture is unlikely to keep pace with food requirements. Alternative sources of energy are required if serious food crisis is to be averted. It is here that mushrooms provide a rich addition to the diet. Their nutritional value lies between that of meat and vegetables. As supplements to vegetarian diets, mushrooms have been called 'vegetable meat', both for their nutritive value and the culinary sophistication. But they do add variety, flavor, along with supplemental protein and vitamins to otherwise inadequate diets. The rarity of using mushrooms as food, the apparently mysterious source of their origin, their texture, and their flavors, combined perhaps with the culinary skill of expert chefs lends it the suspicion of being meat. And this is the reason mushrooms are not yet widely served as food in this country. But gradually the concept of mushroom dishes is definitely catching on. In a non-metropolis one may not get the variety and freshness in different types of mushrooms as in the major cities. But canned mushrooms are available. If freshness is not a criterion, in these days of communication revolution, accessibility is no longer a constraint. Once the mushrooms are used extensively, the demand would increase and the local cultivation and the supply would naturally keep pace.

The number of mushrooms on Earth is estimated at 140,000, yet perhaps only 10 per cent *i.e.* approximately 14,000 named species are known (Wasser and Didukh, 2005) and out of these known species of mushrooms, it was thought that 700 are edible and more than 200 may have medicinal value, although only a small percentage of these mushrooms are available to the consumer (Kendriok, 1985). Tribal members subsist to a great extent on nontraditional food sources, especially wild edible mushrooms, which grow abundantly during monsoon and post-monsoon seasons and are sometimes collected in large quantities for sale in urban markets (Rajak and Rai, 2005). In India more than 200 species of edible mushrooms have already been listed. The artificial cultivation of a few edible mushrooms ensures that mushrooms sold are truly edible. Therefore, there is a need to develop newer varieties of mushrooms by the scientific community and introduce to the population that is interested in consumption of mushrooms due to its culinary and medicinal properties. This could serve them with the improved mushrooms from the biologists' bench.

The health conscious people are turning towards mushroom to a greater extent. The low calorie content and high fiber of mushrooms, as well as lack of sugar and fat when fresh, is a boon for persons on a diet: the obese, the hypertensive and the diabetic. They fill the stomach and give a feeling of satiety; the high fiber slows down absorption of food from the intestines. One can say that mushrooms have now entering mainstream food in India.

Mushrooms are consumed as an energy rich food due to their peculiar property of containing rich proteins, vitamins, and minerals. They are superior to many vegetables and beans in their nutritive value. Mushrooms contain all essential amino acids. The digestibility coefficient of mushroom is also high, about 87 per cent. Their fat content is less than 0.3 per cent. It is less as compared to the fat of meat, egg, and milk. The fat in mushroom is rich in ergosterol, which is involved in the biosynthesis of Vitamin- D in human body. It also contains high proportion of thiamin, riboflavin, niacin, and ascorbic acid. They are also rich in minerals such as Ca, P, Fe, Na, and K. Selenium, an essential mineral, works closely with Vitamin E to produce antioxidants that neutralize the cell-damaging "free radicals" that can increase the risk of cancer and other diseases of aging. It plays an important role in the immune system, the thyroid system and the male reproductive system. *Potassium* is a mineral a human body just can't do without. It helps maintain normal heart rhythm, fluid balance, muscle and nerve function. The U.S. Food and Drug Administration recently gave a nod to its disease-fighting capability by stating: "Diets containing foods that are good sources of potassium and low in sodium may reduce the risk of high blood pressure and stroke." Some mushrooms supply more potassium than foods better known as sources for this mineral. *Copper* is another essential mineral and mushrooms are a good source. We're all aware of iron's role in making red blood cells and delivering oxygen to every part of the body. But the key is that iron can't do its job without copper.

As they have high nutritional value, FAO has recommended dried mushroom as a source of protein (3-4g/100g) in human diet. They are cheaper in price than any other nutritive diet in the market. Thus functional mushrooms deserve further serious investigations. The Indian organic foods industry is expected to witness a boom period. There is a huge export opportunity for the Indian organic farming industry both in niche markets, as well as mainstream markets world over.

Many mushrooms are not strictly pharmaceutical products (real medicines) but represent a novel class of dietary supplements (DSs), functional foods, nutriceutical, nutraceutical, phytochemical, mycochemical, biochemopreventives and designer foods (Chang and Buswell, 1999, 2003; Ziesel, 1999; Wasser *et al.*, 2000 a, b, 2001; Chang and Miles, 2004 and Wasser *et al.*, 2004). DSs are ingredients obtained from foods, plants and mushrooms that are taken without further modification separately from foods for their presumed health-enhancing benefits (McNamara, 1999). Mushrooms are a nutritionally functional food and a rich source of physiologically beneficial medicines.

Mushrooms are valuable health food–low in calories, high in vegetable proteins, iron, zinc, chitin, fiber, vitamins and minerals. Mushrooms also have a long history of use in Traditional Chinese Medicine (Wasser *et al.*, 2004). Their legendary effects on promoting good health and vitality and increasing body's adaptive abilities have been supported by recent studies (Wasser and Didukh, 2005). These studies suggest that Mushrooms are probiotic–they help our body strengthen itself and fight off illness by maintaining physiological homeostasis–restoring our bodies balance and natural resistance to disease. The compounds they contain have been classified as Host Defense Potentiators (HDP) which can have immune system enhancement properties (boost immune system). That is one of the reasons they are currently used as adjuncts to cancer treatments in Japan and China.

The increasing interest in the traditional remedies for various physiological disorders and the recognition of numerous biological activities of mushroom products have led to the coining of the term *mushroom* nutriceutical (Chang and Buswell, 1996, 1999, 2003; Chang, 1999; Wasser *et al.*, 2000 a, b, 2001; Chang and Miles, 2004), not to be confused with *nutraceuticals/functional foods and pharmaceuticals.*

A mushroom nutraceutical is a refined or partially refined extract or dried biomass from either the mycelium or the fruit body of a mushroom, is consumed in the form of capsules or tablets as a DSs and not as a food, and has potential therapeutic applications. Regular intake may enhance the immune response of the human body thereby increasing resistance to disease and in some cases causing regression of the disease state. Acting as immunopotentiators, mushroom preparations modify host biological responses (Hobbs, 1995; Wasser and Weis, 1999a, b; Wasser, 2002) and are also known as *Biological response modifiers* (BRMs).

Several types of culinary and therapeutic formulations of mushrooms available for consumption are like commercially cultivated fruit body powders, alcohol and hot water extracts and their mixtures, dried and pulverized preparations of mycelium, with mushroom primordia, or biomass extracted from the fermentation tank, or naturally grown dried mushroom fruit bodies in capsule or tablet form. Many mushrooms or mushroom preparations traditionally taken as treatments for specific conditions are now marketed for use as prophylactic agents. However, mushrooms are easily vegetatively propagated and thus keep to one clone (Rai *et al.*, 2005).

The safety advantages of using mushroom-based DSs as opposed to herbal preparations are (1) the overwhelming majority of mushrooms used for production of DSs are cultivated commercially and not gathered in the wild, this provides very good chances of proper identification, pre and unadulterated products. It is also genetically uniform. (2) Mushrooms are easily propagated vegetatively and thus are clones. The mycelium can be stored for a long time and the genetic and biochemical consistency may be checked after considerable time.

Pharmacological Potential

In the second half of the 20th century, mushroom-producing technologies have grown enormously. In 2002 the value of world mushroom production was estimated at about $20 billion USD, which is almost the same as the value of coffee production (Chang, 1999, 2001, Wasser *et al.*, 2000a, b, 2001., Wasser 2002, Chang and Buswell, 2003, Chang and Miles, 2004).

Reports indicate the potential of mushrooms as life-saving drugs antibiotics and biologically active substance. It has various industrial uses. It is tempting to say that many mushrooms known today to have medicinal benefits, which arose from observations of their uses in China and Japan, are objects of scientific studies that continue to determine the active components in such mushrooms (Doris *et al.*, 2005). Whereas the documentation of this knowledge is important for the understanding of the sociocultural practices of the Indians, it is equally good for science, because detailed scientific studies of mushroom uses and practices of these people can lead to the discovery of new drugs and nutraceuticals from Indian mushrooms.

A purified compound is very different from the whole mushroom, however, and the inevitable questions that follow are whether eating the whole mushroom has preventive or therapeutic value, and if so, how much mushroom should be consumed and in what form. For shiitake, researchers found that the powdered mushroom fruit bodies given to rats as 10-20 per cent of their diet inhibited transplanted tumors, and small studies have demonstrated lipid-lowering effects consumption of 9 g of dried mushrooms or 90 g of fresh mushrooms (Wasser, 2005).

The content and potency of bioactive ingredients may differ depending on how the mushroom is prepared and ingested. For example, the anticarcinogenic thioproline content varies from undetectable amounts in fresh shiitake, to 134 mg/100 g of dried shiitake, to 843 mg/100 g of boiled shiitake. As is the case for most plants and herbs, the specific strain, growing conditions, and other environmental factors will also significantly affect the taste, form, and substance of the mushroom, as well as affect the bioactive content (Nanba, 1967., Mori *et al.*, 1976., Susuki and Oshirna, 1976 and Royse and Bahler, 1996). Antitumor and immmunostimulating polysaccharides of higher basiomycetes are shown in Table 25.1.

Table 25.1: Antitumor and Immmunostimulating Polysaccharides of Higher Basidiomycetes

Polysaccharides	*Species*	*References*
Glucans		
α-(1→3)-glucan	*Armillariella tabescens*	Kiho *et al.*, 1992a
Linear α-(1→3)-glucan	*Amanita muscaria* *Agrocybe aegerita*	Kiho *et al.*, 1994 Yoshida *et al.*, 1996
α(1→4)-; β-(1→6)-glucan	*Agaricus blazei*	Fujimiya *et al.*, 1998b
α-(1→6)-; α(1→4)-glucan A	*Agaricus blazei*	Mizuno *et al.*, 1990a
β-(1→6)-glucan	*Lycophyllum decastes* *Armilalriella tabescens*	Ukawa *et al.*, 2000 Kiho *et al.*, 1992a
β-(1→6)-; β-(1→3)-glucan	*Agaricus blazei*	Mizuno *et al.*, 1990a
	Grifola frondosa	Nanba *et al.*, 1987
β-(1→6)-; α-(1→3)-glucan	*Agaricus blazei*	Mizuno *et al.*, 1990a
β-(1→3)-glucoronoglucan	*Ganoderma lucidum*	Saito *et al.*, 1989
Mannoxyloglucan	*Grifola frondosa*	Mizuno *et al.*, 1986
Galactoxyloglucan	*Hericium erinaceus*	Mizuno. 1999b
Xyloglucan	*Grifola frondosa*	Mizuno *et al.*, 1986
	Polyporus confluence	Mizuno *et al.*, 1992
	Pleurotus pulmonarius	Zhuang *et al.*, 1993
Xylogalactoglucan	*Inonotus obliquus*	Mizuno *et al.*, 1990a
Mannogalactoglucan	*Pleurotus pulmonarius* *Pleurotus Cornucopiae* *Ganoderma lucidum* *Agaricus blazei*	Gurtirrez *et al.*, 1996 Kim *et al.*, 1994 Cho *et al.*, 1999
Galactomannoglucan	*Flammulina velutipes* *Hohenbuehelia serotina* *Leucopaxillus giganteus*	Ikekawa *et al.*, 1982 Mizuno *et al.*, 1994 Mizuno 1995a

Contd...

Table 25.1–Contd...

Polysaccharides	*Species*	*References*
Arabinoglucan	*Ganoderma tsugae*	Zhang *et al.*, 1994b
Riboglucan	*Agaricus blazei*	Cho *et al.*, 1999
Glycans		
Arabinogalactan	*Pleurotus citrinopileatus*	Zhang *et al.*, 1994a
Glucogalactan	*Ganoderma tsugae*	Wang *et al.*, 1993
Fucogalactan	*Sarcodon asparatus*	Mizuno 2000
α-(1→6)-mannofuco-galactan	*Fomitella fraxinea*	Cho *et al.*, 1998
Fucomannogalactan	*Dictyophora indusiata*	Hara *et al.*, 1993
Mannoaglactofucan	*Grifola frondosa*	Zhuang *et al.*, 1993
Xylan	*Hericium erinaceus*	Mizuno. 1999b
Glucoxylan	*Hericium erinaceus*	Mizuno. 1999b
	Pleurotus pulmonarius	Zhuang *et al.*, 1993
Mannoglucoxylan	*Hericium erinaceus*	Mizuno. 1999b
α-(1→3)-mannan	*Dictyophora indusiata*	Ukai *et al.*, 1983
Glucomannan	*Agaricus blazei*	Hikichi *et al.*, 1999
β-(1→2)-; β-(1→3)-gluco-mannan	*Agaricus blazei*	Tsuchida *et al.*, 2001 Mizuno *et al.*, 1999b
Galactoglucomannan	*Lentinus edodes*	Fujii *et al.*, 1979

Source: Reshetnikov *et al.*, 2001.

It is reported that mushrooms have significant pharmacological effects of homeostasis, regulation of biorhythm, curing of various diseases, and prevention and improvement from life threatening diseases such as cancer, cerebral stroke, and cardiac problems. At the same time it is also being confirmed that mushrooms have effective substances for decreasing the blood cholesterol and possess antihypertension, antihyperlipemia, antidiabetes, antitumor, immunomodulating and other qualities (Chang and Miles, 2004).

Very few agents are effective for both treatment and prevention of disease, but research has shown that certain mushrooms can be used in this way. The fungus *Coriolus versicolor* is found almost worldwide; however, its bioactivity varies depending on the habitat in which it grows (Monro, 2003). To eliminate these variations, Gourmet Mushrooms, Inc. (Sebastopol, California) established the CV-OH1 strain a few years ago. This strain demonstrates rapid and aggressive colonization and far outmatches other isolates in bioactivity and vigor. A mother culture of strain CV-OH1 has been developed and maintained to produce spawn. In-house checks confirm that the mother culture does not alter from the original isolate. The production process involves the inoculation of sterile organic edible grain with spawn from the mother culture. The fungus is allowed to completely colonize the growth medium aseptically. At the correct stage of development–at maximum bioavailability–the living biomass is aseptically air-dried, granulated, and tested microbiologically.

Besides the culinary magics of mushrooms, this review article emphasises the pharmacological properties explored, practiced and accepted widely, of three globally popular mushrooms *viz.*, Lentinus, Ganoderma and Grifola.

Shiitake

At present shiitake is one of the five most cultivated edible mushrooms in the world (Chang, 1999 and Wasser 2005). These mushrooms have excellent nutritional value with water soluble polysaccharides. The mushroom exhibits anticarcinogenic (Chihara *et al.*, 1987) and antitumor (Smith *et al.*, 2002.,Yap and Ng, 2003 and Moriyama 1981) effects, immunomodulating effects (Wasser and Weis 1997 and Nagai and Ng, 2003), cardiovascular effects (Hobbs, 1995., Wasser and Weis 1997., Hobbs, 2000 and Mizuno, 1996), hepatoprotective effects (Przbylowicz and Donoghue, 1990, and Chang, 1999), antiviral, antibacterial and antiparasistic (Wasser and Weis,1997., Hobbs, 2000., Smith *et al.*, 2002 and Ngai and Ng, 2003) effects as well as antifungal activity (Nagai and Ng., 2003).

In 1969, Ikekawa *et al.*, noted that a water extract of shiitake fruiting bodies could inhibit transplanted tumors in mice. Around the same time, Chihara *et al.* (1987) isolated an antitumor polysaccharide from shiitake and named it lentinan. The molecular formula for lentinan is $(C_6H_{10}O_5)n$, and the mean molecular mass is 500 kDa. Lentinan is a D-glucan as shown by electrophoresis, ultracentrifugation, and other instrumental analyses. Its structure was confirmed as (1, 3)-D-glucopyranan with a branched chain of (1,6)-monoglycosyl, showing a right-handed triple helix. Lentinan has been found to activate macrophages, T lymphocytes, and other immune effector cells that modulate the release of cytokines, which may in turn account for its indirect antitumor and antimicrobial properties (Ikekawa *et al.*, 1969., Chihara *et al.*, 1970., Sasaki and Takasuka., 1976; Bluhm and Sarco, 1977 and Hamuro and Chihara, 1985).

Besides the well-studied above mentioned compounds, other potentially beneficial compounds have been found in shiitake. One example is thioproline, which blocks the formation of carcinogenic N-nitroso compounds (Kurashirna *et al.*, 1990).

Ganoderma lucidum

The virtues of another mushroom *Ganoderma lucidum* extracts, handed down from generation to generation, include it as a "cancer cure" and a symbol of happy augury, good fortune, good health, longevity, and even immortality (Wasser, 2005). Medicinal uses of *G. lucidum* in ancient Far East countries included the treatment of neurasthenia, debility from prolonged illness, insomnia, anorexia, dizziness, chronic hepatitis, hypercholesterolemia, mushroom poisoning (antidote), coronary heart disease, hypertension, prevention of altitude sickness, treatment of deficiency fatigue, carcinoma, and bronchial cough in the elderly (Natalia *et al.*, 2005). According to Traditional Chinese Medicine (TCM) different types of *G. lucidum* have different tastes and thus affect different organs. Based on their colors six different types of *G. lucidum* have been classified each with different uses (Table 25.2). The fruiting body, mycelia, and spores of *G. lucidum* contain approximately 400 different bioactive compounds, nucleotides, sterols, steroids, fatty acids, proteins/peptides, and trace elements (Wasser, 2005). It also contains oleic acid, cyclo-octasulfur, an ergosterol peroxide (5, 8-epidioxy-ergosta-6, 22-dien-3-ol) and cerebrosides. Polysaccharides (β-D-glucans, heteropolysaccharides, and glycoprotein) isolated from *G. lucidum* demonstrated antitumor activity against Sarcoma 10 in mice (Doris *et al.*, 2005). Triterpenoids like ganoderic acids T-Z showed cytotoxic activity *in vitro* on hepatoma cells the polysaccharide-mediated potentiation of immune function is thought to be the major mechanism of antitumor action by *G. lucidum*.

Ganoderma has been used as folk medicine since ancient times and it is a popular health food frequently promoted as a cancer cure. *Ganoderma* has been recognized traditionally and scientifically as potentially useful in the treatment of cancer, (Chang, 2001).

Table 25.2: *Ganoderma lucidum* and their Medicinal Properties

Color	Taste	Japanese name	Use
Blue	Sour	Aoshiba	Improves eyesight and liver function, calms nerves
Red[a]	Bitter	Akashiba	Aids internal organs, improves memory, enhances vitality
Yellow	Sweet	Kishiba	Strengthens spleen function, calms the spirit
White	Hot/pungent	Shiroshiba	Improves lung function, gives courage and strong will
Black	Salty	Kuroshiba	Protects kidney
Purple	Sweet	Murasakishiba	Enhances function of ears, joints, muscles, helps complexion

[a] The red colored variety of *G. lucidum* is generally regarded as the most potent and medicinal (Wasser, 2005).

Immunostimulation with Ganoderma Polysaccharides

Nakashima *et al.* (1979) demonstrated T-cell activation by orally administered *Ganoderma* polysaccharides (GP). Subsequently, activation of immune function including the activation of cytotoxic NK cells (Won *et al.*, 1989), and stimulation of cytokines (Chang *et al.* 1988) has also been reported with GP. The B-1, 3 glucan polysaccharide fraction in particular, has been demonstrated to have a broad-based adjuvant stimulatory activity on T-cells and macrophages, and lead to the enhance production of IL-I (Jia *et al.*, 1994), IL-2 (Chang *et al.*, 1988, Zhang *et al.*, 1 993a), and TNF (Zhang *et al.*, 1993b) which have been reported to play a role in antitumor immune surveillance (Lattime and Stutman 1991). Of particular interest is the demonstrated activity of a crude Ganoderma extract on NK cell activity *in vitro* (Zhang *et al.*, 1994) and the effectiveness of a water soluble GP fraction derived from mycelium given by intraperitoneal, intravenous, or oral route in enhancing splenic NK activity in normal mice and restoring depressed NK cytotoxicity in tumor-bearing mice (Won *et al.*, 1989). Other studies demonstrated the ability of GP in activating macrophages (Zhang *et al.*, 1994) and in markedly enhancing the cytotoxicity of CTL (Lei, 1992), both established tumoricidal effector pathways of the host immune system.

Potential of GP Immunostimulation for Prevention of Cancer

Ganoderma has been recognized traditionally and scientifically as potentially useful in the treatment of cancer (Chang 1993). Although triterpenoids and other fractions of *Ganoderma* may have direct cytotoxic activity (Toth *et al.*, 1983, Lin *et al.*, 1997), some evidence supports the notion that major anti-tumor efficacy of *Ganoderma* is host dependent and mediated through GP immune stimulation (Xia *et al.*, 1989, Mizuno 1995).

Ikekawa *et al.* (1968) first reported on the efficacy of soluble extracts from *Ganoderma* in inhibiting transplanted Sarcoma 180 in mice. This host-dependent antitumor activity has been subsequently confirmed to be from the polysaccharide fractions of *Ganoderma* (Sasaki *et al.*, 1911). Multiple similar studies subsequently confirms this observation and antitumor efficacy of *Ganoderma* has been demonstrated from various species, at different stages of growth and using different solvents for extraction and different routes of administration. Antitumor activity has been demonstrated *in vitro* as well as in syngeneic tumor systems in animals. However, no human trials of *Ganoderma* against cancer in peer reviewed journals nor any controlled clinical trials in humans have yet been conducted or published. Since it is now increasingly clear that immunostimulatory bioactivity from most beta-glucan based compounds function via a similar beta-glucan receptor (Czop 1985), it has been possible to hypothesize that *Ganoderma* polysaccharides should function similarly (Chang, 1996). Data from such bioactively comparable compounds all suggest improved quality of life or survival for cancer patients may be possible with *Ganoderma* supplementation.

Standardization in bioactive polysaccharide content and dosages will be necessary to assure its rational use, and clinical trials in selected cancers with defined endpoints will confirm its efficacy. Ultimately, one can believe that integration of the natural, complementary modalities and conventional modern medicine will lead to healing and the saving of lives. The treatment of various ailments through Ganotherapy has been initiated very recently in India and is now under experiment (Rahman *et al.*, 2005). The efforts were intended for promoting alternative medication for curing and maintaining health and at the same time creating social acceptance, adaptation, and affordability of this treatment among a greater segment of people. And it has been found that 80 per cent of the patients were cured and are now leading a better quality of daily life. It may be urged and stressed that a wider scope of clinical research work on Ganotherapy in the country is needed.

Grifola frondosa

Much research has reported that *Grifola frondosa* and its extracts showed remarkable antitumor activities by activating the cellular immune system, enhancing the production of cytokines, or inducing apoptosis. Kawagishi *et al.*, 1990 isolated an N-aceylgalactosamine-specific lectin from fresh fruiting bodies of *G. frondosa*.

Antitumor activity of *G. frondosa* polysaccharide, Grifron D-fraction (GD), on human prostate cancer PC-3 cells *in vitro* was exhibited after an investigation by Fullerton *et al.*, in 2000. Earlier, the anti-HIV activity of *G. frondosa* extract has been recognized by the Japan National Institute of Health (Ishikawa, 1991) and confirmed by the US National Cancer Institute (Screen 1992) that *G. frondosa* extract was able to prevent as much as 97 per cent of HIV-infected T-helper lymphocytes from being destroyed *in vitro*. Kabir *et al.* (1987) and Ohtsuru *et al.* (1999) reported that *G. frondosa* powder lowers the blood pressure in spontaneously hypertensive rats. Whereas in an antidiabetic report diabetic levels of blood glucose were significantly decreased in the rats fed *G. frondosa* (Horio *et al.*, 1995). Kubo *et al.* (1997) reported that *G. frondosa* helps to improve the lipid metabolism, because it inhibits both liver lipid and serum lipid and antiobesity effect of *G. frondosa* was studied by Ohtsuru *et al.*, in 1999. Wu (1994) reported that a proteoglucan from *G. frondosa* was clinically used to treat chronic hepatitis B. Whereas Ochiai (2003) reported that a proteoglucan extracted from *G. frondosa* strongly inhibited the growth of influenza virus.

Adachi *et al.* (1989) and Zhuang *et al.* (1994) reported that the modification of some polysaccharide fractions from the fruiting body or mycelium of *G. frondosa* by Smith degradation and formic acid degradation may increase their antitumor activities (Zhuang and Wasser, 2004).

Need of Molecular Characterization

The vagaries of classical morphological characterization make identification the weak link in research. The use of molecular methods has potential to give greater objectivity to approaches to characterization of species and strains, enabling to look past the influence of habitat on morphology. Mushroom classification and taxonomy is still not an exact science, molecular techniques will help but definitive tools for objective characterization are still a long way off (different methods giving convergent results or comparable ease of utilization).

Improvements can be made by exploiting diversity in wild strains or by using directed molecular breeding. The mushroom genetics program comprises: improvement and exploitation of transformation; molecular analysis of inter- and intra-species relatedness; characterization of developmental genes.

Now-a-days ITS sequencing is being used for identification of species, to establish species relationships within *Agaricus* and develop molecular phylogenetics for the genus (Singh *et al.*, 2006). RAPD markers are also being used as a tool to measure genetic diversity and to aid the analysis of mushroom breeding systems. It's because of these sophisticated techniques of biotechnology that the genetic diversity or any threat to any species can be identified and worked out. Like in *Agaricus*, restricted genetic diversity in cultivated lines represents a risk factor and breeding is needed to incorporate greater variability from wild types.

Analysis of commercial strains of two edible mushrooms, *Pleurotus ostreatus* and *Agaricus bisporus*, using PCR and isozyme electrophoresis techniques lead to differentiate groups of genetically similar and distant strains. Among the commercial strains of *P. ostreatus*, the level of genetic variation was higher suggesting a broader genetic basis employed in breeding of this mushroom. On the other hand, the cultivars and hybrids of *A. bisporus* showed a higher level of homology. The isozyme markers (nonspecific esterase, leucinaminopeptidase, and phosphoglucoisomerase) are recommended for identification of the commercial strains of edible mushrooms (Shnyreva *et al.*, 2003).

Genetic Resources

The collection, molecular characterization and germplasm conservation of wild types becomes critically essential to assure availability of breeding material for research and commercially cultivated mushrooms.

In developing countries, natural mushroom genetic diversity combined with the application/ adaptation of presently available cultivation technologies offers potential for improving productivity of small-scale mushroom growing. Potential advantages that can be obtained from better international coordination in mushroom germplasm include:

- ☆ Generation of better/more complete knowledge of habitat/organism diversity
- ☆ Opportunities to develop appropriate protocols for collecting, identifying and conserving mushroom germplasm
- ☆ Strategic use of scarce resources
- ☆ International collaboration facilitated
- ☆ Opportunities for training for scientists as well as growers.

Challenges

Mushroom genetic resources can contribute significantly to the solution of food supply problems. There is a need for worldwide agreement on how and where to store mushroom germplasm in order to ensure there can be a future for breeding edible mushrooms. Demonstration of serious coordinated pooling efforts on the part of research institutions could be helpful in encouraging industry players and researchers to appreciate the interest for them in participating and helping finance mushroom germplasm collection and conservation work.

Development of high temperature cultivated strains is a major objective in many warm countries and germplasm collection efforts need to be oriented to identifying useful characteristics in wild types. A crash program from time to time to document, collect and conserve wild edible and useful mushroom germplasm is needed in developing countries, especially in India, tapping indigenous knowledge as much as possible.

Research in several Asian countries can collaboratively and usefully focus on identification and domestication of local taxa/strains, with the aim of leading to higher diversity within cultivated mushrooms and reduced vulnerability of the sector. There is a need for training in methods of identification, conservation characterization and utilization of mushroom genetic resources, including training in preparation of high quality spawn.

Strategy for Conservation

Ex situ mushroom germplasm collections–including also associated characterization and evaluation functions–need to be correlated with research and training activities. In India, it is important to harness local peoples' knowledge of edible/useful mushroom habitat and characteristics, and establish local human capacity to survey, characterize and conserve useful mushrooms.

Storage techniques for mushroom strain isolates and cultures needs further work to develop low-cost, feasible, reliable protocols and alternatives that minimize risk of stress-induced degradation. The genomic DNA sequencing can be another advanced technique for germplasm conservation with minimized risk. The group's attention should be focused on macro fungi, in terms of collection, conservation, and characterization of genetic resources. Mushroom genetic resource conservation strategies need elements of cooperation, coordination and strategic planning.

Cooperation among different laboratories is needed to develop molecular techniques as a tool to help species/strain identification and characterization. Responsibility for mushroom genetic resource conservation strategies starts with governments; *ex situ* conservation through mushroom collections at research institutions in each country should be supported by governments and links established with other banks within and among regions. It is necessary and opportune to establish concrete strategic objectives and working arrangements for achieving them first; then address funding issues accordingly.

Mycorrhizal mushrooms are another group of medicinal mushrooms with high therapeutic values and more preferable flavor. Like in other developed countries dedicated task force on research and development of mycorrhizal mushrooms also should be established. In terms of strategic objectives and technical activities to be pursued, the original terms of reference for the mushroom germplasm science network should be retained and updated, *viz.*

- ☆ Collection, characterization and utilization studies on species and strains of edible mushrooms and related fungal organisms.
- ☆ Development of conservation methodologies for mushroom germplasm to protect against degradation or mutation.
- ☆ Development of molecular techniques as tools (to be applied in association with morphological/taxonomic approaches) for characterization and as markers for classification and certification of mushroom strains.
- ☆ Data base establishment and maintenance.
- ☆ It can also be emphasized that the network should promote close cooperation between taxonomists and molecular biologists for identification of macro fungi.

Yet, there are a far greater number of wild edible mushrooms and related fleshy fungi that have not been subject to cultivation. The growing interest in gourmet or exotic mushrooms is the direct result of research. In Asia and in Europe, many species of mushrooms have been eaten and enjoyed for a long period of time. Therefore, the industry has a continuing need for new and improved varieties with well-defined characteristics. International collaborative research and development activity is being encouraged and welcomed on an urgent basis to continue clinical research.

Acknowledgements

The authors are thankful to Department of Science and Technology, New Delhi for providing financial assistance for the mushroom project.

References

Adachi Y., Ohno N., Ohsawa M., Sato K., Oikawa S and Yadomae T. (1989). Physicochemical properties and antitumor activities of chemically modified derivatives of antitumor glucan "Grifolan LE" from *Grifola frondosa*. *Chem Pharm Bull*, 37, 7, 1838-1843.

Anke, T., Oberwinkler, F., Steglich, W. and Schramm, G. (1977) The Strobilurins- new antifungal antibiotics from the basidiomycete *Strobilurus tenacellus* (Pers. ex. Fr.) Sing. *J. Antibiotics*. 30: 806-810.

Anke, T., Werle, A., Bross, M. and Steglich, W. (1990) Antibiotics from basidiomycetes XXXIII, Oudemansin X, a new antifungal *E-?*-Methoxyacrylate from *Oudemansiella radicata* (Rehlan EX FR.) Sing. *J. Antibiotics* 43: 1010-1011.

Anke, T.,Werle, A., Zapf, S., Velten, R. and Steglich, W. (1995) Favolon, a new antifungal triterpenoid from a *Favolaschia* Species. *J. Antibiotics* 48: 725-726.

Arnone, A., Cardillo R., Nasini, G., and Pava, O.V.D. (1993). Cyathiformines A-D, new chorismate-derived metabolites from the fungus *Clitocybe cyathifomis*. *Tetrahedron* 49: 7251–7258.

Arnone, A., Brambilla, U., Nasini, G., and Pava, O.V.D. (1995). Isolation and structure elucidation of Tsugicolines A-D, novel protoilludane sesquiterpines from *Laurilia tsugicola*. *Tetrahedron*. 51: 13357-13364

Arnone, A., Capelli, S., Nasini,G., Meille, S. V., and Pava, O. V. D. (1996) Secondary mould metabolites II Structure elucidation of diatretol–A new Diketopiperzine metabolite from the fungus *Clitocybe diatreata*. Liebigs Ann. 1875-1877.

Atri N.S., Kaur A and Saini S.S. (2000). Taxonomic studies on agarics from Punjab plains. *Indian J. Mush*. 18, 6-14.

Atsumi, S., Umezawa, K., Iinuma, H., Naganawa, H., Nakamura, H.,Iitaka, Y. and Takeuchi, T. (1990). Production, Isolation and Structure Determination of A Novel β- Glucosidase inhibitor, cyclophellitol, from *Phellinus* sp. *J.Antibiotics* 43: 49-53.

Bluhm T.L. and Sarco A. (1977). The triple helical structure of lentinan, β-(1 -3)-D-glucan. *Can J Chem*; 55: 293-9-9

Chang R. (1993). Limitations and potential applications of Ganoderma and related fungal polyglycans in clinical ontology. *First international conference on mushroom biology and mushroom products*: 96.

Chang R. (1996). Functional properties of edible mushrooms, *Nutr Rev*, 54, 11, S91-S93.

Chang S. T and Buswell J. A. (1996). Mushroom nutriceuticals. *World J Microb Biotech*, 12. 473-476.

Chang S. T. (1999). World production of cultivated edible and medicinal mushrooms in 1997 with emphasis on *Lentinus edodes* (Berk.) Sing. In China. *Int. J. Med. Mushr*. 1, 387-409.

Chang S. T. (2001). A 40-year journey through bioconversion of lignocellulosic wastes to mushrooms and dietary supplements. *Int. J. med. Mushr*, 3 299-311.

Chang S. T. and Buswell J. A. (2003). Medicinal mushrooms- a prominent source of nutriceuticals for the 21st century. *Curr Topics Nutraceut res*, 1, 257-280.

Chang S. T. and Miles Ph. G. (2004). Mushrooms. Cultivation, nutritional value, medicinal effect and environmental impact. *CRC Press*, Boca Raton, FL, 451pp.

Chang S.T. and Buswell J. A. (1999). *Ganoderma lucidum* (W.Curt.: Fr.) P. Karst. (Aphyllophoromycetideae)- a mushrooming medicinal mushroom. *Int J Med Mushr*, 1,139-146.

Chang, R. (1993). Limitations and Potential applications of Ganoderma and related fungal polyglycans in clinical ontology; *First International Conference on Mushroom Biology and Mushroom products*: 96

Chihara G., Hamuro J., Maeda Y., Arai Y. and Fukuoka F. (1970). Fractionation and purification of the polysaccharides with marked antitumor activity especially Lentinan, from *Lentinus edodes* (Berk.). Sing., an edible mushroom. *Cancer Res* 30: 2776-81.

Chihara, G., Hamuro, J., Maeda, Y. Y., Shiio, T., Suga, T., Takasuka, N and Sasaki T. (1987). Antitumor and metastasis- inhibitory activities of lentinan as an immuno-modulator: an overview. *Cancer Detect. Rev. Supp.* 1, 423-443.

Cho, S. M., Koshino, H., Yu, S. H. and Yoo, I. D. (1998). A mannufucogalavtan, fomitellan A, with mitogenic effect from fruit bodies of *Fomitella fraxinea* (Imaz.). *Carbohyd. Polym* 37: 31-18.

Cho, S. M., Park, J. S., Kim, K. P., Cha, D. Y. and Yoo, I. D. (1999). Chemical features and purification of immunostimulating polysaccharides from fruit bodies of *Agaricus blazei*. *Korean J. Mycol.* 27: 170-174.

Cuellar, M. J. Giner, R. M., Recio, M. C., Just M. J., Manez, S. and Rios, J. L. (1996). Two Fungal lanostane derivative as Phospholipase A2 Inhibitors. *J. Nat. Prod.* 59: 977 -979.

Czop, J.K., Austen, K.F. (1985). A beta-Glucan inhibitable receptor on human monocytes, *J. Immunol.* 134, 2588-593.

Daferner, M., Anke, T., Hellwig, V., Steglich, W. and Sterner, O. (1998). Strobilurin M, Tetrachloropyrocatechol and Tetrachloropyrocatechol methyl ether: new antibiotics from *Mycena* species. *J. Antibiotics* 51: 816-822.

Doris O. Osagualekhor and J. A. Okhuoya (2005). Sociocultural and ethnomycological uses of mushroom among the Esan people of Nigeria. *Intl J. of Med. Mush.* 3(7)–442-443.

Dufresne, C., Young, K., Pelaez, F., Val, A.G.D., Valentino, D., Graham, A., Platas, G., Bernard, A. and Zink, D. (1997). Illudinic acid, a novel Illudane sesquiterpine antibiotic. *J Nat. Prod.* 60: 188 -190.

Engler, M., Anke, T., Klostermeyer, D. and Steglich, W. (1995). Hydroxystrobilurin A, a new antifungal *E*-β-Methoxyacrylate from a *Pterula* species.*J.Antibiotics* 48: 884 -885.

Erkel,G., Becker, U., Anke, T. and Sterner, O. (1996). Nidulal, a novel inducer of differentiaton of Human Promyelocytic Leukemia Cells from *Nidula candida*. *J.Antibiotics* 49: 1189-1195.

Fujii, T., Ishida, N., Maeda,H., Mizuni, I. and Suzuki, F. (1979). KS-2-A. *Us Patent 4143780*, 8 July 1979.

Fujimiya, Y., Suzuki, Y., Oshima, K. I., Kobori, H., Moriguchi, K., Nakashima, H., Matumoto, Y., Takahara, S., Ebina, T. and Katakura, R.. (1998b). Selective tumoricidal effect of soluble proeoglucan extracted from the basidiomycete, *Agaricus blazei* Murrill, mediated via natural killer cell activation and apoptosis. *Cancer Immunol Immmunother* 46: 147-159.

Fullerton S.A., Smadi A.A., Tortorelis D.G., Choudhury M.S., Mallouh C., Tazaki H. and Konno S. (2000). Induction of apoptosis in human prostatic cancer cells with Beta-glucan (Maitake mushroom polysaccharide). *Molec Urol*, 4, 1, 7-13.

Gan, K. H., Fann, Y-F., Hsu, S-H., Kou, K-W. and Lin, C-N. (1998). Mediation of the cytotoxicity of lanostanoids and steroids of *Ganoderma tsugae* through apoptosis and cell cycle. *J Nat. Prod.* 61: 485-487.

Gutierrez, A., Prito, A., and Martinez, A, T. (1996). Structural characterization of extracellular polysaccharides produced by fungi from the genus *Pleurotus*. *Carbohydr Res* 281: 143-154.

Hamuro J. and Chihara G. Lentinan, (1985). A T-cell oriented immunopotentiator: its experimental and clinical applications and possible mechanism of immune modulation. In: Fenichel RL, Chirigos MA, eds. *Immune Modulation Agents and Their Mechanisms*. New York: Marcel Dekker, 409-36.

Hautzel, R., Anke, H. and Sheldrick, W.S. (1990). Mycenon, A new metabolite from a *Mycena* species TA 87202 (Basidiomycetes) as an Inhibitor of Isocitrate Lyase. *J.Antibiotics*. 43: 1240-1244.

Heim, J., Anke, T., Mocek, U., Steffan, B. and Steglich, W. (1988). Antibiotics from Basidiomycetes XXIX: Pilatin, A new antibiotically active marasmane derivative from cultures of *Flagelloscypha pilatii* Agerer. *J.Antibiotics* 41: 1752-1757.

Hikichi, M., Hiroe, E., and Okubo, S. (1999). Protein polysacchride 0041. *European Patent 0939082*, 9 January 1999.

Hobbs Ch. (1995). Medicinal mushrooms: an exploration of tradition, healing and culture. *Botanica Press*, Santa Cruz, CA, 251.

Hobbs, Ch. (2000). Medicinal value of *Lentinus edodes* (Berk.) Sing. A literature review. *Int. J. Med. Mushr.* 2, 287-302.

Horio H. and Ohtsuru M. (1995). Maitake (*Grifola frondosa*) improves glucose tolerance of experimental diabetic rats. *J Nutr Sci Vitaminol*, 47, 57-63.

Ikekawa T., Uehara N., Maeda Y., Nankinishi M. and Fukuoka F. (1969) Antitumor activity of aqueous extracts of edible mushrooms. *Cancer Res*; 29: 734-5-5

Ikekawa, T., Ikeda, Y., Yoshida, Y., Nikanishi, M., Yokoyama, E., and Yamazaki, E. (1982). Antitumor polysaccharides of *Flamulina velutipes* 2. The structure of EA-3 and further purification of EA-5. *J Pharmacobiol Dyn* 5: 576-581.

Ishikawa K. (1991). Anti-HIV activity in cytopathic effect of proteglucan extracted from Maitake mushroom. *Japan National Institute of Health*, January 23, 1991.

Jia, Y.F., Zhou, XB. Meng, H., and Zhang, (1993). Effects of Ling-Zhi on hemopoietic system in mice–immunopharmacological study (11). In *The research on Ganoderma (part I)*. Zhu S. and Mori M. (eds). Shanghai Med. U. Press, Shanghai, P. 284-288.

Kabir T., Yamaguchi M. and Kimura S. (1987). Effect of Shiitake (*Lentinus edodes*) and Maitake (*Grifola frondosa*) mushrooms on blood pressure and plasma lipids of spontaneously hypertensive rats. *J Nutri Sci Vitaminol*, 33, 341-346.

Kawagishi H., Nomura A., Mizuno T., Kimura A., and Chiba S. (1990). Isolation and characterization of lectin from *Grifola frondosa* fruiting bodies. *Biochem Biophys Acta*, 1034, 247-252.

Kendriok B. (1985). *The Fifth Kingdom*. Waterloo: Mycologue Publication.

Kiho, T., Nagai, Y. S., Sakushima. M. and Ukai, S. (1992a). Polysaccharides in fungi. XXIX. Structural features of two antitumor polysaccharides from the fruiting bodies of *Armillariella tabescence Chem Pharm Bull* (Tokyo) 40: 2212-2214.

Kiho, T., Yoshida, I., Katsuragava, M., Sakushima, M., Usiu, S. and Ukai, S. (1994). Polysaccharides in fungi. XXXIV. Polysaccharides from the fruiting of *Amanita muscaria* and the antitumor activity of its carboxymethylated product. *Biol Pharm Bull* 17: 1460-1462.

Kim, B. K., Kim H.W. and Choi, E.C. (1994). Anti-HIV effects of *Ganoderma lucidum*. In: *Ganoderma*: Systematics, Phytopathology and Pharmacology: Proceedings of Contributed Symposium 59 A, B. 5th International Mycological Congress. Vancouver.

Kubo K. and Nanba H. (1997). Anti-hyperliposis effect of Maitake fruit body (*Grifola frondosa*). *Biol Pharm Bull*, 20, 7, 781-785.

Kubo, I., Kim, M., Wood, W.F. and Naoki, H. (1986). Clitocine, A New Insecticidal Nucleoside from the mushroom *Clitocybe inversa*. *Tetrahedron Letters* 27: 4277-4280.

Kuhnt, D., Anke, T., Besl, H., Bross, M., Herrmann, R., Mocek, U., Steffan, B., and Steglich, W. (1990). Antibiotics from basidiomycetes XXXVII. New inhibitors of cholesterol biosynthesis from cultures of *Xerula melanotricha* Dorfelt. *J. Antibiotics* 43: 1413-1420.

Kurashirna Y., Tsuda M. and Sugimura T. (1990). Marked formation of thiazolidine-4-carboxylic acid, an effective nitrite trapping agent *in vivo*, on boiling of dried shiitake mushroom (*Lentinus edodes*). *J Agric Food Chem* 38: 1945-9-9.

Kuschel, A., Anke, T., Velten, R., Klostermeyer, D., Steglich, W. and Konig, B. (1994). The Mniopetals, New Inhibitors of reverse transcriptases from a *Mniopetalum* species (Basidiomycetes). *J.Antibiotics* 47: 733-739.

Lakhanpal T.N.(1995). Mushroom flora of North West Himalayas. In *Advances in horticulture 13, Mushrooms* (Chandra K.L. and Sharma S.R. Eds.) MPH New Delhi India 351-373.

Lauer, U., Anke, T., Sheldrick, W.,Scherer, A. and Steglich, W. (1989). Antibiotics from basidiomycetes XXXI Aleurodiscal: An Antifungal Sesterterpenoid from *Aleurodiscus mirabilis*. (Berk. and Curt) Hohn. *J. Antibiotics* 42: 875-882.

Lee, I-K., Yun, B-S., Cho, S-M., Kim, W-G., Kim, J-P., Ryoo, I-J., Koshino, H. and Yoo, I-D. (1996). Betulinans A and B, Two Benzoquinone compounds from *Lenzites betulina*. *J. Nat. Prod.* 59: 1090-1092.

Lei J, (1992). Pharmacological study on Cordyceps sinensis (Berk.) Sacc. and ze-e Cordyceps *Chung Kuo Chung Yao Tsa Chih* 17(6), 364-366.

Lin WH, (1997). Dimerization of the N-terminal amphipathic alpha-helix domain of the fungal immunomodulatory protein from *Ganoderma tsugae* (Fip-gts) defined by a yeast two-hybrid system and site-directed mutagenesis. *J Biol Chem* 272(32), 20044-20048.

Manjula B. (1983). A revised list of agricoid and boletoid basidiomycetes from India and Nepal. *Proc. Indian Acad. Sci.* (Plant Sci) 92: 81-213.

Mc Namara H. S. (1999). Dietary supplement legislation. In: *Botonical Medicine*. Eshkinazi D., ed., Mary Ann Liebert, Larchmont, NY. 199-204.

Mizuno T, (1992). Antitumor-active polysaccharides isolated from the fruiting body of *Hericium erinaceum*, an edible and medicinal mushroom called yamabushitake or houtou. *Biosci Biotechnol Biochem* 56(2), 347-348.

Mizuno T. (1995). Bioactive molecules of mushrooms- food, function and medicinal effect of mushroom fungi. *Food RevInt*, 11. 7-21.

Mizuno, M., Minato, K-I, Ito H., Kawade M., Terai H., and Tsuchida H. (1999). Anti-tumor polysaccharide from the mycelium of liquid cultured Agaricus *blazei* Mill. *Biochem. Mol. Biol. Int.* 47: 707-714.

Mizuno, T. (1995a). Shiitake, *Lentinus edodes*: functional properties for medicinal and food purposes. *Food Rev. Int.*, 11(1): 111-128.

Mizuno, T. (1996). A development of antitumor polysaccharides from mushroom fungi. *Food Ingred. J. Jpn.* 167, 69-85.

Mizuno, T. (1999b). Bioactive substances in *Hericeum erinaceus* (Bull.: Fr.) Pres. (Yamabushitake), and its medicinal utilization. *Int J Med Mushr*, 1: 105-119.

Mizuno, T. (2000). Development of an antitumor biological response modifier from *Phellinus linteus* (Berk. et Curt.) Teng (Aphyllophoromycetedeae) *Int J Med Mushr*, 2: 21-33.

Mizuno, T. Ma, Y., Ito, H. and Suzuki, C. (1994). Water insoluble polysaccharides originated in mushroom its production, and antitumor agent mainly comprising the polysaccharide. *Japanese Patent 06-080703*. 22 March 1994.

Mizuno, T., Hagiwara, T., Nakamura, T., Ito, H., Shimura, K., Sumiya, T. and Asakura A. (1990a). Antitumor activity and some properties of water soluble polysaccharides from "Himematsutake" the fruiting body of *Agaricus blazei* Murrill. *Agric Biol Chem.* 54: 2889-2896.

Mizuno, T., Ohsava, K., Hagiwara, N. and Kuboyama, R. (1986). Fractionation and characterization of antitumor polysaccharides from Maitake, *Grifola frondosa*. *Agric Biol Chem* 50: 1679-1688.

Monro. J. A. (2003). Treatment of cancer with mushroom products. *Archives of environmental health.*

Mori K., Toyomasu T., Nanba H. and Kuroda H. (1987). Antitumor activities of edible mushrooms by oral administration. In: Wuest PJ, Royse DJ, Beelman RB, eds. *Proceedings of the International Symposium on Scientific and Technical Aspects of Cultivating Edible Fungi.* Amsterdam: Elsevier, 1-6.

Morita, Y., Hayashi, Y., Sumi, Y., Kodaira, A., and Sibata, H. (1995). Haploporic acid A, a novel dimeric drimane sesquiterpenoid from the basidiomycete *Haploporus odorus*. *Biosci. Biotech. Biochem.* 59: 2008-2009.

Moriyama, M. (1981). Antitumor effect of polysaccharide lentinan on transplanted ascites hepatoma-134 in C3H/He mice. In *Manipulation of host defence mechanisms*, Intl Congress Series 576. Excerpta Media: Amsterdam.

Nagai, P. H. and Ng, T. B. (2003). Lentin, a novel and potent antifungal protein from shiitake mushroom with inhibitory effects on activity of human immunodeficiency virus-1 reverse transcriptase and proliferation of leukemia cells. *Life Sci.* 73, 3363-3374.

Nanba H. (1967). Antitumor action of Shiitake (*Lentinus edodes*) fruit bodies orally administered to mice. *Chem Pharm Bull.* 35: 2459-6-6.

Natalia L., Poyedinok, A. S., Buchalo, O. V., Efremenkova and A. M. Negriyko. (2005). The light factor in biotechnology cultivation of medicinal mushrooms. *Intl J. of Med. Mush.* 3(7)- 448-449.

Natrajan K. and Raman, N. (1983). South Indian agaricales: Today and tomorrow. Printers and Publishers New Delhi 204.

Ochiai H. (2003). The effect of *Grifola frondosa* on influenza virus. In: *The abstract at the 16th annual meeting of the Japanese Biotherapy Association.*

Ohtsuru M., Horio H., Masui H. and Takada I. (1999). Effects of administration of *Grifola frondosa* on blood pressure and body weight in spontaneously hypertensive rats. *Nippon Shokuhin kagaku Kogaku Kaishi,* 46. 12, 806-814.

Pradeep C.K., Vrinda K.B., Mathew, S. and Abraham T.K. (1998). The genus Volvariella in Kerala state, India. *Mushroom Res.* 7, 53-62.

Przbylowicz P. and Donoghue J.(1990). *Shiitake Growers Handbook: The art and Science of mushroom cultivation.* Hunt Publ.Co.: Dubugue, Kendall, 199.

Purkayastha R.P. and Chandra, A. (1985). *Manual of Indian edible mushrooms.* Jagmander Book Agency Deshbandhu Gupta Road New Delhi 267.

Rahman H., Rahman S., Rahman A. and Rahman, K. (2005) Dissemination of case studies on Ganotherapy. *Intl J. of Med. Mush.* 3(7)–456.

Rai M. K. and Tidke G. (2005). Biotechnological potential of mushrooms: drug and dye production. *Intl J. of Med. Mush.* 3(7)- 457.

Rai, M K. (1997). Wild edible mushrooms of tribal areas of Seoni District, Madhya Pradesh, *Mushr. Res.,* 6(2): 107-108.

Rai M. K., Tidke G. and Wasser S. P. (2005). Therapeutic potential of mushrooms. *Natural product radiance.* 246-257.

Razak R. C and Rai M. K. (2005). Edible tribal mushroom resources of Central India and their ethnological aspects. *Intl J. of Med. Mush.* 3(7)- 458.

Reshetnikov S. v., Wasser S. P. and Tan, K.K. (2001). Higher Basidiomycetes as a source of antitumor and immumomodulating polysaccharides (Review). *Int J Med Mushr.* 3, 361-394.

Royse D.J. and Bahler C.C. (1996). Effects of genotype spawn run time and substrate formulation on biological efficiency of shiitake. *Appl Environ Microbial.* 52: 1425-7.

Saito, K., Nishijima, M. and Miyazaki, T. (1989). Studies on fungal polysacchrides: XXXV. Sructural analysis of an acidic polysacchride from *Ganoderma lucidum. Chem Pharm Bull* (Tokyo) 37: 3134-3136.

Saito, T., Akoi, F., Hirai, H., Inagaki, T., Matsunaga, Y., Sakakibara, T., Sakemi, T. S., Suzuki, Y., Watanabe, S., Suga, O., Sujaku, T., Smogowicz, A. A., Truesdell, S.J., Wong, J.W., Nagahisa, A., Kojima, Y., and Kohjima, N. (1998). Erinacine E as a kappa opioid receptor agonist and its new analogs from a basidiomycete, *Hericium ramosum. J. Antibiotics* 51: 983-990.

Sasaki T and Takasuka N. (1976). Further study of the structure of lentinan, an antitumour polysaccharide from *Lentinus edodes. Carbohydr Res.* 47: 99-104.

Sathe A. V. (1979). Agaricology in India-A review of work on Indian Agaricales. *Biovigyanam.* 5: 125-130.

Sathe A. V. and Deshpande S. (1979). Agaricales of Maharashtra In *Advances in Mycology and Plant pathology* (Chattopadhyay S.B. and Samajpati N. eds) 82-88.

Screen A. (1992). Developmental therapeutics program *in-vitro* testing results. National Cancer Institute, January 1992.

Shnyreva A.V., Belokon Y.S. and Belokon M.M. (2003). Differentiation between Commercial Strains of Oyster and Button Mushrooms Using Molecular Markers. *Russian J Genetics*, 39, 11, 1232-1239(8).

Singh S.K., Sharma V.P., Sharma S.R., Satish Kumar and Mugdha Tiwari. (2006). Molecular characterization of Trichoderma taxa causing green mould disease in edible mushrooms. *Current Sci.* 90, 3, 427-431.

Smith, J., Rowan N. and Sulivan, R. (2002). Medicinal mushrooms: Their therapeutic properties and current medical usage with special emphasis on cancer treatment; *special report commissioned by cancer research UK*. The University of Strathelyde in Glasgow, 256.

Stadler, M., Anke, H. and Sterner, O. (1994). New nematicidal and antimicrobial compounds from the basidiomycete *Cheimonophyllum candidissimum* (Berk and Curt) Sing. *J.Antibiotics*. 47: 1284-1289.

Sundin, A., Anke, H., Bergquist, K-E., Mayer, A., Sheldrick, W. S., Stadler, M. and Sterner, O. (1993). The structure determination of Panellon and Panellol, two 14-Noreudesmanes Isolated from *Resupinatus leightonii*. *Tetrahedron* 49: 7519-7524.

Susuki S and Oshirna S. (1976). Influence of Shi-Ta-Ke (*Lentinus edodes*) on human serum cholesterol. *Mushroom Sci* 1 976; 9 (Part 1): 463-7.

Tanimoto,T., Onodera, K., Hosoya, T., Takamatsu, Y., Kinoshita, T., Tago, K., Kogen, H., Fujioka, T., Hamano, K. and Tsujita, Y. (1996). Schizostatin, a Novel Squalene Synthase Inhibitor Produced by the Mushroom, *Schizophyllum commune*. *J. Antibiotics* 49: 617-623.

Toth J.O., Luu B. and Ourission G. (1983). Les acides ganoderiques T a Z: triterpenes cytoxiques de *Ganoderma leucidum* (Polyporaceae). *Tetrahedron Lett.* 24 1081-1084.

Tsuchida, H., Mizuno, M., Taniguchi, Y., Ito, H., Kawade M. and Akasaka K. (2001). Glucomannan separated from Agaricus blazei mushroom culture and antitumor agent containing as an active ingredient. *Japanese Patent 11-080206*, 26 March 2001.

Ukai, S., Kohi, T., Hara, C., Kuruma, I. and Tanaker, Y. (1983). Polysaccharides in fungi: XIV. Antiinflammatory effect of the polysaccharides from the fruit bodies of several fungi. *Journal of Pharmacology Dynamics* 6, 983-990.

Verma R.N., Singh G.B. and Bilgramy K.S. (1987). Fleshy fungal flora of NEH India-I. Manipur and Meghalaya. In *Indian Mushroom Science*: II (Kaul T.N. and Kapoor B.M. Eds.) RRL CSIR Jammu Tawi 414-421.

Vrinda K.B. Pradeep C.K., Mathew S and Abraham T.K. (1999). Agaricales from Western Ghats VII. *Mushroom res.* 8, 9-12.

Wasser S. P. (2002). Medicinal mushrooms as a source of antitumor and immunomodulating polysaccharides. *Appl Microb Biotechnol*, 60, 258-274.

Wasser S. P. (2005). Shiitake (*Lentinus edodes*). Encyclopedia of dietary supplements DOI: 10.1081/E-EDS-120024880.

Wasser, S.P. and Weis A. L. (1999a). Medicinal properties of substances occurring in higher basidiomycetes mushrooms: a modern perspective. *Crit Rev Immunol*, 1965-96.

Wasser, S.P. and Weis A. L. (1999b). Therapeutic effects of substances occurring in higher basidiomycetes mushrooms: current perspectives (Review). *Int J Med Mushr*, 1: 31-62.

Wasser, S.P., Nevo E., Sokolov D., and Timor-Timenetsky M. (2000b). The regulation of dietary supplements from medicinal mushrooms. In: *Science and cultivation of edible fungi.van Griensven*, (ed.) Balkema, Rotterdam. 789-801.

Wasser, S. P., Nevo E., Sokolov D., Reshetnikov S., and Timor-Timenetsky M. (2000a). Dietary supplements from medicinal mushrooms: diversity of types and variety of regulations. *Int. J. Med. Mushr*, 2, 1-19.

Wasser, S. P., Reshetnikov S. V., Solomko E. F., Buchalo A. S and Nevo E. (2002). For higher basidiomycetes mushrooms grown as biomass in submerged culture. *US patent no. 6,372,462 B2*, Publ. Apr. 16, 2002.

Wasser, S. P., Sokolov D., Nevo E., Reshetnikov S., and Timor-Timenetsky M. (2001). Dietary supplements from medicinal mushrooms: how we are going to ensure their quality and safety. *Int. J. Med. Mushr*. 3, 94.

Wasser, S.P. and Didukh M.Y. (2005). Culinary-medicinal higher basidiomycete mushrooms as a prominent source of dietary supplements and drugs for the 21st century. *Fifth international conference on mushroom biology and mushroom products*. 12.20-34.

Wasser, S.P., Didukh M.Y and Nevo E. (2004). Dietary supplements from culinary-medicinal mushrooms: A variety of regulations and safety concerns for the 21st century. *Int J Med Mushr*, 6, 231-248.

Wasser, S. P. (2005). Reishi or Ling Zhi (*Ganoderma lucidum*). *Encyclopedia of dietary supplements DOI*: 10.1081/E-EDS-120022119.

Wasser, S. P., Didukh, M. Y. and Nevo, E. (2004). Dietary supplements from culinary medicinal mushrooms: A variety of regulations and safety concerns for the 21st century. *International J. Med. Mush*, 6- 231-248.

Wasser, S. P., Weis, A. L. (1997). Meidcinal mushrooms. *Lentinus edodes* (Berk) Singer, Nevo, E., Ed.; Peledfus Publ. House: Haifa, Israel. 95.

Weber, W., Anke, T., Steffan, B. and Steglich, W. (1989). Antibiotics from Basidiomycetes XXXII Strobilurin E: A New Cytostatic and Antifungal (E)–Methoxyacrylate Antibiotic from *Crepidotus fulvotomentosus* Peck. *J.Antibiotics* 43: 207-212.

Won, S.J., Lee, SS., Ke, YH., Lin, MT. (1989). Enhancement of splenic NK cytotoxic activity by the extracts of *Ganoderma lucidum* mycelium in mice. *J Biomed Lab Sci* 2: 201-213.

Wood, K.A., Kau, D-A., Wrigley, S.K., Beneyto, R., Renno, D. V., Ainsworth, A.M., Penn, J., Hill, D., Killacky, J. and Depledge, P. (1996). Novel -Methoxyacrylates of the 9- Methoxystrobilurin and Oudemansin Classes Produced by the Basiodiomycete *Favolaschia pustulosa*. *J.Nat. Prod.* 59: 646-649.

Wu S. (1994). Therapeutic effect of Grifola polysaccharides in chronic hepatitis B. In: *the abstracts at International symposium on production and products of Lentinus Mushroom*, Nov 1-3, 1994. China.

Xia, E. and Q. Chen. (1989). Isolation, analysis and biological activities of the polysaccharide of *Tremella Fuciformis*. *ACTA Mycol. Sin.* 7: 166-174.

Yap, A. T., Ng, M. L. (2003). Immunopotentiating properties of lentinan (1-3)-B-D-glucan extracted from culinary- medicinal shiitake mushroom *Lentinus edodes* (Berk) Singer (Agaricomycetideae). *Int. J. Med. Mush.* 5, 352-372.

Yoshida, I., Kiho, T., Usai, S., Sakushima M. and Ukai, S. (1996). Polysacchrides in funji. XXXVII. Immunomodulating activities of carboxymethylated derivatives of linear (1→ 30-alpha-glucans extracted from the fruiting bodies of *Agrocybe cylindrical* and *Amanita muscaria*. *Biol. Pharm. Bull* 19: 114-121.

Zhang J, *et al.* (1994). Antitumor polysaccharides from a Chinese mushroom, "yuhuangmo," the fruiting body of *Pleurotus citrinopileatus*. *Biosci Biotechnol Biochem.*; 58(7): 1195-1201.

Zhang LX, (1993b). Effect of Japanese *Ganoderma Lucidum* on production of interleukin-2 from *Murine splenocytes Chung Kuo Chung Hsi I Chieh Ho Tsa Chih* 13(10), 613-615.

Zhang, J., Wang, g., Li, H., Zhuang, C., Mizuno, T., Ito H., Suzuki, C., Okamoto, H. and Li, J. (1994a). Antitumor Polysaccharides from a Chinese mushroom "Yuhuahgmo" the fruiting body of *Pleurotus citrinopiliatus*. *Biosci Biotechnol Biochem* 58: 1195-1201.

Zhang, J., Wang, g., Li, H., Zhuang, C., Mizuno, T., Ito H., Suzuki, C., Okamoto, H. and Li, J. (1994b). Antitumor activity of protein containing glycans from the Chinese mushroom Songshan Linzhi, *Ganoderma tsugae*, mycelium. *Biosci Biotechnol Biochem* 58: 1202-1205.

Zhang, L. and M. Yu, (1993a). Influence of ling zhi on natural killer cells-Immunopharmacological study (5). From *The research on Ganoderma lucidum (part one)*. Shanghai: Shanghai Medical University Press, pp. 246-253.

Zhuang C., Mizuno T., Ito H and Shimura K. (1994). Chemical modification and antitumor activity of polysaccharides from the mycelium of liquid cultured *Grifola frondosa*. *Nippon Shokuhin Kogyo Gakkaishi*, 41, 10, 733-740.

Zhuang Cun and Wasser S.P. (2004). Medicinal Value of culinary- medicinal Maitake mushroom *Grifola frondosa* (Dicks.: Fr.) S.F. Gray (Aphyllophoromycetodeae). Review. *Int J Med Mushr*, 6, 287-313.

Zhuang, C., Mizuno, T., Shimada, A., Ito, H., Suzuki, C., Mayuzumi, Y., Okamoto, H., Ma, Y. and Li, J. (1993). Antitumor Protein-containing Polysaccharides from a Chinese mushroom Fengweigu or Houbitake, *Pleurotus sajor-caju* (Fr.) Sing *Biosci Biotechnol Biochem* 57: 901-906.

Ziesel S. M. (1999). Regulation of nutraceuticals. *Science*. 285: 1853-1855.

Microbial Biotechnology and Ecology (2011)
Editors: Deepak Vyas, G.S. Paliwal, P.K.Khare and R.K Gupta
Published by: DAYA PUBLISHING HOUSE, NEW DELHI

Pages **472–483**

Chapter 26

Significance of GM Crops in Modern Agriculture

☆ ***Shweta J. Sabannavar[1], H.C. Lakshman[1], Mahesh B. Byatanal[1] and C. Maya[2]***

[1]Post Graduate Department and Research in Botany (Microbiology Lab), Karnataka University, Dharwad – 580 003, Karnataka
[2]Department of Botany, Bangalore University, JB Campus, Bangalore – 560 056

Introduction

Crop improvement was greatly accelerated in the 20th century by the rediscovery of the laws of inheritance. It was by Gregor Johan Mendel in 1865, and after scientists established that the chromosomes contain the information for specific traits encoded in DNA. The rise of molecular biology, starting in the 1950s with the discovery of DNA's structure, led to a series of further discoveries showing how traits are encoded as proteins in the cell and the plants. This understanding and new techniques that allow scientists to manipulates DNA in the laboratory, are revolutionizing plant breeding.

Genetic engineering depends on the fact that the same molecule, DNA, makes up the genes of all organisms. This means that a gene from a fungus (made of DNA) can be inserted in a rice plant's chromosome (also made of DNA) and, with luck and experimental skill, can be induced to function. The ability to transform crops with genes from any other organism opens up the entire community of life as the source for new genes for a crop. Although the process of genetic modification started long ago, only crops that are genetically engineered are referred to as genetically modified (GM) crops. Some writers prefer the term genetically enhanced or improved.

There are several advantages of GM technology over other methods. First and foremost, it is specific: Unlike crosses where many genes are transferred during sexual reproduction, here the scientist transfers only a single gene (or a few genes) to the crop plants. Second, the method is fast; as in any micropropagation technique, many plants can be generated quickly. Finally, the genes themselves are an advantage. Unlike any other breeding methods, plant biotechnology allows a scientist to put virtually any gene from any organism into a crop plant. In practice, scientists create a large number of transformed crop lines for a specific gene and then carry all these lines through to many rounds of conventional plant breeding, to ensure that the introduced characteristic. Thus GM technology does not eliminate plant breeding but supplements it just like other laboratory-based methods.

There is an urgent need to develop techniques in modified crops, which are sustainable from environmental production and socioeconomic points of view. This is to guarantee the sufficient food production in the coming decades. It is beyond critical because modern agricultural production throughout the world does not appear to be sustainable in the long-term FAO (1980), seems to appropriate in this contest.

But while GM crops are now being used widely by farmers in the USA, consumers in the European Union and Japan have reacted strongly against them. Although this has slowed the rate at which GM crops and foods are being introduced, the biotech industry is continuing to push ahead with them. This briefing explains why people should still be concerned about GM crops.

Genetically modified (GM) foods are foods produced from genetically modified organisms (GMO) that had their DNA altered through genetic engineering. GM foods were first put on the market in the early 1990s. The most common modified foods are derived from plants: soybean, corn, canola and cotton seed oil (Maessen, 1997).

Controversies surrounding GM foods and crops commonly focus on human and environmental safety, labeling and consumer choice, intellectual property rights, ethics, food security, poverty reduction and environmental conservation.

GM Foods Currently Used in Development Countries

Currently, there are number of foods which exist in a genetically modified version shown in Table 26.1.

Currently Known GM Crops

Between 1995 and 2005, the total surface area of land cultivated with GMOs had increased, by a factor of 50, from 17,000 km^2 (4.2 million acres) to 900,000 km^2 (222 million acres), of which 55 per cent were Brazil.

Although most GM crops are grown in North America, in recent years there has been rapid growth in the area sown in developing countries. For instance in 2005 the largest increase in crop area planted to GM crops (soybeans) were in Brazil (94,000 km^2 in 2005 versus 50,000 km^2 in 2004.) (Domingo, 2000). There has also been rapid and continuing expansion of GM cotton varieties in India since 2002 (Cotton is a major source of vegetable cooking oil and animal feed.) It is predicted that in 2006/7 32,000 km^2 of GM cotton will be harvested in India (up more than 100 per cent from the previous season). Indian national average cotton yields of GM cotton were seven times lower in 2002, because the parental cotton plant used in the genetic engineered was not well suited to the climate of India and failed. The publicity given to transgenic trait Bt insect resistance has encouraged the adoption of better performing hybrid cotton varieties, and the Bt trait has substantially reduced losses to insect predation. Economic and environmental benefits of GM cotton in India to the individual farmer have been documented (May, Sir R; Halford NCordell and Halford 1999).

Table 26.1: Sowing Genetically Modified Common Food Products Available in Developing Countries

Food	*Properties of the Genetically Modified Variety*	*Trade Name and the company which Produced Initial Version*	*Specific Genetic Modification*	*Percent of Genetically Modified Version Occupies of the Given Food' Agriculture in USA*	*Percent this GMF takes up of agriculture compared to non-GMF version, globally*
Soybeans	Resistant to herbicide	Roundup Ready, Monsanto	Herbicide resistant	TBA	TBA
Corn	Resistance to certain pesticides (tolerating crop spray this way a farmer can use amounts of pesticides which would normally kill the plant, without harming it)	TBA	New gene added/transferred into plant genome	TBA	TBA
Cotton	Pest-resistant cotton	TBA	New gene added/transferred into plant genome	TBA	TBA
Tomatoes	Variety that does not rot (degrade) as fast–the genetically modified tomatos do not produce a substance that normally causes tomatoes to rot	*E.g.* FlavrSavr	First genetically modified tomatoes contained genes that made them resistant to antibiotics. After concern from doctors and the medical community, tomatoes are now genetically modified in an alternative way	TBA	TBA
Rapeseed plants	Resistance to certain pesticides	TBA	New gene added/transferred into plants genome	TBA	TBA
Sugar cane	Resistance to certain pesticides (tolerating crop spray)	TBA	New gene added/transferred into plants genome	TBA	TBA
Sweet corn	Produces its own insecticide (a toxin to insects, so insects, so insect attacks are less likely	*Bt* corn	Insect-killing gene added to the plant. The gene comes from the bacteria *Bacillus thuringiensis*	TBA	TBA
Rice	Genetically modified to contain high amount of Vitamin A (beta carotene)	Golden rice	Three new genes implanted; two from daffodils and the third from a bacterium	TBA	TBA

In 2003, countries that grew 99 per cent of the global transgenic crops were the United States (63 per cent), Argentina (21 per cent), Canada (6 per cent), Brazil (4 per cent), China (4 per cent), and South Africa (1 per cent) (Thompson, 1990). The Grocery Manufacturers of America estimate that 75 per cent of all processed foods in the U.S. contain a GM ingredient (USDA 2006). In particular, Bt corn, which produces the pesticide within the plant itself is widely grown, as are soybeans genetically designed to tolerate glyphosate herbicides. These constitute "input-traits" are aimed to financially benefit the producers, have indirect environmental benefits marginal cost benefits to consumers.

In the US, by 2006, 89 per cent of the planted area of soybeans, 83 per cent of cotton, and 61 per cent maize was genetically modified varieties. Genetically modified soybeans carried herbicide tolerant traits only, but maize and cotton carried both herbicide tolerance and insect protection traits (the latter largely the *Bacillus thuringiensis* Bt insecticidal protein). In the period 2002 to 2006, there were significant increases in the area planted to Bt protected cotton and maize, and herbicide tolerant maize also increased in sown area (Simpson, 1999).

However, several studies have found that genetically modified varieties of plants do not produce higher yields than normal plants.

Transgenic Plants Function as Bioreactor

Plants are easy to grow and can generate considerable biomass. With these features in mind, research has been carried out to determine whether transgenic plants can be used for the production of commercial proteins and chemicals.

Through genetic engineering techniques, compounds of commercial interest that were previously produced only from exotic sources of plants, animal and microbial origin is now produced in domesticated crops. Transgenic plants can act as living bioreactors for the inexpensive production of chemicals and pharmaceuticals, and this is also known as *molecular farming* (Table 26.2). It has been possible to produce carbohydrates, fatty acids, polypeptides, vaccines, industrial enzymes and biodegradable plastics using the molecular farming approach.

GM Crops in Carbohydrates Improvements

Starch is one of the components of plant cells. Tailor-made starches with reduced level o' amylose or increased amount of starch have been developed in potato. Starch precursors have also been rerouted into the biosynthetic pathways of other storage carbohydrates. Nonfructan storing tobacco and potato plants have been transformed with fructosyl trans-'erase gene from *Bacillus subtilis* to accumulate fructan. Production of novel compounds has also been attempted through genetic engineering. Tobacco plants have been transformed with the mannitol-1-phosphate dehydrogenase gene (mf/D) from *E. coli*. These transgenics synthesized more mannitol and were also tolerant to high salinity (Tarczynski *et al.*, 1993). Similarly myo-inositol o-methyl transferase gene from *Mesembryanthemum crystallimum* (ice plant) has been incorporated into tobacco to produce pinnitol a myoinositol derived cyclic sugar alcohol. Trehalose is an additive that improves processed and dried food by making them astier. The plant biotechnological companies MOGEN (Leiden, The Netherlands) and Calgene (Davis, USA) have reported the synthesis of small quantities of trehalose in transgenic tobacco plants.

GM Crops in Lipids

Monounsaturated fatty acid level in plants is desirable so that the nutritional value of oil is enhanced. When a rat desaturase gene was introduced into tobacco, level of palmitoleic acid (16:1) and oleic acid (18:1) levels increased (Grayburn *et al.*, 1992). For the manufacture of detergents and for specialized nutritional applications, thioesterase gene from California bay tree was incorporated into *Arabidopsis* for the accumulation of medium chain 12-carbon fatty acid as storage lipids (Voelker *et al.*, 1992). The first nonfood products of plant bioengineering in commercial production is a genetically engineered rape seed plant variety (Laurical) that was modified to produce lauric acid, a 12-carbon fatty acid used to make soaps and detergents (Table 26.3).

Table 26.2: Some of the Therapeutic Agents Produced in Transgenic Plants

Protein	*Plant(s)*	*Application*
Human protein C	Tobacco	Anticoagulant
Human hirudin variant 2	Tobacco, canola, Ethiopian mustard	Anticoagulant
Human granulocyte-macrophage colony-stimulating factor	Tobacco	Neutropenia
Human erythropoietin	Tobacco	Anemia
Human enkephalins	Thale cress, canola	Antihyperanalgesic by opiate activity
Human epidermal growth factor	Tobacco	Wound repair/control of cell proliferation
Human α-interferon	Rice, turnip	Hepatitis C and B
Human serum albumin	Potato, tobacco	Liver cirrhosis
Human hemoglobin	Tobacco	Blood substitute
Human homotrimeric collagen-I	Tobacco	Collagen synthesis
Human al-antitrypsin	Rice	Cystic fibrosis, liver disease, hemorrhage
Human growth hormone	Tobacco	Dwarfism, wound healing
Human aprotinin	Corn	Tryp: in inhibitor for transplantation surgery
Angiotensin-1-converting enzyme	Tobacco, tomato	Hypertension
α-Tricosanthin	Tobacco	HIV therapy
Glucocerebrosidase	Tobacco	Gaucher disease

GM Crops in Protein Quality

Considerable progress has also been made in the improvement of nutritional quality of legume storage protein by expression of the gene responsible for a methionine-rich protein. The Brazil nut (*Bertholletia excelsa*) seed protein, 2S albumin of Brazil nut under the promoter of phaseolin gene was introduced into tobacco. The accumulation of 2S albumin resulted in a 30 per cent increase in the methionine content in the transgenic tobacco seed (Altenbach *etal.*, 1989). Similarly, expression and accumulation of the Brazil nut 2S albumin protein in transgenic *Arabidopsis*, rapeseed, soybean, French bean\ seeds, and potato have also been reported. Unfortunately, the Brazil nut 2S albumin was found to be allergenic (Nordlee *et al.*, 1996), which raised the safety concern of development of transgenic plants expressing this protein. Sunflower seed albumin, rich in methionine, is not an allergen and has been used for development of transgenic plants, the sunflower albumin gene under the control of the pea vicilin gene promoter has been transferred to lupin, and the, methionine content of seed protein of transgenic plants increased by twofold. Rat feeding experiments demonstrated the superior nutritive value of transgenic lupin (Molvig *et al.*, 1997). Another seed storage protein gene (*Ama1*) isolated from

Table 26.3: The Use of Plants as Bioreactors for the Production of Lipids, Carbohydrates and Proteins

Compound	*Origin of Gene(s)*	*Application*	*Plant Species Used*
		Lipids	
Medium chain fatty acids	California bay tree (*Umbellularia californica*)–Thioesterase	Food, detergent, industrial	Oilseed rape
Mono-unsaturated fatty	Rat-desaturase	Food	Tobacco
		Acids	
Poly-hydroxybutyric acid	*Alcaligenes vutrophus*	Biodegradable plastics	*Arabidopsis*, oilseed rape, soybean.
Saturated fatty acids	*Brassica rapa*	Food, confectioneries	Oilseed rape
γ-Linolenic acid	Desaturase (*Synechocystis*); *Mortierella alpina*	For reducing coronary diseases	Tobacco; canola
Ricinoleic acid	Castor oleate hydroxylase	Nylon paints, varnishes, lubricants	*Arabidopsis*
		Carbohydrates	
Amylose-free starch	*Solarium tuberosutn* (GBSS)	Food, industrial	Potato
Cyclodextrins	*Klebsiella* pnei/mon/ae-Cyclodextrin glucosyl transferase	Food, pharmaceutical	Potato
Fructans	*Bacillus subtilis*-F\jctosyl transferase	Food, Industrial	Tobacco, potato
Increased amount of	*E. coli* (*glgCiG*)	Food, industrial	Potato
		Starch	
Trehalose	*E. coli*	Food stabilizer	Tobacco
Sucrose	Maize sucrose phosphate synthase (SPS)	Sweetner	Tomato
		Proteins	
Alpha-trichsantin	Chinese medicinal plant	Inhibition of HIV replication	*Nicotiana benthamiana*
Angiotensin converting enzyme inhibitor	Milk	Anti-hypersensitive effect	Tobacco, tomato
Antigens I	Bacteria, viruses	Orally administered vaccines	Tobacco, tomato/ potato, lettuce/
Antigens	Pathogens	Subunit vaccine	Tobacco/
Enkephalin	Human	Opiate activity	Oilseed rape, *Arabidopsis*
Hirudin	Synthetic	Thrombin inhibitor	Oilseed rape

Table adapted from Goddjin and Pen *et al.*, 1997). In transgenic plants, sucrose level increased with a concomitant reduction in starch.

Amaranthus is a good candidate for introduction into crop plants as the protein has well-balanced amino acid composition (Raina and Datta, 1992). This gene has been introduced into potato, the level of accumulation of *Ama1* was found to be 0.3 per cent of total soluble protein (Chakraborty *et al.*, 1998). The soybean glycinine gene has been introduced into rice to increase its protein content and to make it more digestible. In addition, some important amino acids, such as lysine, lacking in quantity in normal rice have been replinshed (Momma *et al.*, 1999).

GM Crops in Vitamin and Mineral

Vitamin A content in the diet plays a major role in preventing disorders such as color blindness. Rice, the staple food for billions of people, does not contain any provitamin A in the endosperm. Immature rice endosperm is capable of synthesizing the early intermediate geranyl geranyl diphosphate (GGPP), which can be used to produce the uncolored carotene phytoene by expressing the enzyme phytoene synthase in rice endosperm. The synthesis of ^-carotene requires three additional plant enzymes: phytoene desaturase and x-carotene desaturase, each catalyzing the introduction of two double bonds, and lycopene β-cyclase, encoded by the *lcy*[l] gene. Ye *et al.* (2000) used the *Agrobacterium*-mediated transformation method in rice to introduce the entire p-carotene biosynthetic pathway into the rice endosperm. Plant phytoene synthase (*phy*) gene originated from daffodil {*Narcissus pseudonarcissus*), bacterial phytoene desaturase (*Gt1*) originating from *Erwinia uredovora* placed under the control of endosperm-specific glutelin (Gfi) and the constitutive CaMV35S promoter respectively. The 'phytoene synthase cDNA contained a 5'-sequence coding for a functional transit peptide, and the *crtl* gene contained the transit peptide (fp) sequence of the pea Rubisco small subunit. These two direct the formation of lycopene in the endospeum plastids, the site of geranyl geranyl diphosphate formation. A third gene, lycopene β-cyclase, from *Narcissus pseudonarcissus*, controlled by the rice glutelin promoter; which carried a functional transit peptide allowing piastid import and selectable marker *aphlV*, were introduced. The resulting transgenic rice plants produce sufficient p-carotene converted to vitamin A and rice has been named as "Golden rice".

GM Crops in Commercial Transgenic Crops

Transgenic plant products have now been released as commercial varieties in a range of crops (Table 26.4). By all accounts, 1996 was a critical year in the history of plant biotechnology.

For the first time, farmers planted large areas under transgenic plants. It was in 1995 that potato varieties expressing Bt crystal protein toxic to Colorado potato beetle were made commercially available. In the following year, cotton varieties expressing the *Bt* crystal protein toxic to a number of lepidopteran pests, including the tobacco budworm and cotton bollworm, were introduced. At the same time, Bt corn hybrids with improved resistance to European cornborer became available to the farmers. All these commercial introductions have taken place in USA. *Bt* cotton varieties carrying the same technology as used in USA are being introduced in Australia. Transgenics for herbicide tolerance was the dominant trait in 1997. Transgenics have now been released for various traits from virus resistance to quality and for industrial use.

Transgenics for Quality and Improved Storage

The first approval for commercial sale of a food product was a transgenic tomato "Flavr Savr" with delayed ripening, developed by Calgene, USA in 1994. Improved storage or long shelf life of tomato that is suitable for food processing can be developed by two approaches using (i) antisense RNA technology or (ii) using gene for 1-aminocyclopropane-1-carboxylic acid (ACC; deaminase, which degrades ACC to ethylene. Calgene used antisense RNA against polygalac turonase (PG) enzyme encoding gene. On the basis of PG gene sequence, an antisense PG gene was constructed and tomato plants were transformed. These transgenic tomato plants produced both sense and antisense mRNA for the PG gene resulting in RNA-RNA pairing. This would result in nonproduction of PG gene product, and thus preventing the attack of PG gene upon pectin in the cell wall of ripening fruit and thereby preventing softening of fruit.

Table 26.4: Commercial Releases of Transgenic Plant Varieties

Trait	*Crop*	*Product Bame*	*Organization*
		Insect resistance	
Bt	Cotton	Bollguard	Monsanto Co.
Bt	Cotton	-	Calgene
Bt	Potato	Newleaf	Monsanto Co.
Bt	Maize	Yield Guard	Monsanto Co.
Bt	Maize	Maximizer	Ciba Seeds
Bt	Maize	-	Novartis, Mycogen, Pioneer Hi-Bred
Virus resistance	Squash	Freedom II	Asgrow Seeds, Inc.
Virus resistance	Tobacco, tomato, capsicum	-	(China)
Virus resistance	Cantaloupe	-	Asgrow Seeds, Inc.
Virus resistance	Papaya	Rainbow	-
		Herbicide resistance	
Glufosinate	Maize	Liberty Link	AgrEvo Canada inc.
Glufosinate		Liberty Link	AgrEvo USA Co.
Sethoxydim		-	BASF
Glufosinate		-	DeKalb Genetics Corp
Glyphosate		Roundup Ready	Monsanto Co.
Glufosinate		-	Plant Genetic Systems V
Glufosinate	Oilseed rape, Canola	Innovator	AgrEvo Canada Inc.
Glufosinate		"	AgrEvo USA Co.
Glyphosate		Roundup Ready	Monsanto Co.
Glufosinate		–	Plant Genetic Systems
Bromoxynil		_	Rhone-Poulene
Bromoxynil	Cotton	BXN	Calgene *rz*
Sulfonylurea		-	DuPont
Glyphosate		Roundup Ready	Monsanto Co.
Glyphosate	Soybean	Roundup Ready	Monsanto Co.
Sulfonyl urea	Flax	Triffid	Univ. of Saskatchewan
Glufosinate	Chicory	-	Bejo-Zaden

Contd...

Table 26.4–Contd...

Trait	Crop	Product Bame	Organization
		Quality	
Vine ripened, shelf life	Tomato	Flavr Savr	Calgene
Vine ripened, shelf life	Tomato	Endless Summer	DNA Plant Technology -
Delayed softening, paste Consistency	Tomato	-	Zeneca
Modified starch	Potato		AVEBE
Increased vase life	Carnation		Florigene
Modified flower color	Carnation	-	Florigene
Oil characteristics	Canola	Laurical	Calgene
Male sterility hybrid system	Canola	-	Plant Genetics Systems

More than 4500 GM plant varieties have been tested in the United States, and 50 have been approved for unlimited release. Researchers have been transferred genes to mycorrhizal symbionts of plant roots to confer resistance to pathogens and increase efficiency (Hiremath and Podila, 2000).

Most GM plants target plant protection, including herbicide resistance, insect resistance and disease resistance. There are also many modifications to plant quality including nutrition and chemical content, timing of ripening, increased photosynthesis, and stress tolerance. Plants are also being designed to produce pharmaceuticals, industrial proteins, and biodegradable plastics. Others will remove heavy metals from contaminated soils (Krimsky *et al.*, 1996; Hapgood, 2000).

But regulations will be difficult to enforce. If anybody can produce GM plants, many will. There is no way that every new product can be thoroughly tested for health and environmental safety. Patents can be pirated. Products may be introduced with disclosure of their genetic identity. GM crops produced in foreign countries may cross our borders, and vice-versa. Careless application of marketing rules will lead to debacles such as the recent contamination of taco shells by Starlink corn not approved for human consumption.

Developing nations see great hop in GM plants to help solve their problems. A good example is China (Altman and Watanabe). Chinese scientists have already inserted virus coat proteins into tobacco, tomato, potato, green pepper, chrysanthemum, and rice. The virus coat proteins induce some as-yet unknown mechanism of immunity against virus infection in the host plants. The Chinese have also inoculated more than a million hectares of rice and soybean with recombinant strains of *Rhizobium* bacteria that fix nitrogen more efficiently. Chinese scientists claim a 5-10 per cent increase in yield. Increase cadmium uptake and tolerance, and plan to use the weeds to clean up pollution. They are also working on saline and drought resistance, starch and oil content, and increased protein storage. In area where Chinese growers were spraying pesticides on cotton an average of 15 to 20 times per season, introduction of *Bt* cotton reduced the sprays to near zero in may cases (Cline, Western Farm Press, 2000).

In 1996 the International Food Biotechnology Council convened a panel of allergy experts to develop a standard protocol. First, if transgenes are from a known source of allergy, standard serological and skin prick tests are applied to the new product to check for the known allergen. If the transgenes are from a novel source, they are analyzed for amino acid sequences similar to known allergens, and if some are found, serum antibody tests using the known allergen can be test for reaction to the novel protein. If the researchers find no homologies to known allergens, the novel proteins are submitted to simulated digestion experiments. If they are not digested quickly enough, further tests are needed before marketing or regulatory approval (Lehrer, Samuel, 1999).

Another recent finding is that both plant and animal chromosomes contain large amounts of ancient virus DNA that has become inactivated and lies dormant with the host genome. Ho and her colleagues fear that recombination with CaMV promoter could reactivate some of these provirus segments to form virulent new plant viruses. CaMV (Cauliflower Mosaiç Viral) is related to human hepatitis B virus and retroviruses such as HIV, and some critics hint that CaMV could even recombine to form new virus strains pathogenic to humans, a very scary thought to the public. Of course, GM defenders have rebuttals to all these theories by the critics (Ho *et al.*, 1999).

What are the Concerns About Growing GM Crops?

Farmland is already in severe decline because of intensive, chemical farming. For example, plants which were considered to be arable weeds 40 years ago are now listed as rare or scarce and some are endangered species (Wilson *et al.*, 1990). There is widespread concern that the use of GM herbicide tolerant crops could make this worse.

GM herbicide tolerant crops allow farmers to apply 'broad spectrum' weed killers to their field, which kill all other plants. There is concern that this will continue the decline of farmland wildlife because the use of these GM crops could lead to the removal of weeds from all crops in the normal arable rotation. "Untested introduction of GM crops could be the final blow for such species as the skylark, corn bunting and the linnet, as the seeds an insects on which they feed disappear" (Domingo, 2000).

The GM oilseed rape supplied by Aventis for the farm scale trials in England and Scotland was found to be contaminated with an unauthorized GM variety containing antibiotic resistance markers. The contaminated seed had been plants at more than 20 sites since 1999.

As can be seen, GM contamination is already a problem. The long distance that viable pollen can travel mean that the separation distances between GM and other crops would have to be very large to be effective.

Most GM crops being grown at the moment are destined for markets in rich countries. Such products will not help to feed the poor and hungry of the world. The majority of GM crops are designed for use in intensive farming systems, with single crop in large fields requiring heavy use of chemical inputs. Many farmers in developing countries are small scale, growing many different crops and they often cannot afford the chemicals needed.

Scientists have already raised similar concerns about the feeding of GM in high quantities to both farm animals and babies. Scientists working for the Zambian Government which rejected GM food aid stated that "While it is often said that GM maize is consumed by millions of Americans, it was noted that it is eaten in highly processed form and is not a staple food in the USA. In Zambia maize is the staple food and is usually the only carbohydrate source" (Guest, 1992).

References

Adoption of Genetically Engineered Crops in the U.S. *USDA ERS* July 14, 2006.

Altenbach, S.B., Pearson, K. W., Maker, G., Staraci, L. C., and Sun, S.S.M. (1989) Enhancement of methionine content of seed proteins by the expression of a chimeric gene encoding a methionine rich protein in transgenic plants. *Plant Mol. Biol.* (13): 513-522.

Altman, David w., and Kazuo N. Watanabe (ed.) *Plant biotechnology transfer to developing countries.* R. G. Landes Co. Austin, Texas.

Chakraborty, N., Chakraborty, S., Kesarwan, M., Azam, M and Datta, A. (1998) *Proceedings of IUBS symposium*, Taipei, Taiwan, 1997, pp. 125-131.

Cline, Harry, (2000) *Ag. Biotech quizzing aplenty.* Western Farm Press (Sept, 2, 2000).

Domingo, J. L. (2000) Health risks of GM foods: many opinions but few data. *Science* (288): 1748-9.

Goddjin, O.J.M, and Pen, J (1995) Plants as bioreactors. *TIBTECH* (13): 379-387.

Grayburn, W.S., Collius, G. B. and Hildebrand. D. F. (1992) *Biotechnology*, (10): 675-678.

Guest, G. (1992) *Response to FDA Draft Federal Register Notice on Food Biotechnology.*

Halfore Ncordell, Halford. N (2003). *Genetically modified crops.* Imperial college Press. ISBN 1-86094-353-5.

Hapgood Fred. (2000). Garage biotech is here, or just around the corner. Will genetic modification for fun and profit become a homegrown industry? *Civilization* (April/May 2000): 45-51.

Hiremath, Shivanand, and Gopi Podila. (2000). Development of genetically engineered mycorrhical fungi for biological control. In Podila, Gopi and David Douds, Jr. (ed.) *Current Advanes in Mycorrhizae Research.* APS Press, St. Paul, Minnesota.

Ho, Mae-Wan, Angela Ryan, and Joe Cummins (1999). Cauliflower mosaic Viral Promoter–a recipe for disaster? *Microbial Ecology in Health and Disease* II (4).

Krimsky, Sheldon, and Roger Wrubel. (1996). *Agricultural biotechnology and the environment: Science, policy and social issues.* Univ Illinois Press, Urbana, Illinois.

Lehrer, Samuel, B. (1999). The Potential Health Risks of Genetically Modified Organisms: How can Allergens be Assessed and Minimized? *CGIAR/NAS Biotechnology Conference–October 21-22, 1999.* Univ. Illinois Press, Urbana.

Maessen, G.D.F. (1997). *Genomic stability and stability of expression in genetically modified plants.*

May, Sir. R. (1999) Quote from Sunday Express 14th November 1999.

Mitchell C. Tarazynski, Richard G. Jensen, and Hans J. Bhnert (1993). Stress Protection of transgenic Tobacco by Production of the Osmlyte Mannitol *Science*, (239): 508-510.

Molvig, L., Tabe, L. M., Eggum, B.O., Moore, A.E., Craig, S., Spencer, D. and Higgins, T. J.V. (1997) Enhanced methionine levels and increased nutritive value of seeds of transgenic Lupin (*Lupinus angustifolius*) expressing a sunflower seed albumin gene. *Proc. Natl. Molecular cloning of a gene encoding a seed specific protein with nutritionally balanced amino acid composition from Amaranthus.* Proc. Natl. Acad. Sci. USA (89): 11774-11778.

Momma, K., Hashimoto, W., Ozama, S., Kawai, S., Katsube, T., Takaiwa, F., Kitos, M., Utsumi, S., and Murata, K. (1999) Quality and Safety evaluation of genetically engineered rice with soybean glycinin: analyses of the grain composition and digestibility of glycinin in transgenic rice. *Biosci. Biotechnol. Biochem.* (63): 314-318.

Nordlee, J. A., Taylor, S.L., Townsend, J. A., Thomas, L. A., and Bush, R. K. (1996) Identification of a Brazil nut alhrgen in transgenic soybeans. *New Eng. J. Med.* (339): 688-692.

Raina, A., and Datta, A. (1992) Molecular cloning of a gene encoding a seed specific protein with nutritionally balanced amino acid composition from Amaranthus. *Proc. Natl. Acad. Sci. USA.* (89): 11774-11778.

Simpson, EC *et al.* (1999) Gene flow in genetically modified herbicide tolerant oilseed rape (*Brassicanapus*) in the UK. Gene flow and agriculture: Relevance for Transgenic crops. 1999 *BCC Symposium Proceedings* No.72 pp. 72-81.

Voelker, T. A., Worrell, A. C., Anderson, L., Bleinbaum, J., Fane, C., Hawkins, D.J., Radke, S.E and Davis, H. M. (1992) Fatty acid biosynthesis redirected to medium chains in trangenic oil seed plants. *Science*, (257): 872-874.

Wilson, P.J, Boatman, N.D. and Edwards P.J. (1990) Strategies for the conservation of endangered arable weeds in Great Britain. *Proceedings of the European Weed Research Society Symposium 1990*: Integrated Weed Management in Cereals pp. 93-100. *European Weed Research Society*, Helsinki.

Ye, S., Al-babili, s., Kloeti, A., Zhang, J., Lucca, P., Beyer, P. and Potrykus, I. (2000) Engineering the provitan in A (Beta Carotene) biosynthetic pathway into (Carotenoid free) rich endosperm. *Science* (287): 303-305.

Microbial Biotechnology and Ecology (2011) Pages 484–500
Editors: Deepak Vyas, G.S. Paliwal, P.K.Khare and R.K Gupta
Published by: DAYA PUBLISHING HOUSE, NEW DELHI

Chapter 27

Plant DNA Banking for Biodiversity Assessment and Conservation Research

☆ *D. Thangadurai*[1], *M.A.A. Pinheirho De Car Valho*[2], *D.P. Biradar*[3], *Hemanth K.N. Vasathaiah*[4], *B. Suresh*[5] *and Ganesh R. Hegde*[6]

[1]*Department of Botany, Karnatak University, Dharwad – 580 003*
[2]*ISO Plexis Germplasm Bank, Department of Biology, University of Madeira, Funchal 9000-390, Portugal*
[3]*Department of Agronomy, UAS, Dharwad – 580 005*
[4]*Center for Viticulture and Small Fruit Research, Florida A and M University, 6505 Mahan Drive, Tallahassee, Florida 32317, USA*
[5]*Department of Applied Genetics, Karnatak University, Dharwad – 580 003*
[6]*Department of Botany, Sri Krishnadevaraya University, Anantapur – 515 003*

Introduction

The sequencing of plant genomes opened new frontiers in conservation of their biodiversity and genetic improvement. The advances in gene isolation and sequencing in many plant species allows to envisage that within a few years, gene-bank curators may replace their large cold stores of seeds with plant DNA bank that will be electronically stored (Deutsche Forschungsgemeinschaft, 2008). The characterization of plant genomes will ultimately create a true DNA bank, which should possess a large and accessible gene inventory of today's non-characterized plant gene pools (Willis and van Wyk, 2006). Of course, seed banks of comprehensively investigated stocks should remain because geneticists and plant breeders, the main users of gene banks, will need this germplasm for their work (Klenk, 2008). Genomics may accelerate the utilization of candidate genes available at these gene banks through transformation without barriers across plant species or other living kingdoms (de Vicente and Andersson, 2006). Nonetheless, genetic engineering should be seen as one of the methods of plant breeding that permits the direct alteration and re-building of a crop population. 'Shutting-off' genes coding for undesired characteristics may be another application of transgenics in crop improvement (de Vicente *et al.*, 2006; Moore and Ming, 2008).

There are many areas of basic and strategic research in plant breeding and genetics that are being facilitated by marker-aided analysis (Paterson, 1996). With molecular markers, plant biologists are reviewing crop evolution and gathering new knowledge. Such information should be incorporated into genetic enhancement programmes, especially those with an evolutionary breeding scheme. Likewise, plant ideotypes for each crop should drive the work of plant breeders (Jan Engels and Visser, 2003). Specific plant morphotypes have been defined in rice and wheat based on accumulated knowledge of crop physiology and crop protection (de Vicente and Andersson, 2006). The needed characteristics required to develop improved plant prototypes ensuing from such a 'virtual breeding' approach may be available in gene banks of the crop or in those of other species. Otherwise, breeders may obtain novel transgenes to develop the required ideotype (Zetzsche and Gemeinholzer, 2007).

Nowadays, the finding of new genes that add value to agricultural products seems to be very important in the private agri-business (Dunwell, 2000). Unique gene databases are being assembled by the industry with the massive amount of data generated by genomics research (Jauhar, 2006). A new term 'bioresource' was coined recently to refer to a fast and effective licensed technology of pinpointing genes. With this method, a 'benign' virus infects a plant with a specific gene that allows researchers to observe directly its phenotype (Henry, 2006). Bioresource replaces the standard time-consuming approach of first mapping a gene to subsequently determine its exact function (Sharma *et al.*, 2000). Gene identification in DNA libraries coupled with bioresource technology and an enhanced ability to put genes into plants will be routine for improving crops in the next decade (Li *et al.*, 2001).

Plant DNA banks played a crucial role in restoring crop diversity lost during emergencies in Cambodia, across Africa and in the Middle East. These instances highlight the value and importance of accurate characterization and documentation of DNA bank accessions, so that the right materials can be found quickly and targeted appropriately. Several crops are more difficult to conserve (de Vicente and Andersson, 2006). Potatoes, yams and cassava, for example, are not generally propagated by seed but are grown from tubers or other plant parts. The storage organs of such crops may be kept under cool conditions and at an appropriate humidity (Henry, 2006). But they take up much more space than seed, and must be regenerated (replanted) much more frequently, making it considerably more expensive to conserve such crops than those that can be stored as seeds (de Vicente and Andersson, 2006). Alternatively, root and tuber crops, as well as crops that do not produce seed at all (such as banana and plantain), or that produce seed that dies when it is dried and cooled (such as many tropical fruit species), can be maintained as living collections of plants growing in the field; these are called field gene banks (ETC, 2002; Johnson, 2008). However, such collections are very susceptible to natural hazards–pests, diseases and adverse weather–and it is desirable to also maintain them in more protected conditions (Frankel *et al.*, 1995; Smale, 2000). Thus collections of crops that cannot be stored as seed, are often maintained as DNA. But as the technical complexity of conservation increases, so does the cost (Virchow, 2003).

Modern agriculture entirely depends on the genetic and population diversity of a particular crop. If a new rice disease appears, researchers can search the DNA for resistant varieties. The alleles required to make rice more tolerant of drought, for example, exist within the varieties contained in the collection (Mc Cullum *et al.*, 2003; Purty *et al.*, 2008). The DNA bank contains the genetic diversity helps in identifying such germplasm for genetic improvement purposes. Hence, this article summarizes information on different strategies to plant DNA bank (Henry, 2006).

Diversity and Distribution of Plant Genetic Resources

To exercise national sovereignty over its genetic resources, documentation and characterization of biodiversity based on various approaches, is a prerequisite for any country on the globe. In most instances, genetic diversity is the key to developing crop varieties from wild species. Variability of genetic traits allows some plants in a population to adapt to particular conditions and climates, to be more palatable to humans, or to be more resistant to attacks by pests and disease. Seeds selected from genetically diverse, wild populations performed with varied success in subsequent years. Regional varieties developed as seeds were continuously grown and selected from the same location. When humans began transporting seeds around the globe, regional varieties emerged in diverse regions from diverse cultures (de Vicente and Andersson, 2006). Today for example, we have regional varieties of chiles from Thailand, China, Europe, and even our local improved variety from Araku Valley, all of which derived from a common ancestral gene pool in South America. Human agricultural influence increased genetic diversity within a species by moving it from region to region and propagating it from year to year. Until the twentieth century, it was farmers working with open-pollinated crops who were the plant breeders (Henry, 2006).

During the last century, much has changed with the discovery of genetics and the development of the hybrid seed industry (Griliches, 1991). Hybrids (made from crossing two inbred, open-pollinated varieties) were revolutionary, exhibiting the extreme uniformity advantageous to mechanized farming. Additionally, in certain crops, hybrid varieties exhibited increased vigor compared to some open-pollinates (Peferoen, 1997). Hybrids, however, not only appear uniform, but are genetically extremely uniform, further limiting crop genetic diversity. The first hybrid seed sold to the public was a corn variety developed by Pioneer Seed in the 1920's (Griliches, 1991). Its success came, in part, because corn is one of the crops that benefit most from hybridization (Morrisa *et al.*, 1998). However, due to its success, farmers were quick to adopt hybrid varieties of other crop species that may not have exhibited such improvement. Throughout the 1930s and 40s, hybrids swept the marketplace. As farmers shifted from saving seed to buying from 'professionals', the culture of seed saving dwindled (Pray 2003).

Today, genetic diversity is further reduced by the modern biotechnology industry (Komen and Persley, 1993; Deeds *et al.*, 1997). Rapid reproduction of tissue cultures creates fields of genetically identical plants (de Carolis and Deeds, 1999). The insertion of genetic material in crops places the same genes into each plant. In addition, genetically modified genes pose a threat to our crop species' wild progenitors growing within their regions of origin (Uzogara, 2000). Currently, there is a heated controversy over whether genetically modified genes have been found in land race and wild species of corn growing in Oaxaca, Mexico, modern corn's genetic birthplace (Giesecke, 2000).

The concern is a scrubby wild plant could hold the key to agricultural improvements of enormous value to struggling farmers and the nutrient-deprived poor (Dale, 1992). For example, wild relatives of crops such as the brassicas have great potential to assist in crop improvement. The wild relatives of crops, which include crop ancestors as well as other species more or less closely related to them, have been an important part of crop improvement programme for over 60 years (Raybould and Gray, 1993). Genes from wild relatives have provided crops with resistance to pests and diseases, enhanced tolerance to abiotic stresses and have made possible the production of hybrid varieties and improved quality traits such as protein content (de Vicente and Andersson, 2006). Some successful examples of the use of wild relatives in crop improvement include the introduction of resistance to potato late blight (the disease that caused the Irish famine of the 1800s); the production of rice hybrids, currently planted on 45 per cent of China's rice-growing area; and increased soluble solid content in tomatoes, a trait worth US$240 million per year (Xiao *et al.*, 1998).

A recent study of the presence of genes from crop wild relatives in released varieties of 16 mandate crops of the Future Harvest Centres highlights the successful use of wild relatives in breeding programmes (Hilder and Boulter, 1999; Johnson *et al.*, 2003; Bragdon *et al.*, 2005). While breeding efforts continue to emphasize the use of pest and disease resistance genes, a wider range of characteristics are being introduced from wild relatives than in the past, such as drought tolerance, ability to cope with high or low temperatures, enhanced yield and quality traits such as higher levels of iron (Pasternak, 1987; Plucknett, 1987; Giri and Laxmi, 2000; Smith and Dilday, 2002). Nevertheless, crop wild relatives are still under exploited. Recent advances in molecular technologies and improved interspecies crossing procedures have overcome many genetic and agronomic barriers to using wild relatives in breeding programmes (Jarvis and Hodgkin, 2002). It is hoped that this development will foster greater recognition of the importance and value of using wild relatives in crop improvement (Stewart *et al.*, 2003).

Global Loss of Plant Genetic Resources

The world's biota is under siege with a human population nearing 6 billion places unprecedented pressures on the biosphere (Altieri and Merrick, 1987). Approximately 95 per cent of the terrestrial surface is now occupied by human settlements or ecosystems managed for food and materials production. As a result, natural ecosystems are destroyed and fragmented, species are destroyed or doomed, and global genetic diversity is diminished (Cohen *et al.*, 1991). The scale of this destruction directly threatens human civilization, which is dependent in numerous ways on biological diversity. The enormity of the crisis has stimulated international efforts to conserve biological diversity and to ensure sustainable use of its components (Ellstrand and Elam, 1993).

The world is facing a biodiversity crisis of unprecedented magnitude. Unless there are radical changes in human behavior, we can expect significant and alarming species loss in the near future. For a few reasons, DNA banks have great potential as tools for biodiversity conservation, yet few have been established (Francisco-Ortega *et al.*, 2000). One reason to conserve crop diversity in DNA banks is that it is under threat elsewhere. Habitats continue to be destroyed and with the habitats go the plants. One of the main threats to crop diversity is modern agriculture. As new varieties are taken up by farmers because they offer genuine benefits, they may displace the diversity that was there before (de Vicente and Andersson, 2006). This is especially ironic because all plant breeding is built on existing crop diversity, which makes it imperative that this diversity be conserved and remain available somewhere (Fowler and Hodgkin, 2004). Crop diversity, once lost, is impossible to replace (Henry, 2006).

DNA: The Molecule of Heredity

DNA is a very long, threadlike macromolecule made up of large number of deoxy ribonucleotides, each composed of a base, a sugar and a phosphate group. The bases of DNA molecules carry genetic information, whereas their sugar and phosphate group performs a structural role. This hereditary molecule in recent times can be used to find answers to many unresolved biological questions (Avise *et al.*, 1987). In any given eukaryotic organism, this can be isolated, purified, quantified and maintained for many hundreds of years under controlled conditions (Avise 1991).

The Concept of DNA Banking

The accelerated use of genomic technology in biological research portends a changing pattern in the use of genetic resource collections and fuels the desire among researchers to establish DNA banks. Also, DNA banks are very fundamental in organizing a comprehensive 'Encyclopaedia of Life', as envisioned by E.O. Wilson (2003). DNA sequencing of herbarium sheet specimens, cell cultures and germplasm offers a new approach to studies of gene function, evolution, taxonomy and epidemiology among plants. A catalog of unique genetic sequences 'DNA barcodes' can conceptually unite diverse assemblages of repositories under a common registry of sequence accessions (Armstrong and Ball, 2005; Brower, 2006; Rubinoff, 2006). The challenge for DNA repositories of today is to provide a product that is amenable for uses anticipated in the future. Long-term needs will have a decisive impact on operational organization and repository design and a major limitation involves specimen quality and shelf-life (de Vicente and Andersson, 2006).

For many species that are difficult to conserve by conventional means either as seeds or vegetatively or that are highly threatened in the wild, DNA storage may provide the ultimate way to conserve the genetic diversity of these species and their populations in the short term, until effective methods can be developed (Adams, 1997). As progress in biotechnology advances, numerous techniques are in hand now for conserving germplasm, each with their own advantages and disadvantages (Maxted *et al.*, 1997; Maunder *et al.*, 2004). With the recent developments of Marker Assisted Selection and DNA Barconding of plant genetic resources, DNA extraction and storage are regarded as one of the emerging *ex situ* techniques for plant germplasm conservation, management and further future utilization (Ribaut and Hoisington, 1998).

Loosely, it has been argued that DNA banking is an unrealistic option for germplasm conservation given that DNA cannot resurrect extinct species (Maunder *et al.*, 2004); of course, the DNA extracted from those herbarium specimens of extinct species may provide ample evidences to speculate the speciation and evolutionary significance of such plants. In recent times, DNA is the most frequent and easiest forms of germplasm requested from genebanks for research purpose (de Vicente, 2004) especially for molecular, phylogenetic and systematic research in plants (Henry, 2006).

Approaches of *in situ* conservation have been applied most frequently to cultivated plants, landraces and weedy forms, and not so much for the wild relatives of crops (Kennedy, 2004). Collecting and maintaining representative samples of such wild plant populations in the DNA is crucial, though there has been much debate on how much to collect and from how many populations to ensure the maximum of genetic diversity (Brown and Briggs, 1991; Neel and Cummings, 2003). Today, there has been an increasing global concern towards biodiversity assessment and conservation for future generations (Orr, 2003). There are many approaches exclusively available for this purpose, including *in situ*, *ex situ* and combinations of both techniques. Moreover, when compared to animals, plant conservation activities are inexpensive and less time-consuming. In the late 1980s, efforts were made to encourage groups and institutions to establish repositories of genomic DNA in an attempt to complement other conservation efforts. By 1992, thirty one institutions were participating in a network of DNA banks. In addition, a number of international, national and regional DNA banks have now recently been established (Adams, 1997).

With the advent of traditional plant conservation activities such as the management of *ex situ* living collections in seed banks and botanic gardens, and specimen collections in herbaria and museums, it becomes as easy as to extract and store DNA from such collections for various purposes. It has been estimated in the past that the genetic variation in different plant species is in the range of 1 million to 10 million base pairs and that a DNA bank holding such 10 million species on earth (Mattick *et al.*, 1992). It means that, only very little effort is needed to collect and document such DNA as a genetic resource (Ryder *et al.*, 2000).

A DNA bank is a particular type of genetic resource bank that preserves and distributes the DNA molecule and provides associated information. Existing DNA banks usually support agricultural applications, but may also be necessary to support genomic projects in all species. Material stored at the bank is made available through research groups and individuals making donations of plant material and/or DNA. The DNA is stored at –80°C with the equivalent voucher stored within a herbarium. For example, databased information on DNA stocks and associated data on the source plant species is available as given in the Table 27.1. DNA from plants provides endless information about each species. Researchers that can take advantage of these facilities include phylogenetic, phylogeographic and population studies as well as gene discovery and marker development (Hodkinson *et al.*, 2007).

Table 27.1: Databased Information on DNA Stocks and Associated Data on the Source Plant Species Available at Fairchild Tropical Botanic Garden, Florida, USA for Phoenix DNA Samples

Bank ID	*Accession*	*Family*	*Name*
822	93378A	Arecaceae	Phoenix dactylifera 'Zahidi'
1224	76843F	Arecaceae	Phoenix loureiroi
1221	92263B	Arecaceae	Phoenix loureiroi
990	92263C	Arecaceae	Phoenix loureiroi
1009	95255B	Arecaceae	Phoenix paludosa
1010	99875B	Arecaceae	Phoenix paludosa
1011	89800A	Arecaceae	Phoenix roebelenii
1230	P.129B	Arecaceae	Phoenix roebelenii
1005	88536C	Arecaceae	Phoenix rupicola
1222	88536C	Arecaceae	Phoenix rupicola
996	88536E	Arecaceae	Phoenix rupicola

Many of the world's most valuable food crops–including wheat, rice, maize and many pulses–produce seeds that are relatively easy to store. For conservation purposes, the seeds are cleaned, dried, and placed in a sealed jar or packet. For medium term storage (20 to 30 years), the seeds are maintained at a temperature of about 5°C. For long-term storage (up to 100 years or even more) they are kept in cold rooms, or even domestic deep freezers, at –18 to –20°C. Like plant tissue, isolated plant DNA can be stored, enabling the conservation of the genetic make up of plants like seedless banana varieties that would otherwise be difficult or impossible to maintain (de Vicente and Andersson, 2006).

As methods for extraction, purification and amplification of DNA improve, we actually need very little plant material in order to adequately supply molecular labs. In general, it has been recommended to collect about 3-5 square inches of fresh, young plant material, normally 3-5 leaves or cut parts of larger leaves. It is preferable to remove the midrib from leaf material before putting it into silica gel. Scissors or secateurs can be used to cut plant material. Tearing the material will bruise the leaves, releasing enzymes that will breakdown DNA. The most important protocol to follow when collecting material for DNA is getting the plant material to dry quickly and this is accomplished by increasing the surface area (cutting the leaves into smaller pieces) and using an excess of silica gel. The material is then placed in a reclosable plastic bag with enough silica gel to ensure drying of the material in a couple of hours. Once the material is dry, most of the silica gel can be removed from the sample and dehydrated for future use. Indicator silica gel should be used to help to determine the overall 'dryness' of the sample. Once has to check the sample for signs of mold and add fresh silica gel if necessary. Once dry, the sample can be stored at room temperature without degradation of DNA, although it is preferable to store samples at –20°C (de Vicente and Andersson, 2006).

In general, DNA is extracted using a modification of the CTAB protocol and the DNA banded in cesium chloride. Although more time consuming then the rapid methods available today, the quality of the DNA is very high and the quantity is sufficient that one can share it with many people (Liston *et al.*, 1990; Do and Adams, 1991; Adams, 1997). Leaf material is collected in the field and stored in self-sealing plastic bags at 4°C until processed. Voucher specimens collected are deposited at the local herbarium within the country. All extracted DNA is purified, quantified and maintained at –20°C to –80°C (Nickrent, 1994; Gachet *et al.*, 1998; Porteous *et al.*, 2003).

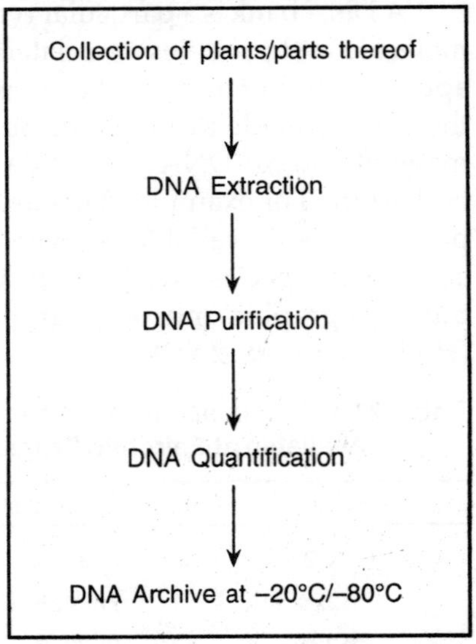

Collection of plants/parts thereof
↓
DNA Extraction
↓
DNA Purification
↓
DNA Quantification
↓
DNA Archive at –20°C/–80°C

Figure 27.1: An Overview of Steps Involved in the Process of Plant DNA Banking at –20°C/–80°C

Plant DNA Banks Around the World

Several international and national efforts have been documented to establish DNA banks worldwide. As plant genes are now being sequenced and barcoded, access to continuous supply of DNA samples from individuals is of great deal in biodiversity and molecular research. Although, DNA banks exist in many countries and in different regions of the world, there is no effective coordination among DNA banks. Also the value of DNA banking to develop conservation and population management strategies is immense. DNA bank also provides the opportunity of analyzing data from the wild and helps in the development of conservation strategies (de Vicente and Andersson, 2006).

In the 1980s, attempts were made to create the plant 'DNA Bank-Net' (Adams, 1988; Adams and Adams, 1992). Unfortunately, the DNA Bank-Net initiative has remained inactive until recently (Ryder *et al.*, 2000; Savolainen and Reeves, 2004). Although there have been more than 1500 genebanks, less than twenty plant DNA banks are operational in various geographical regions of the world, with specific theme of collections of their own country's plant genetic resources and/or exotic germplasm if any (Table 1). Among them, most well known DNA banks are at the Royal Botanic Gardens, UK and the National Herbarium, Netherlands (Adams, 1992). One can deposit and request DNA of a kind of genetic material there are interested to study (Adams *et al.*, 1992). For students and scientists, this will be given at free of cost for research purpose and for others, a nominal charge of around 25USD will be charged for each DNA sample OF 25μL (Adams, 1993; Adams, 1994). These DNA banks will also do DNA extraction for outside people on specific requests (Adams *et al.*, 1999).

Plant DNA Bank: An Indian Scenario

Many of India's natural habitats are under threat and the species within them face potential extinction. Increased pressures from agricultural practices, industry, recreational pursuits and an expanding population has seen India's native flora decline. In order to better manage and preserve our botanical heritage, we need to understand the diversity within our native flora (Harlan, 1975). In this connection, it is necessary to build the research and conservation potential of plant scientists and

Table 27.2: List of Major Plant DNA Banks Around the World

Name of the DNA Bank	*Place and Country*	*Website*
Missouri Botanical Garden	Missouri, USA	http://www.mobot.org/MOBOT/research/diversity dna_banking.htm
Fairchild Tropical Botanic Garden	Florida, USA	www.fairchildgarden.org/
South African National Biodiversity Institute	Capetown, South Africa	http://www.nbi.ac.za/
Kew Royal Botanic Garden	Surrey, Great Britain	http://www.kew.org/data/dnaBank/homepage.html
Australian Plant DNA bank Ltd	Centre for Plant Conservation Genetics, Southern Cross University, Lismore, Australia	http://www.biobank.com
Irish DNA Bank	Trinity College, Dublin, Ireland	www.tcd.ie/
Brazil Plant DNA Bank	Instituo de Pesquisas, Jardim Botanico de Rio de Janeiro, Rio, Brazil	http://www.jbrj.gov.br/pesquisa/div_molecular/ bancodna/index_ing.htm
University of Hawaii	Hawaii	www.hawaii.edu
National Herbarium	Netherlands	www.nationaalherbarium.nl
The Berlin-Dahlem DNA bank	Germany	www.bgbm.org/bgbm/research/dna
NIAS DNA bank	National Institute of Agrobiological Sciences, Ibaraki, Japan	www.dna.affrc.go.jp/
The Plant DNA bank of Korea	South Korea	www.pdbk.korea.ac.kr
DNA Bank	International Rice Research Institute, Philippines	www.irri.org/grc
Italian Plant DNA Bank	Institute of Plant Genetics (CNR), Bari, Italy	http://www.inaav.ba.cnr.it
CATIE DNA Bank	Turrialba, Costa Rica	http://www.catie.ac.cr
RIPF DNA Bank	Pomologiczna, Poland	http://www.insad.pl
CIRAD DNA Bank	Montpellier, France	http://www.cirad.fr

Table 27.3: Potential Centers of Plant DNA Banking Possibilities within India

Institute and Place	*State*	*Special Interest*
National Botanical Research Institute, Lucknow	Uttar Pradesh	Wild plants
NRC for Banana, Trichy	Tamil Nadu	Bananas and Plantains
Central Institute of Medicinal and Aromatic Plants, Lucknow	Uttar Pradesh	Medicinal and Aromatic Plants
Central Drug Research Institute, Lucknow	Uttar Pradesh	Medicinal and Aromatic Plants
Tropical Botanic Garden and Research Institute, Palode	Kerala	Trees, woody lianas, orchids, bamboos, medicinal, aromatic, rare and threatened plants
Indian Institute of Horticultural Research, Bangalore	Karnataka	Wild and cultivated forms of fruit, vegetable, floricultural and horticultural crops
Institute of Forest Genetics and Tree Breeding, Coimbatore	Tamil Nadu	Tree, timber and forest species
Botanical Survey of India	Throughout India	Angiosperms, gymnosperms and the entire Indian flora
Central Potato Research Institute, Shimla	Himachal Pradesh	Potato
GB Pant Institute of Himalayan Environment & Development, Almora	Uttarakhand	Himalayan Species
National Research Centre for Soybean, Indore	Madhya Pradesh	Soybean
National Research Centre for Sorghum, Hyderabad	Andhra Pradesh	Sorghum
National Research Centre for Orchids, Pakyong	Sikkim	Orchids
National Research Centre for Onion and Garlic, Pune	Maharashtra	Onion and garlic
National Research Centre for Medicinal & Aromatic Plants, Boriavi	Gujarat	Medicinal and Aromatic Plants
National Research Centre for Grapes, Pune	Maharashtra	Grapes
National Research Centre for Cachew, Puttur	Karnataka	Cachew
National Bureau of Plant Genetic Resources, Pusa	New Delhi	Agri-horticultural crops
Sugarcane Breeding Institute, Coimbatore	Tamil Nadu	Sugarcane
Indian Institute of Vegetable Research, Varanasi	Uttar Pradesh	Vegetable Crops
Indian Institute of Sugarcane Research, Lucknow	Uttar Pradesh	Sugarcane
Indian Institute of Spices Research, Calicut	Kerala	Spices
Indian Institute of Pulses Research, Kanpur	Uttar Pradesh	Pulses
Indian Grassland and Fodder Research Institute, Jhansi	Uttar Pradesh	Grass and fodder species
Central Tuber Crops Research Institute, Thiruvananthapuram	Kerala	Tuber crops
Central Rice Research Institute, Cuttack	Orissa	Rice
Central Plantation Crops Research Institute, Kasaragod	Kerala	Plantation Crops
Central Institute for Cotton Research, Nagpur	Maharashtra	Cotton
Central Agricultural Research Institute, Port Blair	Andaman & Nicobar Islands	Agri-horticultural crops
National Research Centre for DNA Fingerprinting, Pusa	New Delhi	Agri-horticultural crops and their wild relatives

conservationists in India by setting up a unique archive of plant genetic resources in the form of a DNA bank, and to formulate a policy framework and supporting documents to facilitate its scientific use under strict control and in line with developing CBD policy on access to genetic resources. The establishment of the Indian Plant DNA Bank will provide a repository for DNA samples as a resource to be utilized in plant research by current and future generations. It serves as a historical record of plant diversity and a foundation for conservation genetics and biotechnology. India is one of the 12 megadiverse countries in the world, also provided with two hotspots (Reid, 1998). Hence, our ultimate aim should focus on to preserve representative genetic information from the entire Indian flora. In the field of plant diversity conservation, DNA storage is not very common and little information is available about its practice in India. Moreover, the technical capacity and financial resources for DNA banking are currently very limited in most of the developing countries including India.

Collective efforts have to be made to catalogue, characterize and preserve representative genetic information in the form of genomic DNA from the entire Indian flora, with the aim of facilitating taxonomic and evolutionary studies world-wide by way of inclusion of genetic diversity of plant genetic resources available in the country. By way of honoring the spirit of the Convention on Biological Diversity, emphasis has to be placed over the next few years to extract DNA (and voucher) of all Indian plant species at national institutes and research centers of excellence, universities and of course in botanic gardens. Efforts have also to be made in extracting DNA from the existing herbarium sheets of such extinct/extinct in the wild/endangered species. The focus of an exclusive Indian Plant DNA Bank should be on the collection of India native flora and aims not only to include a representative of each known species but also to capture the within and between species genetic variations.

Of the approximately 17,000 vascular plant species reported to exist in India, nearly 15 per cent are under threat (Ahmedullah, 1999). In Sikkim state of India alone, 60 per cent of the plant species are endemic (Myers, 1988), while 33 per cent of the total Indian flora is endemic to the country (TERI, 2004). With very high and varied diversity of flora, India possesses 11.9 per cent of the recorded world's plants including 49,219 higher plant species and is homeland of 167 cultivated species and 329 wild relatives of crop plants. It has about 30,000 to 50,000 indigenous land races of cultivated plants. In the past three decades, there has been an increasing concern towards the loss of biodiversity due to human and natural factors. Consequently, countrywide efforts have to be made towards conservation of wild and cultivated genetic resources. Since DNA extraction is the routine activity of numerous laboratories working in diverse areas of genetics, biochemistry, molecular biology and biotechnology across the country, DNA of the same can be deposited in any of the authorized DNA repositories in place of voucher specimens of conventional herbariums.

The very purpose of the DNA bank should be to collect, extract and store genomic DNA from all the available plant genetic resources in the country with their wide range of genetic and population diversity. This is in fact can be of special interest for the presence of useful their genes, which can be easily traced from the DNA available in the bank.

The Applications

The plant DNA banks have been solely for the purpose of supporting molecular phylogenetics and can be used only for the study of relationships of plants or for studies aimed at improving our understanding of evolutionary mechanisms. They may not be used for bioprospecting endeavors, screening for genes of interest in agricultural research, or any other commercial application (Henry, 2006). Although, the plant DNA banks can also be used by the scientific community for purposes such as conservation genetics, biodiscovery, plant breeding support, and as quality assurance standards in certain cases. A facility like this will also be advantageous to the research community by reducing the costs often associated with field trips to collect plant specimens. It will also make material from highly protected species available to a wider range of researchers. The DNA bank is one way of saving as many rare plants as possible from extinction (de Vicente and Andersson, 2006).

In course of time, it will become very easier to exchange genetic resources as DNA samples, rather than seed or vegetative propagules, which normally requires time consuming phytosanitary certification procedures and protocols. As molecular analyses are particularly useful in determining bottlenecks and historical events, population structure and phylogenetic and phylogeographic relationships in plants, extraction and storage of DNA is of immense practical value (Brown *et al.*, 1997; Frankham *et al.*, 2002). Herbaria normally maintain only specimens for the purpose of identification and classification based on morphology, whereas a DNA bank keeps tissues for the purpose of DNA extraction and use in molecular based research (de Vicente and Andersson, 2006).

Now a days, plant DNA banks have an enormous potential to collect, conserve and utilize a great deal of information about plant genetic diversity (Mattick *et al.*, 1992). Even more, the assessment of genetic variability within plant populations has made valuable contributions to conservation genetics of rare and threatened species (Byrne, 2005). There are a number of ways by which DNA banks could make an impact in the foreseeable future (de Vicente and Andersson, 2006). Most promising possibilities are to monitor changes in population genetic structure, to assess genetic diversity, to disclose taxonomic relationships, to search for new gene variants, to develop new markers, to identify and to trace typical plant products (Henry, 2006). Moreover, the applications of plant DNA banks on genetic diversity studies, germplasm management, genebank management and germplasm use are of immense practical utility (de Vicente and Andersson, 2006).

Conclusion and Future Prospects

This article focused on the utilitarian value of genetic diversity in terms of plant DNA bank. This is something novel and applicable to our economic and political world in the near future. Certainly the value of genetic diversity is immense, and DNA banking is one example. But some hold that a merely utilitarian view of biodiversity can never succeed in conserving it in that our orientation towards the use of nature is the root cause of the crisis. The refusal by the USA to sign ICBD indicates how a focus on the utility of conservation can hamper cooperation. This point of view has been articulated eloquently by many American thinkers (Thoreau, Leopold, Carson, Abbey and others). Recently, Ehrenfeld asks us to consider conservation not for its utility, but because it is simply the right thing to do.

Interestingly, roughly as many developing as developed countries conserve DNA, although developing countries report greater difficulties in procuring the necessary equipment. Responses from developing countries, in particular, displayed considerable lack of knowledge and insecurity concerning the applications of DNA banking and associated logistical issues. The crucial needs are more and better information about the possible advantages of DNA banking and broader discussion among the scientific community of the opportunities and limitations it provides. Also, issues related to DNA exchange, intellectual property rights and patent laws must be resolved. Policy research is urgently needed in these areas to devise solutions for closing legal gaps and to make DNA storage a more broadly viable crop diversity conservation practice (Correa, 1995; Leskien and Flitner, 1997; Lesser, 1998; Hoisington *et al.*, 1999; Serageldin, 1999; Swanson and Göschla, 2000).

Also, DNA banking is of crucial importance and contributes a pivotal role in the case of critically endangered/threatened species where very few populations or even individuals exist, the entire genepool can be collected and maintained as DNA extracts as one of the measure of *ex situ* collections, in order to represent the maximum available genetic diversity in these collections (Pflieger *et al.*, 2001; Dolezel and Bartos, 2005). However, the management and mobilization of such DNA materials should be well regulated to comply with the provisions of Convention on Biological Diversity and the International Treaty on Plant Genetic Resources for Food and Agriculture (Kate and Laird, 2000; FAO, 2004). Nevertheless, most felt that DNA storage would be very useful for future research, gene/genome conservation and safety duplication. Thus, plant DNA banks are the technology for the near future.

References

Adam, R.P. (1993). The conservation and utilization of genes from endangered and extinct plants: DNA Bank-Net. In: *Gene Conservation and Exploitation* (Ed. Gustafson, J.), pp. 35-52, Plenum Press, New York.

Adams, R.P. (1988). *The preservation of genomic DNA: DNA Bank-Net*. University of California, Davis, USA.

Adams, R.P. (1992). DNA Bank-Net to use DNA technology to save endangered germplasm. *Diversity* 8: 23.

Adams, R.P. (1993). DNA Bank-Net : An international network of DNA banks and *in vitro* storage institutions. *AgBiotech News and Information* 5: 317N-319N.

Adams, R.P. (1994). DNA Bank-Net: An overview. In: *Conservation of Plant Genes II. Utilization of Ancient and Modern DNA* (Eds. Adams, R.P., Miller, J.S, Goldenberg, E.M., Adams, J.E.), pp. 1-13, Missouri Botanical Garden Press, St. Louis.

Adams, R.P. (1997). Conservation of DNA: DNA banking. In: *Biotechnology and Plant Genetic Resources: Conservation and Use* (Eds. Callow, J.A., Ford-Lloyd, B.V., Newbury, H.J.), pp. 163-174, CAB International, Wallingford, UK.

Adams, R.P. (1997). Conservation of DNA: DNA banking. In: *Biotechnology and Plant Genetic Resources* (Eds. Callow, J.A., Ford-Lloyd, B.V., Newbury, H.J.), pp. 163-174, CAB International, Wallingford, UK.

Adams, R.P., Adams, J.E. (1992). Conservation of Plant Genes. *DNA banking and in vitro Biotechnology*. Academic Press, San Diego, USA.

Adams, R.P., Do, N., Gelin, C. (1992). Preservation of DNA in plant specimens from tropical species by desiccation. In: *Conservation of Plant Genes and In vitro Biotechnology* (Eds. Adams, R.P., Adams, J.E.), pp. 135-152, Academic Press, New York.

Adams, R.P., Zhong, M., Fei, Y. (1999). Preservation of DNA in plant specimens: Inactivation and re-activation of DNases in field specimens. *Molecular Biology* 8: 681-684.

Ahmedullah, A. (1999). Country report on red listing of plants in India. In: Using the IUCN red list criteria at the national level: A regional consultative workshop for South and South Asia. http://www.biodiversityasia.org/ebook/html

Altieri, M.A., Merrick, L. (1987). *In situ* conservation of crop genetic resources through maintenance of traditional farming systems. *Journal Economic Botany* 41: 86-96.

Armstrong, K.F., Ball, S.L. (2005). DNA barcodes for biosecurity: Invasive species identification. *Philosophical Transactions of the Royal Society B. Biological Sciences* 360: 1813-1823.

Avise, J.C. (1991). Ten unorthodox perspectives on evolution prompted by comparative population genetic findings on mitochondrial DNA. *Annual Review of Genetics* 25: 45-69.

Avise, J.C., Arnold, J., Ball, R.M., Bermingham, E., Lamb, T., Neigel, J.E., Reeb, CA., Saunders, N.C. (1987). Intraspecific Phylogeography: The Mitochondrial DNA Bridge Between Population Genetics and Systematics. *Annual Review of Ecology and Systematics* 18: 489-522.

Bragdon, S., Fowler, C., França, Z., Goldberg, E. (2005). Law and Policy of Relevance to the Management of Plant Genetic Resources. Learning Module with Review of Regional Policy Instruments, Developments and Trends. 2nd edn. The CGIAR System-wide Genetic Resources Programme (SGRP), the International Plant Genetic Resources Institute (IPGRI) and the International Food Policy Research Institute (IFPRI), IPGRI, Rome, Italy.

Brower, A.V.Z. (2006). Problems with DNA barcodes for species delimitation: 'ten species' of *Astraptes fulgerator* reassessed (Lepidoptera: Hesperiidae). *Systematics and Biodiversity* 4: 127-132.

Brown, A.H.D., Briggs, J.D. (1991). Sampling strategies for genetic variation in *ex situ* collections of endangered plant species. In: Genetics and conservation of rare plants (Eds. Falk, D.A., Holsinger, K.E.), pp. 99-119, Oxford University Press, New York.

Brown, A.H.D., Brubaker, C.L., Grace, J.P. (1997). Regeneration of germplasm samples: Wild versus cultivated plant species. *Crop Sci.* 37: 7-13.

Byrne, C.A. (2005). Genetic variation in plant populations: Assessing cause and pattern. In: *Plant Diversity and Evolution* (Ed. Henry, R.J.), pp. 139-165, CABI Publishing, Wallingford, UK.

Cohen, J.I., Williams, J.T., Plucknett, D.L., Shands, H. (1991). *Ex situ* conservation of plant genetic resources: Global development and environmental concerns. *Science* 253: 866–872.

Correa, C.M. (1995). Sovereign and property rights over plant genetic resources. *Journal Agriculture and Human Values* 12: 58-79.

Dale, P.J. (1992). Spread of Engineered Genes to Wild Relatives. *Plant Physiology* 100: 13-15.

de Carolis, D.M., Deeds, D.L. (1999). The impact of stocks and flows of organizational knowledge on firm performance: an empirical investigation of the biotechnology industry. *Strategic Management Journal* 20: 953–968.

de Vicente, M.C. (2004). The Evolving Role of Genebanks in the Fast-developing Field of Molecular Genetics. Issues in Genetic Resources No. 11, International Plant Genetic Resources Institute (IPGRI), Rome, Italy.

de Vicente, M.C., Andersson, M.S. (2006). DNA banks–providing novel options for genebanks? Topical Reviews in Agricultural Biodiversity. International Plant Genetic Resources Institute, Rome, Italy.

de Vicente, M.C., Carmen de Vicente, M., Andersson, M.S. (2006). DNA banks–providing novel options for genebanks? Bioversity International, Italy.

de Vicente, M.Cl., Andersson, M.S. (2006). DNA banks–providing novel options for genebanks? International Plant Genetic Resources Institute, Rome, Italy.

Deeds, D.L., Decarolis, D., Coombs, J.E. (1997). The impact of firmspecific capabilities on the amount of capital raised in an initial public offering: Evidence from the biotechnology industry. *Journal of Business Venturing* 1: 31-46.

Deutsche Forschungsgemeinschaft. (2008). DFG Biodiversity Research. Wiley-VCH Verlag, Weinheim, pp. 47-52.

Do, N., Adams, R.P. (1991). A simple technique for removing plant polysaccharide contaminants from DNA. *BioTechniques* 10: 162-166.

Dolezel, J., Bartos, J. (2005). Plant DNA flow cytometry and estimation of nuclear genome size. *Annals of Botany* 95: 99-110.

Dunwell, J.M. (2000). Transgenic approaches to crop improvement. *Journal of Experimental Botany* 51: 487-496.

Ellstrand, N.C., Elam, D.R. (1993). Population genetic consequences of small population size: Implications for plant conservation. *Annual Review of Ecology and Systematics* 24: 217-242.

ETC. (2002). GM pollution in the gene bank? *Biotechnology and Development Monitor* 49: 24.

FAO. (2004). The International Treaty on Plant Genetic Resources for Food and Agriculture. Food and Agriculture Organization of the United Nations (FAO), Rome, Italy.

Fowler, C., Hodgkin, T. (2004). Plant genetic resources for food and agriculture: Assessing global availability. *Annual Review of Environment and Resources* 29: 143-179.

Francisco-Ortega, J., Santos-Guerra, A., Kim, S.G., Crawford, D.J. (2000). Plant genetic diversity in the Canary Islands: a conservation perspective. *American Journal of Botany* 87: 909-919.

Frankel, O.H., Brown, A.H.D., Burdon, J.J. James. (1995). The Conservation of Plant Biodiversity. Cambridge University Press, Cambridge.

Frankham, R., Ballou, J.D., Briscoe, D.A. (2002). Introduction to Conservation Genetics. Cambridge University Press, Cambridge, UK.

Gachet, E., Martin, G.G., Vigneau, F., Meyer, G. (1998). Detection of genetically modified organisms (GMOs) by PCR: a brief review of methodologies. *Trends in Food Science and Technology* 9: 380-388.

Giesecke, S. (2000). The contrasting roles of government in the development of biotechnology industry in the US and Germany. *Research Policy* 29: 205-223.

Giri, C.C., Laxmi, G.V. (2000). Production of transgenic rice with agronomically useful genes: an assessment. *Biotechnology Advances* 18: 653-683.

Griliches, Z. (1991). The Search for R and D Spillovers. NBER Working Paper No. W3768. http://ssrn.com/abstract=248593

Griliches, Z. (1991). The search for R and D spillovers. *NBER Working Paper No. W3768.* http://ssrn.com/abstract=248593

Harlan, J.R. (1975). Our vanishing genetic resources. *Science* 188: 617–621.

Henry, R.J. (2006). Plant Conservation Genetics. Food Products Press, New York.

Hilder, V.A., Boulter, D. (1999). Genetic engineering of crop plants for insect resistance–a critical review. *Crop Protection* 18: 177-191.

Hodkinson, T.E., Waldren, S., Parnell, J.A.N., Kelleher, C.T., Salamin, K., Salamin, N. (2007). DNA banking for plant breeding, biotechnology and biodiversity evaluation. *Journal of Plant Research* 120: 17-29.

Hoisington, D., Khairallah, M., Reeves, T., Ribaut, J.M., Skovmand, B., Taba, S., Warburton, M. (1999). Plant genetic resources: What can they contribute toward increased crop productivity? *PNAS* 96: 5937-5943.

Jan Engels, L., Visser, A. (2003). Guide to effective management of germplasm collections. *Bioversity International*, Italy.

Jarvis, D.I., Hodgkin, T. (2002). Wild relatives and crop cultivars: detecting natural introgression and farmer selection of new genetic combinations in agroecosystems. *Molecular Ecology* 8: S159-S173.

Jauhar, P.P. (2006). Modern biotechnology as an integral supplement to conventional plant breeding: The prospects and challenges. *Crop Sci.* 46: 1841-1859.

Johnson, N.L., Lilja, N., Ashby, J.A. (2003). Measuring the impact of user participation in agricultural and natural resource management research. *Agricultural Systems* 78: 287-306.

Johnson, R.C. (2008). Gene banks pay big dividends to agriculture, the environment, and human welfare. *PLoS Biol.* 6: e148.

Kate, K.T., Laird, S. (2000). *The Commercial Use of Biodiversity- Access to Genetic Resources and Benefit-Sharing*. Earthscan Publications, London, UK.

Kennedy, K.L. (2004). The role of Federal Guidance and State and Federal partnership in *ex situ* plant conservation in the United States. In: *Ex situ plant conservation supporting species survival in the wild* (Eds. Guerrant, E.O., Havens, K., Maunder, M.), pp. 67-83, Island Press, Washington DC, USA.

Klenk, H.-P. (2008). DNA-Bank-Netzwerk etabliert. *BIOspektrum* 1: 86.

Komen, J., Persley, G.J. (1993). Agricultural Biotechnology in Developing Countries: A Cross-Country Review. ISNAR Research Report No. 2 (Intermediary Biotechnology Service). International Service for National Agricultural Research, The Hague.

Leskien, D., Flitner, M. (1997). Intellectual Property Rights and Plant Genetic Resources: Options for a Sui Generis System. Issues in Genetic Resources No. 6. International Plant Genetic Resources Institute, Rome, Italy.

Lesser, W. (1998). Intellectual property rights and concentration in agricultural biotechnology. *Ag. Bio. Forum* 1: 56-61. http: / /www.agbioforum.org

Li, Y., Wu, Y.H., McAvoy, R., Duan, H. (2001). Transgenics in crops. *Biotechnol Annu Rev.* 7: 239-260.

Liston, A., Rieseberg, L.H., Adam, R.P., Do, N. (1990). A method for collecting dried plant specimens for DNA and isozyme analyses, and the results of a field test in xinjiang, China. *Ann. Missouri Bot. Gard.* 77: 859-863.

Mattick, J.S., Ablett, E.M., Edmonson, D.L. (1992). The Gene Library: Preservation and analysis of genetic diversity in Australasia. In: Conservation of Plant Genes: DNA Banking and *in vitro* Biotechnology. (Eds. Adams, R.P., Adams, J.E.), pp. 15–35, Academic Press, San Diego, USA.

Maunder, M., Havens, K., Guerrant Jr. E.O., Falk, D.A. (2004). *Ex situ* methods a vital but underused set of conservation resources. In: *ex situ Plant conservation supporting species survival in the wild* (Eds. Guerrant Jr. E.O., Havens, K., Maunder, M.), pp. 3-20, Island Press, Washington DC, USA.

Maxted, N., Ford-Lloyd, B.V., Hawkes, J.G. (1997). *Plant genetic conservation: The in situ approach.* Chapman and Hall, London, UK.

McCullum, C., Benbrook, C., Knowles, L., Roberts, S., Schryver, T. (2003). Application of modern biotechnology to food and agriculture: Food systems perspective. *Journal of Nutrition Education and Behavior* 35: 319–332.

Moore, P.H., Ming, R. (2008). *Transgenics for new plant products, applications to tropical crops, Volume 1, Genomics of tropical crop plants*, Springer, New York.

Morrisa, M.L., Singh, R.P., Pal, S. (1998). India's maize seed industry in transition: changing roles for the public and private sectors. *Food Policy* 23: 55-71.

Neel, M.C., Cummings, M.P. (2003). Effectiveness of conservation targets in capturing genetic diversity. *Conserv. Biol.* 17: 219-229.

Nickrent, D.L. (1994). From field to film: Rapid sequencing methods for field-collected plant species. *Biotechniques* 16: 470-475.

Pasternak, D. (1987). Salt Tolerance and Crop Production-A Comprehensive Approach. *Annual Review of Phytopathology* 25: 271-291.

Peferoen, M. (1997). Progress and prospects for field use of *bt* genes in crops. *Trends in Biotechnology* 15: 173-177.

Pflieger, S., Lefebvre, V., Causse, M. (2001). The candidate gene approach in plant genetics: a review. *Journal Molecular Breeding* 7: 275-291.

Plucknett, D.L. (1987). *Gene Banks and the World's Food.* International Rice Research Institute, Manila, The Philippines.

Porteous, L.A., Seidler, R.J., Watrud, L.S. (2003). An improved method for purifying DNA from soil for polymerase chain reaction amplification and molecular ecology applications. *Molecular Ecology* 6: 787–791.

Pray, C.E. (2003). Public–private sector linkages in research and development: Biotechnology and the seed industry in Brazil, China and India. *American Journal of Agricultural Economics* 83: 742–747.

Purty, R.M., Kumar, G., Singla-Pareek, S.L., Pareek, A. (2008). Towards salinity tolerance in Brassica: An overview. *Physiology and Molecular Biology of Plants* 14: 39-49.

Raybould, A.F., Gray, A.J. (1993). Genetically modified crops and hybridization with wild relatives: A UK perspective. *Journal of Applied Ecology* 30: 199-219.

Reid, W.V. (1998). Biodiversity hotspots. *Trends in Ecology and Evolution* 13: 275-280.

Ribaut, J.M., Hoisington, D. (1998). Marker-assisted selection: new tools and strategies. *Trends in Plant Science* 3: 236-239.

Rubinoff, D. (2006). Utility of Mitochondrial DNA Barcodes in Species Conservation. *Conservation Biology* 20: 1026–1033.

Ryder, O.A., McLaren, A., Brenner, S., Zhang, Y.-P., Benirschke, K. (2000). DNA banks for endangered animal species. *Science* 288: 275-277.

Savolainen, V., Reeves, G. (2004). A plea for DNA banking. *Science* 304: 1445.

Serageldin, I. (1999). Biotechnology and Food Security in the 21st Century. *Science* 285: 387–389.

Sharma, H.C., Sharma, K.K., Seetharama, N., Ortiz, R. (2000). Prospects for using transgenic resistance to insects in crop improvement. *Electronic Journal of Biotechnology*. http://ejbiotechnology.ucv.cl/content/vol3/issue2/full/3/index.html

Smale, M. (2000). *Farmers, Gene Banks and Crop Breeding: Economic Analyses of Diversity in Wheat, Maize, and Rice*. Kluwer Academic, The Netherlands.

Smith, C.W., Dilday, R.H. (2002). *Rice: Origin, History, Technology, and Production*. John Wiley and Sons, Oxford.

Stewart, Jr, N.C., Halfhill, M.D., Warwick, S.I. (2003). Genetic modification: Transgene introgression from genetically modified crops to their wild relatives. *Nature Reviews Genetics* 4: 806-817.

Swanson, T., Göschla, T. (2000). Property rights issues involving plant genetic resources: implications of ownership for economic efficiency. *Ecological Economics* 32: 75-92.

TERI. (2004). Hot spots in India. http://www.teriin.org/biodiv/hotspot.htm

Uzogara, S.G. (2000). The impact of genetic modification of human foods in the 21st century A review. *Biotechnology Advances* 18: 179-206.

Virchow, D. (2003). *Efficient conservation of crop genetic diversity: Theoretical approaches and empirical studies*. Springer, New York.

Willis, C.K., van Wyk, E. (2006). Integrating *in situ* and *ex situ* conservation. *SANBI Biodiversity Series* 1: 35-39.

Wilson, E.O. (2003). The encyclopaedia of life. *Trends Ecol. Evol.* 18: 77-80.

Xiao, J., Lia, J., Grandillo, S., Ahn, S.N., Yuan, L., Tanksley, S.D., McCouch, S.R. (1998). Identification of trait-improving quantitative trait loci alleles from a wild rice relative, *Oryza rufipogon*. *Genetics* 150: 899-909.

Zetzsche, H., Gemeinholzer, B. (2007). Aufbau eines DNA-Bank-Netzwerkes. *GfBS Newsletter* 18: 32-36.

Microbial Biotechnology and Ecology (2011) *Pages* **501–519**
Editors: **Deepak Vyas, G.S. Paliwal, P.K.Khare and R.K Gupta**
Published by: **DAYA PUBLISHING HOUSE, NEW DELHI**

Chapter 28

Progress in Biotechnology of Guava (*Psidium guajava* L.)

☆ *Nasim Akhtar*

Post Graduate and Research Department of Microbiology and Biotechnology, Al-Ameen Arts Science and Commerce College, Bangalore – 560 027

Introduction

Common guava (*Psidium guajava* L.; Family, Myrtaceae) is a diploid species (2n=22), but known to exist in some natural and artificial forms of triploidy (2n=3x=33), thereby giving seedless fruits. It occupies prime position among the furits crops of winter and stands 4th among the most important fruit crops grown in India after citrus, mango and banana (Annon, 1985). Guava is a potent alternative of apple in the tropical world, as it is a rich source of proteins, carbohydrates, fats, vitamins and minerals, and within the reach of a common man and other poorer sections of society, probably that's why it occupies the prime position among the fruit crops and proudly called as the 'poor men's apple'. It is indemic to tropical America, but has been thorougly naturalized throughout the tropics and subtropics from Mexico to Peru to India. It has widespread commercial exploitations in Florida and Hawain islands, Egypt, South Africa, Brazil, Columbia and West Indies (Purseglov, 1968).

The guava plant is a shallow rooted evergreen or subdeciduous large shrub or sometimes a small tree of 3-10 metre height and about 0.9 metre girth. The stem is irregular and fluted when old, branching close to the ground and often produces suckers from root near the base of trunk. Leaves are opposite with oblong to elliptical lamina with variable size (5-15 cm × 3-7 cm). Flowers are epigynous and bisexual (perfect), axillary, solitary or born in 2-3 flowered cyme. Calyx is adnate to bud and persistent. Stamens are numerous and inserted in rows on disc. The anthers are pale yellow in colour dehiscence

* E-mail: nasimakhtar01@yahoo.co.in

longitudinally. Ovary, which is 4-5 locular bears numerous bitegmic ovules in axile placentation. The fruit is a berry, surmounted by calyx lobes and is variable in shape (globose, ovoid or pyriform), skin colour, flesh, taste and flavour. Usually numerous bony, reniform seeds are present in pulp having curved embryos (Purseglove, 1968; Mitra and Bose, 1985; Singh, 1985).

Guava prefers to grow on deep, friable, well drained soil and known to tolerate a soil pH in the range of 4.5 to 8.2, as well as mild conditions of salinity, water-logging and high temepratures, but highly susceptible to low temperature and frost. On comparative ground, it has been found more resistant to drought than other perennial fruit crops. It has been successfully grown in the habitats ranging from tropics to subtropics and from sea level to 5,000 ft; and therefore, can be made adaptable for a wide ranging of agro-climatic zones.

Both self and cross pollination occur in *Psidium guajava* L. The flowers are visited by bees and other insects. Natural cross pollination has been shown to be about 30-35 per cent (Singh, 1985). Fruit setting takes place even in unopen or partially opened flower buds without exposing stigma and anthers conferring self pollination or closed pollination. The flower buds to be cross pollinated are fully opened exposing all floral organs and usually with styles longer than the stamens.

It is cultivated mainly for its delicious sweet, juicy fruits, which are rich in proteins, carbohydrates, minerals, sugars, oils and vitamins (mainly Vitamin-C) and therefore, canned for jams, jellies marmalades, pies, ketchups, chutney and nectar (Annon, 1985).

Guava produces as many as three crops in a year. In a mild tropical climate it can flower and fruit throughout the year continuously. But in regions like northern India where seasons are quite distinct due to variation in temperature or precipitation or both, three flowering seasons *viz.* summer, rainy and autumn with the corresponding harvesting periods as rainy, winter and spring, have been distinctly observed.

Guava cultivars display a great diversity in tree size, bearing habits and yield as well as in fruit shape, size, quality and ripening season. Some of the well grown Indian cultivars are Allahabad safeda, Lucknow-49, Banarsi, Harijha, Chittidar, red/pink fleshed and seedless (Purseglove, 1968; Mitra and Bose, 1985).

Guava cultivation is frequently threatened by wilting syndrome due to *Fusarium, Rhizoctonia,* anthracnos and canker. No definite control measures against the wilt by *F. oxysporum* f. Psidii is reported so far. The wilt (seedling blight) due to *Rhizoctonia bataticola* is equally dreaded. Another disease to which guava succumbs, is its canker caused by *Glomerella psidi, Colletotrichum psidii and Pestalotiopsis psidii.* The bark canker of guava is caused by *Physalospora psidii,* which is also prone to be eaten by a caterpillar *Indarbela queadrinotata;* other serious pests of guava in rainy seasons include mealy scale, *Pulvinaria psidii,* maggots of fruits fly (*Dacus ferrugineus* and *D. zonatus*). The old and neglected orchards of guava are damaged seriously by some partial parasites also (*e.g. Dendrophthaoe falcata*). The plant is also known to attacked by guava mosaic virus.

Traditionally, it has been a cross pollinated perennial fruit crop propagated through seeds (Purseglov, 1968), due to which considerable variabilities exist among its natural populations. It's seedless, triploid and other cultivars have been conventionaly propagated through budding onto the root stocks, inarching or approach grafting to maintain its clonal populations (Menzel, 1985; Singh, 1986).

Despite all these, there has been severe shortage of its suitable planting material that can be vegetatively propagated to get a good harvest of seedless guava having enhanced medicinal and nutritional qualities.

Fruit consumption in India is anticipated to increase by 4 per cent per year according to projected growth rates for income, population, and trends in food preferences. This would result in demand for all fruits reaching 66 million tonnes by 2010, with the bulk of this demand growth for tropical fruit. Mango is by far the most significant tropical fruit produced in India, followed by guava. Mango output was 9.8 million tonnes in 1999, with guava at 1.8 million tonnes. India is the one of the largest and most varied fruit producing nations in the world, accounting for 10 per cent of all fruits and nearly 40 per cent of tropical fruits produced globally. Fruit production in India increased at an average annual growth rate of 5.5 per cent between 1990 and 1999. Fruit tree production contributes 10 per cent on average to the gross value of total agricultural output in India, and 13 per cent of the export earnings attributable to major agricultural products, FAO (2001).

So the demand for good quality guava plants appears to be promising and bears enough potential for domestic and international trade with regards to its wide ranging edible commercial preparations and environment-friendly safe and effective medicinal products. This significance of fruit tree is now being realized globally and recently a few international symposiums have been organized exclusively on guava (Singh *et al.*, 2007); Annonymous (2008).

Breeding and Crop Improvement

Yet, the conventional breeding techniques have been responsible for the development of most delicious cultivar Lucknow-49. But presence of large number of seeds per fruit is a major disadvantage hindering its acceptability (Mitra and Bose, 1985). Only little success was achieved regarding the development of more productive seedless cultivar by corssing Allahabad safeda (a seeded but good quality heavy bearer) with a natural triploid (seedless but very shy bearer). De Cruz and Babu Rao (1962) were the first to isolate two aneuploids with 21 and 31 chromosomes form the progency of a triploid guava strain. Similarly, Majumdar and Mukherjee (1972a, b) have reported 26 diploids, 9 trisomics and 5 tetrasomics (2n+1+1) in the 73 plants raised by crossing the diploids and triploids through conventional breeding techniques.

Among the other conventional breeding work for the improvement of guava, the Fruit Research Stations, Basti, India, have developed 55 hybrid plants of guava by crossing Seedless × Allahabad safeda; Seedless × Lucknow-49; Allahabad safeda × Patillo; Apple coloured × Kothrud and Apple coloured × Red fleshed. The performances of these hybrids have been found promising for the semi-arid tropical areas of Telangana, Rayalseema etc. (Mitra and Bose, 1985). However, retention of their hybrid characteristics during subsequent generations still remained questionable.

The conventional technique of crop improvement for optimum land use, have succumbed to keep-up pace with rapid changes in the natural habitats of horticultural fruit crops, and appears inadequate to comply the demand of fast changing scenario. Biotechnology has opened-up unprecedented opportunities to give authoritative replies to such calamities.

In vitro Progress in Guava Improvements

The improvement of clonally propagated crops through somatic cells have been promising (Litz *et al.*, 1985; Carlson, 1987), which can also be used for guava improvement and its hybrid cultivars development. It bears potentials to incorporate the economically important traits through somatic cell manipulation into existing cultivars to produce improved varieties. Therefore, developing a suitable protocol for the vegetative clonal propagation of biotechnologically raised variants of guava, having better nutritional and medicinal properties in its seedless fruits, and its subsequent release as artificial seeds are the major highlights for the improvement of guava cultivars. In the following section a review of the recent progress in guava biotechnology is presented. The last part of the chapter is discussing the various parameters used in the studies of somatic embryogenesis of guava, followed by discussion on the importance of these parameters for the process in this and other species.

Organogenesis

The culture of excised tissuses of fruit mesocarp *in vitro* for manipulating the somatic cells/ tissues was the first report by Schroeder (1961). Babbar and Gupta (1986a, b) were the first to report the induction of callus and androgenesis in the *in vitro* cultured anthers. In the same year, the *in vitro* proliferation of shoots and plantlet formation from somatic tissues was reported by Jaiswal and Amin, (1986). Soon after, its *in vitro* propagation from shoot tip culture of mature tree was also reported (Jaiswal and Amin, 1987). Guava has been successfully micropropagated through its nodal explants, and it is also possible to obtain the adventitious shoots regenerated from the leaves of already micropropagated *in vitro* grown plantlets (Jaiswal and Amin, 1986, 1987; Amin and Jaiswal, 1987, 1988, 1989a, b). Subsequently, clonal propagation of guava from seedling and grafted plants was reported by Loh and Rao (1989). The very low frequency of regeneration in all these reports was because of high phenolic exudation and media browning. However, Fitchet (1989) has claimed the drying of explants prior to inoculation on the media during the establishment of nodal and shoot tips without oxidative browning. Subsequently, Papadatou *et al.* (1990) reported the rapid multiplication of guava seedlings through *in vitro* shoot tip culture with a success rate of more than 95 per cent, without any oxidative problem of phenolics or necrosis of the explants. Histological analysis of organogenesis in guava cultures was reported for the first time by Amin (1991). Recently, Yasseen *et al.* (1995) of USA have reported the *in vitro* shoot proliferation and propagation of guava from germinated seedlings. The first overview on somatic cell genetic and organogenesis of guava was published by Jaiswal and Amin (1992). Recently direct organogenesis on explants from germinated seddlings of guava has been reported by Singh *et al.* (2002).

The foregoing account on the organogenesis of guava appears to be promising but have almost failed to give any coherent picture of the work done so far on somatic embryogenesis, probably due to the fact that it is basically a highly recalcitrant fruit crop of tropics, and subtropical region of the World.

Somatic Embryogenesis

The first report on induction of somatic embryogenesis as unpublished data of the author and colleague was appreciated (see Jaiswal and Amin (1992). Further published work came out in 1993, when the authors became first in reporting the studies on induction and factors controlling somatic embryogenesis in guava using the zygotic embryo as explants (Jaiswal and Akhtar, 1993). Somatic embryogenesis from zygotic embryo culture of guava had subsequently been reported by the authors (Akhtar, 1996; Akhtar and Jaiswal, 1994, 1995; Jaiswal and Akhtar, 1994). The complete protocol for induction of somatic embryogenesis, dvelopment, maturation and germination of somatic embryos, production of artificial seeds and improvement of guava species had been achieved with commendable success by the author (Akhtar, 1997). Following similar protocols, Ramirez and Salazar (1998) have also reported the induction and development of somatic embryos from the zygotic embryo explant. An overview of the somatic embryogenesis and its applications in guava and other fruit tree species improvement has been overviewed in the recent past (Akhtar *et al.*, 2000; Akhtar and Jain, 2000). Subsequently Jaiswal and Jaiswal (2005) have overviewed the further progress in guava somatic cell genetics. The somatic embryogenesis work on guava is further being perfected at various locations and some new concepts are being published in the recent years by the author and other working on the problem (Chandra *et al.*, 2004; Rai *et al.*, 2007, 2008a, b, c).

The focus of the present report is mainly on recent progress for the improvement of guava species through somatic embryogenesis and development of protocol for micropropogation, artificial seed production.

Salinity Tolerance

As described in the preceding section that induction of somatic embryogenesis had partly been regulated through the stress management. Somatic embryos produced in presence of different concentrations of sodium chloride (NaCl) from both 3 per cent and 5 per cent sucrose containing medium were subjected for germination under the salt stress conditions. Somatic embryos from 75 mM NaCl containing induction and development medium showed better performance in 50 mM NaCl added half strength germination medium. Such plantlets were further grown to 75 and then 100 mM salt containing growth medium. The tolerant plant were subjected to *ex vitro* transfer in artificially made saline condition. As a result guava somatic plant line were selected which were tolerant to 100 mM NaCl containing medium (Akhtar, 1997; Akhtar *et al.*, 2000).

Guava had been found little tolerant to water logging and mild drought conditions. Since induction of water stress condition in the medium by addition of polyethylene glycol in the medium did not support the somatic embryogenesis, the process could not be applied for the selection of drought tolerant lines.

Artificial Seed Production

Various stages of somatic embryos from different week old cultures encapsulated in 2 per cent sodium alginate gel prepared in double distilled water proved to be the best matrix for artificial seeds production. The pH of the gelling medium either 5.8 or 7.0 had no distinct effect of conversion of encapsulated somatic embryos. Sodium alginate gel prepared in quarter or half strength MS medium alone or along with the sucrose had significantly reduced the germination response of artificial seeds. A 3 per cent sodium alginate gel prepared similarly in different medium showed slightly reduced conversion as compared to that encapsulated in 2 per cent sodium alginate gel (Akhtar, 1997; Akhtar *et al.*, 2000).

Artificial seeds encapsulating elongated torpedo stage somatic embryos from 8 weeks old culture showed maximum conversion frequency (Figure 28.1D). Short torpedo stage somatic embryos encapsulated similarly showed only 60-70 per cent conversion frequency. Synthetic seeds with lower (CHG) stages somatic embryos showed much reduced percentage of germination and never converted into plantlets. There was no significant variation in germination frequency of encapsulated and non-encapsulated somatic embryos of different stages (Akhtar, 1997; Akhtar *et al.*, 2000). Recently guava has been regenerated from encapsulated shoot tips of guava (Rai *et al.*, 2008b), alginate encapsulation of segments of guava (Rai *et al.*, 2008c), and encapsulated somatic embryos (Rai *et al.*, 2008a),

Cryopreservation

Cryopreservation as it also referred to freeze preservation or cryogenic storage involves transfer of biological materials for long term storage in liquid nitrogen (LN) (Bajaj, 1995). Cryopresevation of plant tissue culture can eliminate several problems of *in vitro* maintenance of culture in an active state.

There are several reports indicating that cryopreseved cells maintained their biosynthetic and morphogenetic potentials and no phenotypic, genotypic or epigenetic changes have been found as a result of cryopreservation process (Kartha and Engelemann, 1994; Wither and Engelemann, 1998). The cryopreservation studies in citrus and other species was reviewed earlier (Prez, 2000; Akhtar and Jain, 2000).

In case of guava, embryogenesis had been shown as the direct event from the zygotic embryo explants without any callus phase. Substantial efforts have been made in cryogenic preservation of somatic embryos and artificial seeds of guava. Somatic embryogenesis was induced with the average production of 100-150 embryos per zygotic embryo explants in 83.33 per cent culture frequency. Normally about 88–98 per cent elongated and short torpedo stages somatic embryos were converted into plantlets. Zygotic embryo explants (10–weeks post anthesis) treated with 1.0 mg/l of 2,4-D for 8–days in 5 per cent sucrose containing full strength MS medium were used for cryopreservation and regeneration after storage. A slow freezing followed by immersion into liquid nitrogen and subsequent storage at –70 °C of such embryogenic cultures as well as zygotic embryo explants (non induced) was adopted after the cryoprotectant treatment (Grout, 1995; Gupta *et al.*, 1987). Among cryoprotectants highest embryogenesis was observed with 7.5 per cent glycerol followed by in decreasing order by 10 per cent glycerol, 7.5 per cent polyethylene glycol, 10 per cent polyethylene glycol, 7.5 per cent dimethyle sulfoxide, 10 per cent dimethyle sulfoxide along with 5 per cent sucrose dissolved in half strength MS medium. Zygotic embryos pre-exposed to embryogenic treatments showed somatic embryogenesis in 41.67 per cent of cultures with only 25 per cent platlets recovery. Cryopreserved zygotic embryos without embryogenic induction were unsuccessful for somatic embryogenesis irrespective of thawing and induction treatment.

A mixture of cryoprotectant involving dimethylsulfoxide (DMSO) (5-15 per cent) and sucrose at different concentrations (0.1- 1.0 M) have also been used for the cryoprotection of both nacked and encapsulated somatic embryos from 8 week old cultures of guava. The cryoprotectants were added by incubating somatc embryos and synthetic seeds in a series of cryoprotective solution of increasing concentration as described by Gupta *et al.* (1987). Freezing of the material was carried out by dehydrative slow cooling methods of Sakai *et al.* (1991). The material was transferred to cryotubes and incubated first at 4 °C for 30-120 minutes, and then in deep freezer at –35°C for 20–40 minutes prior to direct immersion in liquid nitrogen. The cooling rate was roughly about 2 °C/min. The cryopreserved somatic embryos and artificial seeds were taken out after different periods of storage and thawing was performed by fast warming and immersing the cryotubes in a water bath at 37–40°C (Perez *et al.*, 1997).

The recovery of plantlets from somatic embryos and artificial seeds reduced drastically following the cryopreservation treatment and storage. The best plantlet recovery from somatic embryos and artificial seeds was noted in 28 per cent and 26 per cent frequency, respectively, up till one week of storage in 10 per cent DMSO along with 0.5M sucrose with dehydrative slow cooling and fast thawing procedure. In longer period of storage as well as with slow thawing at room temperature recovery of the plantlets was almost unsuccessful from both encapsulated and non- encapsulated somatic embryos. This very low success in cryopreservation of pretreated and post induced zygotic embryos as well as lower recovery of plantlets from cryopreserved somatic embryos and artificial seeds might be because the guava species is highly susceptible to frost and freezing. The other cryopreservation methods like vitrification could be tried as better alternative for the preservation of guava somatic embryogenesis as it was successful in novel orange (Sakai *et al.*, 1991), wasabi (Matsumoto *et al.*, 1994), strawberry (Hirai *et al.*, 1998).

Protocol of Somatic Embryogenesis in Guava

Material and Methods

Selection of Plant and Preparation of Explant

A 15-20 year old guava trees growing in the botanical garden of Banaras Hindu University were selected for zygotic embryo explants preparation and standardization of various factors for the local cultivar. Development of flower buds were observed regularly in each growing season. Flower buds were tagged and bagged (to ensure self/closed pollination) whenever necessary. Zygotic embryos for other cultivars like pink fleshed, Allahabad safeda, Lucknow-49 were collected from the guava trees growing at various locality of Banaras Hindu University, and subjected similarly to see effect of genotype on induction of somatic embryogenesis. Fruits of a particular age (7-14 weeks after anthesis) were picked up and brought to the laboratory and washed thoroughly under running tap water. The hard green exo- and greenish white mesocarp were removed with the help of a sharp knife or scalpel and the central pulp with seeds was cut into 4-6 vertical lobes. The pulp washed under running tap water for 30 mins and subsequently surface sterilized by gentle shaking in 2 per cent Cetavlon (v/v) with 2-4 drops of Tween-X for about 15-mins. The material then washed under running tap water followed by sterilization under the aseptic condition over a Laminar Flow Hood. Following a Short rinse in 70 per cent ethanol the material was sterilized with 0.05 per cent $HgCl_2$ solution (w/v) for about 20 mins then rinsed 4-5 times with sterile double distilled water.

Dissection of Zygotic Embryos

One of the pulp lobe along with seeds was taken into petridishes in sterile water. Zygotic embryo was dissected by picking up seeds from the pulp one by one. Seeds of guava are more or less J or U shaped with one arm slightly longer than the other. The seed was held with a forceps in left hand over a microscopic slide and a small piece of longer arm was removed with the help of a fine and pointed scalpel. The seed then turned opposite and a small piece of shorter arm was removed similarly. A blunt needle was inserted either through the longer or shorter arm side so that embryo came out of the other end. The embryo was inoculated immediately on the medium in a test-tube with the help of inoculation needle.

Culture Medium

The culture medium consisted of the normal strength of MS basal salts. The initial pH (4.2 ± 0.05) of the medium was raised to 6.2 ± 0.05 with 0.1 N NaOH. The medium was kept on continuous stirring on a magnetic stirrer. After about 1-2 hours the pH of the medium automatically stabilized to 5.8 ± 0.05 or if necessary adjusted with 0.01 N NaOH or HCl. Depending upon the requirement different amount of sucrose dissolved to one litre of medium. The medium was gelled with agar (0.8 per cent, w/v) by heating under pressure. The medium was modified with 0.001, 0.005, 0.01, 0.05, 0.1, 0.5, 1.0, 2.0, 3.0, 5.0, 10.0, 15.0 and 20.0 mg/l of 2,4-D prior to autoclaving. About 8-12 ml of medium was poured to each culture tubes. The medium was autoclave sterilized at 121 °C for 15 mins at 1.1 kg/cm^2 pressure. The medium modified with 2,4- D or any growth regulator(s) were reffered to as induction medium and the other without any growth regulator(s) and used for the development of somatic embryos were reffered to as development medium irrespective of sucrose conditions. All cultures were incubated in an air conditioned culture room maintained at 25 ± 2 °C temperature, 60-65 per cent relative humidity and 16 hrs photoperiod. The cultures were illuminated with 40W white fluorescent tube from a distance of 30-35 cm receiving 30-50 mEm^{-2}s^{-1} light intensity.

Induction of Somatic Embryogenesis

Some of the initial experiments had resulted the conclusions that treatments of zygotic embryos (10 weeks post anthesis) for a minimum of 8 days with 0.5 mg/l of 2,4-D in full strength MS basal medium supplemented with 3 per cent sucrose were the optimum condition for induction of somatic embryogenesis. Later a systematic studies were conducted for the development of efficient regeneration protocols for micropropagation of this species.

Development of Somatic Embryos

Somatic embryos were visible as small watery white transparent globules under stereozoom microscope usually at the end of the third week of culture initiation. In the fourth week of culture several new globular somatic embryos appeared while the older ones increased in size and proceeded in the next stage of development with simultaneous change in the colour from watery white transparent to translucent milksh (Figure 28.1B). In the fifth week of culture some new globular somatic embryos appeared while the older ones continued to grow towards advanced stages of development. After eight weeks of culture initiation most of the somatic embryos were hard solid and milky white irrespective of the developmental morphology.

The number of somatic embryos per explant varied considerably ranging from a single to usually several hundreds, sometimes more than a thousand depending upon the nature of treatment. Usually somatic embryos followed a normal development but sometimes anomalies were also observed as a function of treatment. However, the frequency of anomalous development and the secondary embryogenesis were very low.

Development of somatic embryos was found asynchronous showing 4-5 discernible stages from the same zygotic embryo explants in five weeks and older cultures (Figures 28.1B, C). Depending upon their sizes and post developmental responses *i.e.* response of somatic embryos during maturation, germination and encapsulation, they were grouped into three categories. The most preferred somatic embryos longer than 1.5 mm were called elongated torpedo stage (ET) somatic embryos; slightly less preferred ones ranging from 1.0-1.5 mm in size were termed as short torpedo stage (ST) somatic embryos; the least preferred ones at cotyledonary, heart and globular stages of development and smaller than 1.0 mm were grouped into third category and designated as lower or the CHG stage somatic embryos (Akhtar, 1997; Akhtar *et al.*, 2000).

The fitness of a treatment was calculated based on the six different embryogenic parameters *viz.* i. frequency of embryogenesis, ii. Intensity of embryogenesis *i.e.* average number of somatic embryos produced per explant per treatment, iii. frequency of ET stage somatic embryos, iv. frequency of ST stage somatic embryos, v. frequency of lower or CHG stage somatic embryos, and vi. efficiency of embryogenesis.

Evaluation of Somatic Embryogenesis

The cultures were observed daily and change in zygotic embryo explant were noted after an interval of 1-, 2-, 4-days or weekly. Embryognenic responses were recorded usually 8-10 weeks after culture initiation. Depending upon asynchrony in development and post developmental responses, during maturation germination and in recurrent embryogenesis various stages of somatic embryos were grouped in to three categories (Akhtar, 1997; Akhtar *et al.*, 2000). The results of various treatments has been presented and described under the following headings (Table 28.1).

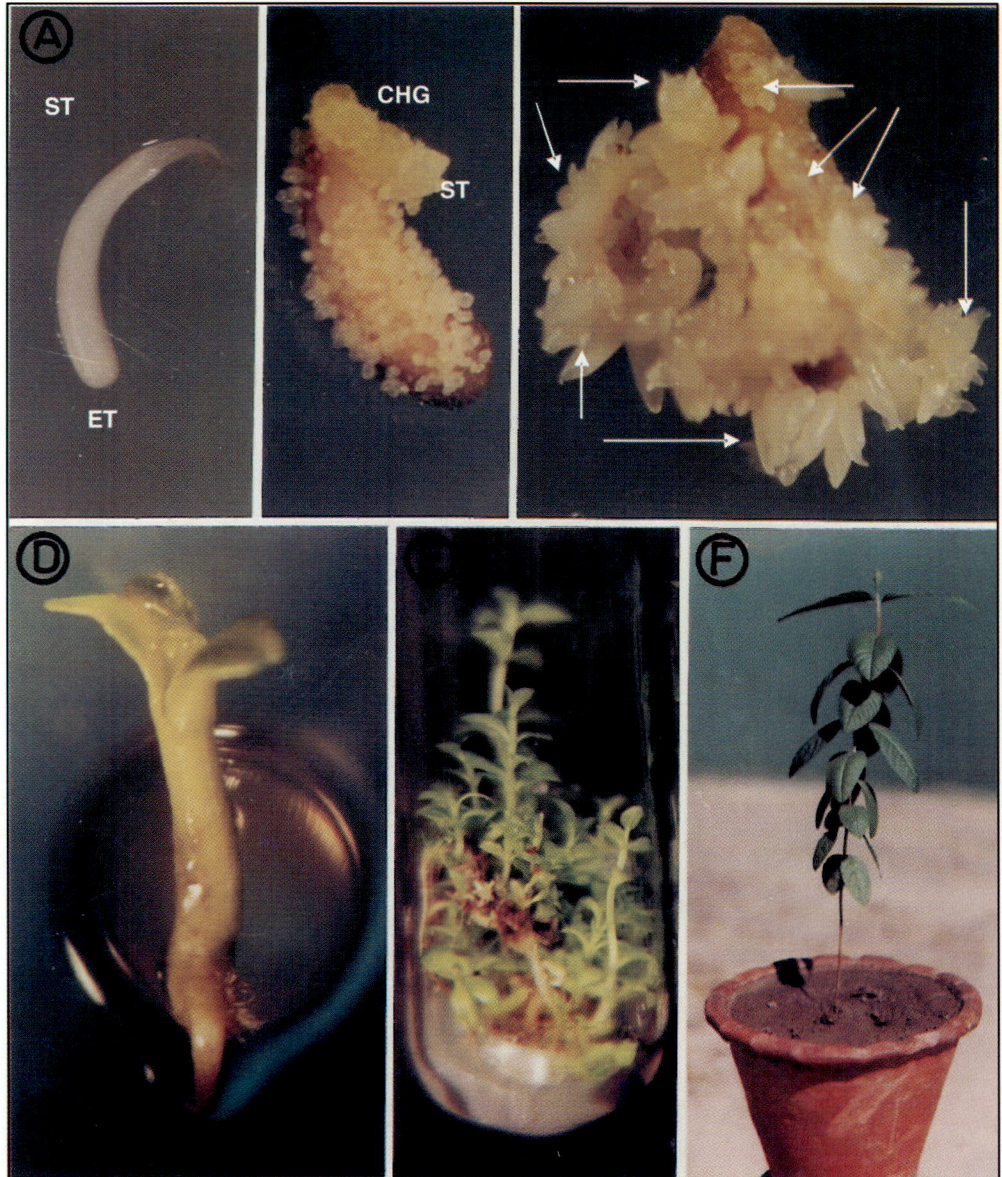

Figure 28.1: Induction of Somatic Embryos from Zygotic Embryos and Regeneration of Plantlet from Somatic Embryos and Artificial Seed of Guava (*Psidium guajava* L.)

(A) Ten weeks post anthesis zygotic embryo used as explants source. (B) Early stages of somatic embryos developing from zygotic embryo explant after four weeks of culture initiation. (C) Advanced stages of somatic embryos developing from zygotic embryo explants after six weeks of culture initiation. (D) A germinating artificial seed (eight weeks old elongated torpedo stage somatic embryos encapsulated in sodium alginate gel matrix) showing the emergence of shoot and root at opposite poles. (E) Germination of different stages of somatic embryo in half strength MS basal medium with 3 per cent sucrose. (F) A six weeks old guava plant (after soil transfer and hardening) regenerated through somatic embryogenesis.

Table 28.1: Induction of Somatic Embryogenesis from Zygotic Embryos of Guava (*Psidium guajava* L.) (Ten week old zygotic embryos of guava were treated continuously with different concentrations of 2,4-D in full strength MS medium added with 3 per cent sucrose. Embryogenic responses were noted after 10 weeks of culture initiation).

Sl. No.	*Conc. of 2,4-D (mg/l)*	*Frequency of Embryogenesis*	*Intensity of Embryogenesis*	*Frequency of Various Stages of Somatic Embryos*			*Efficiency of Embryogenesis*
		FE (per cent)	*IE (ANEPC)*	*ET (per cent)*	*ST (per cent)*	*CHG (per cent)*	*EE (Relative)*
1.	0.000	0.000	0.000	0.000	0.000	0.000	0.000
2.	0.001	9.99 ± 4.75	8.27 ± 5.24	30.21± 6.29	56.42 ± 8.54	13.37 ±11.67	0.65 ± 0.42
3.	0.005	28.97 ± 4.80	13.23 ±1.83	21.26 ± 8.99	47.54 ±12.55	31.30 ±18.50	1.58 ± 0.32
4.	0.01	63.66 ± 2.80	23.80 ± 6.19	10.52 ± 2.07	28.45 ± 6.85	46.50 ± 3.80	13.75 ± 1.02
5.	0.05	30.17 ±7.45	10.39 ± 3.98	6.69 ± 3.20	22.73 ± 10.06	63.03 ± 8.30	2.19 ± 0.52
6.	0.1	17.30 ± 5.09	10.10 ± 5.20	2.89 ± 3.17	8.82 ± 14.80	74.94 ± 13.21	0.39 ± 0.04
7.	0.5	8.33 ± 2.98	8.52 ± 3.65	2.27 ± 5.08	0.000	88.91 ± 19.70	0.18 ± 0.36
8.	1.0	5.55 ± 4.30	6.75 ± 4.16	0.000	0.000	100.00	0.000
9.	1.5	0.000	0.000	0.000	0.000	0.000	0.000
10.	2.0	0.000	0.000	0.000	0.000	0.000	0.000
11.	3.0	0.000	0.000	0.000	0.000	0.000	0.000
12.	4.0	0.000	0.000	0.000	0.000	0.000	0.000
13.	5.0	0.000	0.000	0.000	0.000	0.000	0.000
F (12, 65), *P 0.01*		122.29	19.799	30.215	41.76	21.78	438.702

CHG: Cotyledonary, Heart, Globular Stage Somatic Embryos; 2,4-D: 2,4–Dichlorophenoxy acetic acid; ET: Elongated Torpedo Stage Somatic Embryos; ANEPC: Average number of embryos per culture; ST: Short Torpedo Stage Somatic Embryos; MS: Murashige and Skoog's (1962).

Frequency of Embryogenesis (FE)

It is the proportion of explant showing at least one somatic embryo at any stage of development out of total number of explant inoculated in a particular treatment. It is calculated and presented as percentage of response by the following formula:

$$\text{FE (per cent)} = \frac{\text{Sum of the number of explants showing at least one somatic embryo per treatment}}{\text{Total number of explant inoculated per treatment}} \times 100$$

Intensity of Embryogenesis (IE)

It is the mean number of somatic embryos (irrespective of stage of development) produced per responsive explant in a particular treatment. It is calculated by the following formula and presented as the average number of somatic embryos produced per treatment (ANEPC).

$$\text{IE (ANEPC)} = \frac{\text{Sum of the total number of somatic embryos produced in each of the explant in a particular treatment}}{\text{Total number of explant showing at least one somatic embryo per treatment}} \times 100$$

Since proportion of various stages of somatic embryos varied considerably among different treatments hence, percentage of three different categories of somatic embryos were calculated as per following formulae for every treatment.

Proportion of various stages (categories) of somatic embryos. It is the proportion of a particular stage (category) of somatic embryo developed out of total number of somatic embryos produced in each of the responsive culture in a treatment. It is presented as the percentage of the total number of somatic embryo and calculated separately for each catagory of somatic embryos in the following way:

Proportion of Elongated Torpedo Stage Somatic Embryos (ET)

$$\text{ET (per cent)} = \frac{\text{Sum of the total number of elongated torpedo stage somatic embryos produced in each explant per treatment}}{\text{Sum of the total number of somatic embryos produced per treatmernt}} \times 100$$

Proportion of Short Torpedo Stage Somatic Embryos (ST)

$$\text{ST (per cent)} = \frac{\text{Sum of the total number of short torpedo stage somatic embryos produced in each explant per treatment}}{\text{Sum of the total number of somatic embryos produced per treamernt}} \times 100$$

Proportion of Cotyledonary, Heart and Globular Stage Somatic Embryos (CHG)

$$\text{CHG (per cent)} = 100 - [\, \text{ET (per cent)} + \text{ST (per cent)} \,]$$

Efficiency of Embryogenesis (EE)

This is the most important parameter for induction of somatic embryogenesis in guava which is defined as the potential of a treament to produce somatic embryos at elongated or short torpedo stage or both the stages of development, that are convertible into plantlets. It is entirely relative parameter without any unit and calculated as under:

$$\text{EE (Relative)} = \frac{\text{FE (per cent)} \times \text{IE (ANEPC)} \times [\text{ET (per cent)} + \text{ST (per cent)}]}{10{,}000}$$

Results

Effect of 2,4-Dichlorophenoxy Acetic Acid on Induction of Somatic Embryogenesis

The result of continuous treatment of zygotic embryos with different concentration of 2,4-D in 3 per cent sucrose containing Murashige and Skoog's medium is presented in the Table 28.1. It is clear from the results that 2,4-D had a significant effect on induction of somatic embryogenesis between 0.001–1.0 mg/l concentration as compared to the control culture without any growth regulator. Concentration of 2,4-D higher than 1.0 mg/l had been inhibitory for induction of somatic embryogenesis in continuous presence in 3 per cent sucrose containing full strength MS medium.

The process of somatic embryogenesis in various studies have reported mostly either as frequency or intensity as average number of somatic embryos produced per explant or the both. These parameters however were insufficient to indicate the proportion of convertible somatic embryos. If we consider only frequency and intensity of embryogenesis 0.01 mg/l od 2,4-D showed the maximum response but it did reflect the pproportion of convertible somatic embryos. In addition the convertible somatic embryo (ET + ST), however, showed a decreasing trend in the presence of 2,4-D with maximum number produced in 0.001 mg/l concentration. The proportion of CHG stages somatic embryos showed a positive correlation with 2,4-D concentration. Still there was no clear image to indicate the best inductive treatment of 2,4-D. Hence, it had been imperative to calculate the efficiency of somatic embryogenesis in order to show the potential of each and every treatment of growth regulator (see above). With this single parameter it was easy to find out the potential of any treatment irrespective of types of growth regulators (data not shown). Therefore it is clear from the table that 0.01 mg/l of 2,4-D showed the highest efficiency of somatic embryogenesis with the optimum proportion of convertible embryo which is the utmost requirements for micropropagation of any species.

Growth of Plantlets

Somatic plantlets in liquid as well as agar in solidified germination medium ceased to grow after two weeks of subculture and showed very little percentage of survival upon transfer and hardening to *ex vitro* condition. When subcultured to full strength MS liquid medium with 3 per cent sucrose for an extended growth of two weeks, there was significant improvement of survival frequency. All the plant grew well in this growth medium and attained full height of the culture vessels within 2 weeks of subculture (Akhtar, 1997; Akhtar *et al.*, 2000).

Ex vitro Performance

Plantlets regenerated through somatic embryogenesis in guava could not survive well on non-sterile soil mixture because of fungal infection. Amin (1987) had also encountered such attack of damping off diseases on guava plantlets regenerated through organogenesis. Plantlet from liquid or agar solidified germination medium did not survive even on sterile soil mixture. However, plantlets from liquid growth medium initially required a more porous mixture of sand, soil and compost in a ratio of 5:1:2. Once the root system adjusted to this primary mixture, transfer to a mixture with elevated proportion in a ratio of 1:2:3 of the above component was found beneficial. A regular watering of plantlets at an interval of 1-2 days had resulted in 50-90 cm plant height within 8-10 weeks of soil transplantation (Figure 28.1F). These plants had also performed well in the field and fruited within a period of less than one and a half year.

Discussion

The zygotic embryos had been used as explants material in the present study had also served as the starting explant material for induction of somatic embryogenesis in pea (Stejskal and Griga, 1992), soybean (Barwale *et al.*, 1986, Lazzeri *et al.*, 1987), feijoa (Cruz *et al.*, 1990). There was considerable changes in the explants morphology *in vitro,* reflects the reorganization of structural components of somatic cells in the presence of 2,4-D and other growth regulator (data no shown). The importance of phytohormones in influencing the gene(s) to trigger differentiation of cells in culture has already been reviewed extensively (Vasil 1980, Evan *et al.*, 1983, Bhojwani, 1990, Hobbie *et al.*, 1994, Duddit *et al.*, 1991). The cell size, cytoplasmic content and the type of first division were distinctly different between cell committed to embryogenesis and the cell that form callus tissue (Thorpe, 1988). Asymmetric partition at first division was frequently observed in sub epidermal cell layers of guava zygotic embryo explants among histological preparations (not shown). While, the cells of epidermal layers showed vertical and equal divisions in similar sections resulting into large vacuolated cells with comparatively lesser amount of cytoplasm and developing into callus from the zygotic embryo explants of guava.

Development of somatic embryos among the yellowish or yellowish brown calli at surfaces distal to the medium reflect the formation gradation of growth regulator concentration among different cell layers of the zygotic embryo explants but requires an extensive biochemical investigations. This is further evident why only fraction of cells appears to responds to the embryogenic treatment. Indeed, the detailed comparison between embryogenic and non-embryogenic clones from some genotype of alfalfa has revealed considerably increased sensitivity to 2,4-D in protoplast derived cells or root explants of embryogenic genotype. Embryogenesis in this clone occurs in tissues or colonies grown in the presence of 2,4-D at concentrations that already inhibited the growth of callus tissue (Bogre *et al.*, 1990). Similarly yellowish to yellowish brown calli contributed to embryo formation, in the feijoa (Cruz *et al.*, 1990), potato (Pretoa and Dedicova, 1992), whereas, in soybean (Sellar *et al.*, 1990) almost 95 per cent of zygotic embryos produced calli but somatic embryos produced directly from explants surface than the calli. Although there is no uniformity in the callus, morphology contributing to the embryo formation among various species but their characterization would certainly form the basis for the recognition of cell types for the development of an automated system for the process of somatic embryogenesis.

High frequency of globular stage and embryos showing anomalies in mango (DeWald *et al.*, 1989), feijoa (Cruz *et al.*, 1990), cherry (March *et al.*, 19993) and other systems are linked to long and continuous exposure of explants with auxins. However, frequency of anamolous somatic embryos was invariably low in the present study. The low frequency of anomalies and development of embryos beyond globular stage might be due to the fact that in the present study the culture conditions might maintain the high intracellular concentrations and did not block its polar transport.

Induction of somatic embryogenesis has also been achieved in the presence of other auxins like indole acetic acid, indole butyric acid and naphthalene acetic acid. A minor induction of somatic embryogenesis has been achieved in the presence of cytokinins but presentation of result is beyond the subject of the present study.

In the present study we report the induction of somatic embryogenesis in the presence of broad range of 2,4-D. Evaluation of the process of induction of somatic embryogenesis under several parameters like frequency, intensity and efficiency as well proportions of different stages of somatic embryos have proved beneficial for the analysis of potential of various concentrations of 2,4-D and other growth regulators. This would help to understand the process for high efficiency micropropagation in other species.

Future Prospects

The present work described sufficiently the importance of various parameters on induction of somatic embryogenesis, development, maturation, encapsulation and germination of somatic embryos as well as *ex vitro* performance of regenerated plants for micropropagation of *Psidium guajava* L. species. However, to maintain the clonal fidelity of the cultivar, embryogenesis protocol from somatic tissue like leaves would be beneficial and have yet to develop. Further, a convincing protocol leading to large scale automated commercial production of propagules and their field trial is still lacking and will be the topic for the future research. Indirect production and synchronous development of somatic embryos from callus and cell suspension cultures have to come up to achieve this goals.

The *in vitro* manipulation of somatic cells or tissues for the regeneration of guava plants or for improving its fruit quality, has not been explored sufficiently, and will be the problem for the future research. The problem of large number of seeds per fruits can be minimized in general, by raising the triploid plants through endosperm culture (Johri and Bhojwani, 1977; Wang and Chang, 1978; Bhojwani, 1985; Garg *et al.*, 1996). There is no report available so far on regeneration of guava from endosperm culture in a bid to either induce aneuploidy to get the genetically engineered seedless ones, and hence, will be the focus of future research to get such results.

Somaclonal variations are of common occurrence in various tissue cultures methodologies, which can also be employed in selecting guava variants through different treatment modifications of embryogenic explants. Since the plant regeneration from callus cultures have been suggested to be helpful in selecting the tolerant strains (Jaiswal and Amin, 1992), and the same with embryogenic culture of guava could lead to the development of variants plants resistant to various environmental stress(es) and disease(s). Such developed guava variants can be grown on relatively poor/otherwise problematic soils and may become popular among the poor as a source of monetary earnings from their non-productive wastelands. In any case, it would provide the basis for further investigations on the little explored biotechnological aspects of guava to enrich the intellectual contribution of the Nation.

Isolation and culture of protoplasts offer *direct transformation of plants* through protoplast fusion and somatic hybridization for the generation of somaclonal (protoclonal) variants in fruit crops (Hammerschlag and Litz, 1992). This has led to the development of protoplasts-to-plant protocols in a number of herbaceous and a few woody perennial species (Ochatt *et al.*, 1992). Yet, somatic hybridization occupies the prime position among the aims of protoplast manipulations (Ochatt *et al.*, 1989; 1992), but such reports are not available for the production of somatic hybrids of guava. The isolation of protoplasts from the tissues of embryogenic cultures of existing guava cultivars will be the problem for the future research to produce its somatic hybrids having desired characters.

The improvement of guava for good quality fruits with delayed ripening through the genetic manipulation of somatic cells or tissues is yet to come up. Thus, the genetic transformations using the protoplasts of the embryogenic cultures/calli having high regeneration potential along with the gene(s) of interest are the key components of the future research.

Conclusion

Somatic cell genetic of fruit crops is contingent upon the efficient and reliable regeneration of plants from cell and tissue cultures for clonally selected plants. In our study a number of parameters have been found influencing the induction of somatic embryogenesis, development, maturation, encapsulation and germination of somatic embryos as well as the *ex vitro* performance of regenerated plants for micropropagation of *Psidium guajava* L. species. However, the controlling mechanism underlying the regulation of the process is still missing in this and other fruit species. A better understanding of the process and the factors that influence embryogenesis at molecular level, their interactions couples with the physiological and biochemical studies in guava would probably lead to success in other fruit crops.

The progress in guava somatic embryogenesis described here shows promise as a model system for biotechnological improvement of other fruit tree. Although somatic embryogenesis is a common feature of *in vitro* morphogenesis in many fruit species, this appears to be the first review on somatic embryogenesis for *Psidium guajava* L. Consequently, the establishment of sound protocol for the production of somatic embryos of *Psidium guajava* L. is the first step towards a methodology for production of clonal stocks. Further research should be focused on the development of somatic embryogenesis protocols from tissues of somatic origin like leaves etc. to maintain the clonal propagule in this and other fruit trees.

Acknowledgements

The financial support to the Laboratory of Morphogenesis, Centre of Advanced Study in Botany, Banaras Hindu University, Varanasi, for various research positions under different projects by the University Grant Commission, Council of Scientific and Industrial Research, Central Silk Board, Department of Biotechnology, Department of Science and Technology, Government of India is gratefully acknowledged. The laboratory facilities extended by Jain Institute of Vocational and Advanced Studies, Bangalore and PG Department of Microbiology and Biotechnology, Al-Ameen Arts Science and Commerce College, Bangalore for continuing tissue culture research to the author is gratefully acknowledged.

References

Akhtar, N. (1996). Recurrent embryogenesis as a mean of conservation of guava germplasm. In: *Proc. National Research Seminar in Botany: Environment, Biodiversity and Conservation*, Balaghat (MP), India, p. 17 (Abst.).

Akhtar, N. (1997). Studies on induction of somatic embryogenesis and production of artificial seeds for micropropagation of a tropical fruit tree guava (*Psidium guajava* L.). Unpublished *Ph.D. Thesis*, Banaras Hindu University, Varanasi; 203 pp.

Akhtar, N. and Jain, S. M. (2000). Application of somatic embryogenesis for the improvement of tropical fruit trees. In: *Somatic Embryogenesis in Woody Plants* Vol. 6., (eds). S. M. Jain, P. K. Gupta and R. J. Newton. pp. 215-247. Kluwer Academic Publisher, The Netherland.

Akhtar, N. and Jaiswal, V. S. (1994). Role of somatic embryogenesis and artificial seed production production for micropropagation and improvement of guava (*Psidium guajava* L.). In: *Proc. Symp. on Role of Plant Tissue Culture in Biotechnology in India*, Varanasi, India. p. 2 (Abst.).

Akhtar, N. and Jaiswal, V. S. (1995). Rapid multiplication of *Psidium guajava* L. through recurrent embryogenesis. In: *Proc. All India Symposium on Recent Advances in Biotechnological Application of Plant Tissue Culture*. Mysore, India. p. 49 (Abst.).

Akhtar, N., Kumari, N., Pandey, S., Ara, H., Singh, M., Jaiswal, U., Jaiswal, V. S. and Jain, S. M. (2000). Somatic embryogenesis in tropical fruit trees. In: *Somatic Embryogenesis in Woody Plants* Vol. 6., (eds). S. M. Jain, P. K. Gupta and R. J. Newton. pp. 93-140. Kluwer Academic Publisher, The Netherland.

Amin, M. N. (1987). *In vitro* clonal propagation of guava (*Psidium guajava* L.) and Jackfruit (*Artocarpus heterophyllus* Lamk.). *Ph.D. Dissertation*, Banaras Hindu University, Varanasi.

Amin, M. N. (1991). *Plant Tissue Culture*, 1: 13-18.

Amin, M. N. and Jaiswal, V. S. (1987). Rapid clonal propagation of guava through *in vitro* shoot proliferation on nodal explants of mature trees. *Plant Cell Tiss. Org. Cult.*, 9: 235-243.

Amin, M. N. and Jaiswal, V. S. (1988). Micropropagation as an aid to rapid cloning of a guava cultivar. *Sci. Hort.*, 36 : 89-95.

Amin, M. N. and Jaiswal, V. S. (1989a). *In vitro* propagation of guava (*Psidium guajava* L.): Effects of sucrose, agar and pH on growth and proliferation of shoots. *Bang. J. Bot.*, 18 : 1-8.

Amin, M. N. and Jaiswal, V. S. (1989b). Effects of phloroglucinol, sucrose, pH and temperature on *in vitro* rooting of guava (*Psidium guajava* L.) microcuttings. *Bang. J. Bot.*, 18: 129-139.

Annonymous (1985) : *Publication Information Directorate*, C. S. I. R., New Delhi.

Annonymous (2008). *II International symposium on guava and other Myrtaceae*, Meride Mexico.

Babbar, S. B. and Gupta, S. C. (1986a). Induction of androgenesis and callus formation in *in vitro* cultured anthers of a myrtaceous fruit tree (*Psidium guajava* L.). *The Botanical Magazine*, Tokyo, 99: 75-85.

Babbar, S. B. and Gupta, S. C. (1986b). Embryogenesis in stamen and hypocotyl explants of a myrtaceous fruit tree *Psidium guajva* L. In: *VI. International Congress on Plant Tissue and Cell Culture*. Minneapolis, p. 133. (Abstract).

Bajaj, Y. P. S. (1995). Cryopreservation of somatic embryos. In: *Biotechnology in Agriculture and Forestry. Vol. 30 : Somatic Embryogenesis and Synthetic Seed-I*. Y.P.S. Bajaj (Ed.). Springer Verlag, Berlin, Heidelberg, pp. 221-229.

Benson, E. E., Lynch, P. T. and Stacey, G. N. (1998). Advances in plant cryopreservation technology: current application in crop plant biotechnology. *AgBiotech News and Information*. 10 (5): 133-141.

Bhojwani, S. S. (1985) : In: (Ed.) I.K. Vasil; pp. 258-268, Academic Press London.

Carlson, P. S. (1987) : In : S. Natesh, V. L. Chopra and S. Remohandran (Eds); Oxford and IBH Publishers, New Delhi, Bombay, Calcutta, pp. 85-92.

Chandra, R., Bajpai, A., Gupta, S., and Tiwari, R. K. (2004). Embryogenesis and plant regeneration from mesocarp of *Psidium guajava* L. (guava). *Ind. J. Biotechnol.*; 3: 246- 248.

De'Cruz, R. and Babu Rao, G. (1962). *J. Indian Bot. Soc.*; 41: 316-321.

Doijode, S. D. (2001). Guava: Psidium guajava L. In: *Seed Storage of Horticultural Crops*. (Ed.). Doijode, S.D. pp. 65 -67. Haworth Press, New York.

FAO (2001). Market for Tropical Fruits in India. FAO report on the Second Session on Committee on Commodity Problem: Inter Governmental Groups on Banana and Tropical Fruits, San Jose, Costa Rica: CCP:BA/TF 01/11.

Fitchet, M. (1989). Citrus and Subtropical Fruit Research Institute: *Information Bulletin*; 201: 4-5.

Garg, L., Bhandari, N. N. Rani, V. and Bhojwani, S. S. (1996). *Plant Cell Rep.*, 15 : 855-858.

Grout, B. (Ed.) (1995). *Genetic Preservation of Plant Cells in vitro*: Springer Lab. Manual. Springer- Verlag, Berlin, 169 pp.

Gupta, P. K., Durzan, D. J., and Finkle, B. J. (1987). Somatic polyembryogenic cell masses of *Picea abies* (Norway spruce) and *Pinus taeda* (loblolly pine) after thawing from liquid nitrogen. *Can. J. For. Sci.*, 17: 1130- 1134.

Hammerschlag, F. A. and Litz, R. E. (1992) (Eds). CAB International, Wallingford. UK. 550 pp.

Hirai, D. Shirai, K. Shirai, S. and Sakai, A. (1998). Cryopreservation of *in vitro* grown meristem of strawberry (*Fragaria x ananassa* Duch.) by encapsulation- Vitrification. *Euphytica*; 101:109-115.

Jaiswal, U. and Jaiswal, V. S. (2005). *Psidium guajava. In: Biotechnology of Fruits and Nut Crops* , (Ed.) Litz, RE. pp. 394-401. CAB International, Wallingford, UK.

Jaiswal, V. S. and Akhtar, N. (1993). Studies on induction and factors controlling somatic embryogenesis in guava. In: *Proc. Symp. on Plant Tissue Culture and its Biotechnological Application*, Jaipur, India, p. 48 (Abst.).

Jaiswal, V. S. and Akhtar, N. (1994). Induction of somatic embryogenesis and artificial seed prioduction for micropropagation of guava (Psidium guajava L.). In: *Proc. VIII Int. Cong. Plant Tiss. Cell Cult.* June 12-17, Italy, p. 55.

Jaiswal, V. S. and Amin, M. N. (1986). *In vitro* shoot proliferation and plantlet formation from somatic tissues of guava (*Psidium guajava* L.). *VI International Congress on Plant Tissue and Cell Culture*, Minneapolis, p. 279. (Abstract).

Jaiswal, V. S. and Amin, M. N. (1987). *In vitro* propagation of guava from shoot cultures of mature trees. *J. Plant Physiol*, 130 : 7-12.

Jaiswal, V. S. and Amin, M.N. (1992). Guava and Jackfruit. In: *Biotechnology of Perennial Fruit Crops. Biotechnology in Agriculture*. (Eds.) Hammerschlag, F. A. and Litz, R.E. No. 8. pp. 421-431. CAB International, Wallingford, UK.

Johri, B. M. and Bhojwani, S. S. (1977) : In : J. Reinert and Y. P. S. Bajaj (Eds); Springer-Verlag, Berlin, pp. 398-411.

Kartha, K. K. and Engelmann, F. (1994). Cryopreservation and germplasm storage. NRCS publication no. 32487. In: *Plant Cell and Tissue Culture*. (Eds) I. K. Vasil and T. A. Thorpe. pp. 195-230.

Litz, R. E. (1985). Somatic embryogenesis in tropical fruit trees. In: *Tissue Culture in Forestry and Agriculture*. (Eds.) Henke, R. R., Hughes, K. W., Constantin, M. J. and Hollaender, A. pp. 179-193. Plenum Press, New York,

Loh, C. S. and Rao, A. N. (1989). Clonal propagation of guava (*Psidium guajava* L.) from seedling and grafted plants and adventitious shoot formation *in vitro*. *Sci. Hort.*, 39 : 31-39.

Majumdar, P. K. and Mukherjee, S. K. (1971). *Nucleus*; 14 : 119-131.

Majumdar, P. K. and Mukherjee, S. K. (1972a). *Cytologia*; 34 : 541-548.

Majumdar, P. K. and Mukherjee, S. K. (1972b). *Nucleus*; 15: 42-47.

Matsumoto, T., Sakai, A. and Nako, Y. (1994). Cryopreservation of *in vitro* grown apical meristem of wasabi (*Wasabia japonica*) by vitrification and subsequent high plant regeneration. *Plant Cell Rep.*, 13: 442- 446.

Menzel, C. M. (1985). *Queensland Agri. J.*, 111: 93-98.

Mitra, S. K. and Bose, T. K. (1985). Guava. In : Bose, T. K. (Ed.). *Fruits of India: Tropical and Subtropical.* Naya Prokash, Calcutta, pp. 277-279.

Murashige, T., and Skoog, F. (1962). A revised medium for rapid growth and bioassay with tobacco tissue culture. *Physiol. Plant.*, 15 : 473-497.

Nijjar, G. S. (Ed.) (1977). *Fruit Breeding in India*. Oxford and IBH Publishers, New Delhi, Bombay, Calcutta, 219 pp.

Ochatt, S. J., Patat-Ochatt, E. M. and Power, J. B. (1992). In : F. A. Hammerschlag and R. E. Litz (Eds); CAB International Wallingford, U.K. pp. 77-103.

Ochatt, S. J., Patat-Ochatt, E. M., Rech, E. L., Davey, M. R. and Power, J. B. (1989). *Theo. Appl. Genet.*, 78: 35-41.

Papadatou, P., Pantikis, C. A., Ephtimiadou, E. and Lydaki, M. (1990). Rapid multiplication of guava seedlings by *in vitro* shoot tip culture. *Sci. Hort.*, 45 : 99-103.

Perez, R. M. (2000). Cryostorage of *Citrus* embryogenic cultures. In: *Somatic Embryogenesis in Woody Plants*, Vol. 6. (Eds.) S. M. Jain, P. K. Gupta and R. J. Newton. pp. 687- 705. Kluwer Academic Publisher, The Netherland.

Perez, R. M., Novarro, L. and Duran-Vila, N. (1997). Cryopreservation and storage of embryogenic cullus cultures of several citrus species and cultivars. *Plant Cell Rep.* 17: 44- 49.

Purseglove, J. W. (1968). *Tropical Crops Dicotyledons*. Longman Group Ltd. London, pp. 414-419.

Rai, M. K., Akhtar, N. and Jaiswal, V. S. (2007). Somatic embryogenesis and plantlet regeneration in *Psidium guajava* L. cv. Banarsi Local. *Scientia Horticulturae*; 113: 129 -133.

Rai, M. K., Jaiswal, V. S. and Jaiswal, U. (2008a). Effect of ABA and sucrose on germination of encapsulated somatic embryos of guava (*Psidium guajava* L.). *Scientia Horticulturae*; 117: 302-305.

Rai, M. K., Jaiswal, V. S. and Jaiswal, U. (2008b). Encapsulation of shoot tips of guava (*Psidium guajava* L.) for short term storage and germplasm exchange. *Scientia Horticulturae*; 118: 33- 38.

Rai, M. K., Jaiswal, V. S. and Jaiswal, U. (2008c). Alginate encapsulation of segments of guava (*Psidium guajava* L.) for germplasm exchange and distribution. J. *Horticultural Sci. and Biotechnol.*; 83 (5): 569- 573.

Sakai, A., Kobayashi, S. and Oiyama, I. (1991). Survival by vitrification of nucellar cells of Novel orange (*Citrus sinensis* var. *brasileinsis* Tanaka) colled to–190 °C. *J. Plant Physiol.*; 137: 465-470.

Saxena, Sangeeta, Rajan, S., Chandra, R., Srivastava, N. and Bajpai, A. (2007). Molecular characterization of closely related open pollinated seedling selections in Guava. Proceedings of the First International Guava Symposium. *Acta Horticulturae* No. 735 March 49-55.

Schroeder, C. A. (1961). *Bot. Gaz.* 122: 198-201.

Singh, A. (1986). Kalyani Publishers, New Delhi, pp. 328-331.

Singh, G., Krishnu, R., and Chandra, R. (2007). First International guava symposium, Organized by Society for Development of Subtropical Horticulture and Central Institute for Subtropical Horticulture Lucknow in Collaboration with International Society for Horticultural Science, Nandi Prisad and Agricultural Agricultural Proceesed Food Product Export Authority, at Lucknow. ISHS, ACTA Horticulturae 735 (CDROM).

Singh, R. (1985). *Fruits*. 4th Edition. National Book Trust, India, 213 pp.

Singh, S. K., Meghwal, P. R., Sharma, H. C. and Singh, S. P. (2002). Direct shoot organogenesis on explant from germinated seedlings of *Psidium guajava* L. cv. Allahabad Safeda. *Scientia Horticulturae*; 95: 213–221.

Wang, T. and Chang, C. (1978). In : *Proc. Symp. Pl. Tiss. Cult*, Science Press, Peking, pp. 463-467.

Wilson, C. W. (1980). In : S. Nagy and P. E. Shaw, A. V. I. Publishing, West Port.

Wither, L. A. and Engelmann, F. (1998). *In vitro* conservation of plant genetic resources. *Agricultural Biotechnology*. Marcel Dekker, New York. pp. 57- 88.

Yadav, U. L. (1996). Guava production ij Georgia under cold protection structure. In: *Progress in New Crops*. (Ed.) Janick, J. pp. 451–457. ASHS Arlington, VA.

Yasseen, Y. M., Barringer, S. A., Schnell, R. J. and Splittstoesser, W. E. (1995). *In vitro* shoot proliferation and propagation of guava (*Psidium guajava* L.) from germinated seedlings. *Plant Cell Rep.*, 14: 525-528.

Microbial Biotechnology and Ecology (2011) Pages 520–524
Editors: Deepak Vyas, G.S. Paliwal, P.K.Khare and R.K Gupta
Published by: DAYA PUBLISHING HOUSE, NEW DELHI

Chapter 29

Hepatoprotective Medicinal Plants: A Review

☆ *Siddhartha Singh*, A. Mehta and P. Mehta*

Department of Botany, Dr. H.S. Gour University, Sagar, M.P.

ABSTRACT

Use of herbal drugs in the treatment of liver diseases has a long tradition, especially in Eastern medicine. The chemical compounds present in the plant are responsible for their medicinal properties. The quality and quantity of phytochemicals present in the extract depends upon the solvent used for extraction and the method of extraction. The methanolic extract of *Silybum marianum, Apium graveolens* and *Hygrophila auriculata* seeds, aqueous extract of *Andrographis paniculata* leaves, aqueous and ethanolic extract of bark stem of *Pterocarpus* santalinus, aqueous seed extract of *Cleome viscosa* are some of the examples of hepatoprotective plant extracts. The potential of the active components present in these plant extracts are proved by CCl_4 induced liver damage models in mice.

Keywords: Herbal drugs, Phytochemicals, Extract and Carbon tetrachloride (CCl_4).

Introduction

Medicinal plants play a key role in the human health care. About 80 per cent of the world populations rely on the use of traditional medicine which is predominantly based on plant materials. Liver, the key organ of metabolism and excretion, is constantly endowed with the task of detoxification of xenobiotics, environmental pollutants and chemotherapeutic agents. Thus, disorders associated with this organ are numerous and varied. While a curative agent has not yet been found in modern

* E-mail: siddhartha.research@rediffmail.com

medicine, the current usage of corticosteroids and immunosuppressive agents only brought about symptomatic relief. Furthermore, their usage is associated with risk of relapses and danger of side effects. On the other hand, Ayurveda, an indigenous system of medicine in India, has a long tradition of treating liver disorders with plant drugs. Enhanced lipid peroxidation produced during the liver microsomal metabolism of ethanol may result in hepatitis and cirrhosis. To focus on a more practical and systematic approach towards the development of standardized medicine, many plant derived drugs used in modern medicine are developed by ethnomedical leads and subsequent ethno pharmacological studies. There are more than 100 drugs of known structure that are extracted from higher plants and used in allopathic medicine.

To assess the liver functions, biologists have chosen three basic biochemical parameters which are levels of SGOT, SGPT and serum bilirubin with CCl_4 induced liver damage models of albino rats.

Hepatoprotective Drug Development

Pharmacological validation of each hepatoprotective plant should include efficacy evaluation against liver diseases induced by various agents. Efficacy of the drug against viral hepatitis as well as liver damage induced by hepatotoxic chemicals by oxidative mechanisms or other mechanisms should be determined. Further, the plant drugs have to be evaluated for their effects on liver regeneration and bile secretion, the same drug is unlikely to be effective against hepatic damage caused by various agents.

Medicinal Plant and Hepatoprotection

There are numerous medicinal plants which have shown high efficiency for the hepatoprotective activity and have shown great potential as a natural remedy for the treatment of acute liver diseases and damages. Summary of some of the plants with proven hepatoprotective activity are discussed below.

Silybum marianum

Commonly known as 'Milk thistle' and belongs to family 'Compositae'. It occurs widely in Europe, Canada and South America. In India it is indigenous to Kashmir. Silymarin a flavonoid is an active compound obtained from *S. marianum* with hepatoprotective activity. Silymarin is able to neutralize the hepatotoxicity of several agents, including *Amanita phalloides*, ethanol, paracetamol (acetaminophen) and carbon tetrachloride in animal models. The protection against *A. phalloides* is inversely proportional to the time that has elapsed since administration of the toxin. Silymarin protects against its toxic principle α-amanitin by preventing its uptake through hepatocyte membranes and inhibiting the effects of tumor necrosis factor, which exacerbates lipid peroxidation. The active substances from *S. marianum* also stabilize the cell membrane, exert antioxidant properties and exhibit intrinsic toxicity when tested on primary culture of human hepatocytes.

Andrographis paniculata

It is an annual herb which is commonly called as 'Kalmegh' and belongs to family 'Acanthaceae'. It is widely distributed in Sri Lanka and throughout India especially in Maharashtra, Uttar Pradesh, Madhya Pradesh, Tamil Nadu and Andhra Pradesh. It is another proven hepatoprotective agent. The aqueous extract of which, when given orally to the animals with liver damage induced by hexa-chloro-cyclohexane (BHC) inhibited BHC induced liver toxicity in Swiss male mice as assessed by the biochemical values. The aqueous extract of *A. paniculata* has also role in delaying the hepatic turnerogenic condition by lowering the SGPT, SGOT and alkaline phosphatase level in BHC treated mice.

Apium graveolens and *Hygrophila auriculata*

A.graveolens is a biennial plant found in the regions of Himalaya, Punjab and North Africa. Its common name is 'Celery seeds' and belongs to family 'Umbelliferae'. Pretreatment of rats with 200 mg/kg p.o. of the methanolic extracts of the seeds of *A. graveolens* or *H. auriculata* 24, 48 and 2 h before paracetamol administration exhibited a significant reduction in the paracetamol induced increase in the levels of different SGOT, SGPT and serum bilirubin.

Ginkgo biloba

It is one of the oldest known trees and is widely distributed all over the world, also known as 'Maiden Hair Tree' and belongs to family 'Gingkoaceae'. It is reported that there was a significant increase in the serum hepatic enzyme levels and significant decrease in the TP and Alb levels after CCl_4, which was reversed with *G.biloba.*

Pterocarpus santalinus

P. santalinus belongs to 'Leguminoseae' family and also known by names like 'Bijasal' and 'Indian Kino Tree'. It is mainly found in hilly regions of Gujrat, Madhya Pradesh, Uttar Pradesh and Bihar. It is reported that there was a significant increase in serum levels of bilirubin, alanine transaminase, aspartate transaminase and alkaline phosphatase with a decrease in total protein level, in the CCl_4 treated animals, reflecting liver injury. In the aqueous and ethanol extracts treated animals there was a decrease in serum levels of the markers and significant increase in total protein, indicating the recovery of hepatic cells. Histological study of aqueous extract treated group exhibited moderate accumulation of fatty lobules and cellular necrosis where as ethanol extract treated animals revealed normal hepatic cords without any cellular necrosis and fatty infiltration.

Pergularia daemia

It is a perennial herb grows along the road sides in India and the studies on the hepatoprotective effect of alcoholic extract was carried out using carbon tetrachloride induced liver damage in wistar albino rats. Acetone sub fraction showed significant protective effect by lowering serum levels of various biochemical parameters. These biochemical observations were supplemented by histopathological examination of liver sections. Here, Silymarin was used as positive control. The results justify the use of *P. daemia* as a hepatoprotective agent.

Cleome viscosa

Research suggest that the aqueous seed extract of *C. viscosa* has hepatoprotective activity against carbon tetrachloride (CCl_4) induced liver damage in wistar rats. The aqueous seed extract of *C. viscosa* (200 mg/kg) was administered orally to the animals with hepatotoxicity induced by CCl_4. Silymarin (200mg/kg) was given as reference standard. There was significant reduction in serum enzyme aspartate aminotransferase (AST), alanine aminotransferase (ALT), alkaline phosphatase (ALP), Y-glutamyl transpeptidase and lipid peroxidase and increase in reduced glutathione (GSH). Various pathological changes like centrilobular necrosis and vacuolization observed in CCl_4 treated rats, which were prevented to a moderate extent in groups, treated with *C. viscosa* and Silymarin. It was concluded from the study that aqueous seed extract of *C. viscosa* possesses hepatoprotective activity against CCl_4 induced hepatotoxicity in rats.

Picrorhiza kurrooa

Commonly called as 'Indian Gentian' and 'Kutki'. This perennial herb of family 'Scrophulariaceae' is distributed in upper Himalayas and China and grows naturally in Kashmir and Himachal Pradesh. The hepatoprotective study of *P. kurrooa* was evaluated against alcohol-CCl_4, induced liver damage in rat at the doses of 3, 6 and 12 mg/kg/day, p. o. for 7 days. It showed a significant hepatoprotective activity by lowering of the elevated levels of glutamate oxaloacetate transaminase, glutamate pyruvate transaminase, acid phosphatase, alkaline phosphatase, glutamate dehydrogenase and bilirubin in the serum of alcohol-CCl_4 induced liver damage models.

Discussion

Medicinal plants are of great importance as they have been proven for their effectiveness against various diseases with less or no side effects. Disorders associated with liver are one of the most common problems faced by the human and medicinal plants hold the key for it. The active compounds present in the plant extract are responsible for their hepatoprotective potential. The type and concentration of the phytochemicals present in the extract depends upon the solvent used for extraction and the method of extraction. Flavonoids, diterpinoids, tannins etc. are the most common chemical compounds present in the plant which are responsible for their hepatoprotective potential.

References

Dvorjak, Zdenejk, Kosina, Pavel, Walterova, Daniela, Sjimanek, Vilym, Bachleda, Petr and Ulrichova, Jitka (2003). Primary cultures of human hepatocytes as a tool in cytotoxicity studies: cell protection against model toxins by flavonolignans obtained from *Silybum marianum*. *Toxicology Letters;* 137: 201-212.

Fransworth, N.R. (1990). The role of ethnopharmacology in drug development. In: *Bioactive compounds from plants*. Ciba Foundation Symposium, Chichester, John Wiley and Sons; 154: 2-21.

Fraschini, F., Demartini, G. and Esposti, D. (2002). Pharmacology of Silymarin. *Clin Drug Invest;* 22(1): 51-65.

Handa, S.S., Sharma, A. and Chakraborthi, K.K. (1986). Natural products and plants as liver protecting agents. *Fitoterapia,* LVII (5): 307–351.

Manjunatha, B.K. (2006). Hepatoprotective activity of *Pterocarpus santalinus* L.f., an endangered medicinal plant. *Indian J Pharmacol;* 38: 25-8.

Mitra, S.K., Venkataranganna, M.V., Sundaram, R. and Gopumadhavan, S. (1998). Protective effect of HD-03, a herbal formulation, against various hepatotoxic agents in rats. *Journal of Ethnopharmacology;* 63: 181–186.

Sengottuvelu, S., Duraisamy, R., Nandhakumar, J. and Sivakumar, T. (1998). Hepatoprotective activity of *Cleome viscosa* against Carbon tetrachloride induced hepatotoxity in rats. *Pharmacognosy Magazine,* ISSN: 0973-1296.

Shenoy, K.A. (2001). Hepatoprotective Effects of *Ginkgo biloba* against Carbon Tetrachloride Induced Hepatic injury in Rats. *Indian Journal of Pharmacology;* 33: 260-266.

Singh, A. and Handa, S S. (1995). Hepatoprotective activity of *Apium graveolens* and *Hygrophila auriculata* against paracetamol and thioacetamide intoxication in Rats. *Journal of Ethnopharmacology;* 49: 119-126.

Smuckler, E.A. (1998). Alcoholic drink: Its production and effects. *Fed Proe*; 34: 2038-2044.

Subramoniam, A. and Pushpangadan, P. (1999). Development of Phytomedicines for Liver Diseases. *Indian Journal of Pharmacology*; 31: 166-175.

Sureshkumar, S. V. and Mishra, S. H. (1996). Hepatoprotective activity of extracts from *Pergularia daemia* Forsk. against carbon tetrachloride-induced toxicity in rats. *Pharmacognosy Magazine*, ISSN: 0973-1296.

Tripathi, S.C., Patnaik, G.K. and Dhawan, B.N. (1991). Hepatoprotective activity of Picroliv against Alcohol-Carbon tetrachloride induced damage in Rats. *Indian J Pharmac*; 23: 143-148.

Trivedi, N. and Rawal, U.M. (1998). Effect of Aqueous Extract of *Andrographis Paniculata* on Liver Tumor. *Indian Journal of Pharmacology*; 30: 318-322.

Trivedi, N. and Rawal, U.M. (2000). Effect of *Andrographis paniculata* on Severe Liver Damage. *Indian Journal of Pharmacology*; 32: 288-293.

Microbial Biotechnology and Ecology (2011) Pages 525–543
Editors: Deepak Vyas, G.S. Paliwal, P.K.Khare and R.K Gupta
Published by: DAYA PUBLISHING HOUSE, NEW DELHI

Chapter 30

Cyanobacterial Exploitation in Biotechnology

☆ ***B.D. Kaushik***

Division of Biotechnology
Netaji Subash Institute of Technology, Sector 3, Dwarka, New Delhi – 110078

While writing this chapter I am lost in the sweet memory of late Prof. K.M. Vyas, who dedicated his entire life to up bring the Department of Botany at Sagar University. This lecture is wholly devoted to Prof Vyas.

Introduction

Cyanobacteria are both unicellular and multicellular filamentous. Some of the forms have terminally differentiated specialized structures called heterocyst. The cyanobacteria are self-supporting system and some of the species are capable of fixing atmospheric nitrogen. These are ubiquitous in nature and are next to bacteria in distribution. They grow wherever water, sunlight and limited number of inorganic elements available and rice field ecosystem is the ideal niche for the growth and proliferation of cyanobacteria. Due to their wider occurrence in rice field ecosystem, these organisms have been exploited as a means to provide biologically fixed nitrogen. Some of the cyanobacteria have potential to colonize inhospitable ecosystem *e.g.* salty soils hence are exploited to reclaim such soils. Still some have great economic importance as a source of food, feed and substances of pharmaceutical importance.

Cyanobacteria in Agriculture

Photosynthesis and nitrogen fixation are the two most important biological processes on the earth. Though the atmosphere contains about 79 per cent nitrogen, this form of nitrogen cannot be utilized by most plants, but utilizes nitrogen only in the combined mineral form, such as ammonium

(NH_4^+) or nitrate (NO_3^-). Nutrient nitrogen as such is the most limiting nutrient in soil and use of inorganic nitrogen fertilizers to meet the crop requirements is unavoidable for intensive farming practices. However, the crop utilizes only 30 to 35 per cent of the applied nitrogen and the remaining 65-70 per cent is lost either by volatilization or leaching. These losses are further enhanced due to reduced or almost no use of organic amendments. Under such circumstance microorganisms play significant role in maintaining soil fertility. The dinitrogen reduction so far is confined to prokaryotic cellular forms in nature. Among these prokaryotes, the photosynthetic diazotrophs–cyanobacteria, more commonly known as blue-green algae, are free living as well as symbionts with lichens, ferns and cycads and their contribution in total nitrogen fixation by biological means probably comes next to the legume-*Rhizobium* symbiosis.

Rice is an important food crop as more than 40 per cent of the world's population depends on rice as a major source of calories. In India, rice crop is cultivated in about 44 million hectares with an approximate total production of 81.16 million tonnes. Per hectare rice yield in India is about 1928 kg/ha, which is quite low compare to China (5807 kg/ha) and Japan (6273 kg/ha). Rice crop accounts for the largest share of chemical fertilizers. In tropical rice fields' biological nitrogen fixation is a cyanobacterial process. N-fixing blue-green algae (BGA) have been shown to be the most important in maintaining and improving the productivity of rice fields (Venkataraman, 1979; Kaushik, 1994a). It has been demonstrated that the N fertility of soil is sustained better under flooded conditions than under dry land conditions (Watanbe and Roger, 1984). Favourable conditions for biological N_2 fixation by such BGA is considered to be one of the reasons for the relatively stable yield of rice under flooded condition.

Diazotrophic Cyanobacteria

Cyanobacteria are one of the earliest forms of life on Earth and known to be the primary colonizers in most inhospitable habitats. As early as 1936 (De, 1936) suggested that the fertility of Indian rice field is maintained due to the presence of cyanobacteria, since then large number of forms has been reported from diverse habitats. In Indian rice field soils on an average cyanobacteria accounts to about 33 per cent (Venkataraman, 1975) whereas reports show that up to 50 per cent of the total algae was BGA in some of the southern and eastern states. The aerobic filamentous heterocystous as well as colonial forms represent the common flora of arable lands and are considered to be the important in nitrogen economy of rice cultivation (Table 30.1). The most common filamentous heterocystous species include *Anabaena, Aulosira, Calothrix, Cylindrospermum, Fischerella, Hapalosiphon, Nostoc, Scytonema, Stigonema, Tolypothrix* and *Westiellopsis* (Stewart *et al.*, 1979; Prasanna and Kaushik, 1995) and the unicellular or colonial are the species of *Aphanothece, Gloeothece, Synechoococcus, Synechocystis* and *Xenococcus* (Ripkka *et al.*, 1979; Prasanna and Kaushik, 1994). The non-heterocystous filamentous forms capable of nitrogen fixation are species of *Oscillatoria, Trichodesmium, Microcoleus, Pseudanabaena, Plectonema* and *Lyngbya* (Wyatt and Silvey, 1969).

Nitrogen Contribution

Prasad (1949) estimated *in situ* addition of nitrogen in soils of South Bihar by scrapping encrustations of cyanobacterial mats on soil surface collected from different places and the estimated nitrogen input varied from 12 to 16 kg ha^{-1} after the harvest of the crop. Similarly De and Mandel (1956) estimated nitrogen fixation by cyanobacteria in six rice growing soils of West Bengal and reported values ranging from 13.8 to 44.4 kg ha^{-1} of nitrogen in cropped area. In Japan Watanabe *et al.* (1951) observed addition of 20 kg ha^{-1} nitrogen by *Tolypothrix tenuis*. The water layer with extensive floating colonies of *Gloeotrichia* sp. in Moroccan rice fields has been found to show high rates of nitrogen fixing activity (44 n moles C_2H_4 ml^{-1} hr^{-1}) (Reynault *et al.*, 1975). Using ^{15}N technique, Mac Rae and Castro (1969) demonstrated an addition of 10-15 kg N ha^{-1} in rice fields due to cyanobacteria. Using same technique Yoshida and Ancazas (1993) found an addition of 40-80 kg N ha^{-1}. Even in the temperate soils, nitrogen fixation by algae is substantial. Henriksson (1971) showed annual fixation rate of 15-51 Kg N ha^{-1} yr^{-1} in an agricultural field where *Nostoc* was abundant, and 4.44 Kg N ha^{-1} yr^{-1} in a lakeside meadow containing *Nostoc, Anabaena, Cylindrospermum* and *Calothrix*. The relative contribution of cyanobacteria as a percentage of the total nitrogen fixed in paddy fields varies widely and is mainly dependent on physico-chemical properties of soil, climatic and biotic factors. Quantitative estimations from different countries are: Philippines 18-33 kg/ha (Watanabe and Lee, 1975; Alimango and Yoshida, 1977), India 15-53 kg/ha (De and Biswas, 1952; Singh, 1961; Venkataraman, 1979), Senega 10-30 kg/ha (Renaud and Roger, 1978), Mali 50-80 kg/ha (Traore *et al.*, 1978) and Japan 11-23 kg/ha (Okuda and Yamaguchi, 1955).

Table 30.1: Nitrogen Fixing Genera of Blue-green Algae (Cyanobacteria)

Genera	*Species in India*	*No. of N_2 Fixer*	*Genera*	*Species in India*	*No. of N_2 Fixer*
	Non-heterocystous		*Fischerella*	3	2
	Colonial		*Gloeotrichia*	10	1
Chlorogloea	2	1	*Hapalosiphon*	10	2
Gloeocapsa	23	2	*Mastigocladus*	1	1
Synechocystis	-	1	*Mastigocladopsis*	1	1
	Filamentous		*Nodularia*	1	1
Lyngbya	65	2	*Nostoc*	25	25
Oscillatoria	85	4	*Nostochopsis*	3	1
Phormidium	48	1	*Rivularia*	7	1
Plectonema	11	2	Scytonema	49	2
	Heterocystous		*Scytonematopsis*	2	2
Anabaena	25	25	*Stigonema*	12	1
Anabaenopsis	3	2	*Tolypothrix*	19	1
Aulosira	8	1	*Westiella*	2	1
Calothrix	29	All	*Westiellopsis*	1	1
Cylindrospermum	14	14	*Wollea*	1	1

Higher concentrations of combined nitrogen have been shown to inhibit both the growth as well as the nitrogen fixation ability of the cyanobacteria, and ammonium being toxic at 75 ppm (Stewart, 1964; Mekonnen *et al.*, 2002). Nitrate nitrogen is preferred by the cyanobacteria and is not detrimental even at 100 ppm concentration. There are, however, numerous reports on the beneficial effects of algalization in the presence of nitrogenous fertilizers (Satapathy, 1999). Singh *et al.* (1972) reported that grain yield, when the field was inoculated with algae and 60 kg ha^{-1} urea, was comparable to that obtained with 120 kg nitrogen alone. Similar observations were also made with ammonium sulphate, at nitrogen level as high as 120 kg ha^{-1} (Venkataraman and Goyal, 1963). In an experiment conducted in Haryana, Kaushik (1998) reported about 10-15 per cent increase in rice yield in the presence of fertilizer nitrogen up to 150kg ha^{-1} (Table 30.2). Thus, the response to algalization was generally positive at any level of nitrogen applied in the field, though the response being lower at higher levels.

Table 30.2: Response of Rice to Cyanobacterial Biofertilizer Application– Demonstration Trial 1996-1997 at Farmer's Field in Haryana

Treatments		No. of Trials	Soil Type	Variety	Yield Q ha^{-1}		N-Saving kg ha^{-1}	% Increase
N: P	N: P + BGA				N:P	N: P + BGA		
58:0	29:0	4	Loam	Basmati	45	53	29	17.8
71:35	48:35	6	Loam	Basmati	42	49	23	16.6
80:57	57:57	5	Clay	PR-6	50	60	23	20.0
104:46	76:46	5	Clay	PR-6	45	52	28	15.5
100:35	71:35	5	Loam	Basmati	40	44	29	10.0
108:57	80:57	5	Loam	Basmati	40	45.5	28	13.7
108:57	80:57	5	Loam	PR-6	40	46	29	15.0
115:0	86:0	5	Loam	Terrycot	42	45	29	7.1
124:23	95:23	5	Loam	Basmati	56	62	29	12.7
137:57	109:57	10	Clay	HR-120	48	55	29	14.6
137:57	103:57	5	Clay	HR-120	46.5	52.7	29	13.2
137:57	108:57	5	Clay	Basmati	35	45	29	22.2
Total		65			44.13	50.77	27.83	14.87

Nutrients fixed by algae are released either through exudation or through microbial decomposition after the cells die (Roger and Reynaud, 1979). This fixed nitrogen is partly released extracellularly during growth and remaining through microbial decomposition after death. In paddy fields the death of algae biomass is associated with alternate desiccation and wetting during cultivation cycle or finally after the harvest of the crop. It results in gradual build-up of soil fertility with a residual effect on succeeding crop also. N-uptake studies indicated that 39 per cent of the nitrogen from ^{15}N-labelled *Aulosira* sp. spread on soil and 51 per cent from the algae incorporated into the soil was recovered in the rice crop. It shows that nitrogen fixed through cyanobacteria is readily available to rice (Wilson, 1980).

Growth-Promoting Effect

A large number of researchers have found better growth and germination of seeds of many crop plants after treating them with algal cultures or their extracts. The majority of them observed an enhancement in rice-seed germination, root and shoot growth, weight of rice grains and their protein content (Shukla and Gupta, 1967; Venkataraman and Neelakantan, 1967; Singh and Trehan, 1973; Jacq and Roger, 1977; Misra and Kaushik, 1989a, b); while others found similar stimulatory effects on wheat (Gupta *et al.*, 1967), tomato (Kaushik and Venkataraman, 1979), tomato and radish (Rodgers *et al.*, 1979), peas (Gupta and Gupta, 1972), banana (Ganapathi *et al.*, 1994) etc. Different opinions exist regarding the nature of these substances. Some have described them as hormones, *i.e.* gibberelin-like (Singh and Trehan, 1973), cytokinin-like (Rodgers *et al.*, 1979), auxin-like (Ahmad and Winter, 1968) or abscisic acids (Marsalek *et al.*, 1992); while others have described them either as vitamins particularly vitamin B (Grieco and Desrochers, 1978) or as amino acids (Watanable, 1951), antibiotics and toxins (Metting and Pyne, 1986). However, detailed quantitative and qualitative analyses of these substances produced by different cyanobacterial species were given by Kaushik and coworkers. They reported the different vitamins in the range of ng mg^{-1} biomass: niacin 80-320, pantothenic acid 5-10, folic acid 0.79-1.08 and vitamin B_{12} 3.6×10^{-3} in *Nostoc muscorum* and *Hapalosiphon fontinalis*, and stimulation in the root and shoot growth was observed with folic acid, vitamin B_{12} and pantothenic acid but not with nicotinic acid (Misra and Kaushik, 1989a). Similarly the growth hormones like indole-3-acetic acid and indole-3-propionic acid or 3-Methyl indole were identified and quantified in addition to extracellular sugars and amino acids (Misra and Kaushik, 1989b).

Soil Organic Matter

The most important constituent to determine the fertility of a soil is organic carbon. Soils rich in organic carbon are productive as it helps in better nutrient utilization efficiency and checks the nutrient loss through leaching and volatilization. As early as 1950 (De and Sulaiman, 1950) reported a build up of organic matter due to blue green algal inoculation. Later, a number of workers supported the work. However, a wide variation in the reported values of organic carbon or biomass addition by BGA exists (Table 30.3). A well developed continuous layer of colonies of different species of BGA in rice fields yield a significant amount of biomass. Using ^{15}N, Nekrasova and Aleksandrova (1982) confirmed that algal biomass contributed significantly to humus formation in soils despite the absence of typical lignin in them. Roger *et al.* (1987) indicated that under favourable conditions a good algal bloom in rice fields yields on an average about 6-8 t of fresh biomass. A 0.03 per cent (672 kg ha^{-1}) increased soil organic carbon content was reported due to encouragement of native algal flora alone under laboratory conditions in a six months period (Kaushik, 1985), whereas inoculation of halotolerant cyanobacterial strains to sodic soils led to an addition of 5.3–7.6 t carbon ha^{-1} in a cropping season (Subhashini and Kaushik, 1984).

Table 30.3: Addition of Organic Carbon to Soil Through Blue Green Algae (BGA)

Quantity t/ha	*References*
0.75	Prasad, 1949
6.70	Fuller and Roger, 1952
0.5-1.4	Gollerbach *et al.*, 1956
0.45	Rao and Burns, 1990
41.6	Reynaud and Roger, 1981
3.2-6.8	Das *et al.*, 1991

Improvement in Soil Physical Properties

At the time of puddling before transplanting rice seedlings, the soil structure is completely destroyed. The inoculation of rice fields with BGA may help to quickly regenerate and improve the soil structure (Roychoudhury *et al.*, 1979). BGA are known to excrete extracellularly a number of compounds like polysaccharides, peptides, lipids etc. during their growth in soil (Bertocchi *et al.*, 1990). These compounds possibly diffuse around soil particles, glue and hold them together in the form of microaggregates. Besides these compounds, particularly polysaccharides are made of fibers, which can also entangle clay particles and form clusters. These clusters or microaggregates, in turn, grow and take the shape of macroaggregates and subsequently of larger soil aggregates. The interwoven nature of growing algal filaments may also help in binding the soil particles along with the organic C added through algal biomass. The importance of these compounds in soil-aggregate formation or soil stabilization has been indicated by many workers (Roychoudhury *et al.*, 1979; Schulten, 1985; Rogers and Burns 1994). Some researchers, however, have considered polysaccharides as transient adhesives (Tisdall and Oades, 1982) and or not directly involved in the formation of aggregates, although the products of their microbial degradation like aliphatic and polyphenolic compounds are considered to be responsible for this (Haynes *et al.*, 1991). The quantity and quality of the excreted compounds also vary depending on the species of BGA, their physiological growth stages and also the associated environmental conditions (Saxena and Kaushik, 1992; Roychoudhury *et al.*, 1985). Some species give low yields of excreted compounds (*e.g. Anabaena*), while other give high yields (*e.g. Gloeotrichia, Westiellopsis*). Polysaccharides from different algal species also differ with respect to their protein, uronic acid and sugar composition (Bertocchi *et al.*, 1990) and thus in their stability in soils with respect to microbial and thermal degradation. Kaushik and his co-workers (Kaushik and Krishna Murty, 1981; Subhashini and Kaushik, 1984; Kaushik, 1985) observed significant increases in soil aggregate stability due to an increase in the polysaccharide content of soils as a result of algal inoculation (Table 30.4). Similarly, water-stable aggregates, which are an integral part of good (soil) aggregate formation, have also been shown to increase significantly due to algal inoculation, resulting in an improvement in the water-holding capacity and aeration status of soils (Singh, 1961; Roychoudhury *et al.*, 1979). Such improvement in soil aggregation due to algal inoculation ultimately favoured better seedling emergence of upland crops sown after the paddy harvest (Rogers and Burns, 1994). All these results apparently suggest that the algal species, which liberate higher amounts of complex and thermostable polysaccharides, will possibly be a better choice for inoculation in rice fields for the regeneration of the soil structure. However, such algal species are known to be less efficient N_2 fixers.

Table 30.4: Comparative Effect of Blue Green Algae and *Azolla* on Soil Aggregation and Particle Size Distribution (Roychoudhury *et al.*, 1979)

Treatments	*Particle Size Distribution*		*Per cent Aggregates*		*Per cent Increase > 50 μ Aggregates*
	> 250 μ	*50-250 μ*	*> 250 μ*	*50-250 μ*	
Sand (>50m)	0.5	44.5	-	-	-
Control	1.2	46.8	0.7	2.3	-
BGA	1.5	48.0	1.0	3.5	50
Azolla	1.0	47.0	0.5	2.5	-
60 kg N ha^{-1}	0.7	46.6	0.2	2.1	-
60 kg N ha^{-1}+BGA	1.6	49.0	1.1	4.5	70
60 kg N ha^{-1}+ *Azolla*	0.8	47.2	0.3	2.7	-

Transformation of Soil P

Phosphorus is estimated to be in insufficient amounts in most of the Indian soils as available phosphorus. According to one of the recent compilation, based on about 9.6 million soil tests for available phosphorus in Indian soils, 49.3 per cent area spread in various states is in the low category, 48.8 per cent is of medium and only 1.9 per cent has high phosphorus status (Hasan, 1994). The problem of P management in soil is highly intricate as the applied phosphate through fertilizers is often fixed and becomes unavailable to the crops.

Cyanobacteria, like P-solubilizing bacteria, are known to have the ability to mobilise bound phosphates. They have been shown to solubilise insoluble $(Ca)_3(PO_4)_2$ (Bose *et al.*, 1971), $FePO_4$ (Wolf *et al.*, 1985), $AlPO_4$ (Dorich *et al.*, 1985) and hydroxyapatite $(Ca_5(PO_4)_3OH$ (Cameron and Julian, 1988) in soils, sediments or in pure cultures. There are mainly two hypotheses to explain how cyanobacteria solubilise such bound phosphates. One of the mechanisms may be that cyanobacteria might synthesise a chelator/chelators? Ca^{2+} and drive the following dissolution reaction without changing the pH of the growth medium (Cameron and Julian, 1988; Roychoudhury and Kaushik, 1989):

$$Ca_{10}(OH)_2(PO_4)_6 = 10Ca^{2+} + 2OH^- + 6PO_4^{3+}$$

Others (Bose *et al.*, 1971) were however of the opinion that H_2CO_3 and other organic acids released by cyanobacteria during their growth could solubilise P from Ca sources following the reaction:

$$Ca_3(PO_4)_2 + 2H_2CO_3 = 2CaHPO_4 + Ca(HCO_3)_2$$

A third group (Arora, 1969; Saha and Mandal, 1979; Mandal *et al.*, 1992) believed that the above mechanisms operate simultaneously. Once solubilised, the PO_4^{3-} is taken up by the growing algal cells for their nutrition. After completing their growth cycle, when the cells undergo lysis the cell-bound PO_4^{3-} is released in the growth medium and becomes available to plants on mineralisation. Observance of an initial decrease in the available–P content in soils due to algal growth and an appreciable increase later during biomass decomposition (Saha and Mandal, 1979; Mandal *et al.*, 1992) supported this possible pathway (Table 30.5).

Table 30.5: Changes of Available P mg g⁻¹ Soil Due to Incorporation of Blue Green Algae, *Azolla* and Urea

Days of Flooding	*Control*	*Blue Green Algae*	*Azolla*	*Urea*
7	7.50	7.92	9.37	9.08
14	3.58	3.94	4.89	4.48
21	5.32	13.55	13.97	6.29
28	6.97	14.06	18.45	7.90
35	7.45	10.89	11.62	7.85
LSD at 5 per cent	Treatment mean 1.19	Days mean 1.33	Interaction 2.66	

The solubilising effect of cyanobacteria on bound PO_4^{3-} may also be used for the efficient utilisation of low cost, low grade (in terms of P content) rock-phosphate fertilizers where PO_4^{3-} remains bound as various forms of apatite, like hydroxyapatite, carbonapatite, choloroapatite etc. These rock phosphates are generally used in acid soils as P fertilizer. In fact, Roychoudhury and Kaushik (1989) reported increased solubility of P in rock phosphate due to its inoculation with cyanobacteria.

Fuller and Roger (1952) observed a greater uptake of P by plants from algal materials than from inorganic phosphates when applied in equal amounts. They concluded that: (1) P in algal material is more available to plants than inorganic phosphates over longer periods, (2) chemical fixation is not so important a factor with respect to algal material as with respect to inorganic phosphates, and (3) temporary conversion of available soil or fertilizer P into cell materials by soil algae may be a desirable process from the stand-point of long-term availability. Their proposed hypothesis was that soil algae removed available P from the sphere of chemical fixation by converting it into cell materials for by absorbing it in "luxury" amounts that might be released gradually for crop use through the process of exudation, autolysis or microbial decomposition of old algal cells. Algae also have long been known to take up P in excess of their immediate needs, which may subsequently be released in the form of dissolved organic P (Lean and Nalewajko, 1976).

Technological Developments

The idea of utilizing algal biofertilizer to supplement the nitrogen requirement of rice crop was mooted as early as 1939. However the systematic approach was under taken at IARI and an algal biofertilizer technology was developed (Venkataraman, 1972). The technology was named as rural oriented mass multiplication technology and the application in field was often referred as algalization. In this process cyanobacteria were allowed to grow with soil as carrier and then utilized as inoculum in rice fields. Farmers adopted this all over India because of its simplicity and economic benefits. Depending upon the requirement of algal biofertilizer, the production technology could be scale up to–troughs, pits, and field plots/cemented tanks/polythene layered tanks. It involved -

However the technology could not become popular due to (1) non-availability of inoculum at the time of application, and (2) large variation in inoculum quality. Hence the cyanobacterial biofertilizer of assured quality in terms of known population density; nature of each strain with better compètitiveness was necessary to develop. In view of this, a new technology was developed in which cyanobacteria were grown in a formulated medium in glass/polyethylene house round the year of assured quality (Kaushik, 1998; Prasanna *et al.*, 1998).

Amelioration of Saline and Sodic Soils

Saline and sodic soils constitute a large area of agricultural land in the world. Sodic soils have a high pH, high exchangeable Na, measurable amounts of carbonates and undergo extensive clay dispersion (deflocculation, due to the high zeta potential of active Na^+), leading to poor hydraulic conductivity and reduced soil aeration. While saline soils contain excess amounts of soluble salts imparting high osmotic tension to plant roots for absorption of water and nutrients. Primarily, the reclamation of sodic soils requires the replacement of exchangeable Na with Ca. This is normally done by the application of suitable soil amendments, like gypsum, followed by leaching. The improvement of saline soils, on the other hand, requires leaching of excess soluble salts from the rhizosphere by good quality water. Reports of biological reclamation of these soils through the use of cyanobacteria are available (Singh, 1950; Kaushik, 1989). These methods of reclamation were basically based on the observations of extensive growth of cyanobacteria on alkali soils of India (Singh, 1950) and the USSR (Gollerbach *et al.*, 1956). These observations indicated a considerable tolerance of cyanobacteria to salinity and/or alkalinity stress. Several physiological mechanisms underlying such tolerance have now been identified. Curtailment of Na^+ influx (Subhashini and Kaushik, 1986; Apte *et al.*, 1987) and accumulation of K^+ ion (Jha *et al.*, 1987) or organic (sugar, polyols and quaternary amines etc.) osmoregulators (Blumwald *et al.*, 1983; Reed *et al.*, 1984; Kumar and Kaushik, 1994) are the important mechanisms that provide adequate protection to cyanobacteria against such salt/sodicity stress. Synthesis of salt stress specific fatty acids (Senthil *et al.*, 1993; Venkataraman and Kaushik, 1994) and proteins (Goel *et al.*, 1997) has been detected in several species of algae and cyanobacteria. Cyanobacteria exposed to such salinity/sodicity stress may lose or have diminished nitrogenase activity possibly due to the diversion of their cellular energy towards the biosynthesis of osmoregulators (Apte *et al.*, 1987), while Jha *et al.* (1987) reported enhanced heterocyst frequency in *Westiellopsis prolifica* under salinity suggesting the increased nitrogen demand of organism to overcome the stress. In such cases, the addition of a few kilograms of N, particularly as NO_3^- per hectare together with algal inoculation has been shown to be very effective in protecting them from these stresses and allowing them to establish in the stressed environment, and subsequently enhances their potential as N biofertilizer (Reddy *et al.*, 1989; Fernandes *et al.*, 1993). Once established and subsequently acclimatized to the stress, they may act in ameliorating their surrounding environment. A reduction in electrical conductivity, exchangeable Na and soil pH (Kaushik *et al.*, 1981; Kaushik and Subhashini, 1985) and an increase in the soluble Ca and Mg content of soils (Jain and Kaushik, 1989) have also been reported due to such algalization. The increase in soluble Ca and Mg and decrease in exchangeable Na may ultimately lower the sodium adsorption ratio–an index of alkalinity in soil–of the soils and thus alleviate the negative effects of high sodicity. In fact, Kaushik and his co-workers (Kaushik and Krishna Murthi, 1981; Subhashini and Kaushik, 1981) observed a considerable increase in the hydraulic conductivity of sodic soils due to cyanobacterial inoculation and found that it compared favourably to the use of gypsum in such soils.

A significant reduction in soil salinity (12-35 per cent) due to repeated cultivation of cyanobacteria in soils rendered saline owing to bad farm management has also been reported. The rice yield in saline soils is also less affected when N is given in the form of algal inocula vis-à-vis urea (Antarikanonda and Amarit, 1991). Further, such algal inocula have proved to be almost equally effective in increasing the rice yield in saline soils when compared with gypsum and/or pyrite treatments (Sharma *et al.*, 1989; Kaushik 1994b). Even when irrigated with saline water, cyanobacterial inoculation was found to be useful in minimizing the deleterious effect of the increased salinity on the barley crop (Jain and Kaushik, 1989).

In an alkali soil almost all the problems with respect to rice cultivation are associated with the high concentration and/or activities of Na^+. If somehow its activity is checked, the whole problem is solved. Cyanobacteria secrete organic acids particularly under salt stress (Singh, 1961; Sprent and Sprent, 1990), which can act on $CaCO_3$ to dissolve Ca. They also excrete a number of biologically active compounds, *i.e.* bioflocculants (Jha *et al.*, 1987; Levy *et al.*, 1992), which can flocculate the dispersed clay particles in alkali soils by inactivating/scavenging Na^+. All these effects of cyanobacteria may at least temporarily cause inactivation of Na^+ in alkali soils and make the soil environment favourable to the growth of plants. Successive cultivation of cyanobacteria makes the environment more favourable and after a few years it may help to produce a reasonably good yield of crops as observed in sugarcane and paddy after 3 years of reclamation with cyanobacteria. Although such biological soil amelioration is a time-consuming process, it is considered to be a sustainable approach as compared to reclamation by chemical amendments (Oikarinen, 1996).

Cyanobacteria as a Source of Value Added Products

Spirulina, a filamentous cyanobacterium is one of the extensively exploited micro algae. Its high nutritional value in terms of high protein content *i.e.* about 60-70 per cent of dry weight (Richmond, 1992), high vitamin content (Switzer, 1980) (Table 30.6), presence of unsaturated fatty acids like γ-linoleic acid which do not form cholesterol (Mahajan and Kamat, 1995), low nucleic acid content, easy digestibility due to absence of cellulosic cell wall, confer upon it the status of ideal single cell protein. In addition *Spirulina* is a source of compounds of therapeutic value to treat wounds (Clement *et al.*, 1967), β-carotene known for its anticancer property (Peto *et al.*, 1981). The pigment phycocyanin is used as a natural colour in health food and cosmetic products (Switzer, 1980). Hence, *Spirulina* is commercially cultivated as a source of human food, animal feed, and natural products and for wastewater treatment.

Spirulina Cultivation

In summer possibly high light intensity is found to be the growth regulatory whereas, in winter the low daytime temperature imposes the major limitations (Vonshak *et al.*, 1982). The optimum temperature for photosynthesis for *S. platensis* has been shown to be 35°C and for dark respiration 45°C

(Torzillo and Vonshak, 1994). In India maximum temperature during the summer is about 40°±5°C and in Northern India during winter months the temperature goes down to as low as 2-5°C. While studying the effect of temperature and light intensity on seven strains of *Spirulina* it was observed that all the strains showed maximum growth at 25 Klux light intensity at 30°C temperature, whereas 62-69 per cent growth was reported at 45 Klux light and 20°C temperature and none of the strains survived at 40°C (Basirath and Kaushik, 2002).

Table 30.6: Vitamin Content of *Spirulina* vis-à-vis Other Sources mg kg^{-1} Dry Matter and Meat

Vitamins	*Spirulina*	*Spinach*	*Beef Liver (Fresh)*
Provitamin A	840		
Vitamin E	120	122	10
Thiamine	44	4.9	3
Riboflavin	37	9.7	290
Pyridoxine	3	9.7	7
Cobalamine	7		0.65
Vitamin C	80	2480	310
Biotin	0.3	0.34	1
Inositol	380		
Folic acid	0.4	3.65	2.9
Ca-Pantothenate	13	14.8	73
Nicotinate		29.2	136

The growth of *Spirulina* is also affected by the concentration of sodium bicarbonate and the lowest concentration in which *S. platensis* could be maintained has been reported to be 0.2 M (Vonshak *et al.*, 1983). We observed that a concentration of 8gL^{-1} $NaHCO_3$ (commercial grade) provides biomass statistically equivalent to 16 g L^{-1} as reported earlier.

Natural Colours

A large array of natural products of economic potential may be produced from cyanobacteria. These also represent an attractive source of natural pigments such as phycobiliproteins, amounting to about 20 per cent of total dry weight vis-à-vis phycocyanin and phycoerythrin and *allo*-phycocyanin (Borowitzka, 1988); and carotenoids (Walsh *et al.*, 1997). Phycoerythrins in particular have applications as natural dyes as well as fluorescence microscopy. Some strains of *Anabaena* and *Nostoc* are however, particularly rich in phycoerythrin (Guerrero *et al.*, 1990). These may be used as pigments or colourants in the food industry as well as for cosmetics. The Dai Nippon Inks and Commercial Co. of Japan markets phycocyanin powder under the trade name of "Lina Blue". The product is an odourless, nontoxic blue powder with slight sweetness and has a brilliant blue with faint reddish fluorescence in water. The blue pigment from *Spirulina* is being used for eye shadow, eyeliner and lipsticks. A preparation of *Spirulina* chlorophyll in a mixture containing iron oxide and a higher alcohol was patented as a strong deodorant (Yamaguchi, 1981). Carotenoids have the widest commercial application *e.g.* food colouring, feed additives to enhance flesh colour of salmonoid fish, as well as the colour of the egg yolk. Also these improve the health and fertility of cattle (Borowitzka, 1988).

The blue pigment phycocyanin given orally to mice injected with liver tumor cells showed that the survival rate of treatment group was significantly higher than that of controls (Iijima *et al.*, 1982). They suggested that phycocyanin might generally stimulate the immune system providing protection against a variety of diseases. It was possible to prevent experimental oral cancer in rats by extracts of *Spirulina* (Schwartz *et al.*, 1986). Relatively high β-carotene of *Spirulina* was suggested to reduce certain cancer risks when ingested in suitable amounts (Schwartz *et al.*, 1986).

Recently (Kaushik, 2000) forty one species of cyanobacteria including unicellular, colonial, non-heterocystous and heterocystous filamentous were screened for the phycobilin pigments. *Lyngbya versicolor* ARM 348 which produced 10.2 per cent total phycobilins including c-phycocyanin 74.37 mg g^{-1} of dry biomass was superior to other unicellular *Anacystis nidulans* ARM 336, *Synechocystis* sp. ARM 340, or colonial *Gloeocapsa rupestris* ARM 338, *Aphanocapsa pulchra* ARM 341 and *Chlorogloea fritschii* ARM 342. The twenty one species of *Calothrix* showed greater diversity and produced as low as < 1 per cent to as high as 18.21 per cent by *Calothrix brevissima* ARM 114. The other heterocystous forms *Anabaena variabilis* ARM 310, *Aulosira fertilissima* ARM 68, *Hapalosiphon* sp. ARM 419 and *Tolypothrix tenuis* ARM 76 are the probable cyanobacterial species these can be exploited as the source of natural phycobilin content which varied from 14.72 to 17.52 per cent. From a total of six heterotrichous forms examined barring *Hapalosiphon* sp. ARM 419 (14.72 per cent phycobilin) all produced very little quantity of pigments.

Transgenic Cyanobacteria

Growing of genetically modified algae (or other organisms) is still not popular, as it is feared that the artificially engineered organisms could be unsafe and harmful for the environment due to spread of the foreign gene to unmodified organisms. But, genetically modified organisms are specially created for introducing useful traits not existing in their natural counterparts and many genetically modified organisms have a revolutionary impact on the agricultural sector.

A large number of genes have been cloned in cyanobacteria, *e.g. cat* (Friedberg, 1988), *lac* Z (Subramanian and Kaushik, 2001) and *lux* A and B (Schmetterer *et al.*, 1986) that catalyze the production of chloramphenicol, acetyl transferase, β-galactosidase and luciferase, respectively. Cyanobacterial colonies expressing *lac* Z when treated with the indicator 5-bromo-chloro-3-indolyl-β-D-galactoside (X-Gal) turn from green to turquoise surrounded by the blue halos. The *lux* operon has been originally derived from the bacterium *Vibrio fischeri* and *V. harveyi*, and the *luc* operon from the American firefly *Photinus pyralis*. Cells containing luciferase produce light on addition of the aldehyde and the resultant light emission is quantified. Subramanian and Kaushik (2001) have used the technique of cloning of the *lac* Z and *luc* genes in cyanobacteria *Anacystis cylindrica* ATCC 29414 and *Synechocystis* sp. ARM 340 to assess the growth and establishment of inoculated species under field conditions as well as the stability of these reporter genes in soil microcosm.

Most insecticides currently used are chemicals, but there are successful biological insecticides also. Resistance to chemical insecticides has occurred in several insect species. Management of such resistance remains a challenge, and new methods of controlling such species are needed. Various proteins have been identified as possessing insecticidal activities, *e.g.* α-amylase, lectins and insecticidal proteins from *Bacillus* species. The proteins produced by the *Bacillus* species possess the most potent insecticidal activities. Use of transgenic cyanobacteria to control insects is a new technology. *Bacillus thuringiensis* subsp. *israelensis* has been widely used as a biological pesticide to control mosquitoes and black flies, which are vectors for infectious human diseases, without adverse effects on other organisms. The larvicidal activity of this organism is due to the production of d-endotoxin. The applications of *B. thuringiensis israelensis* for mosquito control are limited by the short half-life of existing preparations under field conditions. This problem can be overcome by the cloning of d-endotoxin genes into cyanobacteria, which inhabit the breeding zones of mosquitoes and are used by them as a food source. Several attempts have been made to produce transgenic mosquitocidal cyanobacteria (Soltes-Rak *et al.*, 1995) and some success has been achieved in expressing single *cry* genes in unicellular strains, but the transformed cells displayed lower levels of mosquito-larvicidal activity than the level required for effective and practical use as bioinsecticides in natural aquatic environment. Various combinations of the genes *cry* IVA, *cry* IVD and p20 from *Bacillus thuringiensis israelensis* were introduced into *Anabaena* sp. strain PCC 7120, which displayed toxicity against third-instar larvae of *Aedes aegypti* at levels greater than any level previously reported for transgenic cyanobacteria (Xiaoqiang *et al.*, 1997).

Conclusion

A yield improvement of rice of between 5 per cent and 25 per cent was found when fields were inoculated with cyanobacteria even in the presence of 100-150 kg N ha^{-1} as fertilizer.

Cyanobacteria bring about, directly or indirectly, certain changes in the physical, chemical and biological properties of the soil and soil-water interface in rice fields, which are of agronomic importance. The extracellular organic compounds liberated by the algae and the O_2 released due to photosynthesis during their active growth period, and the subsequent addition of biomass after their death, are likely to cause some important changes in the physico-biochemical properties of soil.

The work done at Indian Agriculture Research Institute, New Delhi can be summarised as: (*a*) in areas where chemical nitrogen fertilisers are not used for various reasons, algal application as biological input can give to the rice farmers the benefit of applying 20-30 kg N/ha, (*b*) where fertilisers are used, the dose can be reduced by 30kg N/ha by algal supplementation, and (*c*) even with high levels of nitrogen fertilisers, the yield per unit input can be increased by 10-15 per cent through algal complementation.

Saline and alkali soils can be effectively reclaimed by the use of specific salt tolerant cyanobacteria along with gypsum is amply demonstrated in the work done at author's laboratory.

These mosquitocidal cyanobacterial strains could be efficiently grown in the production tanks as well as in the rice fields without any application of the insecticides thus reducing the pollution effect in the environment.

Blue green algal biomass has been considered since long as an alternative source of protein that could supplement conventional food and feed production. Other practical uses include the reclamation of wastewater, and the production of variety of commercial chemicals on a renewable basis as lipids, polysaccharides, pigments, vitamins and other compounds of industrial and pharmaceutical interest. Besides this, cyanobacteria are also useful in the production of different bioactive compounds (antibiotics, enzymes, cell growth promoters, toxins etc.). The interest in these organisms as generators of pharmacologically active compounds has been stimulated by recent results from the group of workers related to anti-cancer and immuno-stimulation properties of phycobiliproteins, as well as to the inhibition by the blue green algal sulfolipids of cytopathic effects of the human immuno-deficiency viruses (HIV).

References

Ahmad, M.R. and Winter, A. (1968). Studies on the hormonal relationship of algae in pure culture. 1. The effect of indole-3-acetic acid on the growth of blue-green and green algae. *Planta*, 78: 277-286.

Alimango, B.V. and Yoshida, T. (1977). *In situ* acetylene-ethylene assay of biological nitrogen in lowland rice soils. *Plant and Soil*, 47: 239-244.

Antarikanonda, P. and Amarit, P. (1991). Influence of blue-green algae and nitrogen fertilizer on rice yield in saline soils. *Kasetsart J. Nat. Sci.*, 25: 18-25.

Apte, S.K., Reddy, B.R. and Thomas, J. (1987). Relationship between sodium influx and salt tolerance of nitrogen-fixing cyanobacteria. *Appl. Environ. Microbiol.*, 53: 1934-1939.

Arora, S.K. (1969). The role of algae on the availability of phosphorus in paddy fields. *Riso* 18: 135-138.

Basirath, R. and Kaushik, B.D. (2002) Influence of light and temperature on mass multiplication of *Spirulina* strains. *Indian J Plant Physiology*, 7: 52-55.

Bertocchi, C., Navarini, L., Cesarp, A. and Anastasio, M. (1990). Polysaccharides from cyanobacteria. *Carbohydr. Polym.*, 12: 127-153.

Blumwald, E., Mehlhorn, R.J. and Packer, L. (1983). Studies of osmoregulation in salt-adaptation of cyanobacteria with ESR spin-probe techniques. *Proc. Natl. Acad. Sci.* USA, 80: 2599-2602.

Borowitzka, M.A. (1988). Vitamins and fine chemicals from micro algae. In: *Micro-algal biotechnology* (M.A. Borowitzka and L.J. Borowitzka eds) pp.153-196, Cambridge University Press, Cambridge.

Bose, P., Nagpal, U.S, Venkataraman, G.S. and Goyal, S.K. (1971). Solubilisation of tricalcium phosphate by blue-green algae. *Curr. Sci.*, 40: 165-166.

Cameron, H.J, and Julian, G.R. (1988). Utilisation of hydroxyapatite by cyanobacteria as their sole source of phosphate and calcium. *Plant Soil*, 109: 123-124.

Clement, G., Robellar, M. and Zarrouk, C. (1967). Wound treating medicaments containing algae. *Fr. Med.* pp. 5279.

Das, S.C., Mandal, B. and Mandal, L.N. (1991). Effect of growth and subsequent decomposition of blue green algae on the transformation of iron and manganese in submerged soils. *Plant Soil*, 138: 75-84.

De, P.K. (1936). The problem of nitrogen supply of rice: Part I. fixation of nitrogen in the rice soils under waterlogged conditions. *Indian J Agr Sci*, 6: 1237-1242.

De, P.K. and Biswas, N.R.D. (1952). Fixation of nitrogen in rice soils in the dry period. *Indian J agric Sci.*, 22: 375-388.

De, P.K. and Mandal, L.N. (1956). Fixation of nitrogen by algae in rice. *Soil Sci* 81: 453-458.

De, P.K. and Sulaiman, M. (1950). The influence of algal growth in the rice fields on the yield of crops. *Indian J Agric Sci*, 20: 327-342.

Dorich, R.A., Nelson, D.W. and Sommers, L.E. (1985). Estimating algal-available phosphorus in suspended sediments by chemical extraction. *J. Environ Qual*, 14: 400-405.

Fernandes, T.A., Iyer, V. and Apte, S.K. (1993). Differential responses of nitrogen-fixing cyanobacteria to salinity and osmotic stresses. *Appl. Environ. Microbiol*, 59: 899-904.

Friedberg, D. (1988). Use of reporter genes in cyanobacteria. *Methods Enzymol.* 167: 736-747.

Fuller, W.H. and Roger, R.N. (1952). Utilisation of the phosphorus of algal cells as measured by the Neubauer technique. *Soil Sci*, 74: 417-429.

Ganpati, T.R., Suprasanna, P., Bapat, V.A. and Rao, P.S. (1994). Stimulatory effect of cyanobacterial extract on banana shoot tip cultures. *Trop Agric* (Trinidad), 71: 299-302.

Goel, S., Mamta, M. and Kaushik, B.D. (1997). Nitrogen fixation and protein profile of halotolerant *Nostoc muscorum*-R strain isolated from rice fields and ARM 221 strain. *Indian J exptl Biol.*, 35: 746-750.

Gollerbach, M.M., Novichkova, L.A. and Sdubrikova, N.Y. (1956). The algae of takyrs. In: *Takyrs of western Turkmenia and routes of their agricultural conquest. Nauk. Moscow*, pp. 22-29.

Grieco, E. and Desrochers, R. (1978). Production de vitamine B_{12} parune algae belue. *Can J. Microbiol*, 24: 1562-1566.

Guerrero, M.G., Vargas, A.M., Rivas, J., Rodriguez, H., Moreno, J. and Losada, M. (1990). Cultivation of nitrogen fixing micro-algae for the generation of products with commercial interest. In: *From genes to bioproducts*. (Ed. Organizing Committee of Biotech.) 90. 91-97, PPU DM, MURACIA.

Gupta, A.B. and Gupta, K.K. (1972). Effect of *Phormidium* extract on growth and yield of *Vigna catjang* (cowpea) T.5369. *Hydrobiologia*, 40: 127: 132.

Gupta, A.B., Agarwal, V. and Kushwaha, A.S. (1967). The effect of algal growth-promoting substances on wheat. *Proc. Natl. Acad. Sci.* India, 37B: 349-355.

Hasan, R. (1994). In: *Phosphorus research in India*. (Edt. G. Dev) *Proc Group Discussion* at IARI-PPICIP Gurgaon, India. Pub 7.

Haynes, R.J, Swift, R.S. and Stephen, R.C. (1991). Influence of mixed cropping rotations (pasturearable) on organic matter content, water-stable aggregation and cold porosity in a group of soils. *Soil Till Res*, 19: 77-87.

Henriksson, E. (1971). In: *Biological nitrogen fixation in natural and agricultural habitats*. (Edd. T.A. Lie and E.G. Mulder) pp. 415. *Plant and Soil*, Special Volume.

Iijima, N., Fugii, I., Shimamatsu, H. and Katoh, S. (1982) Anti-tumor agent and method of treatment therewith. U S Patent pending, ref. No. P1150-726-A 82679.

Jacq, V. and Roger, P.A. (1977). Decrease of losses due to sulphate reducing processes in the spermosphere of rice by pre-soaking seeds in a culture of blue-green algae. *Cah ORSTOM Ser Biol*, 12: 101-108.

Jain, B.L. and Kaushik, B.D. 1989. Effect of algalization on crop response under saline irrigation. *J. Indian Soc Soil Sci.*, 37: 382-384.

Jha, M.N., Venkataraman, G.S. and Kaushik, B.D. (1987). Response of *Westiellopis prolofica* and *Anabaena* sp. to salt stress. *Mircen J. Appl. Microbiol Biotechnol*, 3: 307-317.

Kaushik, B.D. (1985). Effect of native algal flora on nutritional and physico-chemical properties of sodic soils. *Acta Bot Indica*, 13: 143-147.

Kaushik, B.D. (1989). Reclamative potential of cyanobacteria in salt-affected soils. *Phykos*, 28: 101-109.

Kaushik, B.D. (1998). Use of cyanobacterial biofertilizer in rice cultivation: A Technology Improvement. *In*: Cyanobacterial Biotechnology (edt) G Subramanian, BD Kaushik, GS Venkataraman, pp. 211-222, Science Publs. Inc. USA.

Kaushik, B.D. (1994a). Blue green algae and sustainable agriculture. In: *Natural Resource Management for sustainable Agriculture and Environment*, (edt. DL Deb) Angkor Publishers, New Delhi, pp.404-416.

Kaushik, B.D. (1994b). Algalization of rice in salt-affected soils. *Ann.Agril. Res.*, 15: 105-106.

Kaushik, B.D. (2000). Screening of cyanobacterial strains for natural colours. *Indian Hydrobiology*, 3: 81-84.

Kaushik, B.D. and Krishna Murti, G.S.R. (1981). Effect of blue green algae and gypsum application on physico-chemical properties of alkali soils. *Phykos*, 20: 91-94.

Kaushik, B.D., Krishna Murti, G.S.R. and Venkataraman, G.S. (1981). Influence of blue-green algae on saline alkali soils. *Sci. Cult.*, 47: 169-170.

Kaushik, B.D. and Subhashini, D. (1985). Amelioration of salt affected soils with blue green algae. II. Improvement in soil properties. *Proc Indian natn Sci Acad*. B 51: 386-389.

Kaushik, B.D. and Venkataraman, G.S. (1979). Effect of algal inoculation on the yield and vitamin C content of two varieties of tomato. *Plant and Soil*, 52: 135-137.

Kumar, H. and Kaushik, B.D. (1994). Response of *Calothrix brevissima* to salt. *Indian J Microbiol.*, 34: 38-41.

Lean, D.R.S. and Nalewajko, C. (1976). Phosphate exchange and organic phosphorus excretion by freshwater algae. *J. Fish Res. Bd Can.*, 33: 1312-1323.

Levy, N., Magdassi, S. and Baror, Y. (1992). Physico-chemical aspects in flocculation of bentonite suspensions by a cyanobacterial bioflocculant. *Water Res.*, 26: 249-254.

Mac Rae, I.C. and Castro, T.F. (1969). Nitrogen fixation in some tropical rice soils. *Soil Sci* 103: 277.

Mahajan, G. and Kamat, M. (1995). Gamma-linolenic acid production from *Spirulina platensis. Appl. Microbiol. Biotechnol.* 43: 466-469.

Mandal, B., Das, S.C. and Mandal, L.N. (1992). Effect of growth and subsequent decomposition of blue-green algae in the transformation of phosphorus in submerged soils. *Plant Soil*, 143: 289-297.

Marsalek, B., Zahradnickova, H. and Hronkova, M. (1992). Extracellular abscisic acid produced by cyanobacteria under salt stress. *J. Plant Physiol.*, 139: 506-508.

Mekonnen, A.E., Prasanna, R and Kaushik, B.D. (2002). Cyanobacterial nitrogen fixation in presence of nitrogen fertilizers. *Indian J Experimental Biol.*, 40: 854-857.

Metting, B. and Pyne, J.W. (1986). Biologically-active compounds from microalgae. *Enzyme Microbial Technol.*, 8: 386-394.

Misra, S. and Kaushik BD. (1989a). Growth promoting substances of cyanobacteria.I. Vitamins and their influence on rice plant. *Proc Indian natn Sci Acad*, B55: 295-300.

Misra, S. and Kaushik, B.D. (1989b). Growth promoting substances of cyanobacteria. II. Detection of amino acids, sugars and auxins. *Proc Indian natn Sci Acad*, B55: 499-504.

Nekrasova, K.A. and Aleksandrove, I.V. (1982). Participation of *Collembola* and earthworm in the transformation of algal organic matter. *Sov Soil Sci.*, 14: 31-39.

Okuda, A. and Yamaguchi, M. (1955). Nitrogen fixing microorganisms in paddy soils. I. Characteristics of the nitrogen fixation in paddy soils. *Soil and Plant Food*, 1: 102-104.

Oikarinen, M. (1996). Biological soil amelioration as the basis of sustainable agriculture and forestry. *Biol Fertil Soils*, 22: 342-344.

Peto, R., Doll, R., Bukley, J.D. and Sporn, M.B. (1981). Can dietary Beta-carotene materially reduce human cancer rates? *Nature* 290: 201-208.

Prasad, S. (1949). Nitrogen recuperation by blue green algae in soils of Bihar and their growth on different types. *J. Proc. Inst. Chem India*, 21: 135-140.

Prasanna, R. and Kaushik, B.D. (1994). Physiological and molecular genetic aspects of nitrogen fixation in non-heterocystous cyanobacteria. *Ind J Exptl Biol*, 32: 248-251.

Prasanna, R. and Kaushik, B.D. (1995). Nitrogen fixation and *nif* gene organization in branched heterocystous cyanobacteria; variation in the presence of *xis*A. *Folia Microbiol*, 40: 176-180.

Prasanna, R., Sharma, B.K., Sharma, R.K. and Kaushik, B.D. (1998). Standardization of growth parameters and formulation of medium for cyanobacterial biofertilizer strains. *Indian J Microbiol.*, 38: 211-215.

Rao, D.L.N. and Burns RG. (1990). Use of blue Green algae and bryophyte biomass as a source of nitrogen for oilseed rape. *Biol Fertil Soils*, 10: 61-64.

Renaud, P.A. and Roger, P.A. (1978). Nitrogen fixing algal biomass in Senegal rice fields. *Ecol Bull.* Stockholm, 26: 148-157.

Reynaud, P.A. and Roger, P.A. (1981). Seasonal variations of algal flora and of nitrogen fixing activity in a waterlogged sandy soils. *Rev Ecol Biol Sol*, 18: 9-27.

Reynault, J., Sasson, A., Pearson, H.W. and Stewart, W.D.P. (1975). Nitrogen fixing algae in Morocco. In: *Nitrogen fixation by free living microorganisms* (WDP Stewart ed.) p 229-248, London, Cambridge Univ. Press.

Reddy, B.R., Apte, S.K. and Thomas, J. (1989). Enhancement of cyanobacterial salt tolerance by combined nitrogen. *Plant Physiol.*, 89: 204-210.

Reed, R.H., Richardson, D.L., Warr, S.R.C. and Stewart, W.D.P. (1984). Carbohydrate accumulation and osmotic stress in cyanobacteria. *J. Gen Microbiol.*, 130: 1-4.

Richmond, A. (1992). *Spirulina.* In: Microalgal Biotechnology. Borowitzka MA and Borowitzka LJ (eds.) pp. 85-121. Cambridge University Press, Cambridge.

Rippka, R., Deruelles, J., Waterbury, J.B, Herdmann, M. and Stanier, R.Y. (1979). Generic assignment, strain histories and properties of pure culture of cyanobacteria. *J Gen Microbiol*, 111: 1-61.

Rodgers, G.A., Bergman, B., Henriksson, E. and Udris, M. (1979). Utilisation of blue-green algae in biofertilizers. *Plant Soil*, 52: 99-107.

Roger, P.A. and Reynaud, P.A. 1979. Ecology of blue green algae in paddy fields. p.289-309 *In*: International Rice Res. Institute. *Nitrogen and Rice*. Los Banos, Philippines.

Roger, P.A., Grant, I.F., Reddy, P.M. and Watanabe, I. 1987. The photosynthetic aquatic biomass in wetland rice fields and its effect on nitrogen dynamics. In: *Efficiency of nitrogen fertilizers for rice.* IRRI, Manila, pp. 43-68.

Rogers, S.L. and Burns, R.G. 1994. Changes in aggregate stability nutrient status indigenous microbial populations and seedling emergence following inoculation of soil with *Nostoc muscorum*. *Biol Fertil. Soils*, 18: 209-215.

Roychoudhury, P. and Kaushik, B.D. (1989). Solubilization of Mussorie rock phosphate by cyanobacteria. *Curr Sci*, 58: 569-570.

Roychoudhury, P., Kaushik, B.D., Krishna Murty, G.S.R. and Venkataraman, G.S. (1979). Effect of blue green algae and *Azolla* application on the aggregation status of soil. *Curr Sci.*, 48: 454-455.

Saha, K.C. and Mandal, L.N. (1979). Effect of algal growth on the availability of P, Fe and Mn in rice soils. *Plant Soil*, 52: 139-149.

Satapathy, K.B. (1999). Comparative efficiency of blue-green algae, *Azolla* and other biofertilizers on growth of rice. *Indian J Plant Physiol* 4: 100-104.

Saxena, S. and Kaushik, B.D. (1992). Polysaccharides (biopolymers) from halotolerant cyanobacteria. *Indian J exptl Biol.*, 30: 433-434.

Schmetterer, G., Wolk, P. and Elhai, J. (1986). Expression of luciferases from *Vibrio harveyi* and *Vibrio fischeri* in filamentous cyanobacteria. *J Bacteriol* 167: 411-414.

Schulten, J.A. (1985). Soil aggregation by cryptogams of a sand prairie. *Am J. Bot.*, 72: 1657-1661.

Schwartz, J., Scklar, G. and Suda, D. (1986). Inhibition of experimental oral carcinogenesis by β-carotene. Harvard School of Dental Medicines. *Carcinogenesis*, 7: 711-715.

Senthil, C., Roychoudhury, P. and Kaushik, B.D. (1993). Lipid profile of halosensitive *Calothrix marchica bharadwajae*. *Indian J Microbiol.*, 33: 281-285.

Sharma, M.L., Bhardwaj, G.S. and Chauhan, Y.S. (1989). Study on the effect of biofertilizer, pyrite and gypsum on paddy in the salt-affected soils. *Indian J Agron.*, 34: 129: 130.

Shukla, A.C. and Gupta, A.B. (1967). Influence of algal growth-promoting substances on growth, yield and protein contents of rice plants. *Nature*, 213: 744.

Singh, D.N., Venkataraman, G.S., Rao, S.B.P., Bhattacharya, A. and Goyal, S.K. (1972). Effect of algal inoculation on jaya rice variety under field condition. *Labdev J Sci Technol*, 10B: 107-108.

Singh, R.N. (1950). Reclamation of "usar" lands in India through blue-green algae. *Nature*, 165: 325-326.

Singh, R.N. (1961). Role of Blue green algae in nitrogen economy of Indian agriculture. Indian Council of Agricultural Research, New Delhi. p.175.

Singh, V.P. and Trehan, T. (1973). Effect of extracellular products of *Aulosira fertilissima* on the growth of rice seedlings. *Plant Soil*, 38: 457-464.

Soltes-Rak, E., Kushner, D.J., Williams, D.D. and Coleman. J.R. (1995). Factors regulating *cry* IVB expression in the cyanobacterium *Synechococcus* PCC 7942. *Mol Gen Genet* 246: 301-308.

Sprent, J.I. and Sprent, P. (1990). Nitrogen fixing organism–pure and applied aspects. *Chapman and Hall*. London. pp. 256.

Stewart, W.D.P. (1964). Nitrogen fixation by Myxophyceae from marine environment. *J Gen Microbiol* 36: 415-422.

Stewart, W.D.P., Rowell, P., Ladha, J.K. and Sampio, M.J.A. (1979). Blue-green algae (cyanobacteria)–some aspects related to their role as source of fixed nitrogen in paddy soils. In: *Nitrogen and Rice*, International Rice Research Institute, Los Banos, Philippines, p. 263.

Subhashini, D. and Kaushik, B.D. (1981). Amelioration of sodic soils with blue-green algae. *Aust. J. Soils Res.*, 19: 361-367.

Subhashini, D. and Kaushik, B.D. (1984). Amelioration of salt affected soils with blue green algae. I. Influence of algalization on the properties of saline alkali soils. *Phykos*, 23: 273-277.

Subhashini, D. and Kaushik, B.D. (1986). Uptake of sodium and potassium by blue green algae (cyanobacteria). *Zbl fur Mikrobiol.*, 141: 177-180.

Subramanian, S. and Kaushik, B.D. (2001). Development of genetic markers in cyanobacteria and stability of genetically marked strains in soil. *World J. Microbial Biotech*, 17: 535-544.

Switzer, L. (1980). *Spirulina*–The whole food Revolution. Los Angeles, CA: Bantan Books.

Thomas, J. (1977). Biological nitrogen fixation. *Nucl India*, 15 : 2-8.

Tisdall, J.M. and Oades, J.M. (1982). Organic matter and water stable aggregates in soils. *J. Soil Sci.*, 33: 141-163.

Torzillo, G. and Vonshak, A. (1994). Effect of light and temperature on the photosynthetic activity of the cyanobacterium *Spirulina platensis*. *Biomass Bioenergy*. 6: 399-403.

Traore, T.M., Roger, P.A., Renaud, P.A. and Sasson A. (1978). Nitrogen fixation by blue green algae in paddy field in Mali. *Cab ORSTOM Ser Biol*, 13: 181-185.

Venkataraman, G.S. (1972). Algal biofertilizer and rice cultivation. Today and Tomorrow's publ., New Delhi.

Venkataraman, G.S. (1975). The role of blue green algae in tropical rice cultivation. In: *Nitrogen fixation by free living microorganisms*. (Edt. W.D.P. Stewart) Cambridge Uni Press, p.207-268.

Venkataraman, G.S. (1979). Algal inoculation of rice fields. *In*: International Rice Res. Institute. *Nitrogen and Rice*. Los Banos, Philippines, 311-321.

Venkataraman, G.S. and Goyal, S.K. (1963). Role of blue-green algae in nitrogen economy of Indian soils. *Agric Res* New Delhi. 3: 9.

Venkataraman, G.S. and Neelakantan, S. (1967). Effect of cellular constituents of nitrogen fixing blue-green alga *Cylindrospermum* on root growth of rice plants. *J. Gen. Appl. Microbiol.*, 13: 53-62.

Venkataraman, S. and Kaushik, B.D. (1994). Fatty acid profile of a marine *Nostoc calcicola* under saline and non-saline conditions. *Curr Sci.*, 67: 120-122.

Vonshak, A., Abelovich, A., Boussiba, S., Arad, S.M. and Richmond, A. (1982). Production of *Spirulina* biomass: Effects of environmental factors and population density. *Biomass* 2: 175-185.

Vonshak, A., Boussiba, S., Abelovich, A. and Richmond, A. (1983). Production of Spirulina biomass: Maintenance of monoalgal cultures outdoors. *Biotechnology and Bioengineering* 25: 341-349.

Walsh, K., Jones, G.J. and Dunstan, R.H. (1997). Effect of irradiance on fatty acid, carotenoid, total protein composition and growth of *Microcystis aeruginosa*. *Phytochemistry* (UK) 44: 817-824.

Watanabe, A. (1951). Production in cultural solution of some amino acids by the atmospheric nitrogen fixing blue-green algae. *Arch Biochem. Biophys.*, 34: 50.

Watanabe, A. (1973). On the inoculation of paddy fields in the pacific area with nitrogen fixing blue-green algae. *Soil Biol Biochem* 5: 161-162.

Watanabe, A., Nishigzaki, S. and Konishi, C. (1951). Effect of nitrogen fixing blue green algae on the growth of rice plants. *Nature* 108: 748.

Watnable, I. and Roger, P.A. (1984). Nitrogen fixation in wet land rice fields. In: *Current development in biological nitrogen fixation*. (Edt. N.S. Subba Rao) Oxford IBH New Delhi, pp. 237-276.

Wilson, J.T. (1980). In Blue green algae and Rice. PA Roger and SA Kulasooriya. International Rice Research Institute, Los Banos, Philippines.

Wyatt, J.T, and Silvey, J.K.G. (1969). Nitrogen fixation by *Gloeocapsa. science*, 165: 908-909.

Yoshida, T. and Ancazans, P.R. 1993. *Soil Sci Soc Amer Proc* 37: 42.

Wolf, A.M., Baker, D.E., Pionke, H.B. and Kunichi, H.M. 1985. Soil test for estimating labile, soluble and algal available phosphorus in agricultural soils. *J. Environ. Qual.*, 14: 341-348.

Xiaoqiang W, Vennison SJ, Huirong L, Ben-Dov E, Zaritsky A and Boussiba S 1997 Mosquito larvicidal activity of transgenic *Anabaena* strain PCC 7120 expressing combinations of genes from *Bacillus thuringiensis* sub. sp. *israelensis. Appl Enviro. Microbiol* 63: 4971-4975.

Yamaguchi, T. (1981). Strong Deodorant. *Japanese Patent*, 79 JP-116131.

Microbial Biotechnology and Ecology (2011) *Pages* **544–552**
Editors: **Deepak Vyas, G.S. Paliwal, P.K.Khare and R.K Gupta**
Published by: **DAYA PUBLISHING HOUSE, NEW DELHI**

Chapter 31

Effect of Herbicides on Mitosis, Nucleic Acids and Protein Contents in *Corchorus* and Soybean Plants

☆ ***A.K.S. Chouhan and S.K. Yadav***

Department of Botany, Dr. H.S. Gour Vishwavidyalaya, Sagar – 470 003, M.P.

ABSTRACT

Effects of three herbicides, *viz.*, Fluchloralin, Butachlor and Pendimethalin in varying concentrations (200, 400, 600, 800 and 1000 ppm) was studied on mitotic cell division, nucleic acids, (DNA and RNA) and protein contents of leaves of soybean crop and *Corchorus olitorius* Lin. a dominant weed of soybean field. All the three herbicides reduced cell division (Miotic Index) significantly in *Corchorus* root meristem at all the test concentrations. Further, the reduction of miotic index increased with the increase in the concentration of herbicides. In soybean lower concentrations of these herbicides showed no effect, where as higher concentrations reduced mitotic index significantly. No significant chromosomal abnormalities were observed in our experiment, however few abnormal cell showing sticky and eroded chromosoms were seen in both the plant samples treated with 1000 ppm concentration of fluchloralin.

All the three herbicides affect the DNA, RNA and protein contents of leaves in Soybean and *Corchorus* plants, but the magnitude of effect vary for the plants as well as for herbicides. Fluchloralin was found to be the most effective herbicide. It decreased DNA, RNA and protein contents considerably in both the plants, and the amount of these biomolecules decreased with the increase in treatment concentration. Butachlor and pendimethalin also decreased nucleic acids and protein contents considerably in *Corchorus* but with less efficiency as compared to fluchloralin. Lower concentrations of these herbicides *i.e.* 200 and 400 ppm showed a vary little or no effect on nucleic acids and protein in Soybean where as, higher concentrations reduced the amount of these molecules considerably. It is suggested that for the control of weeds in the crop field, lower concentrations of herbicides should be used to avoid the damage of crop plants.

Introduction

The continuous, consistent and indiscriminate use of agrochemicals for maximizing the crop yield is leading to senseless chemical saturation of environment and creating a vary serious human health as well as environmental problem (Odum 1971).

Herbicides are important agrochemicals used for controlling weeds in the crop. The use of these chemicals are increasing tremendously all over the world and a large number of them are being added annually to the market under different brand names. A survey of available literature on chemical weed control reveals that much of the work done so far pertains mostly on the morphological and anatomical aspects of the weeds as well as the crop plants. Workers like Sawamura (1964), Strove (1973), Amer and Ali (1974), Skorupaska (1975), Tomkins and Grant (1976), Sikka and Sharma (1976), Mousa (1982), Reddy and Rao (1982), Hess (1983), Soheir *et al.* (1989), Badr (1983), Soupuri and Mishra (1993), studied the effects of different herbicides on cell division in different plants and have reported various types of chromosomal aberrations and reduction in the number of dividing cells. A very few records are available on the biochemical effects of herbicides in weed and crop plants. Workers like West *et al.* (1960), Key and Hanson (1961), Key *et al.* (1966), Moreland *et al.* (1969), Chen *et al.* (1972), Bell *et al.* (1976), Chouhan and Yadav (2007). Kolhe (1979) have investigated the effect of different herbicides on nucleic acids and protein contents in different plants. Some of them observed increase and some of them observed decrease in nucleic acid and protein contents.

The forgoing reports indicate that several herbicides used in the control of unwanted weeds have the ability to inhibit cell division and induced chromosomal abnormalities. Chromosomal aberrations have been considerd as reliable indicators of mutagenic activity (Mohandas and Grant 1972) and there have been evidences for a correlation between chromosomal damage and toxic effects of a number of herbicides (Gichner *et al.*, 1968; Tomkins and Grant, 1976; Delcourt and Deysson 1976). Neilson *et al.* (1968) stated rightly that any new drugs or chemicals must be tested for their toxic effects on cell at cellular level before they are released for general use. For better and safe use of herbicides for increasing the agricultural productivity study of mode of action of these chemicals at cellular level is pre-requisite. Fluchloralin, Butachlor and Pendimethalin are the common herbicides, widely used for weed control in Soybean fields in this region. So for as the authers are aware these herbicides were not studied for their cytological and biochemical effects. It is with this view the present problem was undertaken to investigate the effects and the mode of action of these herbocides on cell division and nucleic acids and protien contents in *Corchorus* weed and Soybean crop.

Materials and Methods

Effect of these herbicides, *viz.*, Fluchoralin, Butachlor and Pendimethalin in five different concentrations (200, 400, 600, 800 and 1000ppm) on cell division, nucleic acids and protien contents in *Corchorus* and Soybean plants was studied. The details of methods are as follows:

Effect on Cell Division

Seeds of *Corchorus* and Soybean were treated with different concentrations of the test herbicides for 24 hours. Then they were washed thoroughly with water and kept for germination on moist filter paper in petridishes in a germination incubator at 27°±2°C. For control the seeds were soaked in water for 24 hours. Root tips of about 48 hours old germinating seeds were used for this study.

Roots in each case were examined to note the extent of cell division process and chromosomal abnormalities. Root squashes were made in 2 per cent acetoorcein following the method described by Sharma and Sharma (1965). The data obtained were analysed statisticaly and expressed as mean ±

standard error to gather with 't' significance test for mitotic index and as percentage of chromosomal abnormalities.

Effect on Nucleic Acids and Protein Contents

The plants of *Corchorus* and Soybean were sprayed with different concentrations of herbicides. The leaves were collected when morphological symptoms of the herbicides were seen on leaves.

Preliminary Extraction of Leaves

Leaves weighing one gram fresh weight were taken for estimation of nucleic acids and proteins. For extraction, the procedure of Nieman and Poulsan (1963) was followed with slight modification.

The Frozen samples were homogenized in chilled 10 ml of 95 per cent of ethanol. The homogenate was rinsed into a centrifuge tube with another 5 ml of cold ethanol and centrifuged. All centrifuging were done at room temperature at 3500 rpm. The supernatant was discarded each time. The sediment was extracted successively by suspending and centrifuging with 12 ml of each of the following reagents.

1. 95 per cent of ethanol at room temperature: Once
2. 50 per cent ethanol adjusted to pH 4.5 with glacial acitic acid at room temperature: Twice.
3. Chilled (4°C 0.2 N perchloric acid (PCA): Twice : The suspension was held at 4°C for 20 minutes before centrifuging.
4. 95 per cent ethanol at room temperature: Once.
5. Boiling absolute ethanol at room temperature: Once.
6. Ether at room temperature: Once.

Separation of Nucleic Acids and Proteins

The leaf powder obtained in the above procedure was suspended with 10 ml of 0.3N NaOH and held at 30°C for 18 hours. The sediment was removed by centrifuging and washed once with 5 ml of 0.3N NaOH. The extract and the wash were combined and made to 15 ml with 0.3N NaOH. Eight ml (8.0ml) aliquot, reserving 7 ml for protein estimation, was acidified to pH 1 with 15 per cent PCA, held at 4°C for 40 minutes and then centrifuged. The supernatant equals RNA fraction. The DNA-protein sediment was resuspended with 2 ml of water followed by 2 ml of 1 N PCA. The suspension was held at 4°C for 20 minutes, then centrifuged and the supernatant was added to the RNA fraction. The final RNA extract was made to 15 ml with water.

The DNA-protein was suspended with 3 ml of 0.5 N PCA, heated at 70°C for 15 minutes and centrifuged. The supernatant equals the DNA fraction. The protein sediment was washed with 2 ml of 0.5 N PCA and centrifuged and the wash added to the DNA fraction. The final DNA extract was made to 5 ml with 0.5 N PCA.

Estimation of Nucleic Acids

DNA

The samples of separated DNA from the extract ranging from 0.6 to 1.5 ml were taken in different test tubes and the volume was made to 2 ml with distilled water. Blank was prepared using 2 ml distilled water. Each tube was added with 4 ml of freshly prepared diphenylamine reagent and the mixture was heated for 5 minutes in boiling water bath. They were cooled to room temperature and read at 600 nm on spectrophotometer (UV 108 spectrophotometer). The DNA content of the samples was calculated from standard graph of calf-thymus DNA. The total DNA content was calculated on per gram-dry weight basis.

RNA

The samples of separated RNA from the extract ranging from 0.1 to 0.5 ml were taken in clean dry test tubes and the volume was made 2 ml with distilled water. Blank was prepared taking 2 ml distilled water only. In each test tube 5 ml of ferric chloride-hydrochloric acid was added, followed by 0.3 ml orcinol reagent. The tubes were placed in boiling waterbath for 20 minutes. The tubes were allowed to cool to room temperature and read at 660 nm on spectrophotometer. The RNA content in sample was calculated using standard graph of yeast RNA. The total RNA content was calculated on per gram dry weight basis.

Estimation of Proteins

The samples of proteins ranging between 0.1 to 0.4 ml were taken in clean dry test tubes and the volume was made to 1.2 ml with distilled water. Each tube was added with 6 ml freshly prepared alkaline copper solution. After 10 minute 0.3 ml Follin Ciacaltue's phenol reagent was added mixed thoroughly. Percent transmittance was read at 500 nm on spectrophotometer after 30 minutes. The protein content in the sample was calculated using a standard graph of egg albumin protein and one per gram dry weight basis.

Results and Discussion

The experimental data obtained after the treatment of plants were analysed in terms of following parameters:

1. Mitotic Index (MI) comparison between treated and control and 't' significance test.
2. Induced mitotic abnormalities–any abnormality in the dividing cells at chromosomal level.
3. Percentage increase or decrease in the amount of nucleic acids and protein contents after herbicidal treatment.

Effect on Cell Division

The results indicate that all the test herbicides inhibited cell division process significantly in *Corchorus* weed as well as in Soybean crop. Moreover, in *Corchorus* the inhibitory effect increased gradually with the increase in the concentration of herbicides, but in Soybean lower concentrations showed no effect where as higher concentrations of these herbicides reduced cell division (mitotic index) significantly. Fluchloralin was found to be the most effetive in both the plants followed by Butachlor and Pentimethalin. No significant chromosomal abnormalities were observed in our investigation, however, few abnormal cells showing sticky and eroded chromosomes were seen in both the plant samples treated with 1000 ppm of fluchloralin (Table 31.1).

Reduction in number of dividing cells due to herbicidal treatment has been reported by number of workers. Ryland (1948) observed a general inhibition of cell division in young root tips of *Allium* and *Narcissum* with the treatment of 2, 4-D. Kolhe (1979) studied the cytological effets of 2,4-D, Hyvar X and Gramoxone on farm weeds. He observed different chromosomal abnormalities and reduction in number of dividing cells in root tip by these herbicides. Many other workers also noticed similar observations in different weed species treated with different herbicides (Sawamura, 1964; Khosla, 1967; Bakale, 1972; Amar and Ali, 1974; Tomkins and Grant, 1976; Sikka and Sharma, 1976; Njagi and Gopalan, 1981; Mousa, 1982; Reddy and Rao, 1982). All these investigators noted changes in the mitotic stages with herbicides.

Table 31.1: Miotic Indices in Root Meristem of *Corchorus olitorius* and Soybean Treated with Different Concentrations of Herbicides

Species	*Herbicides*	*Concentration of Herbicides (ppm)*					
		Control	*200*	*400*	*600*	*800*	*1000*
Corchorus oliterius	F	1.83±0.36	1.12±0.18 (4.84)**	0.61±0.12 (8.03)**	0.48±0.09 (9.42)**	0.40±0.13 (8.48)**	0.33±0.15 8.39)**
	B	1.83±0.36	1.49±0.19 (2.01)	0.59±0.13 (7.94)**	0.42±0.12 (9.67)**	0.52±0.15 (8.08)**	0.58±0.20 (7.31)**
	P	1.83±0.36	1.18±0.11 (4.53)**	0.85±0.08 (7.13)**	0.59±0.06 (9.38)**	0.49±0.22	0.74±0.35 (4.27)**
Glycin max	F	2.34±0.41	2.02±0.22 (1.65)	1.91±0.12 (2.13)	1.69±0.15 (3.35)**	1.48±0.19 (5.84)**	0.62±0.18 (9.51)**
	B	2.34±0.41	2.18±0.08 (1.98)	2.04±0.30 (2.02)	1.94±0.24 (2.29)*	1.87±0.26 (2.88)*	0.93±0.13 (6.45)**
	P	2.34±0.41	2.08±0.31 (1.92)	1.95±0.17 (3.63)**	1.88±0.17 (3.63)**	1.64±0.31 (4.02)**	1.08±0.22 (5.98)**

*: Significant at P > 0.05 : 18 df values given in poven these one 't' value.

**: Significant at P > 0.01 18 df value.

An agent can disrupt the mitotic cycle in three ways (*i*) by inhibiting the process of cell division (*ii*) by disturbing the normal functioning of mitotic spindle and (*iii*) by producing chromosomal abnormalities. In this study reduction in percentage of dividing cells (MI) and increase in pre-metaphase/Postmetaphase ratio (Table 31.2) due to test herbicides indicate that the herbicides have some antimitotic activity and they are acting at both interphase and pre-metaphase levels affecting some vital functional units of the cell and the normal functioning of spendle mechanism respectively.

Effect on Nucleic Acids and Protein Contents

All the three herbicides affect the DNA, RNA and protein contents of leaves in Soybean and *Corchorus*, however the magnitude of effect vary for the plants as well as for herbicide (Table 31.3). Fluchloralin was found to be the most effetive herbicide. It decreased the DNA, RNA and protein contents (biomolecule) considerably in both plants. Further, the decrease in biomolecule contents was increased with the increase in concentration of this herbicide. Butachlor and pendimenthalin also decreased the amount of DNA, RNA and protein in *Corchorus* but with less efficiency as compared to fluchloralin. Lower concentrations of these herbicides showed a very little or no effect on biomolecule contents in Soybean, where as higher concentrations reduced the amount of these biomolecules considerably in Soybean also.

It is evident from the results that fluchloralin was the most effective herbicide as it caused maximum redution of biomoleule contents in both the plants followed by butachlor and pendimethalin. Some workers have studied the effect of different herbicides on DNA, RNA and protein contents in different weed and crop species. Key *et al.* (1966) reported inrease in DNA and protein contents in soybean seedling after spray with 2,4-D. Chen *et al.* (1972) also reported incrase in DNA and protein in cucumber and wheat seedling by 2,4-D. Inhibition of DNA synthesis by paraquat in *Vicia faba* seedling was reported by Bell *et al.* (1976). Decrease in DNA content in *Taphrosia hamiltonii* after treatment with 2,4-D and gramoxone was reported by Kolhe (1979). West *et al.* (1960) reported in corn and cucumber tissue that with one exception, low concentration of 2,4-D decreased and high concentrations increased the level of RNA. Moreland *et al.* (1969) studied the effects of 22 different herbicides on RNA and protein synthesis in maize mesocotyle and soybean hypocotyle and found that 14 of the herbicides used, inhibited RNA and protein synthesis *in vivo*. Similar results were also reported by other workers (Chrispeels and Hanson, 1962; Shannon *et al.*, 1964; Gulifoyle and Hanson, 1974; Bakale, 1972; Chouhan and Yadav, 2007).

Table 31.2: Premetaphase (A) and Post-metaphase (B) Ratio in Root Meristem of *Corchorus olitorius* and Soybean Treated with Various Concentration of Herbicides

Herbicides	*Concentration (ppm)*	*Corchorus olitorius*			*Glycine max*		
		A	*B*	*A/B Ratio*	*A*	*B*	*A/B Ratio*
Control	–	38	13	2.92	68	32	2.13
	200	18	10	1.80	42	24	1.75
	400	08	02	4.00	15	04	3.75
	600	05	01	5.00	13	03	4.33
	800	03	01	3.00	12	02	6.00
	1000	03	00		09	01	9.00
	200	27	09	3.00	51	15	3.40
	400	10	03	3.33	23	06	3.83
	600	07	01	7.00	18	03	6.00
	800	07	01	7.00	15	03	5.00
	1000	06	01	6.00	16	04	4.00
	200	18	12	1.50	38	17	2.24
	400	12	05	2.40	28	09	3.11
	600	07	01	7.50	18	05	3.60
	800	06	00	–	13	03	4.33
	1000	03	00	–	15	03	5.00

Table 31.3. Amount of nucleic acids and protein (mg/g) in *Corehorus* and soybean after spraying with different concentrations of Fluchloralin (F), Butachlor (B) and Pendimethalin (P)

Corchorus

Concentration (ppm)	*DNA*			*RNA*			*Protein*		
	F	*B*	*P*	*F*	*B*	*P*	*F*	*B*	*P*
Control	160.00	160.00	160.00	168.00	168.00	168.00	240.00	240.00	24.00
200	144.00 (–100.00)	148.00 (–07.00)	160.00 (00.00)	148.00 –11.91	156.00 –07.15	160.00 –04.77	167.00 (–30.21)	200.00 (–16.67)	202.50 (–15.53)
400	124.00 (–22.50)	140.00 (–12.50)	140.00 (–12.50)	132.00 (–21.43)	140.00 (–16.67)	140.00 (–16.67)	130.00 (–45.84)	175.00 (–27.09)	182.00 (–24.19)
600	112.00 (–30.00)	142.00 (–23.75)	125.00 (–21.88)	112.00 (–33.34)	120.00 (–28.58)	120.00 (–56.25)	105.00 (37.50)	150.00 (37.50)	157.00 (–34.59)
800	110.00 (–31.25)	110.00 (–31.25)	120.00 (–25.00)	92.00 (–45.24)	112.00 (–33.34)	110.00 (–34.53)	67.00 (–72.09)	132.00 (–45.00)	132.50 (–44.80)
1000	80.00 (–50.00)	108.00 (–32.50)	100.00 (–37.50)	64.00 (–61.95)	92.00 (–45.24)	92.00 (–45.24)	57.00 (–76.25)	120.00 (–50.00)	114.50 (–52.30)

Contd...

Table 31.3–Contd...

Soybean

Concentration (ppm)	DNA			RNA			Protein		
	F	B	P	F	B	P	F	B	P
Control	200.00	200.00	200.00	192.00	192.00	192.00	412.50	412.50	412.00
200	188.00 (–06.00)	200.00 (00.00)	200.00 (00.00)	160.00 (–16.67)	168.00 (–12.50)	168.00 (–12.50)	377.50 (–08.49)	382.50 (–07.28)	407.50 (–01.22)
400	152.00 (–24.00)	200.000 (00.00)	200.00 (00.00)	116.00 (–39.59)	132.00 (–31.25)	152.00 (–20.84)	340.00 (–17.58)	362.50 (–12.13)	382.50 (–07.28)
600	128.00 (–36.00)	160.00 (–20.00)	180.00 (–10.00)	100.00 (–47.92)	108.00 (–43.75)	120.00 (–37.50)	282.00 (–31.52)	330.00 (–20.00)	325.00 (–21.22)
800	100.00 (–50.00)	140.00 (–30.00)	160.00 (–20.00)	80.00 (–58.34)	88.00 (–54.17)	112.00 (–41.67)	200.00 (–51.52)	250.00 (–39.40)	300.00 (–27.48)
1000	84.00 (–58.00)	120.00 (–40.00)	140.00 (–30.00)	52.00 (–72.92)	68.00 (–64.59)	100.00 (–47.92)	119.00 (–70.16)	160.00 (–63.22)	272.00 (–33.94)

Values given in Parenthesis are increase (+) or decrease (–) above and below control level.

In many cases the herbicidal effects noted on protein and nucleic acids synthesis may be indirectly due to limitation of photosynthetic energy supply by reducing ATP synthesis (Moreland, *et al.*, 1969). It is known that approximately 90 per cent of all the ATP generated in the cell are used to produce macromolecules such as DNA, RNA and proteins. The treatment of cell with toxic substances at sublethal dose affects the enzyme system of cell (Dustin, 1947) and presence of organic compound in a cell may exert some fundamental effects on enzyme system (Wuu and Grant 1966a) might be resulting in disturbance of homeostasis of the cell by genetic variability induced by herbicides.

The forgoing results and discussions indicate that all the three test herbicides possessed the potential to inhibit the process of cell division and the synthesis of nucleic acids and protein in *Corchorus* and Soybean. The possible explanation and interpretation for the mechanism of action of these herbicides may be derived from the above observations. In all possibilities as the enzyme system of biochemical pathways leading to the generation of ATP and synthesis of macromolecules, are impaired, these herbicides may act as metabolic inhibitors. Metabolic disturbance due to these chemicals may generally effect the synthesis of nucleic acids and proteins, consequently resulting in decrease in rate of cell division and so also in the miotic index.

Acknowledgement

The authors are grateful to Head, Department of Botany, Dr. H.S. Gour Vishwavidyalaya, Sagar for providing necessary lab facilities.

References

Amar, S.M. and Ali, E.M. (1974). Cytological effects of pesticides V. effects of some herbicides on *Vicia faba. cytologia* 39: 633-643.

Badr, A. (1983). Mitodepressive and Chromotoxic activities of two herbicides in *Allium cepa. Cytologia* 48 : 451-457.

Bakale, V.L. (1972). Effect of Weedicides on cytomorphology of weeds. *Althernanthera polygonides var. erecta, Cressa cretica* and *Xanthium strumarium. Ph.D. Thesis*, Bombay University.

Bell, S.L., Schwarz, O.J. and Hughes, K.W. (1976). Studies on the herbicide paraquat, I. Effects on the cell cycle and DNA synthesis in *Vicia faba*. *Can. J. Genet. Cytol.* 18: 93-99.

Chen, L.G., Switzer, C.M. and Fletcher, R. 1972). Nucleic acid and protein changes induced by auxin like herbicides. *Weed Sci.*, 20: 53-55.

Chouhan, A.K.S. and Yadav, S.K. (2007). Effect of three herbicides on the nucleic acids and protein content in wheat crop. *J. Bot. Univ. Sagar*, 42: 12-19.

Chrispeels, M.S. and Hanson, J.B. (1962). The increase in RNA content of cytoplasmic particulates of soybean hypocotyl indued by 2,4-D. *Weeds* 10: 123-125.

Delcourt, A. and Daysson, G. (1976). Effet of trifluraline on the root meristem of *Allium sativum*. *Cytologia* 41(1): 75-89.

Dustin, P. (1947). Some new aspects of mitotic poisoning, *Nature*. 159: 794-796.

Gichner, T., Goul, H. and Omura, T. (1968). The influence of post treatment washing and redrying of barley seeds on the mutagenic activity of N-methyl N nitroso urea and N-ethyl N-nitroso urea. *Radiation Botany* 8: 499-537.

Gulifoyle, T.J. and Hanson, J.B. (1974). Greater length of ribonucleic acid synthesized by chromatin-bound polymerase from auxin-treated soybean hypocotyls. *Plant Physiol.* 110-113.

Hess, F.D. (1983). Mode of action of herbicides that affect the cell division. In :Pesticide chemistry, Human health welfare and environment Eds. J. Miyamoto and P.C. Kervey, Pergaman Press, Ltd., Headington, Hill Hall Oxford : 420-425.

Key, J.L. and Hanson, J.B. (1961). Some effects of 2,4-D on soluble nucleotides and nucleic acids of soybean seedlings. *Plant Physiol.* 36: 145-152.

Key, J.L., Lin, C.Y., Gifford, E.M. (Jr) and Dengler, R. (1966). Relation of 2,4-D induced growth aberrations to changes in nucleic acid metabolism in soybean seedlings. *Bot. Gaz.* 127: 87-94.

Khosla, S.N. (1967). Effect of herbicides on the cytomorphology of weeds. Ph.D. thesis, Bombay University.

Kolhe, R.L. (1979). Effect of herbicides on the cytomorphology of farm weeds. Ph.D. thesis, Nagpur University, Nagpur.

Mohandas, T. and Grant, W.F. (1972). Cytogenetic effects of 2,4-D and amitrole in relation to nuclear volume and DNA content in some higher plants. *Can. J. Genet. Cytol.*, 14: 773-783.

Moreland, D.E., Malhotra, S.S., Gruenhagen, R.D. and Shokraii, E.H. (1969). Effects of herbicides on RNA and protein synthesis. *Weed Sci.*, 17: 556-563.

Mousa, M. (1982). Effects of some herbicides on mitotic activity and mitotic aberrations in root tips of onion. *Egyption J. Gemet. Cytol.*, 11: 193-2007.

Neilson, J.W., Friedrich and Tsuboi, T. (1968). Chromosome abnormalities and Psychotropic drugs. *Nature*. 218: 488-489.

Nieman, R.H. and Poulsen, L.L. (1962). Spectrophotometric estimation of nucleic acid of plant leaves. *Plant. Physiol*, 38: 31-35.

Njagı, C.D.E. and Gopalan, H.N.B. (1981). Mutagenicity testing of herbicides fungicides and insecticides I. Chromosome aberration in *Vicia Faba*. *Cytologia*, 46: 169-172.

Odum, E.P. (1971). *Fundamentals of Ecology*. W.B. Saunders Co. Phildelphia, London.

Reddy, S.S. and Rao, G.H. (1982). Cytogenetic effects of agricultural chemicals II. Effects of herbicides 'Lasso' and 'Bassagram' on chromosomal mechanism in relation to yield in chilli : (Capsicum annum L.). *Cytologia*, 47: 257-267.

Ryland, A.G. (1948). A cytological study of the effect of colchicine, indoleacetic acid, potassium cynide and 2,4-Dichlorophenoxy acetic acid on plant cells. *J. Elisha Mitchell Sci. Soc.*, 64: 117-125.

Sawamura, S. (1964). Cytological studies on the effects of herbicides on plant cells *in vivo*. I. Hormonic herbicides. *Cytologia*, 29: 86-102.

Shannon, J.C., Hanson, J.B. and Wilson, C.M. (1964). Ribonuclease levels in the mesocotyl tissue of *Zea maize* as a function of 2,4-D application. *Plant Physiol.*, 39: 804-809.

Sharma, A.K. and Sharma, A. (1965). Chromosome Techniques: Theory and Practice, Butterworth and Co. Ltd. London.

Sikka, K. and Sharma, A.K. (1976). The effects of some herbicides on plant chromosome. *Proc. Indian Nat. Sci. Academy*, (B) 42: 299-307.

Skorupska, H. (1975). Radioimmetic effect of herbicides on the progress of mitosis in pea in comparison with those of chromomutagens and gamma rays. *Genetica Polonica*. 16: 301-311.

Sohier El-Khodary. Antoinette Habıt and Atif Haliem (1989). Cytological effects of the herbicide Garlon-4 on root mitosis of *Allium cepa*. *Cytologia*, 54: 465-472.

Sonpuri, A.K. and Mishra, S.K. (1993). Cytological effects of starthene (Acephate) in root meristems of *Allium cepa*. *Biome*: 6(2): 102-104.

Strove, V.S. (1973). The cytogenetic activity of the herbicides atrazine-chloro-LPC and Paraquat. *Sov. Genet*. 6: 293-297.

Tomkins, D.J. and Grant, W.F. (1976). Monitorning natural vegetation for herbicides induced chromosomal aberrations *Mut. Res*. 36: 73-83.

West, S.H., Hanson, J.B. and Key, J.L. (1960). Effect of 2,4-D on nucleic acid and protein content of seedling tissue. *Weeds*. 8: 333-340.

Wuu, K.D., Grant, W.F. (1966a). Morphological and somatic chromosomal aberrations induced by pesticides in barley (*Hordeum vulgare*) *Can. J. Genet. Cytol*. 8: 481-501.

Microbial Biotechnology and Ecology (2011)
Editors: **Deepak Vyas, G.S. Paliwal, P.K.Khare and R.K Gupta**
Published by: **DAYA PUBLISHING HOUSE, NEW DELHI**
Pages **553–570**

Chapter 32

Biotechnological Potential of Cyanobacteria

☆ ***Surendra Singh****

Centre of Advanced Study in Botany,
Banaras Hindu University, Varanasi – 221 005, U.P.

ABSTRACT

Cyanobacteria are ubiquitous in nature and considered to be next to bacteria as far as their distribution is concerned. This large and diverse group of Gram negative prokaryote having traditional applications, is now being utilized and further exploited for biotechnological development. These organisms also possess immense potentials for application towards human welfare. However, except for the use of *Spirulina* as a health food, there are no other major products from cyanobacteria in India and elsewhere. This is due to the limitations in the economic production of cyanobacterial products in low quantity. Furthermore, mass cultivation technology has not yet been evolved for such potential organisms and in many cases the methods of industrial extraction are not even optimized. Intensive research is thus warranted to understand many of the basic aspects pertaining to the production of a metabolite with the concurrent evolution of applied research towards the large scale production of the product.

In recent years people throughout the world are focusing their attention towards cyanobacteria for their possible use for the photobiological production of biofuel, ammonia, amino acids, various metabolites, vitamins, toxins, therapeutic substances, aqua or animal feed. Various chemicals including restriction enzymes, pharmacological probes and labeled compounds for research, as well as fluorescent probes for clinical diagnostics are now commercially available. Potentially useful compounds, including pharmaceuticals and industrial chemicals, have been identified and are

* E-mail: surendrasingh.bhu@gmail.com

currently being developed. This review summarizes the biotechnological potentials of cyanobacteria, and highlights various areas of applications mainly nutraceutical, pharmaceutical and bioactive potential.

Introduction

Cyanobacteria are oxygenic photosynthetic prokaryotes, which have long been recognized as having potential in biotechnology. These organisms have been evolved nearly about three billion years ago and have been responsible for the initial oxygenation of the Earth's atmosphere. They are the large and diverse group of prokaryotic organism occupying unique taxonomic position. They combine an autotrophic mode of nutrition that is common to eukaryotic algae and plant cells with a metabolic system that is generally regarded as bacterial rather than the plant like. These prokaryotic organisms thus offer the growth potential of microbial cells growth with the light harvesting capabilities of plant cells, making them ideal candidates for biosolar energy conversion programs. Another advantage of cyanobacteria over eukaryotic organisms is the capacity of several strains to fix atmospheric nitrogen (N_2). Cyanobacteria perform various metabolic functions like other prokaryotic bacteria. Similarly they are also exposed to diverse conditions in their natural habitats and hence have evolved alternate metabolic pathways and elegant regulatory mechanisms for adaptation.

Cyanobacteria are now increasingly attracting the attention of the biologists in view of their importance in agriculture, industry, environmental pollution abatement, conservation, biodiversity and pharmaceutical markets. Cyanobacteria in general are one of the richest sources of known and novel bioactive compounds including toxins with wide pharmaceutical applications (Becker 1994; Patterson 1996). This has led to the systematic screening of cyanobacterial strains both to test their potential pharmaceutical applications and also to know their general effects on animal systems. In recent years people throughout the world are focusing their attention towards cyanobacteria for their possible use for the photobiological production of biofuels, ammonia, amino acids, various metabolites, vitamins, toxins, therapeutic substances and aqua or animal feed (Singh 1992, 1993; Mohanthy 1996). Although, the screening of cyanobacterial strains having the ability to produce novel compounds with antimicrobial and antineoplastic activities were started as early as 1970 (Moore 1981; Rinehart *et al.*, 1981), the systematic screening for therapeutic substances from micro-algae particularly cyanobacteria has, however, received greater attention recently.

Pharmaceuticals

Microorganisms play a significant role in medical sciences as they not only cause infections, but also produce organic substances that can cure infections. The discovery of penicillin in 1929 heralded the era of antibiotics and led to the realization that microorganisms can be considered as a rich source of clinically useful natural products. Since then several natural products with bioactive potentials have been discovered from microorganisms. The tremendous rate of discovery is a testament to the inherent ability of microorganisms to produce bioactive metabolites.

However, despite many discoveries, the pharmaceutical industries have focused their attention on the same group of microorganisms, mainly the actinomycetes as their primary source for new drugs. Although actinomycetes continue to be studied extensively, it is clear that the rate of discovery of novel metabolites from this group is decreasing and hence new sources of bioactive natural products must be explored. One such resource is cyanobacteria, which are recently being exploited for their potential as producers of biomedically efficient metabolites.

Cyanobacterial bioactive compounds will contribute significantly to drug development either directly or as models for developing analogs for increased activity and as research tools for studying physiological processes and diseases. Pharmacological evalutions of cyanobacterial products have been revolutionized over the past two decades, beginning with the early investigation of toxins, followed by studies of cytotoxic and antitumor activity, to the present where a myriad of activities based on whole animal models and receptor binding assays are being pursued.

Antimicrobials

Any compound, natural, synthetic or semi synthetic (*i.e.*, chemically derived from natural substances) that is clinically used for the treatment of microbial infections is generally known as antimicrobials. These antimicrobials include antibacterials, antifungals and antialgals and antivirals.

Antibacterials

The antibacterial activity of cyanobacteria in general has been poorly studied (Reichelt, and Borowitzka 1984; Moore *et al.*, 1988).The cell-extract fractions from *Spirulina subsalsa* resulted in the complete inhibition of the growth of a clinical isolate of *Pseudomonas aeruginosa*, which is considered to be one of the difficult pathogens to treat (Sundararaman 1992). *Nostoc muscorum* also produces an antibacterial agent having broad-spectrum activity (Bloor and England 1991). The chloroform-methanol extracts of several *Oscillatoria* species inhibit the Gram-positive bacterial pathogen, *Staphylococcus aureus.* Whereas, the compounds obtained from *Phormidium angustissimum* and *Lyngbya* sp. were found to be effective against Gram negative and Gram positive pathogenic bacteria, the compounds obtained from *S. subsalsa* were, however, found to possess antibacterial activity against Gram negative organisms only (Sundararaman 1992). Similarly, the crude extracts of *P. angustissimum* and *Lyngbya* sp. were found to be potential sources of new broad-spectrum antibacterial compounds (Sundararaman 1992).

Antifungals

A large number of cyanobacteria are reported to possess the ability to produce the compounds which exhibit the antifungal activity. The cyanobacterial extracts that inhibit the proliferation of tissue cultured mammalian cells also inhibit the fungal growth, indicating that the mechanism of inhibition involves a function similar to eukaryotic cells. Scytophycin, a potent bioactive metabolite from cyanobacteria also exhibited antifungal activity (Ishibashi *et al.*, 1986; Patterson and Carmeli 1992). Tjipanazoles, N-glycosides of indole-carbazoles isolated from the cyanobacterium *Tolypothrix tjipanasensis* exhibited significant fungicidal activity against phytopathogenic fungi (Bonjouklian *et al.*, 1991). The laxaphycins are a large family of cyclic undeca and dodecapeptides responsible for antifungal activity caused by crude extracts of *Anabaena laxa*. The laxaphycins structurally and biologically resemble to a group of cyclic peptides known as hormothamnins, which have recently been isolated from the *Hormothamnion enteromorphoides* (Gerwick *et al.*, 1989). Extracts of *Synechococcus elongatous*, *P. corium* and *Dichothrix baueriana* were found to be active against *Candida* species (Sundararaman 1992). A compound, presumably a methoxylated disaccharide, purified from *Oscillatoria latevirens* exhibited anti-*Candida*, anti-*Mucor* and antibacterial activity (Deth 1999).

Antialgals

One hundred and ninety-eight cyanobacterial strains, isolated mainly from diverse habitats in Australia, Indonesia, Nepal, Thialand and Vietnam, were screened for their antibiotic activity against green algal species of the genera *Coelastrum*, *Scenedesmus* and *Monoraphidium* (Schlegel *et al.*, 1999). Out of these, ten strains of *Fischerella*, seven strains of *Nostoc* and three strains of *Calothrix* produce antialgal compounds with a broad spectrum activity. Some of these bioactive cyanobacteria are reported to inhibit the growth of *Coelastrum, Scenedesmus* and *Monoraphidium*, whereas others inhibited the growth of either two or one algae (Schlegel *et al.*, 1999). *P. valderianum* completely eliminated a dense population of marine diatoms inducing the extracellular production of antidiatom compound.

Antivirals

To discover a new antiviral agent from cyanobacteria, extracts from cyanobacteria were screened for anti-HIV properties (Boyd 1988). Cellular extracts of *Lyngbya langerhimii* and *Phormidium tenue* protected human lymphoblastoid T cells from the cytopathic effect of HIV- 1 infection. With the use of an *in vitro* anti-HIV-1 assay, a new class of HIV-1 inhibitory compound, the sulfonic acid containing glycolipids was isolated (Gustafson *et al.*, 1989). Recently a tetrazolium based microculture assay was developed to screen the extracts of cultured cyanobacteria for inhibition of the cytopathic effects of HIV (Gustafson *et al.*, 1989). At non-cytotoxic concentration, pure cyanobacterial compounds were found to be active against HIV-1 in cultured human lymphoblastoid T cell-lines (Gustafson *et al.*, 1989).

An aqueous extract of *Spirulina platensis* inhibits HIV-1 replication in human derived T-cell lines and in human peripheral blood mononuclear cells. The extracts also blocked Raucher Murine Leukemia Virus (RLV) induced plaque (Ayehunie *et al.*, 1998). The aqueous extract of *Spirulina* also exhibited a dose- dependent inhibition of the replication of *Herpes simplex* virus type 1 (HSV-1) in Hela cells within the concentration range of 0.08-50 mg ml^{-1}. However, this extract does not show any virucidal activity and could not even interfere the adsorption of the virus to the host cells (Hayashi *et al.*1993). Bioactivity-directed fractionation of a hot water extract from *S. platensis* led to the isolation of a novel sulfated polysaccharide, calcium spirulan (Ca-SP), as an antiviral principle. This polysaccharide was composed of rhamnose, ribose, mannose, fructose, galactose, xylose, glucose, glucuronic acid, galacturonic acid, sulfate and calcium. Ca-SP was found to inhibit the replication of several enveloped viruses, including *Herpes simplex* virus type 1 (HSV 1), Human Cytomegalo Virus (CMV), Measles Virus, Mumps Virus, Influenza A Virus and HIV 1. Ca-SP also selectively inhibits the penetration of viruses into the host cells. Retention of the molecular conformation by chelation of calcium ion with sulfate groups was suggested to be indispensable to its antiviral effect (Hayashi *et al.*1996).

A large number of cyanobacterial extracts also exhibited antiviral activity against *Herpes simplex* virus II (HSV-2) (Rinehart *et al.*, 1981). Whereas 10 per cent of the cyanobacterial extracts showed anti HSV-2 activity, 2.5 per cent of them, however, exhibited activity against respiratory syncytial virus (Patterson *et al.*, 1993). When antiviral activity of lipophilic and hydrophilic extracts of cyanobacteria against three pathogenic viruses were examined, a significant reduction in cytopathic effect normally associated with viral infection was recorded (Patterson *et al.*, 1993). Sulfoglycolipids isolated from cyanobacteria also exhibit strong antiviral properties. In *in vitro* studies, Helper T cells exposed to cyanobacterial sulfoglycolipids were protected from HIV-1 infection (Gustafson *et al.*, 1989). *P. valderianum, Plectonema terebrans* and *Pseudanabaena schimidelei* also exhibited HbsAg-clearing activity (Sundararaman 1992), indicating their potential use against Hepatitis B virus.

Cyanovirin derived from the cultures of the freshwater cyanobacterium *Nostoc ellipsosporum* binds to GP-120 protien of HIV and thus inhibits its replication. *N. ellipsosporum* producing cyanovirin-N and cyanovirin-V is also capable of inhibiting the growth of HIV-I and HIV-II (Chauhan *et al.*, 2004). Recently, allophycocyanin, a red fluorescent protein isolated from *S. platensis* is found to inhibit enterovirus 71-induced apoptosis, which may have a significant impact on protecting hosts from severe consequences associated with infection with enterovirus 71 (Shih *et al.*, 2003).

Other Potential Drugs

The hypoglycemic effect of *Spirulina* in non-insulin dependent diabetes mellitus (NIDDM) patients has been reported (Venkataraman, 1983). A significant reduction in the fasting and postprandial blood and urine sugar level has been reported following the uptake of about 2g of *Spirulina* (Venkatraman 1983). This has also been confirmed in experiments using albino rats with allaxan-induced diabetes. The reduction in the sugar level following *Spirulina* uptake has been attributed to the possible stimulation of prostaglandins. However, more studies on the similar lines are necessarily required not merely to establish the levels of *Spirulina* tablets, but also to understand the mechanisms of its action (Venkataraman, 1983). β–carotene as a dietary supplement has been reported to inhibit the development of 7, 12 dimethyl benzanthrazene (DMBA)-induced salivary gland carcinomas in rats.

Nutraceuticals

Cyanobacteria have found many tradition applications. However, its biotechnological applications have recently been recognized. *Spirulina*, a filamentous and non-heterocystous cyanobacterium has been used as food and food supplement and considered to be the major product from cyanobacteria (Puniya *et al.*, 1995). The high contents of protein, vitamin B_{12}, iron, β-carotene, iodine and γ-linolenic acid make the *Spirulina* protein as " naturally made" promising dietary substitute that could provide significant nutritional input to the Third World (Puniya *et al.*, 1995). A number of different cyanobacteria, mostly *Nostoc* strains have traditionally been used as food or food supplements, however, these strains are not extensively exploited (Jassby *et al.*, 1988).

Protien Efficiency Ratio (PER) of *Spirulina* protein has been reported to be higher than vegetables, cereals and soya proteins. The digestibility coefficient and biological values of *Spirulina* protein are only marginally lower than the milk protein, casein. Supplementation of *Spirulina* with cereals like rice and wheat on isoproteinic levels improved the protein quality (Venkataraman 1983). The bioavailability of total carotenes and in particular β-carotene from *Spirulina* was found to be comparable to the values reported for carotenes from other plant sources like leafy vegetables and carrots (Annapurna *et al.*, 1991). *Spirulina* is also a good source of vitamin A and hence it can be used as a source of vitamin A in the diet (Annapurna *et al.*, 1991). *Spirulina* is the most extensively researched food microalga documented in numerous books, journals, articles and periodicals.

Phycobiliproteins

Cyanobacteria in general possess all the known phycobiliproteins: phycocyanin, phycoerythrin, phycoerythrocyanin and allo-phycocyanin. Among them, phycocyanin and phycoerythrin are commercially valuable. 'Linablue' a phycocyanin product from Dainippan ink and Chemicals Inc, Japan is an odourless, non-toxic blue powder and used for colouring candy, ice cream, dairy products and soft drinks (Cohen 1986). Phycocyanin is also obtained in a water insoluble form from *Spirulina* and used in eye shadow, eyeliner and lipstick preparations (Dainippon Patent 1980). The blue or red chromophores are isolated by enzymatic or acid hydrolysis of the protein to yield more concentrated pigment which is used in cosmetics (Dainippon Patent 1981). Fhycoerythrin from *Spirulina* and other cyanobacteria is used as a food colour for products like icecream, yoghurt and it could also be used in cosmetics.

C-phycocyanin is a major biliprotein of *S. platensis*, the cyanobacterium having antioxidant (Upasani, *et al.*, 2001), anti-arthritic, and anti-inflammatory properties (Ramirez *et al.*, 2002). Phycocyanin acts as a hepatoprotective agent and as a hydroxyl radical scavenger (Madhava *et al.*,

2000). This pigment also inhibits oxidative damage in DNA and hence may be used as a therapeutic agent (Bhat and Madyastha 2001). However, the mechanism of its action is not yet clearly understood.

C-phycocyanin, which has been shown to be a selective COX-2 inhibitor, induces dose-dependent apoptosis in BC- 8 cells with a concomitant decrease in cell viability. However, BC-8 cells transfected with Bcl-2 gene were found to be resistant to phycocyanin mediated apoptosis. These observations were further confirmed by staining of these cells with Annexin-V. Annexin-V staining is observed in BC-8 cells after treatment with phycocyanin, which was, however, not observed in Bcl-2-transfected cells. These observations clearly demonstrate the phycocyanin-induced apoptotic death in BC-8 cells and its inhibition by Bcl–2 (Bobbili *et al.*, 2003).

β-Carotene

The β-carotene level in *Spirulina* at over 300 mg per cent is perhaps the highest content available from any other natural sources (Venkataraman, 1983). The β-carotene content of *Spirulina* is more than 18 times greater than carrot, which is the normally known source of β-carotene. Furthermore, the natural β-carotene of *Spirulina* is different from the synthetic β-carotene, since it contains a higher percentage of 9-cis-isomer as compared to over 47 per cent of all trans in the synthetic form. β-carotene as a dietary supplement has been reported to inhibit the development of DMBA-induced salivary gland carcinomas in rats and UV-induced skin cancer in hairless mice. Based on epidemiological studies, it has been suggested that β-carotene can also reduce the chances of occurrence of cancer in human (Normal and Temple 1988).

Amino Acids

Overproduction of amino acids is common feature of microbial resistance to analogs of amino acids. In general, the overproducing organisms are heterotrophic and production of metabolites is supported by the organic sources supplied with the medium. To our knowledge, such a phenomenon has been reported rarely for obligate photoautotrophs, a category which includes most cyanobacteria. Cyanobacteria liberate small quantities of amino acids into their medium (Fogg 1971; Fogg *et al.*, 1973). The most abundant amino acids liberated by cyanobacteria were phenylalanine, threonine, glutamate and glycine, irrespective of the nitrogen source available on which the cells were grown. Amino acid production was obtained with the mutant strains of *Anabaena variabilis*, which liberated alanine as the major abundant amino acid along with phenylalanine and tyrosine (Kerby *et al.*, 1987). Anolog-resistant mutants of *S. platensis* also produce the corresponding amino acids (Riccardi *et al.*, 1981). Continuous photobiological production of amino acids was achieved following immobilization of the mutant cells in calcium alginate gel (Kerby *et al.*, 1988). However, the effective isolation of strains for commercial production of amino acids is dependent on our knowledge of transport and metabolism of amino acids. Characterization of such strains can increase our basic knowledge thus permitting further strain improvement. Advances are being made in both fundamental and applied aspects by use of mutant strains of cyanobacteria. Recent advances in cyanobacterial molecular genetics can be expected to have a major impact in this field.

Ammonia

One of the biotechnological aspects receiving considerable interest, especially by using cyanobacteria, is the photobiological production of ammonia. Light-driven synthesis of ammonia at the expense of N_2 and water via photosynthesis is a photobiological process for the conversion of solar energy into chemical energy, namely ammonia which can be used as fertilizer. Since, cyanobacteria in natural conditions release limited or no fixed-N (ammonia), attempts are being made to generate strains which can fix N_2 at higher rate and release most of the fixed-N in the form of ammonia. In symbiosis about 50-90 per cent of the N_2-derived ammonia is liberated by the cyanobiont (Rai 1990). Attempts have also been made for the photobiological production of ammonia at the expense of N_2 and nitrate by using L-Methionine -DL-sulphoximine (MSX), a glutamate analogue and an irreversible inhibitor of GS (Vincenzini *et al.*, 1986; Singh and Rai 1989; Musgrave *et al.*, 1982; Guerrero *et al.*, 1982; Ramos *et al.*, 1987; Singh 1992, 1993). However, this approach seems to be impractical because MSX rapidly leads to deficiency of glutamine and other vital nitrogenous compounds with cessation of ammonia production and finally lysis of the cells. An alternative approach is to select mutant strains particularly deficient in GS activity which would liberate ammonia resulting from N_2 fixation into the medium. Mutant strains of *A. variabilis* and *Nostoc* ANTH fixed N_2 and liberated most of the fixed N_2 in the form of ammonia into the external medium (Singh 1992, 1993). Following immobilization in calcium alginate gel, sustained photoproduction of ammonia was obtained in reactors. The rate of ammonia production was comparable to the rate of its MSX-treated freely suspended wild type counterpart.

Fatty Acids

Fatty acids, in general, are of commercial value and many are pharmaceutical agents. Fatty acid of *Spirulina* possesses palmitic acid, γ-linolenic acid (GLA), linolenic acid and oleic acid predominantly. The concentration of GLA ranged between 8 to 31.7 per cent of the total fatty acids. Since, *Spirulina* is one of the best sources of GLA, a rare essential fatty acid and the key to good health, efforts are being made to produce GLA from other cyanobacterial strains.

Furthermore, the presence of essential fatty acids in *Spirulina* is very important. Essential fatty acids protect the cell membranes from destruction by short wave length electromagnetic radiations, carcinogens, bacteria and viruses (Horrobin 1990). Essential fatty acids decrease the aggregation of blood platelets and coronary thrombosis and also inhibit the salt-induced hypertension (Horrobin 1990). Essential fatty acids are also recommended for the prevention and treatment of multiple sclerosis (Horrobin 1990).

In diabetes mellitus, essential fatty acids reduce the diabetic retinopathy. Diabetes induces the capillary permeability and fragility whereas essential fatty acids increase the membrane intregrity. Because of their fortifying action in cellular membranes, essential fatty acids are important in the control of gastrointestinal, connective tissue and skin disorders (Horrobin 1990).

Vitamins

Although, a number of cyanobacteria are known to be rich source of vitamins and many are known even to excrete them into their milieu (Borowitzka and Borowitzka 1988), no report is, however, available on the commercial exploitation of these organisms for vitamin production. Some of the marine cyanobacteria appear to be the potential source of vitamin B complex group and vitamin E (Sundararaman 1992). *Spirulina* is considered to be the potential source of vitamin B_{12}, which is essential for healthy nerves and tissues especially for vegetarians (Henrikson 1997). Studies among preschool children in India have demonstrated *Spirulina fusiformis* to be an effective source of dietary vitamin A (Annapurna *et al.*, 1991).

Cyanobacteria as a Source of Polysaccharides

The exploitation of cyanobacteria as polysaccharides is emerging as new area of biotechnological application for the human welfare. The polysaccharides of microbial origin show advantages over the polysaccharides extracted from plants or macroalgae. The cyanobacteria have been considered for polysaccharide production due to their capability to excrete mucilaginous material with potential useful properties. In fact, most of the cyanobacterial strains possess additional surface structures, mainly of a polysaccharide nature, that comprise of sheaths, capsules and slimes. During cell growth in batch cultures aliquots of the polysaccharides material of both capsules and slimes may be released as water soluble material into the surrounding medium.

Bioactive Compounds

The discovery of new sources of bioactive natural products are of paramount importance to assure the supply of new drugs needed to treat those infectious diseases that have become resistant to currently available drugs and also to combat newly emergent diseases. Considerable efforts have been made in the past to identify interesting bioactive compounds from different sources including cyanobacteria (Table 32.1). The potential impact of this field on cyanobacterial biotechnology is immense (Patterson 1996). The wide array of cyanobacterial strains and the range of habitats that they occupy guarantee statistically to predict success in finding a valuable compound.

Table 32.1: Bioactive Compounds from Cyanobacteria (Burja *et al.*, 2001)

Organisms	*Compounds*	*Activity*
Microcystis aeruginosa	Aeruginosin, Kawaguchipeptin, microcystilide, microcystin micropeptin, microviridin	Enzyme inhibitor, cytotoxic, cell-differentiation, hepatotoxin, promoter, endotoxic, tumor antibiotic, anticancer
Microcystis viridis	Cyanoviridin RR	Toxic
Synechocystis trididemni	Didemnin	Anticancer, antiviral, Immunosuppressive
Lyngbya langerheimii	Sulfolipid	Anti–HIV activity
Lyngbya majuscula	Antillatoxin, aplysiatoxin, Aparamide, barbamide, Sulfolipid, lyngbyatoxin	Anticancer, anti-inflammatory, antiviral, anti-HIV, antimicrobial, cytotoxic, toxin
Oscillatoria acutissima	Acutiphycin	Anticancer activity
Oscillatoria agardhii	Agardhipeptin, microcystin	Enzyme inhibitor, hepatotoxin
Oscillatoria nigroviridis	Oscillatoxin	Anticancer
Phormidium tenue	Sulfolipid	Anti-HIV activity
Plectonema radiosum	Radiosumin, tubercidin	Enzyme inhibitor
Spirulina platensis	Calcium spirulan, poly-β-hydroxybutyrate, phycocyanin	Anticancer, anti-HIV activity, free-radical scavenger
Anabaena basta	Bastadin, bastadin *O*-sulfate esters	Antibiotic, anti-inflammatory, cytotoxicity
Anabaena circinalis	Circinamide, microcystin	Enzyme inhibitor, toxic
Aphanizomenon flos-aquae	Aphanorphine, siatoxin	Antibiotic, anticancer toxic
Nostoc commune	Nostodione, microsporine, diterpenoid	Antifungal, antibiotic, antimitotic, cytotoxic, suncreen pigment
Nostoc ellipsosporum	Cyanovirin	Anti-HIV, antiviral
Nostoc muscorum	Muscoride	Antibiotic
Nostoc sphaericum	Staurosporine, indolecarbazole	Antiviral, cytotoxic
Tolypothrix nodosa	Tolyporphin	Antibiotic
Tolypothrix tenuis	Toyocamycin, tubercidin	Antifungal, cytotoxic

Screening for a wide variety of potentially useful bioactivities, including cytotoxic, multi-drug resistance reversal, anti-fungal and antiviral effects, has led to the discovery and identification of numerous novel bioactive compounds or secondary metabolites possessing unprecedented structures. Structural novelty can be combined with exceptionally high incidence of biological activity.

Enzymes

Microbial enzymes have been used in various industries for many centuries. Recently, with the advent of biotechnology, there has been a growing interest and demand for enzymes with novel properties. Cell bound and extracellular phosphatase activities of cyanobacterial isolates have also been reported (Whitton *et al.*, 1991). A number of studies have been conducted on the detection of cyanobacterial enzymes including phosphatase, arylsulfatase, chitinase, L-asparginase, L-glutaminase, amylase, protease, lipase, cellulase, urease and lactamase (Chandrasekaran 1997). Freely-suspended and immobilized cells of *Anacystis nidulans* contain amino acid oxidase activity, which is further increased by illumination with red light (Wikstrom *et al.*, 1982). Superoxide dismutase exists in all aerobic organisms and has been purified from *Spirulina*.

Restriction Enzymes

Although more than 500 restriction enzymes with at least 100 different site specificities have been reported (Roberts 1985), enzymes with new specificities are continuously sought to increase the possibilities of DNA manipulation. Many species of cyanobacteria, both filamentous and unicellular, appear to be a promising source of such enzymes (Table 32.2).

Table 32.2: Important Restriction Enzymes Identified in Cyanobacteria (Ciferri *et al.*, 1989)

Organisms	*Enzymes*	*Isoshizomer of*	*Recognition Sequence*
Anacystis nidulans	Ani I	–	CCNNGG
Anabaena variabilis	Ava I	–	C ↓ PyCGPuG
	Ava II	—	G ↓ G(A/T)CC
	AvaIII	–	ATGCAT
Anabaena cylindrica	Acy I	–	Gpu ↓ CGPyC
Nostoc sp. 6705	Nsp BI	AsuII	TTCGAA
	Nsp BII	–	C(G/C)G ↓ C(T/G)G
Nostoc sp. 8009	NspMACI	BglII	A ↓ GATCT
Nostoc sp. 7413	NspHI	Nsp(7524)I	PuCATG ↓ Py
	NspHII	AvaII	GG(A/T)CC
Spirulina platensis	SplI	–	C ↓ GTACG
	SplII	TthIIII	GACNNNGTC
	SplIII	HaeIII	GGCC
Tolypothrix tenuis	TtnI	HaeIII	GGCC

Cyanobacteria contain different endonucleases in different combinations, some of which are isoschizomers even in unrelated strains. For example, the isoschizomers *Aqu* I and *Ava* I, that recognize and cleave the sequence CPyCGPuG are produced by a unicellular cyanobacterium *Synechococcus* and a filamentous cyanobacterium *Anabaena*. Similarly, besides other restriction endonucleases, *Fremyella* and *Nostoc* contain enzymes with the same specificity as *Ava* II (Whitehead and Brown 1985), the enzyme which was first identified in *Anabaena*. This is not unusual as the same restriction enzyme has been found in different bacterial genera (Roberts 1985). Such findings may indicate that some of the activities are plasmid or phage-borne, although, at the moment, there is no evidence correlating restriction activity and presence of plasmids or phages.

Immunomodulators

Spirulina is commercially produced for human consumption as well as for feed ingredients. Recently, whole *Spirulina* and cell extracts were found to enhance immunity in animals by increasing phagocytic activity. The whole cells of cyanobacteria and lipopolysaccharides (LPS) isolated from cyanobacterial cells were shown to stimulate the production of macro and micro globulin antibodies (Rathore *et al.*, 2004).

C-phycocyanin and polysaccharides isolated from *Spirulina* was found to possess high erythropoeitin (EPO) activity. Effect of these compounds on peripheral blood and bone marrow hematopoietic stem and progenitor cell in normal, irradiated and anemic mice showed the unique capacity of C-phycocyanin and polysaccharide to influence the differentiation and proliferation of committed hematopoietic progenitor cell. In addition to this, they also lower the anemic degree of mice combined with gamma-ray irradiation and Benz hydrazine hydrochloric acid and peritoneri injection (Zhang-Chang-Wu 1994).

Mice fed with *Spirulina* diet showed increased numbers of spleenic antibody producing cells in the primary immune response to sheep red blood cells (SRBC). *Spirulina* enhances the immune response, particularly the primary response by stimulating the macrophages function, phagocytosis and IL-1 production (Hayashi *et al.*, 1994).

Bronchoalveolar lavage macrophages isolated from cats, when cultured on a glass cover slip with water-soluble extracts of *S. platensis* in a concentration range of 0-60 mg ml^{-1} for 2 h could not cause significant macrophage cytotoxicity over untreated controls. The *S. platensis* extract enhances macrophage phagocytic fuction which implies that *Spirulina* supplementation might improve the disease resistance potential in cats (Qureshi *et al.*, 1996).

The exposure of chicken macrophage to *S. platensis* extract enhances selected effector functions of cells of the chicken immune system. However, the ability of spleenic natural killer cells to kill tumour cell targets was not affected by *Spirulina* treatment. Macrophage cultures exposed to *Spirulina* produced a factor in their culture supernatant with tumoricidal potential, which was similar in reactivity to the factor produced by macrophage following exposure to lipopolysaccharide (Qureshi *et al.*, 1995).

Chicken macrophage exposed to water soluble extracts of *Spirulina* showed enhanced phagocytic activity *in vitro*, suggesting activation of mononuclear phagocytic system function. Furthermore, dietary supplemention of *Spirulina* (1,000 to 10,000 ppm), improved thymic weights, enhanced CBH response, increased tumor cell killing by NK cells and doubled the macrophage phagocytic potential over chickens fed a basal diet. *Spirulina* enhances several immunological end points in chickens both during *in vitro* and in *in vivo* exposures (Qureshi *et al.*, 1995). *Spirulina* consumption lowers the amount of igE in the blood, which in turn normalizes and reduces allergies in the body without any side effect (Evets *et al.*, 1994). *Spirulina* also shows the immunomodulatory and biomodulatory effects (Rathore *et al.*, 2004).

Anticancer/Antitumer/Anti-Proliferative and Cytotoxic Compounds

Micro algae in general and cyanobacteria in particular have been identified as the most significant group of organisms from which new anticancer type natural products have been isolated (Moore *et al.*,

1988). Many of these bioactive compounds possess unprecedented structures. Structural novelty is combined with exceptionally high incidences of biological activity.

The extracts of some cultured cyanobacteria exhibited good anticancer activity (Barchi *et al.*, 1983). Ethanolic extract of cultured *Tolypothrix byssoideae* was found to show significant inhibitory activity *in vitro* against KB and NIH/3T3 cells and *in vivo* against P-388 lymphocytic leukemia in mice (Barchi *et al.*, 1983). Bioassay directed isolation and identification of the active constituent (tubericidin) have also been reported from *T. byssoideae* (Barchi et *al.*, 1983).

Bioassay directed fractionation of extract of *Phormidium tennue* led to the isolation of three classes of glycolipids *viz.* monogalactosyl diacylglycerols (MGDGs) as antitumor factors. Among 17 tested MGDGs and digalactosyl diacylglycerols (DGDGs), three of the DGDGs showed more potent inhibitory activity towards tumor proliferation than the others (Shirahashi *et al.*, 1993).

The extract of *Lyngbya majuscula* was found to have strong cytotoxic effect against a Vero cell line ATCC CCI 81 (Gerwick *et al.*, 1994). The extract was also found to be toxic to brine shrimp (LC 50=25ng ml^{-1}). Using the brine shrimp assay to guide fractionation, a unique metabolite was isolated (8-10 per cent of the crude extract) which was found to be responsible for the potent brine shrimp toxicity (LC 50=3ng ml^{-1}) and mammalian cell antiproliferative activity (IC 50=6.8ng ml^{-1}) in the Chinese hamster Aux B1 cell line.

Bioassay guided fractionation of the organic extract of *L. majuscula* led to the isolation of a new lipid, curacin A, with exceptional brine shrimp toxic and tumor antiproliferative activities. Pure curacin A is an antimitotic agent (IC 50 values in three cell lines ranging from 7-200 nm) that inhibits microtubule assembly and the binding of colchicines to tubulin (Gerwick *et al.*, 1994).

In discovering new efficient drugs for the treatment of solid tumors in clinical conditions, Corbett *et al.* (1992) developed a rapid inexpensive disk diffusion assay to find agents that exhibit greater cytotoxicity against tumour cells than leukemia cells. Aulosirazole, the major cytotoxin of *Aulosira fertillissima* shows solid tumor selective activity in the Corbett assay. Its structure has been determined to be 5-hydroxy-3 methoxinapthol (2,3-d) 1,2-Thiazole-4,9-dione (Startman *et al.*, 1994).

The recently discovered antiproliferative agents cryptophycin-A, curacin A (Gerwick *et al.*, 1994) and notodion A (Kobayashi *et al.*, 1990) produced by *Nostoc* sp., *L. majuscula,* and *Nostoc commune*, respectively, inhibit microtuble assembly function and show promise as potentially useful anticancer agents.

The extracts of *Spirulina-Dunaliela* in which β- carotene is a major component inhibited the growth and destroyed oral cancer cells *in vitro* (Schwartz *et al.*, 1988). β- carotene, a nontoxic carotenoid had a cytostatic and cytotoxic dose-dependent effect on hamster and human oral squamous cell carcinoma cell lines (Schwartz and Shklar 1987). The chemo preventative activity of *Spirulina* (1g day^{-1} for 12 months) in reversing oral leukoplakia in pan tobacco chewers in Kerala, India showed complete regression of lesions in evaluable subjects supplemented with *Spirulina* (Mathew *et al.* 1995).

Polysaccharide of *Spirulina* can inhibit the proliferation of ascetic hepatoma cells of mice at a concentration of 200 mg Kg^{-1}. It can inhibit the incorporation of H-thymidine, H-uridine and H-leucine into DNA, RNA and protein synthesis of sarcoma 180 and ascetic hepatoma cells during the period of 24 h after exposure *in vitro*. The degree of inhibition increases with the increase in incubation time. Polysaccharide of *Spirulina* can inhibit DNA synthesis of Sarcoma 180 and ascetic hepatoma cells. The inhibition is due to the alteration in DNA metabolism (Lisheng *et al.*, 1991).

An extract of *Spirulina-Dunaliella* was shown to prevent tumor development in hamster buccal pouch when a solution was applied topically three times weekly for 28 weeks (Schwartz *et al.*, 1988). Anti-cancer properties and antineoplastic activity have also been demonstrated using compounds from marine cyanobacteria (Murray and Mitsui 1982).

Antitoxin

Mercury induced kidney toxicity in rats was suppressed by feeding *Spirulina*. Para aminophenol and cisplatin induced renal toxicity in rats was significantly reduced by phycocyanin extract of *Spirulina*. (Fukino *et al.*, 1990). Thus, phycocyanin plays a major role in the protective effect of *Spirulina* against mercury and pharmaceutical drugs induced renal failure and that *Spirulina* might be applicable to the reduction of general renal dysfunction (Fukino *et al.*1990).

Radioprotection

The radioprotective effect of *Spirulina* extract was studied using the micronucleus test in polychromatic erythrocytes of bone marrow in mice. The extract caused a significant reduction of the micronucleus frequencies induced by gamma radiation (Qishen *et al.*, 1989).

Spirulina reduces urine radioactivity levels by 50 per cent within 20 days. Use of *Spirulina* also decreases radiation load received from food contaminated with radio nucleotides, Cesium-137 and Strontium-90. *Spirulina* is favourable for normalizing the adaptive potential of children's bodies in conditions of long lived low dose radiation (Loseva and Dardynskaya 1993). The intake of easily digestible micro and macro elements of *Spirulina* also has a positive influence on many functions of the immune system (Loseva 1999).

Reproductive Modulators

Carotenoids are used to improve the health and enhance the fertility of cattle (Jackson 1981). Crude ethanolic extract of *Oscillatoria willei* causes abnormal changes in the sperm of mouse (Thirunalasundari and Subramanian 2000). An immune potentiating property coupled with murine antifertility activity, without being toxic to other systems in mice models was exhibited by the extracts of *O. willei* (Krishnaprema 1996; Jagdeshwari 1998; Ansarudin 1999) and *O. late-virens* (Deth 1999).

Conclusion

Cyanobacteria are oxygenic, photosynthetic prokaryotes which have long been recognized as having potential in biotechnology as biofertilizers, amino acid production, fuel production, antibiotic production, single cell protein production and for the production of other secondary metabolites and pigments used in food industries. These interesting features have fascinated the Scientists all over the world to understand and explore in detail the basic mechanisms involved for the biotechnological exploitation of cyanobacteria for the betterment of mankind.

The traditional use of cyanobacteria including food, energy source and biofertilizers flourish today and are beginning to reap the benefits of modern molecular biology to enhance their performance. The first generation of high value added byproducts produced by cyanobacteria, including phycoflours are currently available in the market and is quite popular. However, only a few cyanobacterial strains producing intresting compounds have so far been exploited commercially. Screening programs must therefore identify useful products and the cyanobacterial strains having the ability to produce the products in significant amounts should be cultured in mass. Projection for future research on pharmaceutical potential of cyanobacteria includes discovery of novel bioactive metabolites, investigation of the pathways by which selected metabolites are synthesized and regulated and a precise elucidation of the mechanism by which these novel compounds exert their biological effects.

Acknowledgements

I am thankful to Dr. Narendra Kumar and Mr. Pawan Kumar for their help in preparation of the manuscript.

References

Annapurna, V., Shah, N., Bhaskaram, P., Bamji, M.S. and Reddy, V. (1991). Bioavailability of *Spirulina* carotene. *Journal of Clinical Biochemistry and Nutrition* (10). : 145–151.

Ansarudin, P.A. (1999). Bioactive compound from a marine cyanobacterium *Oscillatoria willei* BDU 130511. *M.Sc. Thesis*, Bharthidasan University, Tiruchirappalli, India.

Ayehunie, S., Belay, A., Baba, T.W. and Ruprecht, R.M. (1998). Inhibition of HIV-1 replication by an aqueous extract of *Spirulina platensis* (*Arthrospira platensis*). *Journal of Acquired Immune Deficiency Syndromes and Human Retrovirology* (18): 7-12.

Barchi, J.J., Norton, T.R., Furusawat, E., Patterson, G.M. and Moore RE (1983). Identification of a cyatotoxin from *Tolypothrix byssoideae* as tubericidin. *Phytochemistry* (22). : 2851-2855.

Becker, E.W. (1994). Microalgae. In: *Biotechnology and Microbiology*. Cambridge University Press, Cambridge, U.K.

Bhat, V.B. and Madyastha, K.M. (2001). Scavening of peroxynitrite by phycocyanin and phycocyanobilin from *Spirulina platensis*: protection against oxidative damage to DNA.. *Biochemical and Biophysical Research Communications* (285): 262-266.

Bloor, S. and England, R. R. (1991). Elucidation and optimization of the medium constituents controlling antibiotic production by the cyanobacterium *Nostoc muscorum*. *Enzyme Microbial Technology* (13): 76-81.

Bobbili, V. V., Pardhasaradhi, A., Mubarak Ali, A., Kumari, L., Reddanna, P. and Khar, A. (2003). Phycocyanin-mediated apoptosis in AK-5 tumor cells involves down-regulation of Bcl-2 and generation of ROS. *Molecular Cancer Therapy* (2): 1165–1170.

Bonjouklian, R., Smitra, T.A., Doolin, L.E., Molly, R.M., Debono, M., Shaffer, S.A., Moore, R.E., Stewart, J.B. and Patterson, G.M.L. (1991). Tjipanazoles, new antifungal agents from the blue-green alga *Tolypothrix tjipanasensis*. *Tetrahedron*. (47): 7739-7740.

Borowitzka, M.A. and Borowitzka, L.J. (1988). *Microalgal Biotechnology*. Cambridge University Press, Cambridge, U.K.

Boyd, M.R. (1988). Strategies for the identification of new agents for the treatments of AIDS: A national program to facilitate development of new drug candidates for clinical evaluation. In : *AIDS Etiology, Diagnosis, Treatment and Prevention*. (Eds. V.J. De Vita Jr., S. Hillman and S.A. Rosenberg). pp. 305-315, Philadelphia, Lippincott.

Burja, A. M., Banaigs, B., Mansour, E.A., Burgess, J.G. and Wright, P.C. (2001). Marine cyanobacteria– a prolific source of natural products. *Tetrahedron* (57). : 9347-9377.

Chandrasekaran, M. (1997). Industrial enzymes from marine microorganisms: The Indian Scenario. *Journal of Marine Biotechnology* (5): 86-89.

Chauhan, V. S., Singh. B., Singh, S. and Bisen, P.S. (2004). Screening of cyanobacterial strains producing cyanovirin–N and cyanovirin–V, protein capable of inhibiting growth of HIV-I and HIV-II. In: *Proceedings of the International Conference on Recent Advances in Biomedical and Therapeutic Sciences*, pp. 247, Bundelkhand University, Jhansi, India.

Ciferri, O., Tiboni, O. and Sanangelantoni, A.M. (1989). The genetic manipulation of cyanobacteria and its potential uses. In: *Algal and Cyanobacterial Biotechnology*. (Eds. R.C. Cresswell, T.A.V., Rees and N. Shah). pp. 239-262, Longman Group, UK.

Cohen, Z. (1986). Products from microalgae In: *CRC Handbook of Microalgal Mass Culture*. (Eds. A. Richmond). pp. 421-454, CRC Press, Boca Raton, Florida, USA.

Corbett, T.H., Valeriote, F.A., Polin, L.C., Pugh, S. and White, K. (1992). Models and concepts for discovery and development. In : *Cytotoxic Anticancer Drugs*. (Eds. F.A. Valeriote, T.H. Corbett and L.H. Baker). pp. 35-41, Kluwer Academic Publishers. Norwell.

Dainippon Ink and Chemicals Inc. (1981). Cosmetics containing water soluble phycocyanin. *Japanese Patent* (79). : 138755.

Dainippon Ink and Chemicals Inc. (1980). Production of highly purified alcoholophilic phycocyanin. *Japanese Patent* (80). : 77890.

Deth, S.K. (1999). Antimicrobial compound from marine cyanobacteria with special reference to the bioactivity of a purified compound from *Oscillatoria latevirens*. *Ph.D. Thesis*, Bharthidasan University, Tiruchirappalli, India.

Evets, L.B., Belookaya, T., Lyalikov, S., Orehov, S.D. and Shipulin, E. (1994). Means to normalize the levels of immnoglobulin E. Russian Federation Committee of Patents and Trade. Patent Number (19). RU (11)20005486 C1 (51). 5 A 61K35/80.

Fogg, G.E. (1971). Extracellular products of algae in freshwater. *Archives of Hydrobiology* (5): 1-25.

Fogg, G.E., Stewart, W.D.P., Fay, P. and Walsby A.E. (1973). *The Blue Green Algae*. Academic Press, London.

Fukino, H., Takagi, Y. and Yamane, Y. (1990). Effect of *Spirulina* (*S. platensis*). on the renal toxicity induced by inorganic mercury and cisplatin. *Eisei Kagaku* (36): 5.

Gerwick, W.H., Mrozek, C., Moghaddam, M.F. and Agrawal, S.K. (1989). Novel cytotoxic peptides from the tropical marine cyanobacterium *Hormothamnion enteromorpoides*. 1. Discovery, isolation and initial chemical and biological characterization of the hormothamnins from wild and cultural material. *Experientia* (45). : 115-117.

Gerwick, W.H., Proteau, P.J., Nagle, D.G., Hamel, E., Blokhin, A. and Slate, D.I. (1994). Structure of curacin A, a novel antimitotic, antiproferative and brine shrimp toxic natural product from the marine cyanobacterium *Lyngbya majuscula*. *Journal of Organic Chemistry* (59): 1243-1247.

Guerrero, M.G., Ramos, J.L. and Losada, M. (1982). Photosynthetic production of ammonia. *Experientia* (38): 53-55.

Gustafson, K.R., Cardellina, J.H. II, Fuller, R.W., Weslow, O.S., Kiser, R.F., Snader, K.M., Paterson, G.M. and Boyd, M.R. (1989). AIDS-antiviral sulfolipids from cyanobacteria (blue-green algae). *Journal of National Cancer Institute* (81): 1254-1258.

Hayashi, K., Hayashi, T. and Morita, N. (1993). An extract from *Spirulina platensis* is a selective inhibitor of *Herpes simplex* virus type 1 penetration into HeLa cells. *Phytotherapy Research* (7): 76-80.

Hayashi, K., Hayashi, T. and Kojima, I. (1996). A natural sulfated polysaccharide, calcium spirulan, isolated from *Spirulina platensis*: *in vitro* and *ex vivo* evaluation of anti-*Herpes simplex* virus and anti-human immunodeficiency virus activities. *AIDS Research and Human Retroviruses* (12): 1463-1471.

Hayashi, O., Katoh, T. and Okuwaki, Y. (1994). Enhancement of antibody production in mice by dietary *Spirulina platensis. Journal of Nutritional Science and Vitaminology* (40): 431-441.

Horrobin, D.F. (1990). *Omega-6 Essential Fatty acids : Pathophysiology and Roles in Clinical Medicine.* Wiley-Liss, New York.

Ishibashi, M., Moore, R., Patterson, G.M.L., Xu, C. and Clardy, J. (1986). Scytophycins: cytotoxic and antimycotic agents from the cyanophyte *Scytonema pseudohojmanni. Journal of Organic Chemistry* (51): 5300-5305.

Jackson, P.S.A. (1981). Note on a possible association between plasma β-carotene levels and conception rate in a group of winter housed dairy cattle. *Animal Production* (32): 109-112.

Jassby, A., Lembi, C.A. and Waaland, J.R. (1988). *Algae and human affairs.* Cambridge University Press, Cambridge, UK.

Jagdeshwari (1998). Effect of purified compound from *Oscillatoria willei* BDU 130511 on the testis and accessory reproductive organs of swiss albino mice. *M.Sc. Thesis,* Bharthidasan University, Tiruchirappalli, India.

Kerby, N.W., Niven, G.W., Rowell, P. and Steward W.D.P. (1987). Photoproduction of amino acids by mutant strains of N_2- fixing cyanobacteria. *Applied Microbiology and Biotechnology* (25): 547-552.

Kerby, N., Niven, G., Rowell, P., Steward, W.D.P. (1988). Ammonia and amino acid production by cyanobacteria. In: *Algal Biotechnology.* (Eds T. Stadler, J. Mollion, M.C.Verdus, Y. Karamanos, H. Morvan and D. Christiasen). pp. 277-283, Elsevier Applied Science, London, New York.

Kobayashi, J., Ishibashi, M., Murayama, J., Takamatsu, M., Iwamura, M., Ohizumi, Y. and Sasaki, T. (1990). Amphidinolide-E, a novel antileukemic 19-membered microlide from the cultured symbiotic dinoflagellate *Amphidinium* sp. *Journal of Organic Chemistry* (55): 3421-3425.

Krishnaprema, K. (1996). Effect of the crude ethanolic extract of *Oscillatoria willei* BDU 130511 on male BALB C mice. *M.Sc. Thesis,* Bharthidasan University, Tiruchirappalli, India.

Lisheng, L., Baojiang. G., Jihong. R., Guangquan, Q. and Botang, Wu (1991). Inhibitive effect and mechanism of polysaccharide of *Spirulina platensis* on transplanted tumor in mice. *Marine Science* (5): 33-38.

Loseva, L.P. and Dardynskaya, I.V. (1993). *Spirulina*- natural sorbent of radionucleides. In : *Proceedings of 6th International Congress of Applied Algology,* Czech Republic, Belrus.

Loseva, L.P. (1999). *Spirulina patensis* and specialties to support detoxifying pollutants and to strengthen the immune system. In : *Proceedings of 8th International Congress of Applied Algology,* Italy, Republic, Belrus.

Madhava, C., Reddy, J., Bhat, V. B., Kiranmai, G. M., Reddy, S., Reddanna, P. and Madyastha, K. M. (2000). Selective Inhibition of cyclooxygenase-2 by C-phycocyanin, a biliprotein from *Spirulina platensis. Biochemical and Biophysical Research Communications* (277): 599-603.

Mathew, B., Sankaranarayanan, R., Nair, P.P., Varghese, C., Somanathan, T., Amma, B.P., Amma, N.S. and Nair, M.K. (1995). Evaluation of chemoprevention of oral cancer with *Spirulina. Nutrition and Cancer* (24). : 197-202.

Mohanthy, P. (1996). Cyanobacterial photosynthesis: concepts and applications. *Journal of Scientific and Industrial Research* (55). : 553-570.

Moore, R.E. (1981). Constituents of blue- green algae. In: *Marine Natural Products : Chemical and Biological Perspectives* (Eds. P.J. Scheuer). Academic Press, New York.

Moore, R.E., Patterson, G.M.L. and Carmichael, W.W. (1988). New pharmaceuticals from cultured blue green algae. In : *Biomedical Importance of Marine Organisms.* (Eds. D.G. Fautin). pp. 143-146, California Academy of Sciences.

Murray, R.L. Jr and Mitsui, A. (1982). Growth of hybrid Tilapia fry fed nitrogen fixing marine blue green algae in sea water. *Journal of World Mariculture Society* (13): 198-203.

Musgrave, S.C., Kerby, N.W., Codd, G.A. and Stewart, W.D.P. (1982). Sustained ammonia production by immobilized filaments of the nitrogen-fixing cyanobacterium *Anabaena* 27893. *Biotechnology Letters* (4): 647-52.

Normal, J. and Temple, I. (1988). Does β-carotene prevents cancer : a critical appraisal. *Nutrition Research* (8): 685-690.

Patterson, G.M.L., Baker, K.K., Baldwin, C.L., Bolis, C.M., Caplan, F.R., Larson, L.K., Levine, I.A., Moore, R.E., Nelson, C.S., Tschappat, K.D. and Tuang, G. (1993). Antiviral activity of cultured blue-green algae (cyanophyta). *Journal of Phycology* (29): 125-130.

Patterson, G. M. L. and Carmeli, S. (1992). Biological effects of toly-toxin (6-hydroxy-7-O-methyl-scytophycin B), a potent bioactive metabolite from cyanobacteria. *Archives of Microbiology* (157): 406-411.

Patterson, G. M. L. (1996). Biotechnological application of cyanobacteria. *Journal of Scientific and Industrial Research* (55). : 669-679.

Puniya, A.K., Singh, S., Ganeshkumar, C. and Singh, K. (1995). Single cell protein : a promising dietary substitute. *Indian Journal of Experimental Biology* (33). : 545-551.

Qishen, P., Baojiang, G. and Kolman, A. (1989). Radioprotective effect of extract from *Spirulina platensis* in mouse bone marrow cells studied by using the micronucleus test. *Toxicology Letters* (48): 165-169.

Qureshi, M. and Ali, R. (1996). *Spirulina platensis* exposure enhances macrophage phagocytic function in cats. *Immunopharmacology and Immunotoxicology.* (18). : 457-463.

Qureshi, M.A., Kidd, M.T. and Ali, R.A. (1995). *Spirulina platensis* extract enhances chicken macrophage functions after *in vitro* exposure. *Journal of Nutritional Immunology* (3): 35-44.

Qureshi, M.A., Garlich, J. and Kidd, M. (1996). Dietary *Spirulina platensis* enhances humoral and cell-mediated immune function in chickens. *Immunopharmacology and Immunotoxicology* (18): 465-476.

Rai, A. N. (1990). *Handbook of Cyanobacteria.* CRC Press Boca Raton, Florida, USA.

Ramirez, D., Gonzalez, R., Merino, N., Rodriguez, S. and Ancheta, O. (2002). Inhibitory effects of *Spirulina* in zymozan-induced arthritis in mice. *Mediators of Inflammation.* (11): 75-79.

Ramos, J. L., Guerrero, M.G. and Losada, M. (1987). Factors affecting the photoproduction of ammonia from dinitrogen and water by the cyanobacterium *Anabaena* sp. Strain ATCC 33047. *Biotechnology and Bioengineering* (29): 566-571.

Rathore, N.K., Singh, S. and Singh, V. (2004). *Spirulina* as immuno- enhancer and biomodulator. *Journal of Immunology and Immunopathology* 6 (2): 1-10.

Riccardi, G., Sora, S. and Cifferi, O. (1981). Production of amino acids by analog-resistant mutants of the cyanobacterium *Spirulina platensis*. *Journal of Bacteriology* (147): 1002-1007.

Rinehart, K. L. Jr, Shaw, P. D., Shield, L. G., Gloer, J. B., Harbour, G. C. and Koker, M. E. S. (1981). Marine natural products as sources of antiviral, antimicrobial and antineoplastic agents. *Pure and Applied Chemistry* (53). : 795-799.

Reichelt, J. L. and Borowitzka, M.A. (1984). Antibiotics from algae: results of a large scale screening programme. *Hydrobiologia* (116/117). : 143-147.

Roberts, R. J. (1985). Restriction and modification enzymes and their recognition sequences. *Nucleic Acids Research* (13): 2165-2200.

Schwartz, J. and Shklar, G. (1987). Regression of experimental hamster cancer by beta-carotene and algae extracts. *Journal of Oral Maxillofacter Surgery* (45). : 510-515.

Schwartz, J., Shklar, G., Reid, S. and Trickler, D. (1988). Prevention of experimental oral cancer by extracts of *Spirulina-Dunaliela* algae *Nutrition and Cancer* (11): 127-134.

Schlegel, I., Thanh Doan, N., Nola de, C. and Smith, G. D. (1999). Antibiotic activity of new cyanobacterial isolates from Australia and Asia against green algae and cyanobacteria. *Journal of Applied Phycology* (10). : 471-476.

Shih, S. R., Tsai, K. N., Li, Y. S., Chueh, C. C. and Chan, E. C. (2003). Inhibition of enterovirus 71-induced apoptosis by allophycocyanin isolated from a blue-green alga *Spirulina platensis*. *Journal of Medical Virology* (70): 119–125.

Shirahashi, H., Murakami, N., Watanabe, M., Nagatsu, A., Sakakibara, J., Tokuda, H., Nishino, H. and Iwashima, A. (1993). Isolation and identification of antitumour promoting principle from freshwater cyanobacterium *Phormidium tunne*. *Chemical and Pharmaceutical Bulletin* (41): 1664-1667.

Singh, S. (1992). Photobiological production of ammonia by an L-methionine-DL-Sulfoximine -resistant mutant of the cyanobiont *Nostoc* ANTH. *Indian Journal of Experimental Biology* (30): 284-287.

Singh, S. (1993). Immobilization-caused physiological and biochemical changes in the cyanobiont *Nostoc* ANTH. *Indian Journal of Experimental Biology* (31): 446-449.

Singh, S. and Rai, A.K. (1989). Methionine sulphoximine induced changes in the cyanobacteria *Anabaena doliolum* and *Anacystis nidulans*. *Indian Journal of Experimental Biology* (27): 227-229.

Startman, K., Belli, J., Jensen, C.M., Moore, R.E. and Patterson, G.M.L. (1994). Aulosirasole, a novel solid tumor selective cytotoxin from the blue green alga *Aulosira fertilissima* *Journal of Organic Chemistry* (59): 6279-6285.

Sundararaman, M. (1992). Intra and extra cellular substances in marine cyanobacteria. *Ph.D. Thesis*, Bharathidasan University, Tiruchirappalli, India.

Thirunalasundari, T. and Subramanian, G. (2000). Antifertility compound from marine cyanobacterium. In: *Proceedings of International Conference of Reproductive Biology*. 9th French- Czech- Slovak Colloquium. Slovak Academy of Sciences, Stara Lesna.

Upasani, C.D., Khera, A. and Balaraman, R. (2001). Effect of lead with vitamin E, C or *Spirulina* on malondialdehyde, conjugated dienes and hydroperoxides in rats. *Indian Journal of Experimental Biology* (39): 70-74.

Venkataraman, L.V. (1983). *Spirulina* in India. In : *Proceedings of National Seminar on Cyanobacterial Research-Indian Scene* (Eds. G. Subramanian). pp. 92, National Facility of Marine Cyanobacteria, Tiruchirappalli.

Vincenzini, M., De Philippis, R., Ena, A. and Florenzano, G. (1986). Ammonia photoproduction by *Cyanospira rippkae* cells "entrapped" in dialysis tube. *Experientia* (42): 1040-43.

Whitehead, P.R. and Brown N.L. (1985). Three restriction endonucleases from *Anabaena flos-aquae*. *Journal of General Microbiology* (131): 951-958.

Whitton, B. A., Grainger, S. L. J., Hawley, G. R. W. and Simon, J. W. (1991). Cell bound and extracellular phosphatase activities of cyanobacterial isolates. *Microbial Ecology* (21): 85-98.

Wikstrom, P., Szwajcer, E., Brodelius, P., Nilsson, K. N. and Mosbach, K. (1982). Formation of alpha keto acids from amino acids using immobilized bacteria and algae. *Biotechnology Letters* (4): 153-156.

Zhang-Chang-Wu (1994). Effects of polysaccharides and phycocyanins from *Spirulina* on peripheral blood and haemopoietic system of bone marrow in mice. In: *Proceedings of Second Asia Pacific Conference on Algal Biotechnology*. pp. 58, University of Malasiya.

Microbial Biotechnology and Ecology (2011)
Editors: **Deepak Vyas, G.S. Paliwal, P.K.Khare and R.K Gupta**
Published by: **DAYA PUBLISHING HOUSE, NEW DELHI**

Pages **571–576**

Chapter 33

Plants and Rhizobium Techniques

☆ *Pooja Agrawal*

Department of Applied Microbiology and Biotechnology,
Dr. H.S. Gour University, Sagar – 470 003, M.P.

Soils are the excellent culture media for the growth of different groups of microorganisms *e.g.* bacteria, virus, fungi, algae and actinomycetes. The number and kinds of soil microorganism found in a habitat, depends upon its nature, chemical composition, temperature, pH etc.

Maximum microbial growth and activity in the soil is found around the roots of plants (Hiltner, 1904). This region is called *Rhizosphere.* Practically all the interactions such as symbiosis, syntrophism, antagonism, synergism and commensalisms between plants and microorganisms and among different microorganisms are operative in this region. Their interactions may be favourable, indispensable, unfavourable or can be lethal. The most important functions of soil microflora is to decompose various kinds of organic matter and to mineralize them into inorganic/mineral constituents.

Some soil microorganisms are supporting the plant growth and are called "plant growth promoting rhizobacteria" or PGPR. These bacteria are generally found in symbiotic association with the leguminous plants (Pea, Gram, Mung, Soybean, Arhar and many other) and possess ability to fix atmospheric nitrogen.

The root nodule symbiosis with leguminous plant is generally developed by *Rhizobium, Bradyrhizobium* and *Azorhizobium* belonging to *Rhizobiaceae* family (Elkan, 1984). Bousingault (1834) proved that nodules on legume roots are responsible for fixing atmospheric nitrogen. Based on our knowledge of known leguminous plants it has been proved that not all the legumes bear nodules on their roots, only 10-12 per cent of legumes has been so far examined for nodulation. Beside this, some of the non-leguminous plants also bear nodule and has the ability to fix atmospheric nitrogen *e.g. Parasponia* (Trinick, 1973). *Rhizobium* is the well known genus known for fixing atmospheric nitrogen in symbiotic association with leguminous plants by way of forming nodules on the plant roots. Apart from legumes nodulated by genus *Rhizobium*, roots of some plants belonging to different families also nodulated by member's of actinomycetes classified in the genus, *Frankia*.

The *Rhizobium* is the most exploited genus of bacteria known for the development of bioinoculant. The genus has 7 known species *i.e. R. leguminosarum, R. phaseoli, R. trifoli, R. japonicum, Rhizobium* spp., *R. meliloti, R. lupini* forming cross inoculation groups with Pea group, Bean group, Clover group, Soyabean group, Cowpea group, Alfalfa group, Lupini group. (The cross-inoculation groups are based on the classical studies of Fred *et al.*, 1932). The principal of cross inoculation grouping is based on the ability of an isolate of *Rhizobium* to form nodules in a limited genera of species of legumes *i.e. Pisum, Phaseolus, Trifolium, Glycine, Vigna, Arachis, Melilotus, Lupinus* related to one another.

Nodulation and Mechanism of Nitrogen Fixation

The nodules formed on plants are agronomically significant as they provide an alternative to the use of expensive ammonium fertilizer's. Symbiotic nitrogen fixation takes place in a specialized structure called nodule that originate in a root as a consequence of microsymbiont infection. During nodulation the bacteria are transformed into bacteriods which are able to carry out transformation of nitrogen to ammonia ($N_2 \rightarrow NH_3$) later the ammonia is incorporated to the plant metabolism, is called nitrogen metabolism (Dilworth, 1991).

Symbiotic nitrogen fixation is that which occurs by the symbiosis of both plant and bacteria *e.g. Rhizobium* that can fix atmospheric nitrogen only when it gets associated with roots of leguminous plants. Some microorganisms are also capable of fixing nitrogen non-symbiotically *i.e. Azotobacter, Cynobacteria, Azospirullum and Clostridium.*

The reduction of nitrogen to ammonia requires a valency change *i.e.* from initial oxidation state 0 to –3 oxidation state. Six electrons are required to reduce one mole of nitrogen to Ammonia.

$$N_2 + 6H^+ + 6e^- \longrightarrow 2NH_3$$

This requires the break up of nitrogen bonds. It is agreed that the atoms of oxygen are separated in the biological oxidation state through the change in the valency of metal ion (Fe^{++}) in the enzyme, Cytochrome oxidase and that the atoms of nitrogen are separated through the change in the valency of metal ion Molybdenum (Mo^{+2}), bound to the enzyme involved in the reduction of nitrogen. The main enzyme involved in the nitrogen fixation is nitrogenase, it binds to nitrogen and converts it into free ammonium ions. It consist of two component, component I consist of Mo-Fe protein while component II consist of Fe protein, combination of two component reconstitute nitrogenase activity. If no suitable electron acceptor is available nitrogenase forms molecular hydrogen which generates ATP and consequently improves the efficiency of nitrogen fixation (Pawar and Dagniwala, 2002). While moving on to the genetic level and searching for the genes required for nodulation, *Rhizobium* species that nodulate the legumes were studied and it was proposed that genes for nodulation (nod) genes and genes for nitrogen fixation (nif) are clustered on large symbiotic plasmid. Nif genes are found in clustered form in a particular region of DNA. They are not found in scattered form (Roberts, 1978). The genes represent host range specificity.

Isolation and Characterization of *Rhizobium*

Beijernick (1888) was the first to isolate and cultivate a microorganism from the nodules of leguminous plants. He named it as *Bacillus radicicola*. Later on Frank in 1889 renamed the nodulated bacteria as *Rhizobium*. It is now placed in Bergey's manual of determinative bacteriology under the genus *Rhizobium*. *Rhizobium* falls under Rhizobiaceae family which consist of four genera, two of which include the symbiotic nitrogen fixing bacteria *Rhizobium* and *Bradyrhizobium*. *Rhizobia* is a non spore forming free living bacteria found in soil. Bergey's manual described rhizobia as cells without endospore, normally rod shaped, motile, aerobic and gram negative.

Rhizobia contains one polar, subpolar or peritrichous flagella. It produces extracellular slime on carbohydrate containing media. It can survive at low temperature and can tolerate temperatures upto 50°C. Rhizobia cells are generally bacilli, some times coccobacilli and formed poly-β-hydroxy granules which are also visible under the light microscope.

Yeast Extract Mannitol Agar (YEMA) is the specific medium for the culture of *Rhizobium* (Date, 1974). Vitamins such as thiamine and biotin are required for *Rhizobium* growth. *Rhizobium* produces white, translucent, glistening, elevated and comparatively smaller colonies with entire margin.

Method of Isolation

Collection of Roots of the leguminous plants will be done carefully. The process of isolation of *Rhizobium* from root nodules includes many steps which are described in the following text.

Surface Sterilization of Nodules

Healthy, unbroken, large and pinkish nodules should be preferred from the plant roots after thorough washing with the tap water. Nodules will be washed with sterile water. The nodules will then immersed in 3 per cent H_2O_2 for about 5 minutes to surface sterilize them. There after the nodules will washed in sterilized water to get rid of sterilizing agent. The nodules will then placed in 70 per cent ethyl alcohol for 2-3 minutes and then again washed with distilled water, these nodules will crushed with the help of glass rod in 1 ml of sterile distilled water. This suspension will then used for the isolation of bacteria using YEMA medium having congo red.

Preparation of Medium

Yeast extract mannitol agar (YEMA) with congo red (as differential reagent) should prepared using following ingradients as suggested by Subbarao (1995).

Mannitol	10.0 gm
K_2HPO_4	0.5 gm
$MgSO_4.7H_2O$	0.2 gm
NaCl	0.1 gm
Agar	20.0 gm
Yeast extract	1.0 gm
Distilled water	1000 ml
Congo red 1 per cent solution	2.5 ml

The media without congo red will be autoclaved at 121°C for 20 minutes. 1 per cent cango red solution will be prepared and sterilized separately. 2.5 ml of this will be added to 1000 ml sterile medium before pouring into the petriplates.

Isolation of Bacteria

The isolation of *Rhizobium* will be carried out by serial dilution of the nodule suspension followed by a streak plate method (Waksman, 1927; Vincent, 1970). Serial dilutions of the nodule suspension have to prepare in sterile distilled water. The suspension will dilute upto 10^{-5} and this dilution was used for streaking. The plates having YEMA medium with congo red will streaked with a loopful suspension using disposable plastic loops. The plates were then incubated at 37°C and were observed after 24 hours for bacterial growth. The colonies with typical *Rhizobium* growth (small, white, translucent, glistening) were picked up on a separate medium for further examination.

Purification

All the colonies picked up for the isolation of *Rhizobium* were purified. Purification was done by adopting a streak plate technique in which a particular colony will be picked up from the streaked plates showing bacterial colonies, using a loop and then streake onto a plate containing YEMA with congo red (Waksman, 1927). These plates are then incubated at 37°C to obtain the pure culture or specific colonies of *Rhizobium*.

Preservation

The purified cultures obtained during the isolation will be preserved and maintained on agar slants having YEMA medium. These should keep in a refrigerator at 4°C for future use.

Morphological Characterization

To study the morphological characteristics, each isolate was studied for gram staining and carbol fuchsin staining. The procedure adopted for gram staining and carbol fuchsin staining are as follows:

Gram's Staining

The gram stain procedure is the most widely used differential staining procedure in bacteriology. The gram positive bacteria appears violet since they retain the primary stain and gram negative bacteria appears red or pink.

The stained slide was then examined under the oil immersion objective to determine which organism is gram positive and which is gram negative.

Carbol Fuchsin Staining

A loop full of the suspension of selected bacterium is spread on a microscopic slide in a drop of water and allowed to dry in air. The slide is then passed through the top position of the flame of a Bunsen burner to heat fix the bacteria. The slide is then allowed to cool, and then flooded with dilute carbol fuchsin stain for 10-20 seconds. The slide is then washed in running water and allowed to dry. It is then examined under microscope for the presence or absence of poly-β-hydroxy butyrate granules.

Lactose-Agar Test

This test is used to differentiate *Agrobacterium* from *Rhizobium*. *Agrobacterium* utilize lactose to form a reduced product ketolactose, when Benedict's reagent is poured over Agar medium containing lactose on which nodule bacteria are growing, the development of yellow colour due to Cu_2O around the colony indicates the presence of *Agrobacterium*. The medium used was having following composition:

Lactose	10.0 gm
K_2HPO_4	0.5 gm
$MgSO_4.7H_2O$	0.2 gm
NaCl	0.1 gm
Yeast	1.0 gm
Distilled water	1000 ml
Agar	20.0 gm

Citrate Utilization Test

This Test is used to differentiate bacteria on the basis of ability to utilize citrate or ferment citrate as a sole carbon source. The utilization of citrate depends on the presence of an enzyme citrate permease produced by the organism that helps its transport into the cell. The composition of the medium used for testing the citrate utilization was as follows:

K_2HPO_4	1 gm
$NH_4H_2PO_4$	1 gm
NaCl	5 gm
Sodium citrate	2 gm
Magnesium sulphate	0.2 gm
1.5 per cent Bromothymol blue	10.0 ml
Distilled water	1000 ml
Agar	20 gm
pH	6.8

Root nodulating bacteria (*Rhizobium*) has been classified based on their growth on definite substrate as (i) Fast grower's and (ii) Slow grower's (Elkan, 1984). Fast grower include rhizobia associated with clover, alfalfa, pea and bean while slow grower include soybean and cowpea rhizobia. Fast grower are acid producing (Vincent, 1970) contains peritrichous flagella and generally called as *Rhizobium* while slow grower's are alkali producing, contain sub-polar flagella and are generally called as *Bradyrhizobium*. *Rhizobium* consist of five species *R. leguminosarum, R. meliloti, R. loti, R. galegae* and *R. fredii.* (Elkan, 1984).

A new genus called *Azorhizobium* has also been officially recognized (Dreyfus *et al.*, 1988). This bacterium was first isolated from the stem nodules of *Sesbania rostrata* and was found to be phenotypically and genotypically different from the other two genera *i.e., Rhizobium* and *Bradyrhizobium*. *Azorhizobium* consist of the species *A. caulinodans* which falls into taxa different from slow and fast growing *Rhizobium*. A unique photosynthetic *Rhizobium* is also known and named as *Photorhizobium* (Hardy, 1989).

Mass Production of *Rhizobium* Bioinoculant

Rhizobial broth is grown on YEM medium in large flasks on a shaker for small requirements or in fermenters for large requirements. The powdered carrier (passing through 100 mesh sieve) is neutralized with $CaCO_3$ and autoclaved at 15 lbs pressure for 4 hours. After cooling, a high count broth is mixed so as to attain a 40 per cent moisture holding capacity of the carrier. The carrier and the broth are mixed either manually or by means of a mechanical mixer, cured in trays for 2-5 days and packeted in polythene bags.

References

Beijernick, M.W. (1888). Die bacterien der popilionaceen knollchen. *Bot. Ztg*, 46 : pp. 726-804.

Bergey's Manual of discriminative bacteriology Vol. 1 (1984). pp. 261-267.

Boussingault, J. B. (1834). The nitrogen cycle. *Proceedings of American Philosophical Society*, Vol. 114, No. 6, pp. 435-479.

Date, R.A. (1974). Principles in Rhizobium strain selection. In: *Symbiotic Nitrogen Fixation in Plants*. Ed. P.S. Nutman Cambridge University, pp. 137-150.

Dilworth, H.J. (1991). Biology and biochemistry of nitrogen fixation. *Biochem. Biophys*, pp. 127, 285-294.

Dreyfus, B.L. (1981). Nitrogen fixing nodules induced by Rhizobium on stem of tropical legumes *S. rostrata*. *FEMS Microbial, Lett.*, pp. 313-317.

Elkan, G.H. (1984). Taxonomy and metabolism of Rhizobium and its genetic relationship in biological. *Nitrogen*, pp. 1-38.

Fred, E.B. Baldwin, I.L. and McCoy, E. (1932). *Root Nodule Bacteria and Leguminous Plants*. Univ. Wisconsin, Madison.

Hardy, R.W.F., Burns R.C and Parshall, G.W. (1971) . The biochemistry of nitrogen fixation. In: *Advances in Chemistry*, pp. 218-247.

Hellriegel, H. and Wilfarth, H. (1896). Die Lendwirtchaftlichen versuchs stationen Bd.46, S- 1-8. (Mil Bild Und verzeichris der wichtingsten vero foentlichugen).

Hiltner, L. (1904). Iifer neuere Erfahrungen iind probleme aufodem gebiet der Bodenbakteriologie iind unter besonderer Berucksichtingung der Griindiinging iind Brache, Art.Dtsch., Landw. Ges; 98, pp. 58-78.

Pawar, C.B. and Daginawala, H.F. (2000). *General Microbiology*, Ed. 2, pp. 520-540.

Roberts, D. G. (1978). RRS discovery cruise 90-20, institute of oceanographic science, Cruise report, Vvormeley, U.K., 68.

Subba Rao, N.S. (1993). *Biofertilizer's in Agriculture and Forestry*, Ed. 3, pp. 1-40.

Subba Rao, N.S. (1995). *Soil Microorganism and Plant Growth*, Ed. 3, pp. 170-190.

Trinick, J.J. (1973). Symbiosis between Rhizobium and non Legume, Trema aspera. *Nature*, London, pp. 224, 459-460.

Vincent, J.M. (1970). *A Manual for the Practical Study of the Root Nodule Bacteria*. IBP, Handbook No. 15, Backwell scientific publication, Oxford.

Waksman, S.A. (1927). *Principles of Soil Microbiology*. Williams and Wilkins Co., Baltimore.

Microbial Biotechnology and Ecology (2011) *Pages* **577–590**
Editors: **Deepak Vyas, G.S. Paliwal, P.K.Khare and R.K Gupta**
Published by: **DAYA PUBLISHING HOUSE, NEW DELHI**

Chapter 34

Quest for a Novel Tuberculosis Vaccine: A Global Endeavor

☆ ***Umesh Dutta Gupta[1]*, Vijender Singh[2] and Pushpa Gupta[1]***

[1]*National JALMA Institute for Leprosy and Other Mycobacterial Diseases, Agra – 282 001*
[2]*Institute of Microbial Technology, Chandigarh – 160 036*

Tuberculosis (TB): A Global Health Problem

Tuberculosis (TB) is an archaic scourge that has distressed mankind for millennia and *Mycobacterium tuberculosis*, the causative agent, is one of the oldest and most successful of human pathogens (Collins, 1997). The etiological agent for TB was discovered by Robert Koch in the last of 19th century, is a gram-positive bacterium known as tubercle bacilli or *Mycobacterium tuberculosis.* In 1993, the World Health Organization (WHO) has declared TB as 'a global emergency'. Despite a more than a half century of extensive vaccination, TB claims a high burden of morbidity and mortality throughout the world (Korenromp *et al.*, 2009) (WHO 2009). Estimates of PPD skin-test indicate that tubercle bacilli infect a one-third of the world's population, leading to approximately 8.9 new cases of the disease and 1.7 million casualities each year (Korenromp *et al.*, 2009). Despite the worldwide efforts to control TB, the worldwide problem of TB is deteriorating, particularly in developing countries. Further the situation exacerbated by HIV-TB co-infection and the global emergence of multidrug-resistant strains of *M. tuberculosis* (WHO 2009). Although drug-susceptible TB can be effectively treated by current chemotherapy with a 6-month regimen which involves three or four drugs (WHO, [Directly Observed Treatment and Short-course drug therapy] DOTS strategy, with >95 per cent cure rate) (Acheson *et al.*, 2000) but for a definite control and elimination of this disease, there is a serious need and challenge for scientific community to develop a novel and effective vaccine against TB.

* E-mail: gupta.umesh95@gmail.com

Epidemiology of Tuberculosis

On the basis of surveillance and survey, WHO has reported approximately 9.2 million new cases of TB occurred in 2007. Out of these 9.2 million new cases, about 44 per cent (~ 4.1 million) account for new smear positive cases. India, China, Indonesia, Nigeria, and South Africa order first to fifth in terms of the total number of incidences. Among all global cases Asia responsible for 55 per cent and the African region for 31 per cent. The American, European and Eastern Mediterranean regions are accountable only for small fractions of global cases. The African region is at the rank first with 13 countries out of total 15 countries with the highest estimated TB incidence rates. This phenomenon is directly linked to high rates of HIV co-infection. In 2007 amongst total 9.2 million incident cases of TB, 1.37 million (14.8 per cent) were estimated as HIV-positive. The African region accounted for most (79 per cent) HIV-positive TB cases, where South Africa alone responsible for 31 per cent of cases in the African region. The occurrence of HIV-positive TB cases in the South-East Asia Region (mainly India) is about 11 per cent of total cases. Globally, around 0.5 million cases of MDR-TB were found, of which 0.3 million were among people not previously treated for TB and 0.2 million were among previously treated TB patients. Indian and China are at top among all countries with the largest number of cases of MDR-TB (WHO 2009).

The total numbers of global cases are still escalating in an absolute terms due to population growth. There is anticipated occurrence of new 9.8 million cases of TB in 2010, more than in any previous year in history. About 80 per cent of the cases will be found in the highest-burden countries like India and China which will be account for one third of 80 per cent cases (Dye *et al.*, 2009). Nonetheless, due to various strategies of WHO like based on Directly Observed Treatment and Short-course drug therapy (DOTS) which was reinforced by Stop TB strategy in 2006, the number of incident cases per capita is falling globally at an estimated 1 per cent per year (WHO 2009).

Pathogenesis of the Tuberculosis

Various observations from human TB infection and experimental animal models give raise the pattern of various events that start with the infection with mycobacterium (Flynn and Chan, 2005; Russell, 2007). The droplet nuclei containing virulent *M. tuberculosis* enters the lungs via the aerosol route on inhalation. The bacteria in inhaled droplets are engulfed primarily by resident alveolar macrophages which trigger innate and adaptive immune response in the host. This leads to the induction of a local inflammatory response that resulted in to recruitment of mononuclear cells from neighboring blood vessels. These cells are the basic ingredient of the granuloma, which is the characteristic pathological feature of this disease. In the initial stage, the granuloma is an unstructured mass of macrophages, monocytes, and neutrophils. In granuloma the macrophages also differentiate into several specialized cell types, like multinucleated giant cells, epithelioid macrophages and foamy macrophages. With the arrival of lymphocytes during acquired immune response, the granuloma acquires a more structured and stratified structure. In a classical granuloma, the macrophage rich center is surrounded by a layer of lymphocytes which may be restricted within a fibrous sheath that marks the periphery of the structure. The arrival of mycobacterium-specific lymphocytes which takes about 2 to 3 weeks post-infection, check the rapid bacterial multiplication and set a containment state which is in mice, characterized, by relatively stable bacterial numbers. At this particular stage, the extensively vascularization of granuloma results in to active recruitment of cells at the site of infection. The pathology results as disease progress; the fibrous cuff at the periphery of granulomas becomes more firms and blood vessels that penetrate granuloma diminish and vascularity of the granuloma reduces to minimum. Next, number of foamy macrophages also increase, which may be accountable for the caseous debris in the center of the granuloma (Russell *et al.*, 2009). In the next stage of progression, the caseous center of the granuloma becomes hypoxic (Via *et al.*, 2008). This condition can induce a state of persistence with non-replicative state of *M. tuberculosis*. In the last stage, active granulomas exhibit extensive pathology which ultimately lead to the rapture of the granuloma and liberate thousands of viable, infectious bacilli into the airways (Kaplan *et al.*, 2003) and a productive cough develops, in human that facilitates aerosol spread of infectious bacilli ready to infect healthy hosts.

Host Response to Tuberculosis

M. tuberculosis primarily infects macrophages of the lungs. This bacillus is an enormously successful pathogen that has evolved numerous mechanisms for evading elimination by the host immune response. After infection, mycobacteria persist within macrophages in early phagosomes and escape from the immune system notably by preventing phagosome acidification, arresting phagosome maturation and fusion with lysosomes (Russell, 2003).The immunological control of *M. tuberculosis* infection is a complex and multi-faceted. However, given the intracellular nature of the pathogen, the role of cellular immunity in the control of *M. tuberculosis* infection has been established beyond doubt. T-lymphocytes play a central role in the protection against TB. The protection against TB critically depends on T-helper 1 (Th1) type CD4 T cells which secrete the key cytokines IFN-g and TNF-α (Quesniaux, Jacobs *et al.*, 2010) Moreover, IFN-g and TNF-α are the important cytokines which activate macrophages to control bacterial multiplication by increasing fusion of the phagosome with the lysosome (Schaible *et al.*, 1998; MacMicking *et al.*, 2003). In addition, CD8 T cells also contribute to by secreting similar cytokines and by producing effector molecules like perforin and granulysin, which not only kill *M. tuberculosis* infected macrophages but also directly attack on the mycobacteria (Woodworth *et al.*, 2008).

During tuberculosis infection, in addition to the conventional CD4 T cells and CD8 T cells, CD1-restricted unconventional T cells are also give specific response against glycolipids of *M. tuberculosis* (Ulrichs *et al.*, 2003). Recent evidence also indicated the contribution of newer T cell subset, T-helper 17 (Th17) which secrete IL-17. These T cells mainly attract monocytes to the site of *M. tuberculosis* replication where they activate them. It has been also shown that Th17 cells are recruited to the lungs after immunization and rapidly respond to TB infection by increasing the enrolling Th1 cells into the lung (Khader *et al.*, 2007). Recent studies also showed that presence of regulatory T cells (Treg) can diminish an effective T-cell response required for protection against TB (Kursar *et al.*, 2007). Hence for novel vaccination strategy, restriction of Tregs cells and enrichment of IL-17 producing Th17 cells may help in generation of effective Th1 response for the control of TB infection.

Bacillus Calmette-Guerin (BCG): The Current Vaccine

Albert Calmette and Camille Guerin, in 1908 isolated *Mycobacterium bovis* from cattle suffering from tuberculous mastitis. They made an attenuated strain from this isolated mycobacterium (*M. bovis*) which a close relative of *M. tuberculosis*, by growing it for 13 years and 230 subcultures until it lost the ability to cause disease in inoculated individuals (Huebner 1996).Today more than 3 billion people have vaccinated with BCG, which makes this vaccine the most widely used throughout world. Further, in 1992, approximately 100 million newborns and children vaccinated with BCG through the World Health Organization (WHO)/United Nations Children's Emergency Fund (UNICEF) expanded program for immunization (Andersen *et al.*, 1995) (WHO 1992). At present, BCG is the only vaccine available for prevention of TB and estimated that it prevent only 5 per cent of the all vaccine preventable fatalities due to TB (Bishai and Mercer, 2001). In spite of the fact that BCG is the most widely administered of all vaccines, TB still continues to scourge the human life. It is however, been shown to be protective against the meningeal TB in young children (Udani, 1994). Nevertheless, its efficacy in preventing adult pulmonary TB, that is responsible for the major burden of morbidity and mortality, varies dramatically as revealed by carefully conducted studies throughout the world from 0 per cent in Chinglepet, India to approximately 80 per cent in the UK (Fine, 1995).

Although, first BCG vaccine has been administered successfully in human in 1921(Sakula 1983), yet TB continues to kill approximately 2 million people annually (Korenromp *et al.*, 2009).

Although BCG is enough good vaccine but due to number of unidentified host as well as environmental factors badly affect its protective efficiency (Smith *et al.*, 2000). There are many hypotheses that can be explained the insufficient protective efficiency of BCG against pulmonary tuberculosis and probable new strategies for its improvement. Some of the probable reasons for inadequate efficacy of the BCG are directly related to the vaccine itself like a number of genes related to protective immunity had been lost during attenuation procedure (Behr, 2002); inappropriate treatment, storage and also inadequate strains of BCG are few more direct correlates (Fine, 1995). In addition, other hypotheses suggest defects in basic immunological character. As discussed various T cells play an important role in immunity to TB; failure of BCG to stimulate all required T cells types effectively also had been suggested (Behr *et al.*, 1999).

Besides probable reasons mentioned above, many others also have been attributed like methodology of clinical trials, genetic difference within and among population and pre-sensitization of host immune response by environmental mycobacteria. Further, the comparative genomic analysis of different strains of BCG has shown a lot of variability among all six BCG vaccine sub-strains (Copenhagen-1331, Pasteur-1173P, Glaxo-1077, Tokyo-172, Russian, Moreau) and this genetic variability may contribute to the disparity in protective efficacy in different geographic regions of the world (Behr, 2001).

Nevertheless, as several reports indicated that neonatal vaccination with BCG is effective in reducing the incidence of childhood TB in endemic regions and reducing the rate of complications from disseminated TB (Fine, 2001). The protection imparted by BCG in children indicates that it expresses antigenic repertoire necessary to defend against TB. In contrast, its failure to protect against pulmonary TB in adults signifies that BCG cannot induce the generation of long-lasting memory response (Brewer and Colditz, 1995; Orme *et al.*, 2001; Triccas and Nambiar, 2009). Thus, the development of more effective novel vaccines and immunization strategies should be designed to protect against primary infection and also to boost waning BCG-induced protective immune responses are of urgent need to facilitate world-wide control of tuberculosis.

Novel Vaccines and Vaccination Strategies

To reduce the global burden of TB, new vaccination strategies against *M. tuberculosis* need to induce a more efficient immunity than that attained with BCG vaccine, not only in infants but also in adolescents and adults. With the emergence of understanding about BCG vaccine ineffectiveness in protecting adult form of TB has impelled a major global effort to develop new candidate vaccines (Izzo *et al.*, 2005; Orme, 2005; Orme, 2006).

Present Vaccine Candidates

The crucial fundamental mechanism of action of present vaccine candidates is stimulation of Th1 cells, which activate macrophages capacities for antimycobacterial activity (Kaufmann, 2006; Kaufmann *et al.*, 2006). The multifunctional memory T cells that produce several cytokines concomitantly especially, IFN-γ, TNF-α, and IL-2 are of central importance (Foulds *et al.*, 2006). In addtion, CD8 T cells that can directly attack *M tuberculosis* by perforin and granulysin (Stenger *et al.*, 1998) and Th17 cell support Th1 responses (Khader *et al.*, 2007) are also play a very considerable role.

Live Vaccines

Live vaccines are based either on improvement of BCG vaccine through addition of protective genes or on deletion of virulence genes of *M. tuberculosis.*

Recombinant BCG Vaccines

The protective efficacy of BCG vaccine against TB was always a matter of dispute. But some basic features of BCG for instance, enough immunogenic nature, can be given at the time of birth and single dose is enough. These factors have encouraged many investigators to focus their efforts on approaches based on recombinant DNA technology to modify BCG into a recombinant BCG vaccine against TB.

Two superior recombinant BCG (rBCG) vaccines have already started initial clinical evaluation. In the preclinical studies in different animal models, the potency and safety of both rBCG vaccines was found to be superior to the currently used BCG vaccine (Grode *et al.*, 2005; Tullius *et al.*, 2008). The rBCG30 that overexpresses Ag85B, a secretory and immunogenic protein of *M. tuberculosis* and BCG was the first vaccine candidate that showed substantially greater protection than parental BCG in different animal models (Horwitz *et al.*, 2000; Horwitz and Harth, 2003). In Phase I clinical trial which was conducted over 30 healthy adult volunteers, no significant safety issues was observed and also compared to parent BCG strain an enhanced immunogenicity was reported (Hoft, 2005).

The second vaccine, rBCGΔureC:Hly, is a recombinant BCG strain that secretes listeriolysin (of *Listeria monocytogenes* origin which is a cytolysin pores froming protein) which punches holes in the endosome and allows some leakage of BCG into the cytoplasm of infected host cells (Hess *et al.*, 1998; Grode *et al.*, 2005). Because optimal activity of Hly requires an acidic environment, urease gene (*ureC*) of the BCG, which facilitates mycobacteria to block the acidification of the early phagosome was also deleted in the construct (Grode *et al.*, 2005). In addition to CD4 T cells, protective immunity against *M. tuberculosis* infection seems to also involve both CD8 T cells, so antigens must be presented by MHC class I. Perforation of the phagosomal membrane probably promotes antigen translocation into the cytoplasm and facilitates cross-priming and stimulation of Th17 cells (Winau *et al.*, 2006; Torchinsky *et al.*, 2009). In preclinical studies in mice, a better efficacy of rBCGΔUreC:Hly than the BCG strain was observed (Grode *et al.*, 2005). The Aeras Global TB Vaccine Foundation (a non-profit Product Development Partnership) constructed different rBCG strains by utilizing pH-independent perfringolysin (rBCG-pfo), instead of Hly (Portnoy *et al.*, 1992), with overexpression of several immunodominant antigens including Ag85A, Ag85B and TB10.4 (Sadoff, 2005).

Attenuated *M. tuberculosis* Vaccines

Alternatively, *M. tuberculosis* that contains above 120 (some are directly related to virulence) genes that were deleted in BCG during development, can be attenuated by the genetic manipulation (Behr *et al.*, 1999; Gordon *et al.*, 1999; Salamon *et al.*, 2000). MTBVAC01 vaccine was constructed by disruption of the transcriptional regulator *phoP* gene associated with *M. tuberculosis* virulence) and the *fadD26* genes (Martin *et al.*, 2006; Verreck *et al.*, 2009). Other attenuated *M. tuberculosis* vaccine candidates includes *M. tuberculosis* deleted mutants ΔRD1ΔpanCD (Sambandamurthy *et al.*, 2006). Some of these live vaccines probably enter in clinical trials in the next few years (StopTB Partnership Working Group on New TB Vaccines).

Subunit and Live Vector-Based Vaccines for Prime-Boost Strategy

Numerous vaccines for prime-boost strategy have been used to enhance the immune response evoked by primary BCG vaccine. The main desirability from the heterologous prime–boost approach is that it should preferentially expand TB-reactive pre-existing memory T cells against common antigens of the prime and booster vaccines. Subunit vaccine candidates are based on antigens of *M. tuberculosis* that trigger T cells in infected humans (cured or latently infected) and experimental animals are believed better vaccine candidates.

Subunit vaccine candidates were recognized by various biochemical techniques. Initially, major secretary proteins of *M. tuberculosis* like Ag85 complex, MPT32, PhoS, DnaK, GroES, MPT46, MPT53, MPT63 and the 19-kDa lipoprotein were identified (Andersen and Hansen, 1989; Nagai *et al.*, 1991; Young and Garbe, 1991). Next, low molecular mass antigens in the range of 6–10 kDa (ESAT-6 family) and 26–34 kDa (Ag85B and MPT59) were defined (Andersen *et al.*, 1995; Skjot *et al.*, 2000). Other important immune-dominant antigens like Mtb32 and Mtb39 (Skeiky *et al.*, 1999) were recognized by T-cell and serological expression cloning (Alderson *et al.*, 2000; Dillon *et al.*, 2000; Skeiky *et al.*, 2000). Potential antigen like Rv3407 (Mollenkopf *et al.*, 2004) was identified by proteomic approach (Covert, *et al.*, 2001; Mattow *et al.*, 2003).

Two kinds of candidates have been developed for boosting primary immune response generated by BCG vaccine: (*i*) recombinant fusion proteins consisting of two or three immuno-dominant *M. tuberculosis* or BCG protective antigens; (*ii*) live viral vectors that express one or several mycobacterial proteins. The fusion proteins needs an adjuvant that enhances Th1 immune responses and can be given repeatedly while live viral vector vaccines do not require an adjuvant but pre-sensitization of the vector can clear the construct. These vaccine candidates induced a dominated T helper-1 (Th1) immune response to the expressed heterologous antigen and also generate Cytotoxic T cells (CD8 T cells) responses. In preclinical studies in mice and guinea pigs model of tuberculosis, almost all prime-boost candidate vaccines exhibited a similar level of protection from TB, obtained with BCG vaccine. In addition, several vaccine candidates found to be protective in non-human primates (Verreck *et al.*, 2009).

Recombinant fusion proteins based candidate vaccines were selected by their strong recognition by immune cells of experimentally vaccinated or infected animals and infected individuals. Following fusion proteins either with appropriate adjuvant or live virus vector were employed as vaccine candidates for testing against TB.

Ag85B-ESAT-6 (Hybrid 1)

Early secreted antigen target (ESAT-6) which is absent from all BCG, but present in *M. tuberculosis* strains. Mycobacterium reactive T cells from infected individuals or in animal models of TB recognized this protein very strongly. The second major protein secreted by *M. tuberculosis* is Ag85 complex, which is a mycolyltransferase consist of three closely related proteins, Ag85A, Ag85B and Ag85C. Among, Ag85A and Ag85B are the most potent antigens and main targets of *M. tuberculosis* specific T cell in human (Huygen *et al.*, 1996; Baldwin *et al.*, 1998). A fusion protein of two antigens was given with IC31 (by Intercell, Vienna, Austria) which is a strong Th1 adjuvant and its potency was assessed in two phase 1 clinical trials (Dietrich *et al.*, 2006; Lingnau *et al.*, 2007). This vaccine candidate was well tolerated and found to be very immunogenic in human volunteers without any adverse effects (Aagaard *et al.*, 2009).

Ag85B-TB-10.4 (H4, AERAS-404)

Alternatively, TB10.4 which also a strong immuno-dominant protein in BCG vaccinated donors was fused with Ag85B to minimize the interference with ESAT-6-based diagnostic assays (Skjot *et al.*, 2002; Dietrich *et al.*, 2005). This fusion protein elicited comparable protection against TB to Ag85B-ESAT-6 and BCG vaccine.

Mtb72

A hybrid protein of two TB antigens, Mtb32 and Mtb39 which is formulated in an adjuvant system consist of monophosphoryl lipid A and QS21 to strengthen the immune response required for protective immunity again TB (Skeiky *et al.*, 2004). This vaccine candidate also had reasonable acceptability and induced required T-cell responses in healthy adults (van Dissel *et al.*, 2010).

MVA85A

It is a recombinant, modified Vaccinia Ankara virus (replication-deficient vaccinia), that expresses Ag85A. Priming with BCG and then boosting with MVA85A regimen, induced a enhance level of both CD4 and CD8 T cells. Protection imparted this regimen was found better that either BCG or MVA85A alone (Goonetilleke *et al.*, 2003). In phase I clinical trials in human beings (immunized with BCG from 6 months to 36 years earlier), MVA85A boosting showed persisting CD4 T cells which secrete high level of IFN-γ. In contrast, only transient response was observed in case of BCG or MVA85A alone (McShane *et al.*, 2004; Sander *et al.*, 2009). Prior exposure with vaccinia virus might diminish the effectiveness of vaccines based on this viral vector (Rooney *et al.*, 1988).

Ad35 or AERAS-402 and AdAg85A

These vaccine constructs are based on replication deficient (E1-deleted) recombinant adenoviruses (Santosuosso *et al.*, 2006; Radosevic *et al.*, 2007).

Adenoviral vectors are potent delivery vehicles for recombinant vaccines but prior natural exposure with homologous or cross-reacting strain might hamper the required responses (Bangari and Mittal, 2006). The elicitation of superior CD8 T-cell responses is the main feature of vaccine constructs. Mice immunized by intranasal route with AdAg85A (recombinant Adenovirus 5 expressing Ag85A) exhibited substantial protection (mediated by bothCD4 and CD8T cells) compared to BCG (Wang *et al.*, 2004). Highly prevalence of Adenovirus 5 in human populations can affect the potency of vaccine due to preexisting antibodies. Adenovirus 35 based vaccines might be attractive choice because of it low sero-prevalence (5 per cent–20 per cent in different geographical regions). Areas Global TB Vaccine Foundation and Crucell (a global biopharmaceutical company) together constructed various vaccine candidates with non-replicating Ad35 vectors expressing Ag85A, Ag85B and TB10.4. Single immunizations of with rAd35-TB construct conferred protection against TB (Radosevic, 2006). In a prime-boost study this construct responded with enhanced level of mycobacterium specific CD4 and CD8 T-cell responses compared with rAd35-B or BCG alone immunized mice.

Novel Tuberculosis Vaccines in Clinical Trials

New vaccines are urgently needed to reach the ultimate goal of reducing global incidence of tuberculosis considerably by 2050 (Young and Dye, 2006). Promising finding of various vaccine candidates in pre-clinical testing in various animal models of tuberculosis, stipulate for their extension for approval in initial phase I (safety) by regulatory authority for testing in human subjects. The first objective of initial clinical trials for new tuberculosis vaccines is to assess their safety in a small study group including healthy, PPD-negative individuals (usually adults). Populations at risk of TB-HIV co-infection should be considered particularly during trials with live vaccines. Additional Phase I trials may be include PPD+ individuals, children, infants, or other groups for which the vaccine may be given ultimately. Usually these trials are combined with a phase IIA trial in which generation of immunological responses to the vaccine was studied. Biomarkers to assess the immunity generated by the vaccine like assays measuring T-cell responses to peptide epitopes contained within the vaccine should be checked at this stage. Unfortunately, present biomarker assays are not directly correlates with protective efficiency of vaccines. The demonstration of safety in phase I and immunogenicity in phase II are prerequisites for any new TB vaccine candidate to go forward into phase III (efficacy) trials. Table 34.1 lists the novel TB vaccines, which are currently at various levels of clinical trials in human being.

Table 34.1: Novel Tuberculosis Vaccines at Different Steps in Clinical Trials

Candidate	*Description*	*Clinical Trail Stage*	*Sponsor or Funding Agency*
H1-CAF01	Recombinant fusion protein of Ag85B-ESAT-6 in CAF01 adjuvant	Phase 1 continuing	Statens Serum Institute, Tuberculosis Vaccine Initiative
AdAg85A	Ag85A expressing Ad5 (Non-replicating)	Phase 1	McMaster University
AERAS-402	Ag85A, Ag85B, and TB10.4 expressing Ad35 (Non-replicating)	Phases 1 and 2 continuing	Aeras
H4-IC31 (AERAS-404)	Recombinant fusion protein of Ag85B-TB10.4 in IC31 adjuvant	Phase 1 completed	Statens Serum Institute, Aeras
rBCGΔUreC:Hly (VPM1002)	BCG with an endosome escape	Phase 1 completed	Tuberculosis Vaccine Initiative, Max Planck Institute
H1-IC31	Recombinant fusion protein of Ag85B-ESAT-6 in IC31 adjuvant	Phase 1 completed	Statens Serum Institute, Tuberculosis Vaccine Initiative
M72	Recombinant fusion protein of Mtb39 and Mtb32 in AS02 and AS01 adjuvants	Phases 1 and 2 completed	GlaxoSmithKline, Aeras, Tuberculosis Vaccine Initiative
rBCG30	Ag85B over-expressing BCG	Phase 1 completed	University of California, Los Angeles; Aeras
MVA85A	Attenuated vaccinia expressing Ag85A	Phase 1 completed and phase 2 continuing; phase 2b in infants started	Wellcome Trust, Aeras, Emergent BioSolutions
RUTI	Detoxified *M. tuberculosis* in liposomes	Phase 1 completed	Archivel Farma
M. vaccae	Inactivated *M. vaccae*	Phase 3 completed	National Institutes of Health

Ag: Antigen; ESAT-6: Early secretory antigenic target-6; CAF: Cationic adjuvant formulation; Ad: Adenovirus; Hly: Haemolysin; AS: Adjuvant system; MVA: Modified vaccinia Ankara.

Challenges Continues

TB vaccine research has gained impetus in recent years; still there are some major barriers. The efficacy of novel TB vaccines must be greater than current BCG and importantly should be safe enough so can be used in HIV-endemic countries. Although, several subunit vaccines are in various phages of clinical trials but they could not show better efficacy than BCG in pre-clinical studies in various animal models, which is the reason to considered them as a booster but rather than a replacer for BCG. In addition, the safety issue of various recombinants BCG and attenuated *M. tuberculosis* strains remains in question. As WHO has recommend that BCG should not be given to HIV-positive children, even if they are asymptomatic, because of high risk of BCG-induced disseminated disease in immune-compromised individuals with HIV infection.

Regulatory authorities of developing nations should actively participate in both product and clinical assessment to tested TB vaccines within their country. But many developing countries do not have their regulatory authorities. So some global systems are considered necessary for sharing information among regulatory authorities of all countries engaged in the production and clinical evaluation of candidate vaccines. To the surprise, till the date there is no comprehensible global regulatory pathway for new TB vaccine candidates; hence a "regulatory plan" should be developed before the start of phase III of clinical trials. So there is a need for global competent and efficient local and national ethics and regulatory authorities for all countries engaged in TB vaccine development.

On the basis of outcome of Phase II of clinical trials the promising TB vaccine candidates may enter in phase III of clinical trials which require a large number (10 000, or more) of individuals to check the efficacy to vaccines candidates. These clinical trials should be done in various geographical regions of the world so the generated data can be translated to other countries with genetically, culturally, and environmentally diverse populations. This is the main obstacle for the development of a site for the assessment of new tuberculosis vaccine candidates.

In addition, there is paucity of distinct surrogate bio-markers for the assessment of protective efficacy of vaccine candidates. So, clinical studies are crucial to ascertain the efficacy of vaccine candidates. This needs continuous follow-up, high cohort maintenance, and especially good surveillance systems. Scientific research is an indispensable but inadequate facet in the reduction or elimination of TB. Any successful vaccine needs to be accompanied by strong political determination, clear policies and objectives, a facilitative regulatory authority, and sufficient funding, to considerably reduce the disease.

References

Aagaard, C., J. Dietrich, *et al.* (2009). "TB vaccines: current status and future perspectives." *Immunol Cell Biol* 87(4): 279-86.

Acheson, D., G. A. Alleyne, *et al.* (2000). "Round table discussion. Health inequalities and the health of the poor." *Bull World Health Organ* 78(1): 75-85.

Alderson, M. R., T. Bement, *et al.* (2000). "Expression cloning of an immunodominant family of Mycobacterium tuberculosis antigens using human CD4(+) T cells." *J Exp Med* 191(3): 551-60.

Andersen, A. B. and E. B. Hansen (1989). "Structure and mapping of antigenic domains of protein antigen b, a 38,000-molecular-weight protein of Mycobacterium tuberculosis." *Infect Immun* 57(8): 2481-8.

Andersen, P., A. B. Andersen, *et al.* (1995). "Recall of long-lived immunity to Mycobacterium tuberculosis infection in mice." *J Immunol* 154(7): 3359-72.

Baldwin, S. L., C. D'Souza, *et al.* (1998). "Evaluation of new vaccines in the mouse and guinea pig model of tuberculosis." *Infect Immun* 66(6): 2951-9.

Bangari, D. S. and S. K. Mittal (2006). "Development of nonhuman adenoviruses as vaccine vectors." *Vaccine* 24(7): 849-62.

Behr, M. A. (2001). "Correlation between BCG genomics and protective efficacy." *Scand J Infect Dis* 33(4): 249-52.

Behr, M. A. (2002). "BCG–different strains, different vaccines?" *Lancet Infect Dis* 2(2): 86-92.

Behr, M. A., M. A. Wilson, *et al.* (1999). "Comparative genomics of BCG vaccines by whole-genome DNA microarray." *Science* 284(5419): 1520-3.

Bishai, D. M. and D. Mercer (2001). "Modeling the economic benefits of better TB vaccines." *Int J Tuberc Lung Dis* 5(11): 984-93.

Brewer, T. F. and G. A. Colditz (1995). "Relationship between bacille Calmette-Guerin (BCG) strains and the efficacy of BCG vaccine in the prevention of tuberculosis." *Clin Infect Dis* 20(1): 126-35.

Collins, F. M. (1997). "Tuberculosis research in a cold climate." *Tuber Lung Dis* 78(2): 99-107.

Covert, B. A., J. S. Spencer, *et al.* (2001). "The application of proteomics in defining the T cell antigens of Mycobacterium tuberculosis." *Proteomics* 1(4): 574-86.

Dietrich, J., C. Aagaard, *et al.* (2005). "Exchanging ESAT6 with TB10.4 in an Ag85B fusion molecule-based tuberculosis subunit vaccine: efficient protection and ESAT6-based sensitive monitoring of vaccine efficacy." *J Immunol* 174(10): 6332-9.

Dietrich, J., C. Andersen, *et al.* (2006). "Mucosal administration of Ag85B-ESAT-6 protects against infection with Mycobacterium tuberculosis and boosts prior bacillus Calmette-Guerin immunity." *J Immunol* 177(9): 6353-60.

Dillon, D. C., M. R. Alderson, *et al.* (2000). "Molecular and immunological characterization of Mycobacterium tuberculosis CFP-10, an immunodiagnostic antigen missing in Mycobacterium bovis BCG." *J Clin Microbiol* 38(9): 3285-90.

Dye, C., K. Lonnroth, *et al.* (2009). "Trends in tuberculosis incidence and their determinants in 134 countries." *Bull World Health Organ* 87(9): 683-91.

Fine, P. E. (1995). "Variation in protection by BCG: implications of and for heterologous immunity." *Lancet* 346(8986): 1339-45.

Fine, P. E. (2001). "BCG: the challenge continues." *Scand J Infect Dis* 33(4): 243-5.

Flynn, J. L. and J. Chan (2005). "What's good for the host is good for the bug." *Trends Microbiol* 13(3): 98-102.

Foulds, K. E., C. Y. Wu, *et al.* (2006). "Th1 memory: implications for vaccine development." *Immunol Rev* 211: 58-66.

Goonetilleke, N. P., H. McShane, *et al.* (2003). "Enhanced immunogenicity and protective efficacy against Mycobacterium tuberculosis of bacille Calmette-Guerin vaccine using mucosal administration and boosting with a recombinant modified vaccinia virus Ankara." *J Immunol* 171(3): 1602-9.

Gordon, S. V., R. Brosch, *et al.* (1999). "Identification of variable regions in the genomes of tubercle bacilli using bacterial artificial chromosome arrays." *Mol Microbiol* 32(3): 643-55.

Grode, L., P. Seiler, *et al.* (2005). "Increased vaccine efficacy against tuberculosis of recombinant Mycobacterium bovis bacille Calmette-Guerin mutants that secrete listeriolysin." *J Clin Invest* 115(9): 2472-9.

Hess, J., D. Miko, *et al.* (1998). "Mycobacterium bovis Bacille Calmette-Guerin strains secreting listeriolysin of Listeria monocytogenes." *Proc Natl Acad Sci U S A* 95(9): 5299-304.

Hoft, D. F. (2005). "Results of the 1st Phase I trial of a recombinant BCG TB vaccine (rBCG30." Presented at US–Japan Cooperative Medical Science Program; *40th Tuberculosis and Leprosy Research Conference*. (Seattle, Washington).

Horwitz, M. A. and G. Harth (2003). "A new vaccine against tuberculosis affords greater survival after challenge than the current vaccine in the guinea pig model of pulmonary tuberculosis." *Infect Immun* 71(4): 1672-9.

Horwitz, M. A., G. Harth, *et al.* (2000). "Recombinant bacillus calmette-guerin (BCG) vaccines expressing the Mycobacterium tuberculosis 30-kDa major secretory protein induce greater protective immunity against tuberculosis than conventional BCG vaccines in a highly susceptible animal model." *Proc Natl Acad Sci U S A* 97(25): 13853-8.

Huebner, R. E. (1996). "Bacillus of Calmette and Guerin (BCG) vaccine." In *Tuberculosis* (W. N. Rom, S. Garay, eds.), New York, Little, Brown and Company: 893–904.

Huygen, K., J. Content, *et al.* (1996). "Immunogenicity and protective efficacy of a tuberculosis DNA vaccine." *Nat Med* 2(8): 893-8.

Izzo, A., L. Brandt, *et al.* (2005). "NIH pre-clinical screening program: overview and current status." *Tuberculosis* (Edinb) 85(1-2): 25-8.

Kaplan, G., F. A. Post, *et al.* (2003). "Mycobacterium tuberculosis growth at the cavity surface: a microenvironment with failed immunity." *Infect Immun* 71(12): 7099-108.

Kaufmann, S. H. (2006). "Envisioning future strategies for vaccination against tuberculosis." *Nat Rev Immunol* 6(9): 699-704.

Kaufmann, S. H. (2006). "Tuberculosis: back on the immunologists' agenda." *Immunity* 24(4): 351-7.

Kaufmann, S. H., S. Baumann, *et al.* (2006). "Exploiting immunology and molecular genetics for rational vaccine design against tuberculosis." *Int J Tuberc Lung Dis* 10(10): 1068-79.

Khader, S. A., G. K. Bell, *et al.* (2007). "IL-23 and IL-17 in the establishment of protective pulmonary CD4+ T cell responses after vaccination and during Mycobacterium tuberculosis challenge." *Nat Immunol* 8(4): 369-77.

Korenromp, E. L., A. L. Bierrenbach, *et al.* (2009). "The measurement and estimation of tuberculosis mortality." *Int J Tuberc Lung Dis* 13(3): 283-303.

Kursar, M., M. Koch, *et al.* (2007). "Cutting Edge: Regulatory T cells prevent efficient clearance of Mycobacterium tuberculosis." *J Immunol* 178(5): 2661-5.

Lingnau, K., K. Riedl, *et al.* (2007). "IC31 and IC30, novel types of vaccine adjuvant based on peptide delivery systems." *Expert Rev Vaccines* 6(5): 741-6.

MacMicking, J. D., G. A. Taylor, *et al.* (2003). "Immune control of tuberculosis by IFN-gamma-inducible LRG-47." *Science* 302(5645): 654-9.

Martin, C., A. Williams, *et al.* (2006). "The live Mycobacterium tuberculosis phoP mutant strain is more attenuated than BCG and confers protective immunity against tuberculosis in mice and guinea pigs." *Vaccine* 24(17): 3408-19.

Mattow, J., U. E. Schaible, *et al.* (2003). "Comparative proteome analysis of culture supernatant proteins from virulent Mycobacterium tuberculosis H37Rv and attenuated M. bovis BCG Copenhagen." *Electrophoresis* 24(19-20): 3405-20.

McShane, H., A. A. Pathan, *et al.* (2004). "Recombinant modified vaccinia virus Ankara expressing antigen 85A boosts BCG-primed and naturally acquired antimycobacterial immunity in humans." *Nat Med* 10(11): 1240-4.

Mollenkopf, H. J., L. Grode, *et al.* (2004). "Application of mycobacterial proteomics to vaccine design: improved protection by Mycobacterium bovis BCG prime-Rv3407 DNA boost vaccination against tuberculosis." *Infect Immun* 72(11): 6471-9.

Nagai, S., H. G. Wiker, *et al.* (1991). "Isolation and partial characterization of major protein antigens in the culture fluid of Mycobacterium tuberculosis." *Infect Immun* 59(1): 372-82.

Orme, I. M. (2005). "Current progress in tuberculosis vaccine development." *Vaccine* 23(17-18): 2105-8.

Orme, I. M. (2005). "Tuberculosis vaccines: current progress." *Drugs* 65(17): 2437-44.

Orme, I. M. (2006). "Preclinical testing of new vaccines for tuberculosis: a comprehensive review." *Vaccine* 24(1): 2-19.

Orme, I. M., D. N. McMurray, *et al.* (2001). "Tuberculosis vaccine development: recent progress." *Trends Microbiol* 9(3): 115-8.

Portnoy, D. A., R. K. Tweten, *et al.* (1992). "Capacity of listeriolysin O, streptolysin O, and perfringolysin O to mediate growth of *Bacillus subtilis* within mammalian cells." *Infect Immun* 60(7): 2710-7.

Quesniaux, V. F., M. Jacobs, *et al.* (2010). "TNF in host resistance to tuberculosis infection." *Curr Dir Autoimmun* 11: 157-79.

Radosevic, K., C. W. Wieland, *et al.* (2007). "Protective immune responses to a recombinant adenovirus type 35 tuberculosis vaccine in two mouse strains: CD4 and CD8 T-cell epitope mapping and role of gamma interferon." *Infect Immun* 75(8): 4105-15.

Radosevic, K. (2006). "Presented at TB vaccines for the world (April 19–21, Vienna, Austria)."

Rooney, J. F., C. Wohlenberg, *et al.* (1988). "Immunization with a vaccinia virus recombinant expressing herpes simplex virus type 1 glycoprotein D: long-term protection and effect of revaccination." *J Virol* 62(5): 1530-4.

Russell, D. G. (2003). "Phagosomes, fatty acids and tuberculosis." *Nat Cell Biol* 5(9): 776-8.

Russell, D. G. (2007). "Who puts the tubercle in tuberculosis?" *Nat Rev Microbiol* 5(1): 39-47.

Russell, D. G., P. J. Cardona, *et al.* (2009). "Foamy macrophages and the progression of the human tuberculosis granuloma." *Nat Immunol* 10(9): 943-8.

Sadoff, J. (2005). "Public private partnership approach to vaccine development." *Presented at New Approaches to Vaccine Development*. (Sept. 8–10, Berlin, Germany).

Sakula, A. (1983). "BCG: who were Calmette and Guerin?" *Thorax* 38(11): 806-12.

Salamon, H., M. Kato-Maeda, *et al.* (2000). "Detection of deleted genomic DNA using a semiautomated computational analysis of GeneChip data." *Genome Res* 10(12): 2044-54.

Sambandamurthy, V. K., S. C. Derrick, *et al.* (2006). "Mycobacterium tuberculosis DeltaRD1 DeltapanCD: a safe and limited replicating mutant strain that protects immunocompetent and immunocompromised mice against experimental tuberculosis." *Vaccine* 24(37-39): 6309-20.

Sander, C. R., A. A. Pathan, *et al.* (2009). "Safety and immunogenicity of a new tuberculosis vaccine, MVA85A, in Mycobacterium tuberculosis-infected individuals." *Am J Respir Crit Care Med* 179(8): 724-33.

Santosuosso, M., S. McCormick, *et al.* (2006). "Intranasal boosting with an adenovirus-vectored vaccine markedly enhances protection by parenteral Mycobacterium bovis BCG immunization against pulmonary tuberculosis." *Infect Immun* 74(8): 4634-43.

Schaible, U. E., S. Sturgill-Koszycki, *et al.* (1998). "Cytokine activation leads to acidification and increases maturation of Mycobacterium avium-containing phagosomes in murine macrophages." *J Immunol* 160(3): 1290-6.

Skeiky, Y. A., M. R. Alderson, *et al.* (2004). "Differential immune responses and protective efficacy induced by components of a tuberculosis polyprotein vaccine, Mtb72F, delivered as naked DNA or recombinant protein." *J Immunol* 172(12): 7618-28.

Skeiky, Y. A., M. J. Lodes, *et al.* (1999). "Cloning, expression, and immunological evaluation of two putative secreted serine protease antigens of Mycobacterium tuberculosis." *Infect Immun* 67(8): 3998-4007.

Skeiky, Y. A., P. J. Ovendale, *et al.* (2000). "T cell expression cloning of a Mycobacterium tuberculosis gene encoding a protective antigen associated with the early control of infection." *J Immunol* 165(12): 7140-9.

Skjot, R. L., I. Brock, *et al.* (2002). "Epitope mapping of the immunodominant antigen TB10.4 and the two homologous proteins TB10.3 and TB12.9, which constitute a subfamily of the esat-6 gene family." *Infect Immun* 70(10): 5446-53.

Skjot, R. L., T. Oettinger, *et al.* (2000). "Comparative evaluation of low-molecular-mass proteins from Mycobacterium tuberculosis identifies members of the ESAT-6 family as immunodominant T-cell antigens." *Infect Immun* 68(1): 214-20.

Smith, D., E. Wiegeshaus, *et al.* (2000). "An analysis of some hypotheses related to the Chingelput bacille Calmette-Guerin trial." *Clin Infect Dis* 31 Suppl 3: S77-80.

Stenger, S., D. A. Hanson, *et al.* (1998). "An antimicrobial activity of cytolytic T cells mediated by granulysin." *Science* 282(5386): 121-5.

Torchinsky, M. B., J. Garaude, *et al.* (2009). "Innate immune recognition of infected apoptotic cells directs T(H)17 cell differentiation." *Nature* 458(7234): 78-82.

Triccas, J. A. and J. K. Nambiar (2009). "Challenge of developing new tuberculosis vaccines to generate life-long protective immunity." *Expert Rev Vaccines* 8(7): 823-5.

Tullius, M. V., G. Harth, *et al.* (2008). "A Replication-Limited Recombinant Mycobacterium bovis BCG vaccine against tuberculosis designed for human immunodeficiency virus-positive persons is safer and more efficacious than BCG." *Infect Immun* 76(11): 5200-14.

Udani, P. M. (1994). "BCG vaccination in India and tuberculosis in children: newer facets." Indian J Pediatr 61(5): 451-62.

Ulrichs, T., D. B. Moody, *et al.* (2003). "T-cell responses to CD1-presented lipid antigens in humans with Mycobacterium tuberculosis infection." *Infect Immun* 71(6): 3076-87.

van Dissel, J. T., S. M. Arend, *et al.* (2010). "Ag85B-ESAT-6 adjuvanted with IC31 promotes strong and long-lived Mycobacterium tuberculosis specific T cell responses in naive human volunteers." *Vaccine* 28(20): 3571-81.

Verreck, F. A., R. A. Vervenne, *et al.* (2009). "MVA.85A boosting of BCG and an attenuated, phoP deficient M. tuberculosis vaccine both show protective efficacy against tuberculosis in rhesus macaques." *PLoS One* 4(4): e5264.

Via, L. E., P. L. Lin, *et al.* (2008). "Tuberculous granulomas are hypoxic in guinea pigs, rabbits, and nonhuman primates." *Infect Immun* 76(6): 2333-40.

Wang, J., L. Thorson, *et al.* (2004). "Single mucosal, but not parenteral, immunization with recombinant adenoviral-based vaccine provides potent protection from pulmonary tuberculosis." *J Immunol* 173(10): 6357-65.

WHO (1992). "*World Health Organization. Expanded program for immunization: program report.*" Geneva: World Health Organization."

WHO (2009). "World Health Organization, Tuberculosis fact sheet number 104, March 2010. Available at http://www.who.int/mediacentre/factsheets/fs104/en/index.html. Accessed on June 14, 2010".

Winau, F., S. Weber, *et al.* (2006). "Apoptotic vesicles crossprime CD8 T cells and protect against tuberculosis." *Immunity* 24(1): 105-17.

Woodworth, J. S., Y. Wu, *et al.* (2008). "Mycobacterium tuberculosis-specific CD8+ T cells require perforin to kill target cells and provide protection *in vivo.*" *J Immunol* 181(12): 8595-603.

Young, D. and C. Dye (2006). "The development and impact of tuberculosis vaccines." *Cell* 124(4): 683-7.

Young, D. B. and T. R. Garbe (1991). "Lipoprotein antigens of Mycobacterium tuberculosis." *Res Microbiol* 142(1): 55-65.

Microbial Biotechnology and Ecology (2011) *Pages* **591–605**
Editors: **Deepak Vyas, G.S. Paliwal, P.K.Khare and R.K Gupta**
Published by: **DAYA PUBLISHING HOUSE, NEW DELHI**

Chapter 35

Silver Nanoparticles: A New Generation of Antimicrobial Agents

☆ ***Mukesh K. Upadhyay*, Devendra Jain, Abhijeet Singh, Sushma Rishi and Narayan Rishi***

School of Life Sciences, Jaipur National University, Jaipur – 302 025, Rajasthan

ABSTRACT

Nanotechnology is gaining tremendous impetus in the present century due to its capability of modulating metals into their nanosize, which drastically changes the chemical, physical and optical properties of metals. Silver has been in use since ancient time in the form of metallic silver, silver nitrate, silver sulfadiazine for the treatment of burns, wounds and several infections. Nanosilver has developed as a potent antibacterial, antifungal, anti-viral and anti-inflammatory agent. Due to the outbreak of the infectious diseases caused by different pathogenic microorganisms developing antibiotic resistance, the pharmaceutical companies and the researchers are searching for new antibacterial agents. In the present scenario, nanoscale silver has emerged as novel antimicrobial agents. Hence, silver nanoparticles have emerged up with diverse medical applications ranging from silver based dressings, silver coated medicinal devices, such as nanogels, nanolotions etc.

Introduction

Silver is a naturally occurring pre-historic element. It has been positioned as the 47th element in the periodic table having an atomic weight of 107.8. For centuries silver has been in use for the treatment of burns and chronic wounds. It's use for medicine or local antibacterial agents was not

* E-mail: mukeshfungi@gmail.com

recognized until the 19th century (Oloffs *et al.*, 1994). Since then the antimicrobial property of silver has been investigated and employed more extensively than any other inorganic antibacterial agent (Russell and Hugo, 1994). Ag is known to attack a broad range of biological processes in microbes including the alteration of cell membrane structure and functions (Pal *et al.*, 2007). Ag inhibit expression of proteins associated with ATP production (Yamanaka *et al.*, 2005) although it's specific antimicrobial mechanism are still not completely understood. Micromolar doses of Ag are sufficient to kill bacteria in water (Liu *et al.*, 1994) while Ag can be toxic at high doses to mammals (Conrad *et al.*, 1999), freshwater and marine organisms (Morgan *et al.*, 2005). Such micromolar concentrations of Ag have no harmful effects on humans (Berger *et al.*, 1976) hence Ag is widely used for development of many biological and pharmaceutical products and coating materials for medical devices (Raad and Hanna, 2002). With the emergence and increase of microbial organisms resistant to multiple antibiotics, and the continuing emphasis on health care costs, many researchers have tried to develop new, effective anti-microbial reagents free of resistance and with reduced cost. Ag has long been known to exhibit a strong toxicity to a wide range of microbes (Liau *et al.*, 1997), for this reason silver based compounds have been used extensively in many bactericidal applications (Nomiya *et al.*, 2004). Silver nanoparticles show efficient antimicrobial property compared to other salts due to their extremely large surface area (Song and Kim, 2008), which provides better contact with microorganisms. The nanoparticles get attached to the cell membrane and also penetrate inside the bacteria. The bacterial membrane contains sulfur-containing proteins and the silver nanoparticles interact with these proteins in the cell as well as with the phosphorus containing compounds like DNA. When silver nanoparticles enter the bacterial cell it forms a low molecular weight region in the centre of the bacteria to which the bacteria conglomerates thus, protecting the DNA from the silver ions (Song *et al.*, 2006). The nanoparticles preferably attack the respiratory chain, cell division finally leading to cell death. The nanoparticles release silver ions in the bacterial cells, which enhance their bactericidal activity. Therefore, this review is emphasized for the development of silver nanoparticles as new generation medicine.

Nanotechnology

The term nanotechnology was coined by Professor Norio Taniguchi of Tokyo Science University in 1974 (Taniguchi, 1974). Nanotechnology is not a single thing rather a collective term that implies capacity to work with materials at nanoscale level. Nanotechnology enables us to expand the surface area of silver particles markedly. It is emerging as a rapidly growing field with its application in science and technology (Albrecht *et al.*, 2006). Nanotechnology involves the creation and manipulation of materials at nanoscale levels (1–100 nm) to create products that exhibit novel properties. Till recent times nanotechnology has been a domain of physics, chemistry, electrical engineering and material sciences, there has been a considerable progress in the visualization, construction and manipulation of material at nanometer scale. It is creating a growing sense of excitement in life sciences especially bio-medical devices and biotechnology.

Nanoparticles

Nanoparticles are clusters of atoms with a size up to 100 nm. They have high surface area to volume ratio (Song *et al.*, 2008). Specific surface area is relevant for catalytic activity and other related properties such as antimicrobial activity in silver nanoparticles. Their unique size dependent properties make these materials superior and indispensable as they show unique physical, chemical and biological properties. Use of nanoparticles is gaining impetus in the present century as they posses defined chemical, optical and mechanical properties. The metallic nanoparticles are the most promising as they show good antibacterial properties.

Biomimetics

A number of approaches are available for synthesis of silver nanoparticles for example reduction in solution, thermal decomposition of silver compounds, chemical and photochemical reactions in reverse micelles, ultrasonication irradiation etc. but these methods are proving harmful for the environment hence, it is our need to learn about the secrets inherently present in the nature and it's products, led to the development of biomimetic approaches for the growth of advancements in the synthetic process of nanoparticle synthesis (Song and Kim, 2008). Biomimetics is a technology in which we use biological systems such as yeast, fungi, bacteria and plants for the synthesis of nanostructures. This technology is an advancement over chemical methods as it is cost effective and eco-friendly (Singh *et al.*, 2010).

Metallic Silver

Silver is inert in its metallic state but reacts with the moisture in the skin and the fluid of the wound and gets ionized. The ionized silver is highly reactive, as it binds to tissue proteins and brings structural changes in the bacterial cell wall and nuclear membrane leading to cell distortion and death. Silver also binds to bacterial DNA and RNA by denaturing and inhibits bacterial replication (Castellano *et al.*, 2007).

Silver as an Antimicrobial Agent

The use of silver for medicine or local antibacterial agent was not recognized until the nineteenth century. Since then the antimicrobial property of silver has been investigated and employed more extensively than any other inorganic antibacterial agent. As early as 1000 B.C. silver was used to make water potable. Silver nitrate was used in its solid form for the treatment of venereal diseases, fistulae from salivary glands, and bone and perianal abscesses (Klasen, 2000; Landsdown, 2002). In the19th century granulation tissues were removed using silver nitrate to allow epithelization and promote crust formation on the surface of wounds. Varying concentrations of silver nitrate was used to treatment of fresh burns (Castellano *et al.*, 2007; Klasen, 2000). In 1881, Carl S. F. Crede cured opthalmia neonatorum using silver nitrate eye drops. Crede's son, B. Crede designed silver impregnated dressings for skin grafting (Klasen, 2000; Landsdown, 2002). In the 1940s, after penicillin was introduced the use of silver for the treatment of bacterial infections minimized (Hugo and Russell, 1982; Demling and DeSanti, 2001; Chopra, 2007). Silver again came in picture in the 1960s when Moyer introduced the use of 0.5 per cent silver nitrate for the treatment of burns. He proposed the antibacterial property of silver against *Staphylococcus aureus*, *Pseudomonas aeruginosa* and *Escherichia coli* (Moyer *et al.*, 1965; Bellinger and Conway, 1970). In 1968, silver nitrate was combined with sulfonamide to form silver sulfadazine cream, which served as a broad-spectrum antibacterial agent and was used for the treatment of burns. Silver sulfadazine is effective against bacteria like *E. coli*, *S. aureus*, *Klebsiella* sp., *Pseudomonas* sp. Due to the increasing bacterial resistance to classic antibiotics, the investigations on the antibacterial activity of silver nanoparticles have increased.

Nanosilver Synthesis

The biosynthesis of nanoparticles emerging as an highlight of the combination of nanotechnology and biotechnology has received increasing attention. Increasing attention due to a growing need to develop environmentally benign technologies in material synthesis (Huang *et al.*, 2007). Silver nanoparticles can be synthesized through an array of methods like chemical, biological etc. like spark discharging, electrochemical reduction, solution irradiation and cryochemical synthesis.

Chemical Synthesis

Chemical reduction is the most frequently applied method for the preparation of silver nanoparticles (AgNPs) as stable, colloidal dispersions in water or organic solvents as stable, colloidal dispersions in water or organic solvents. Kazachenko *et al.* (2000) investigated the synthesis and antimicrobial activity of silver complexes with histidine and tryptophan. The toxicity of silver complexes of tryptophan and histidine was tested on a group of white mongrel mice. The histidine complex with silver compound showed good antimicrobial activity against Gram-negative bacteria while, the tryptophan complex with silver compound showed higher antimicrobial activity and broad spectrum of action. Panigrahi *et al.* (2004) synthesized different metal nanoparticles (Au, Ag, Pt, Pd) using sugars like glucose, fructose and sucrose as reducing agents. Song *et al.* (2006) reported the synthesis of nano-sized Ag colloid using silver nitrate dissolved in ammonia, water, formaldehyde as a reducing agent and polyvinyl pyrrolidone (PVP) as the stabilizing agent. Nanoparticles around 5 nm in size were obtained. They showed excellent antibacterial activity against *S. typhi, E.coil, P. aeruginosa, S. aureus* and *M. tuberculosis*. Andreescu *et al.* (2007) prepared silver nanoparticles by reducing silver diamine ions $[Ag(NH_3)^2]^+$ with D-glucose in the presence of a stabilizing agent. Uniform Ag nanoparticles ranging in size from 30 to 120 were obtained. Kim *et al.* (2007) reported the use of silver nanoparticles for the control of infections occurring due to microorganisms. The silver nanoparticles were synthesized using silver nitrate and sodium borohydride (reducing agent). The antimicrobial efficiency of silver nanoparticles was tested against yeast and bacteria isolated from *Bovine mastitis*. The silver nanoparticles showed absorption band at ~391 nm which is typical for spherical nanoparticles. Shape and size distribution of the silver nanoparticles was studied using TEM, which depicted the presence of monodisperse particles in the size range of 13.5 nm. The synthesis of silver nanoparticles with different sizes (7, 29, and 89 nm mean values) using gallic acid in an aqueous chemical reduction method was reported by various researchers and the nanoparticles were characterized using TEM, dynamic light scattering (DLS), XRD, and UV–Vis absorption spectroscopy. The antibacterial activity of these nano silver particles was assessed using the standard microdilution method (Kim *et al.*, 2007; Kim *et al.*, 2008). From the microscopies studies (TEM) it was observed that silver nanoparticles have spherical (7 and 29 nm) and pseudospherical shape (89 nm) with a narrow size distribution. Das *et al.* (2009) reported the preparation of stable, uniform silver nanoparticles by reduction of silver ions by ethanol. Samples were characterized by (XRD) and (TEM), which revealed that the particles are mostly spherical in shape and have an average size of 16 nm. The UV-Vis. spectra showed an absorption peak at 410 nm.

Drawback of Chemical Methods

These are energy intensive processes and a large amount of capital is involved. The use of hazardous chemicals such as hydrazine eliminates the method from being an eco-friendly one. Moreover, nanoparticles produced by these methods exhibit aggregation with time, there compromising with the size factor upon storage (Mukherjee, 2008). The growing need to develop clean, non-toxic and eco-friendly methods for the synthesis of nanoparticles has resulted in the use of biological systems such as bacteria, fungi, plants etc.

By Bacteria

Biosynthetic methods employing either biological microorganisms or plant extracts have emerged as a simple and viable alternative to chemical synthetic procedures and physical methods (Saifuddin *et al.*, 2009). Although it is known that microorganisms such as bacteria play an important role in remediation of toxic metals through reduction of the metal ions, this was considered interesting as nanofactories very recently. Some bacteria reduce Fe^{3+} oxides by producing and secreting small, diffusible redox compounds that can serve as electron shuttle between the microbe and the insoluble iron substrate. This extracellular enzyme shows an excellent redox properties and it can act as an electron shuttle in the metal reduction. It was evident that electron shuttles or other reducing agents (e.g. hydroquinones) released by bacteria is capable of reducing ions to nanoparticles. However, biological nanoparticles synthesis generates nanoparticles at a much slower rate. In the studies synthesis of silver nanoparticles using the cell mass of bacteria or their leached cell components, the time required completing the reaction ranged from 24 to 120 h; this lengthy reaction is the one major drawback of the biological synthesis. Biological synthesis would have greater commercial viability if the nanoparticles could be synthesis more rapidly and in the large production scale. Shahverdi *et al.* (2007) investigated the combination effects of silver nanoparticles with antibiotics. The silver nanoparticles were synthesized using *Klebsiella pneumoniae* and evaluated its antimicrobial activity against *S. aureus* and *E. coli*. From the experimental work it was observed that the antibacterial activity of antibiotics like penicillin G, amoxicillin, erythromycin, clindamycin and vancomycin increased in the presence of silver nanoparticles against *E. coli* and *S. aureus*. The highest activity was observed with erythromycin against *S. aureus*. Minaeian *et al.* (2007) produced nanoparticles by *Klebsiella pneumoniae, Escherichia coli, Enterobacter cloacae, Staphylococcus aireus, Bacillus subtilis, Lactobacillus acidophilus* and *Candida albicans*. The silver nanoparticles were characterized by scanning electron microscopy and UV-visible spectroscopy. Saifuddin *et al.* (2009) described a novel combinatorial synthesis approach for the synthesis of metallic nanostructures of noble metals such as silver (Ag), by using a combination of culture supernatanant of *Bacillus subtilis* and microwave (MW) irradiation in water in absence of a surfactant or soft template. It was found that exposure of culture supernatanant of *Bacillus subtilis* and microwave irradiation to silver ion lead to the formation of silver nanoparticles. The silver nanoparticles were in the range of 5-60 nm in dimension. The nanoparticles were examined using UV-Visible Spectroscopy, and Transmission Electron Microscopy (TEM). The formation of nanoparticles by this method was extremely rapid, requires no toxic chemicals and the nanoparticles are stable for several months. Pugazhenthiran *et al.* (2009) synthesized AgNPs by *Bacillus* sp. TEM and energy dispersive X-ray (EDX) analyses confirmed that silver nanoparticles of 5–15 nm in size were deposited in the periplasmic space of the bacterial cells. Natarajan *et al.* (2010) demonstrated a simple biotechnological process for the intracellular and extracellular synthesis of silver nanoparticles using *E.coli*. The formation of nanoparticles using different basal medium was also investigated; the LB medium has the ability to maximize the synthesis of silver nanoparticles than NB medium. The characterization of silver ion exposed to microbial strain and the reduction of silver nitrate to silver nanoparticles was confirmed by UV-visible spectroscopy. Natarajan *et al.* (2010) also investigated that maximum synthesis of silver nanoparticles is proportional to bacterial biomass which occurred in the stationary phase of incubation period. It revealed that the particles formed from the distinct basal medium were associated with growth. The extracellular formation of silver nanoparticles was more expressed than intracellular formation.

By Fungi

Mukherjee *et al.* (2001) synthesized silver nanoparticles using the fungus *Verticillium*. Exposure of the fungal biomass to aqueous Ag^+ ions resulted in the intracellular reduction of the metal ions and formation of silver nanoparticles of dimensions 2.5 -12 nm. Fungal cells exposed to Ag^+ ions show broad absorption band at 450 nm. Electron microscopy analysis of thin sections of the fungal cells indicated that the silver particles were formed below the cell wall surface. The metal ions were not toxic to the fungal cells and the cells continued to multiply after biosynthesis of the silver nanoparticles.

Kowshik *et al.* (2002) synthesized silver nanoparticles in the size range of 2–5 nm extracellularly by a silver-tolerant yeast strain MKY3. Optical absorption, transmission electron microscopy, X-ray diffraction and X-ray photoelectron spectroscopy investigations confirmed that metallic (elemental) silver nanoparticles were formed. Duran *et al.* (2005) carried out the extracellular production of metal nanoparticles by several strains of the fungus *Fusarium oxysporum*. It was found that aqueous silver ions when exposed to several *F. oxysporum* strains are reduced in solution, thereby leading to the formation of silver hydrosol. The silver nanoparticles were in the range of 20–50 nm in dimensions. The reduction of the metal ions occurs by a nitrate-dependent reductase and a shuttle quinone extracellular process. The silver nitrate solution incubated with SMS changed to a yellow color from 24 hr onward, indicating the formation of silver nanoparticles. The purified solution yielded the maximum absorbance at 436 nm. X-ray analysis of the freeze-dried powder of silver nanoparticles confirmed the formation of metallic silver. Transmission electron microscopic analysis of the samples showed a uniform distribution of nanoparticles, having an average size of 30nm. These silver nanoparticles showed excellent antibacterial activity against two representative bacteria, *Staphylococcus aureus* and *Klebsiella pneumoniae.* Durán, *et al.* (2005) performed the extracellular production of silver nanoparticles by *F. oxysporum* strain and studied its bactericide effect in cotton and silk cloth against *S. aureus*. To incorporate silver nanoparticles in the cloth, these were immersed in the filtrate fungal, centrifuged and dried. The reduction of metal ions occurred by a nitrate dependent reductase and quinone extracellular process. Antibacterial activity was observed when silver nanoparticles were incorporated in cotton cloth. However, in silk cloth this activity was not observed demonstrating a low incorporation of the silver nanoparticles possibly due to the size of the silk pores. Their work demonstrated the possible use of biologically synthesized silver nanoparticles and its incorporation in cloths leading them to sterilization. Mukherjee *et al.* (2008) for the first time reported a biosynthetic route for the formation of nanocrystalline silver particles by using cell-free aqueous filtrate of a non-pathogenic and commercially viable biocontrol agent *Trichoderma asperellum*. The kinetics of the reaction was studied using UV–Vis spectroscopy. An intense surface plasmon resonance band at 410 nm in the UV–Vis. spectrum clearly revealed the formation of silver nanoparticles. The size of the silver particles using TEM and XRD studies was found to be in the range 13–18 nm. These nanoparticles were highly stable and even after prolonged storage for over 6 months they do not showed significant aggregation. Ingle *et al.* (2008) investigated the use of *Fusarium accuminatum*, isolated from infected ginger, for the synthesis of silver nanoparticles. The antibacterial activity of silver nanoparticles was checked against *E. coli, S. aureus, Salmonella typhi, S. epidermis.* The UV–Vis. spectra showed absorption at 420 nm, which is characteristic for spherical nanoparticles. The spherical shape of the nanoparticles was confirmed by the TEM study and the size of the nanoparticles ranged from 5–40 nm. Gade *et al.* (2008) exploited *Aspergillus niger* for the synthesis of silver nanoparticles. The silver nanoparticles were detected with the help of UV–Vis spectrophotometer while, the characterization was done using TEM. The antibacterial activity of silver nanoparticles was assessed against *E. coli* and *S. aureus*. The UV–Vis spectra denoted a peak at 420 nm. The TEM study of silver nanoparticles confirmed the presence of spherical shaped nanoparticles in the size range of 20 nm. The silver nanoparticles showed efficient antibacterial activity against *E. coli* and *S. aureus,* which, was also analyzed using TEM. The electron microscopic study demonstrated presence of silver nanoparticles in the cell membranes of test bacteria. The synthesis of nanoparticles from some fungi is summarized in Table 35.1.

By Plants

Synthesis of nanoparticles by plant extracts is at present under exploitation as some researchers worked on it (Prabhu *et al.*, 2009; Jain *et al.*, 2009; Singh *et al.*, 2010). The employ of *Azadirachta indica*

(Neem), *Medicago sativa* (Alfalfa), *Aloe vera, Jatropha curcas* (Ratanjoot) and *Emblica officinalis* (Amla, Indian Gooseberry) has previously been reported (Chandran *et al.*, 2006; Bar *et al.*, 2009). Consistent with preceding reports, the polyol components and the water-soluble heterocyclic components are largely accountable for the reduction of Ag ions and the stabilization of the nanoparticles, respectively. There are also reports on reductases and polysaccharides as factors involved in biosynthesis and stabilization of the nanoparticles, respectively (Bar *et al.*, 2009). Singh *et al.* (2010) states that some factors jointly conclude the nanoparticle synthesis, as well as the plant source, the organic compounds in the crude leaf extract, the concentration of Ag nitrate, the temperature and other than these, even the pigments in the leaf extract. The Ag is only characterized by UV-Vis spectroscopy, TEM, and atom force microscopy (AFM). TEM and AFM of the sample showed uniform and monodispersive particle distribution in the colloids. The synthesis of metal nanoparticles synthesized from some plants are summarized in Table 35.2.

Table 35.1: List of Metal Nanoparticles Synthesized from Different Fungi (Gade *et al.*, 2009)

Sl.No.	*Name of Organism*	*Nanoparticle Synthesized*	*Intracellular/Extracelluar*	*Size (nm)*
1.	*F. oxysporum*	Silver	Extracellular	5–15
2.	*F. oxysporum*	Silver	Extracellular	20–50
3.	*Trichothecium* sp.	Gold	Intracellular and Extracellular	–
4.	*F. oxysporum*	Silica and Titania	Extracellular	5–15
5.	*Colletotrichum* sp.	Gold	Extracellular	20–40
6.	*F. oxysporum f.* sp. *lycopersici*	Platinum	Intracellular and Extracellular	10–100
7.	*F. oxysporum*	Magnetite	Extracellular	20–50
8.	*Schizosaccharomyces* pombe	CdS	Intracellular	2–2.5
9.	*Torulopsis* sp.	PbS	Intracellular	2–5
10.	*Verticillium* sp.	Silver and Gold	Intracellular	2–20

Table 35.2: List of Metal Nanoparticles Synthesized from Different Plants (Kumar and Yadav, 2008)

Sl.No.	*Plants*	*Silver/Gold/Copper*	*Shape*	*Size (nm)*
1.	*Medicago sativa*	Silver	Spherical	6–20
2.	*Medicago sativa*	Gold	fcc tetrahedral, hexagonal platelets, icosahedral multiple twinned, decahedral multiple twined and irregular shaped.	15–200
3.	*Brassica juncea*	Silver, gold, copper	Triangular, spherical	2–20
4.	*Azadirachta indica*	Silver, gold and Ag core–Au shell	Polydisperse, flat, plate-like spherical, peculiar core–shell structure	5–35
5.	*Cinnamommum camphora*	Silver and gold	Triangular, spherical	55–80
6.	Rice paper plant stem	Silver	–	Below 100
7.	*Triticum aestivum*	Gold	fcc tetrahedral, hexagonal platelets, irregular shaped, rod shaped	10–30
8.	*Pelargonium graveolens*	Gold	Spherical rods, flat, sheets and triangular	21–70
9.	*Aloe vera*	Silver and gold	Triangular, spherical	6–20
10.	*Argemone mexicana*	Silver	Polygonal	20-30

Prabhu *et al.* (2009) made the first attempt of introducing silver herbal nanoparticle isolation and antimicrobial assessment. The herbal leaves like *Ocimum sanctum* and *Vitex negundo* were included to analyze the productivity of nanoparticles. The silver phyto nanoparticles were collected from each herbal plant and tested their antibacterial activity. The test cultures included in this study were *Staphylococcus aureus, Vibrio cholerae, Proteus vulgaris* and *Pseudomonas aeruginosa.* The antibacterial activities of all the herbal nanoparticles obtained from *Ocimum sanctum* showed maximum inhibitory rate using 150μg of these plants extract compared with *Vitex negundo.* The silver nanoparticles from herbal leaves showed a good antibacterial activity than the plants used. Parashar *et al.* (2009a) described the synthesis of silver nanoparticles using *Parthenium* leaf extract. UV-Vis spectroscopy was used to investigate shape and size of nanoparticles Transmission electron microscopy analysis of these particles showed that they are ~50 nm in size and very irregular in shape. SAED pattern indicate that the silver nanoparticles were single crystalline in nature. Chandran *et al.* (2006) synthesized gold nanotriangles and spherical silver nanoparticles by a simple procedure using *Aloe vera* leaf extract as the reducing agent. The kinetics of gold nanotriangle formation was followed by UV-Vis-NIR absorption spectroscopy and transmission electron microscopy (TEM). The effect of reducing agent concentration in the reaction mixture on the yield and size of the gold nanotriangles was studied using transmission electron microscopy. It was observed that the slow rate of the reaction along with the shape directing effect of the constituents of the extract are responsible for the formation of single crystalline gold nanotriangles. Reduction of silver ions by *Aloe vera* extract however, led to the formation of spherical silver nanoparticles of 15.2 nm. X-ray diffraction analysis showed that the nanoparticles were of face centered cubic structure. A comparison of radius of nanoparticles obtained from HRTEM image with the optimized cavity radius of the cyclic peptides present within the latex revealed that the particles having radius 10–20 nm are mostly stabilized by the cyclic peptides. Jain *et al.* (2009) for the first time synthesized nanoparticles using plant fruit extract. Extract of papaya fruit was used as reducing and capping agent. Nanoparticles were characterized using UV–Vis absorption spectroscopy, FTIR, XRD and SEM. Further these biologically synthesized nanoparticles were found to be highly toxic against different multi drug resistant human pathogens.

Parashar *et al.* (2009 b) and Farooqui *et al.* (2010) synthesized silver nanoparticles from leaf extracts of *Mentha piperita* and *Clerodendrum inerme.* They observed a rapid reduction of silver ions leading to the formation of stable crystalline silver nanoparticles in the solution. Nanoparticles were analysed by TEM and UV-Vis Spectroscopy. Atomic force microscopy (AFM) analysis of the nanoparticles revealed differences in sizes for the nanoparticles synthesized from different leaf conditions.

Mechanism of Action

The exact mechanism of action of silver on the microbes is still not known but the possible mechanism of action of metallic silver, silver ions and silver nanoparticles have been suggested according to the morphological and structural changes found in the microorganisms.

Mechanism of Action of Silver/Silver Ions

The mechanism of action of silver is linked with its interaction with thiol group compounds found in the respiratory enzymes of bacterial cells. Silver binds to the bacterial cell wall and cell membrane and inhibits the respiration process (Klasen, 2008). In case of *E. coli,* silver acts by inhibiting the uptake of phosphate and releasing phosphate, mannitol, succinate, proline and glutamine from *E. coli* cells (Yamanaka *et al.,* 2005). The mechanism for the antimicrobial action of silver ions is not properly understood however, the effect of silver ions on bacteria can be observed by the structural and morphological changes. It is suggested that when DNA molecules are in relaxed state the replication of DNA can be effectively conducted. But when the DNA is in condensed form it loses its replication ability hence, when the silver ions penetrate inside the bacterial cell the DNA molecule turns into condensed form and loses its replication ability leading to cell death. Also, it has been reported that heavy metals react with proteins by getting attached with the thiol group and the proteins get inactivated (Feng *et al.*, 2000).

Mechanism of Action of Silver Nanoparticles

The silver nanoparticles show efficient antimicrobial property compared to other salts due to their extremely large surface area, which provides better contact with microorganisms. The nanoparticles get attached to the cell membrane and also penetrate inside the bacteria. The bacterial membrane contains sulfur-containing proteins and the silver nanoparticles interact with these proteins in the cell as well as with the phosphorus containing compounds like DNA. When silver nanoparticles enter the bacterial cell it forms a low molecular weight region in the center of the bacteria to which the bacteria conglomerates thus, protecting the DNA from the silver ions. The nanoparticles preferably attack the respiratory chain, cell division finally leading to cell death. The nanoparticles release silver ions in the bacterial cells, which enhance their bactericidal activity (Feng *et al.*, 2000; Sondi and Salopek-Sondi, 2004; Morones *et al.*, 2005; Song *et al.*, 2006).

Effect of Size and Shape on the Antimicrobial Activity of Nanoparticles

The size of the nanoparticle implies that it has a large surface area to come in contact with the bacterial cells and hence, it will have a higher percentage of interaction than bigger particles (Kreibig and Vollmer, 1995; Mulvaney, 1996; Morones *et al.*, 2005; Pal *et al.*, 2007). The nanoparticles smaller than 10 nm interact with bacteria and produce electronic effects, which enhance the reactivity of nanoparticles. Thus, it is corroborated that the bactericidal effect of silver nanoparticles is size dependent (Raimondi *et al.*, 2005; Morones *et al.*, 2005). The antimicrobial efficacy of the nanoparticle depend on the shapes of the nanoparticles also, this can be confirmed by studying the inhibition of bacterial growth by differentially shaped nanoparticles (Morones *et al.*, 2005) (Figure 35.1). According to Pal *et al.* (2007) truncated triangular nanoparticles show bacterial inhibition with silver content of 1 µg. While, in case of spherical nanoparticles total silver content of 12.5 µg is needed. The rod shaped particles need a total of 50 to 100 µg of silver content. Thus, the silver nanoparticles with different shapes have different effects on bacterial cell.

Nanosilver as a Potent Bactericidal Agent

Microorganisms (bacteria, yeast and fungi) play an important role in toxic metals remediation through reduction of metal ions. Silver nanoparticles have been known to have inhibitory and bactericidal effect (Chu *et al.*, 1988 Deitch *et al.*, 1987; Margraff and Covey, 1977; Silver, 2003; Atiyeh *et al.*, 2007; Law *et al.*, 2008). The combined effect of silver nanoparticles with antibiotics has proven to be productive. Such effects were first observed in *Staphylococcus aureus* and *E. coli* using disc diffusion method. The antibacterial activities of penicillin G, amoxicillin, erythromycin, clindamycin, and vancomycin increased in the presence of AgNPs against both test strains. The same effect was not observed in the case of antibiotics tested. The effects of AgNPs on the antibacterial activity of the above mentioned antibiotics for *E. coli* were lower than *S. aureus*. In contrast, the most synergistic activity was observed with erythromycin against *S. aureus* (Hope *et al.*, 1989).

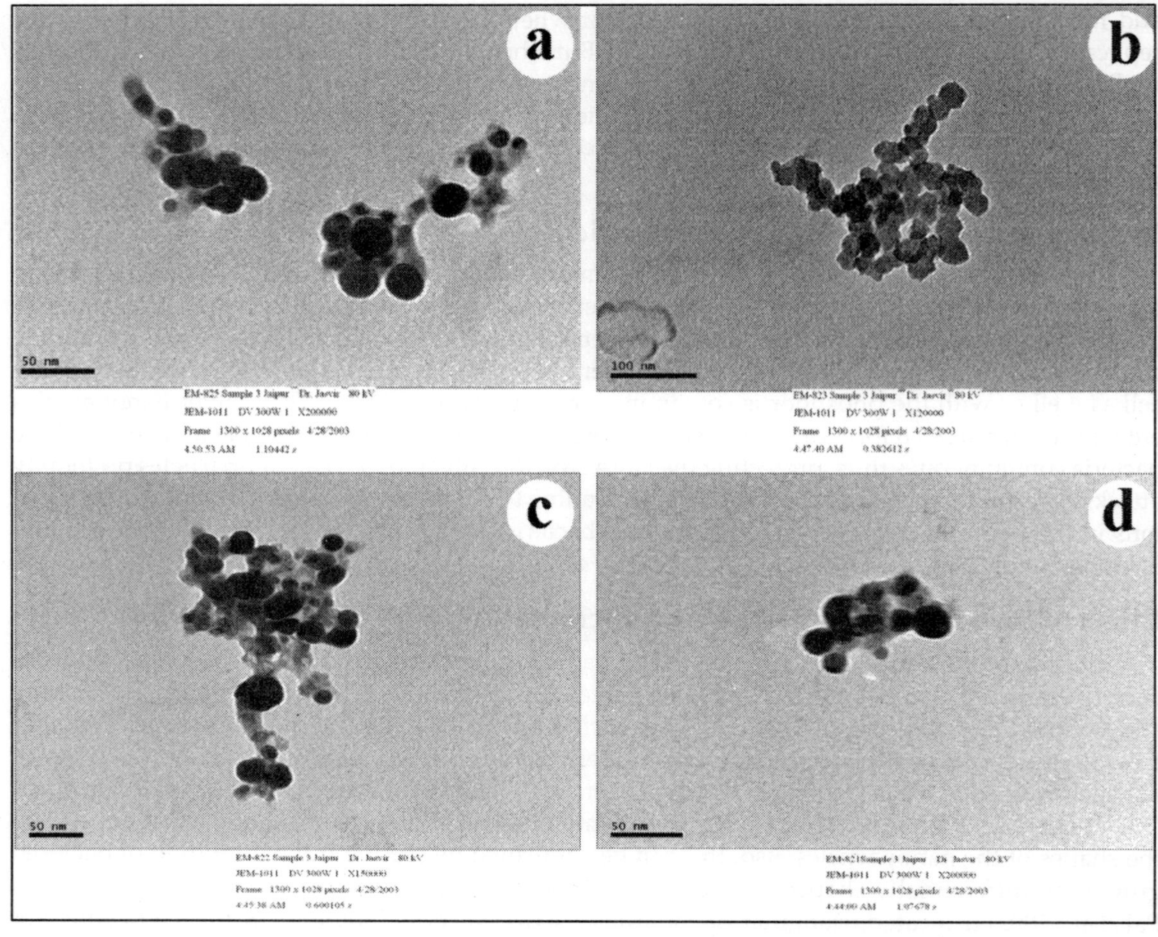

Figure 35.1: a,b,c and d are Different Shape of Nanoparticles

Nanosilver as an Antifungal Agent

Fungal infections have become more common in the recent years. In particular, fungal infections are more frequent in patients who are immunocompromised because of cancer chemotherapy, or organ or human immunodeficiency virus infections (Groll *et al.*, 1996). The availability of the antifungal drugs is limited because prophylaxis with antifungals may lead to the emergence of resistant strains. By 1980, members of the four major classes of antifungal agents–polyenes, azoles, morpholines, and allylamines–had been identified, yet the only new drug introduced for the treatment of systemic fungal infections was oral ketoconazole (Kauffman and Carver, 1997). The development of new antifungal drugs is creating new potential combination therapies. Amphotericin B, an antifungal agent used to treat serious systemic infections was used as a positive control to compare with AgNPs (Hartsel and Bolard, 1996). AgNPs showed significant antifungal activity against *T. mentagrophytes* and *Candida* species. Towards all fungal strains, AgNPs exhibited similar activity with amphotericin B, but more potent activity than fluconazole. However, this compound exhibited less potent activity than amphotericin B for *C. parapsilosis* and *C. krusei*. The ability of AgNPs to disrupt the fungal envelope structure was documented using Transmission Electron Microscope. The treated fungal cells showed significant damage, which was characterized by the formation of a "pit" in their cell walls and pores in their plasma membrane.

Nanosilver as an Antiviral Agent

Silver nanoparticles have been used to exhibit the antimicrobial efficacy against viral particles. They have been shown to exhibit promising cytoprotective activities towards HIV-infected T-cells; however, the effects of these nanoparticles towards other kinds of viruses remain largely unexplored. The research on the nanoparticles HIV-1 interaction demonstrated that silver nanoparticles inhibited HIV-1 infectivity *in vitro* by binding to the disulfide bond regions of the CD4 binding domain within the gp120 glycoprotein subunit. Binding of these nanoparticles to the gp120 subunit appeared to be size dependent as particles greater than 10 nm were not observed attached to the viral envelope (Elechiguerra *et al.*, 2005).

Conclusion

Numerous synthetic methods for Ag NPs using inexpensive biological materials were summarized and experimental approaches under different conditions which are responsible for morphology and size of the Ag particles. Rapid and green synthetic methods using extracts of bio-organisms have shown a great potential in Ag NP synthesis. However, understanding the mechanism by which the biomolecules of these systems are involved in nano material synthesis is still lacking.

References

Albrecht, M.A., Evan, C.W. and Raston, C.L. (2006). Green chemistry and the health implications of nanoparticles. *Green Chem*. 8: 417–432.

Andreescu, D., Eastman. C., Balantrapu, K. and Goia, D.V. (2007). A simple route for manufacturing highly dispersed silver nanoparticles. *J Mater Res*. 22(9): 2488-2496.

Atiyeh, B.S., Costagliola, M., Hayek, S.N. and Dibo, S.A. (2007). Effect of silver on burn wound infection control and healing: review of the literature. *Burn*. 33: 139–148.

Bar, H., Bhui, D.K., Sahoo, G.P., Sarkar, P. and De, S.P. and Misra, A. (2009). *Colloids and Surfaces A: Physicochemical and Engineering Aspects*. 339: 134–139.

Bellinger, C.G. and Conway, H. (1970). Effects of silver nitrate and sulfamylon on epithelial regeneration. *Plast Reconstr Surg*. 45: 582–505.

Berger, T.J., Spadaro, J.A., Chapin, S.E. and Becker, R.O. (1976). Electrically generated silver ions: Quantitative effects on bacterial and mammalian cells. *Antimicrob. Agents Chemother*. 9: 357-358.

Castellano, J.J., Shafii, S.M., Ko, F., Donate, G., Wright, T.E. and Mannari, R.J. (2007). Comparative evaluation of silver-containing antimicrobial dressings and drugs. *Int Wound J*. 4(2): 114-122.

Chandran, S.P., Chaudhary, M., Pasricha, R., Ahmad, A. and Sastry. M. (2006). Synthesis of gold nanotriangles and silver nanoparticles using *Aloe vera* extract. *Biotechnology Progress*. 22(2): 577-583.

Chopra I. (2007). The increasing use of silver-based products as antimicrobial agents: a useful development or a cause for concern? *J Antimicrob Chemother*. 59: 587–590.

Chu, C.S., McManus, A.T., Pruitt, B.A. and Mason, A.D. (1988). Therapeutic effects of silver nylon dressing with weak direct current on *Pseudomans aeruginosa* infected burn wounds. *J Trauma*. 28: 1488–92.

Das, R., Nath, S.S., Chakdar, D., Gope, G. and Bhattacharjee, R. (2009). Prepration of silver nanoparticles and their characterization. *Journal of Nanotechnology Online*. 10: 1343-1348.

Deitch, E.A., Marin, A., Malakanov, V. and Albright, J.A. (1987). Silver nylon cloth: *in vivo* and *in vitro* evaluation of antimicrobial activity. *J Trauma*. 27: 301–4.

Demling, R.H. and De Santi, L. (2001). Effects of silver on wound management. *Wounds*. 13: 4.

Duran, N., Marcato, P.D., Alves, O.L., D'Souza, G. and Esposito, E. (2005). Mechanistic aspects of biosynthesis of silver nanoparticles by several *Fusarium oxysporum* strains. *J Nanobiotechnol*. 3: 8–14.

Elechiguerra, J.L., Burt, J.L., Morones, J.R., Bragado, A.C., Gao, X. and Lara, H.H. (2005). Interaction of silver nanoparticles with HIV-1. *J Nanobiotechnol*. 3: 1-10.

Farooqui, M.D., Chauhan, P.S., Krishnamoorthy, P. and Shaik. J. (2010). Extraction of Silver nanoparticles from the leaf extract of Clerodendrum inerme. *Digest Journal of Nanomaterials and Biostructures*. 5(1): 577-583.

Feng, Q.L., Wu, J., Chen, G.Q., Cui, F.Z., Kim, T.N. and Kim, J.O. (2000). A mechanistic study of the antibacterial effect of silver ions on *Escherichia coli* and *Staphylococcus aureus*. *J Biomed Mater*. 52(4): 662–668.

Groll, A.H., Shah, P.M., Mentzel, C., Schneider, M., Just-Nuebling, G. and Huebner, K. (1996). Trends in the postmortem epidemiology of invasive fungal infections at a University Hospital. *J Infect*. 33: 23–32.

Hartsel, S. and Bolard, J. (1996). Amphotericin B: new life for an old drug. *Trends Pharmacol Sci*. 17: 445–9.

Hope, P.G., Kristinsson, K., Norman, P. and Elson, R.A. (1989). Deep infection of cemented total hip arthroplasty caused by coagulase-negative staphylococci. *J Bone Jt Surg Br*. 71: 851–5.

Huang, J., Li, Q., Sun, D., Lu, Y., Su, Y. and Yang, X. (2007). Biosynthesis of silver and gold nanoparticles by novel sundried *Cinnamomum camphora* leaf. *Nanotechnology*. 18:104. 1045.

Hugo, W.B. and Russell, A.D. (1982). Types of antimicrobial agents. In: *Principles and practice of disinfection, preservation and sterilization*. 106-108.

Ingle, A., Gade, A., Pierrat, S., Sonnichsen, C. and Rai, M. (2008). Mycosynthesis of silver nanoparticles using the fungus *Fusarium accuminatum* and its activity against some human pathogenic bacteria. *Curr Nano*. 4: 141–144.

Jain, D., Daima, H.K., Kachhwaha, S. and Kothari, S.L. (2009). Synthesis of plant mediated silver nanoparticles using papaya fruit extract and evaluation of their antimicrobial activities. *Digest Journal of Nanomaterials and Biostructures*. 4(3): 557-563.

Kauffman, C.A. and Carver, P.L. (1997). Antifungal agents in the 1990s: current status and future developments. *Drugs*. 53: 539–49.

Kazachenko, A.S., Legler, T.A.V., Peryanova, T.O.V. and Vstavskaya, Y.A. (2000). Synthesis and antimicrobial activity of silver complexes with histidine and tryptophan. *Pharm Chem J*. 34(5): 34–35.

Kim, J.S., Kuk, E., Yu, K.N., Kim, J.H., Park, S.J. and Lee, H.J. (2007). Antimicrobial effects of silver nanoparticles. *Nanomed Nanotechnol Biol Med*. 3: 95-101.

Kim, K.J., Sung, W.S., Suh, B.K., Moon, S.K., Choi, J.S. and Kim, J.G. (2008). Antifungal activity and mode of action of silver nano-particles on *Candida albicans*. *Biometals*. 22(2): 235-242.

Klasen, H.J. (2008). A historical review of the use of silver in the treatment of burns. Part I early uses. *Burns*. 30: 1–9.

Kreibig, U. and Vollmer, M. (1995). *Optical properties of metal clusters*. Berlin, Germany: Springer.

Landsdown, A.B.G. (2002). Silver I: its antibacterial properties and mechanism of action. *J Wound Care*. 11: 125–138.

Law, N., Ansari, S., Livens, F.R., Renshaw, J.C. and Lloyd, J.R. (2008). The formation of nano-scale elemental silver particles via enzymatic reduction by *Geobacter sulfur reducens*. Appl Environ *Microbiol*. 74: 7090–3.

Liau, S.Y., Read, D.C., Pugh, W.J., Furr, J.R. and Russell, A.D. (1997). Interaction of silver nitrate with readily identifiable groups: relationship to the antibacterial action of silver ions. *Lett. Appl. Microbiol*. 25: 279-283.

Liu, Z., Stout, J.E., Tedesco, L., Boldin, M., Hwang, C., Diven, W.F. and Yu, V.L. (1994). Controlled evaluation of copper-silver ionization in eradicating *Legionella pneumophila* from a hospital water distribution system. *J. Infect. Dis*. 169: 919-922.

Margraff, H.W. and Covey, T.H. (1977). A trial of silver–zinc-allantoine in the treatment of leg ulcers. *Arch Surg*. 112: 699–704.

Minaeian, S., Shahverdi, A.R., Nohi, A.S. and Shahverdi, H.R. (2008). Extracellular biosynthesis of silver nanoparticles by some bacteria. *JSIAU*. 17(66) :1-4

Morgan, T.P., Guadagnolo, C.M., Grosell, M. and Wood, C.M. (2005). Effects of water hardness on toxicological responses to chronic waterborne silver exposure in early life stages of rainbow trout (Oncorhynchus mykiss). *Environ. Toxicol. Chem*. 24: 1642-1647.

Morones, J.R., Elechiguerra, J.L., Camacho, A. and Ramirez, J.T. (2005). The bactericidal effect of silver nanoparticles. *Nanotechnology*. 16: 2346--53.

Moyer, C.A., Brentano, L., Gravens, D.L.,Margraf, H.W. and Monafo, W.W. (1965). Treatment of large human burns with 0.5 per cent silver nitrate solution. *Arch Surg*. 90: 812–867.

Mukherjee, P., Ahmad, A., Mandal,D., Senapati, S., Sainkar, S.R. and Khan, M.I. (2001). Fungus-mediated synthesis of silver nanoparticles and their immobilization in the mycelial matrix: A novel biological approach to nanoparticle synthesis. *Nano Lett*. *1*: 515–609.

Mukherjee, P., Roy, M., Mandal, B.P., Dey, G.K., Mukherjee, P.K. and Ghatak, J. (2008). Green synthesis of highly stabilized nanocrystalline silver particles by a non-pathogenic and agriculturally important fungus *T. asperellum*. *Nanotechnology*. 19: 7.

Mulvaney, P. (1996). Surface plasmon spectroscopy of nanosized metal particles. *Langmuir*. 12: 788–800.

Natarajan, K., Selvaraj, S. and Murty, V.R. (2010). Microbial production of silver nanoparticles. *Digest Journal of Nanomaterials and Biostructures*. 5(1): 135-40.

Nomiya, K., Yoshizawa, A., Tsukagoshi, K., Kasuga, N.C., Hirakawa, S. and Watanabe, J. (2004). Synthesis and structural characterization of silver(I), aluminium(III) and cobalt(II) complexes with 4-isopropyltropolone (hinokitiol) showing noteworthy biological activities. Action of silver(I)-oxygen bonding complexes on the antimicrobial activities. *J. Inorg. Biochem.* 98: 46-60.

Oloffs, A., Grosse-Siestrup, C., Bisson, S., Rinck, M., Rudolph, R. and Gross, U. (1994). Biocompatibility of silver-coated polyurethane catheters and silver-coated Dacron® material. *Biomaterials.* 15: 753-758.

Pal, S., Tak, Y.K. and Song, J.M. (2007). Does the antibacterial activity of silver nanoparticles depend on the shape of the nanoparticle? A study of the Gram-negative bacterium *Escherichia coli*. *Appl. Environ. Microbiol.* 73: 1712-1720.

Panigrahi, S., Kundu, S., Ghosh, S.K., Nath, S. and Pal, T. (2004). General method of synthesis for metal nanoparticles. *Journal of Nanoparticle Research.* 6: 411-14.

Parashar, V., Parashar, R., Sharma, B. and Pandey, A.C. (2009 a). Parthenium mediated synthesis of silver nanoparticles: A novel approach towards weed utilization. *Digest Journal of Nanomaterials and Biostructures.* 4(1): 45-50.

Parashar, U.K., Saxena, P.S. and Srivastava, A. (2009 b). Bioinspired Synthesis of Silver nanoparticles. *Digest Journal of Nanomaterials and Biostructures.* 4(1): 159–166

Prabhu, N., Raj, D.T., Yamuna, G. K., Ayisha, S.S., Joseph, P. and Innocent, D. (2010). Synthesis of Silver phytonanoparticles and their antibacterial efficacy. *Digest Journal of Nanomaterials and Biostructures.* 5(1): 185-189.

Pugazhenthiran, N., Anandan, S., Kathiravan, G., Prakash, N.K.U., Crawford, S. and Kumar, M.A. (2009). Microbial synthesis of silver nanoparticles by *Bacillus* sp. *J Nanoparticle Research.* 11: 1811-15.

Raad, I.I. and Hanna, H.A. (2002). Intravascular catheter-related infections: New horizons and recent advances. *Arch. Intern. Med.* 162: 871-878.

Raimondi, F., Scherer, G.G., Kotz, R. and Wokaun, A. (2005). Nanoparticles in energy technology: examples from electochemistry and catalysis. *Angew. Chem., Int. Ed.* 44: 2190–209.

Russell, A. D. and Hugo, W.B, (1994). Antimicrobial activity and action of silver. *Prog. Med. Chem.* 31: 351-370.

Saifuddin, N., Wong, C.W. and Nuryasumira, A.A. (2009). Rapid biosynthesis of silver nanoparticles using culture supernatant of bacteria with microwave irradiation. *E-J Chem* 1149. 6: 61–70.

Silver. S. (2003). Bacterial silver resistance: molecular biology and uses and misuses of silver compounds. *FEMS Microbiol Rev.* 27: 341–53.

Sondi,I. and Salopek-Sondi, B. (2004). Silver nanoparticles as antimicrobial agent: a case study on *E. coli* as a model for Gram-negative bacteria. *J Colloid Interface Sci.* 275: 177- 182.

Song, H.Y., Ko, K.K., Oh, L.H. and Lee, B.T. (2006). Fabrication of silver nanoparticles and their antimicrobial mechanisms. *Eur Cells Mater.* 11: 58.

Song,J.Y. and Kim, B.S. (2008). Rapid biological synthesis of silver nanoparticles using plant leaf extracts. *Bioprocess Biosystem Engineering.* 32: 79-84.

Taniguchi, N. (1974). On the Basic Concept of Nano-Technology. *Proc. Intl. Conf. Prod. Eng. Tokyo, Part II*. Japan Society of Precision Engineering.

Vigneshwaran, N., Kathe, A.A., Varadarajan, P.V., Nachane, R.P. and Balasubramanya, R.H. (2007). Silver Protein (Core-Shell) Nanoparticle Production Using Spent Mushroom Substrate. *Langmuir*. 23: 7113-117.

Yamanaka, M., Hara, K. And Kudo, J. (2005). Bactericidal actions of a silver ion solution on *Escherichia coli*, studied by energy-filtering transmission electron microscopy and proteomic analysis. *Appl. Environ. Microbiol*. 71: 7589-93.

Microbial Biotechnology and Ecology (2011) *Pages* **606–615**
Editors: **Deepak Vyas, G.S. Paliwal, P.K.Khare and R.K Gupta**
Published by: **DAYA PUBLISHING HOUSE, NEW DELHI**

Chapter 36

Phenolic Quantification and Anti-Aging Activity of *Morchella esculenta*

☆ ***Javed Ahmad Wagay*, Ashok Shukla, Anjuli Choubey, Poonam Dehairya and Deepak Vyas***

*Lab of Microbial Technology and Plant Pathology,
Department of Botany, Dr. H.S. Gour Central University, Sagar – 470 030, M.P.*

ABSTRACT

The present investigation was designed for the analysis to determine the *in vitro* antioxidant potential of a pharmaceutically important mushroom (*Morchella esculenta*). Four basic test systems *viz.*, DPPH (1,1-diphenyl-2-picrylhydroxyl radical) free radical scavenging, nitric-oxide scavenging activity, super-oxide scavenging activity and total phenolic compounds were used. Among all the scavenging tests a significant correlation existed between concentrations of the extract and per cent inhibition of free radicals. Measurement of total phenolic content of the extract was achieved using Folin-Ciocalteau reagent containing 23.42±0.89mg g^{-1} of phenolic content, which was found significantly higher when compared to reference standard gallic acid. DPPH scavenging activity of methanolic mushroom extract showed highest per cent inhibition value, which was found to be 70.8±0.89, followed by super oxide scavenging activity (52.9±0.76). The least value was found to be that of nitric oxide *i.e.* 49.04±0.23.

Keywords: DPPH, Phenols, Gallic acid, Antioxidant, Morchella esculenta.

Introduction

Morchella esculenta (Guchi or sponge mushroom) belongs to family Helvellaceae. The most therapeutic and highly priced mushroom found in Himalayan ranges of extreme north western

* E-mail: ufaq07@rediffmail.com/javediqbal49@gmail.com

extremity of Indian subcontinent–Kashmir (J and K).The state is located between 32°-17 and 37°-5 North latitude and 73°-26 and 80°-30 East longitude and its average height from the mean sea level varies from 300 to 7200 meters with average rain fall 150 cm. The temperature range is between –5°C to 28°C as minimum and maximum in January and June. Due to suitable environmental conditions, the region is rich in mushroom diversity particularly different species of *Morchella*. Its growing season is usually from 15-March to July and is mostly used as food and ethenomedicine after sun dried by the tribals of Kashmir.

Majority of the diseases/disorders are mainly linked to oxidative stress due to free radical formation (Gutteridgde, 1995). Free radicals are fundamental to any biochemical process and represent an essential part of aerobic life and metabolism (Tiwari, 2001). The most common reactive oxygen species (ROS) include superoxide, anion, hydrogen peroxide (H_2O_2), peroxyl (ROO-) radicals, and reactive hydroxyl (OH-) radicals. The nitrogen derived free radicals are nitric oxide (NO_2) and peroxynitrite anion (ONOO). ROS have been implicated in over a hundred of diseases which range from arthritis and connective tissue disorders to carcinogenesis, aging, physical injury, infection and acquired immunodeficiency syndrome (Joyce, 1987). In treatment of these diseases, antioxidant therapy has gained an immense importance. Current research is now directed towards finding naturally occurring antioxidants of plant origin. Antioxidants have been reported to prevent oxidative damages by quenching free radical formation, and may prevent the occurrence of diseases such as, cancer and aging which are directly related to reactive free radical production. It can interfere with the oxidation process by reacting with free radicals, chelating catalytic metals, and also by acting as oxygen scavengers (Buyukokuroglu, 2001). Mushrooms are being used as a source of medicine since long. The medicinal properties of mushrooms have been investigated in the recent scientific developments throughout the world, due to their potent antioxidant activities, no side effects and have economic viability (Auudy, 2003). Phenolic compounds widely distributed in mushrooms which have been reported to exert multiple biological effect, including antioxidant, free radical scavenging abilities, anti-inflammatory, anti-carcinogenic etc. (Miller, 1996). They were also suggested to be a potential iron chelators (Boyer, 1998; Harsteen, 1983). The antioxidative and free radical scavenging properties of the phenolic content of mushroom methanolic extracts have been reported, suggesting possible protective roles of these compounds, due to their ability to capture metals, inhibit lipoxygenase and scavenge free radicals (Mau, Chang, Huang, and Chen, 2004). Recently, Valentao *et al.* (2005) identified the presence of six phenolic compounds (3-, 4- and 5-O-caffeoylquinic acid, caffeic acid, p-coumaric acid and rutin) and five organic acids (citric, ascorbic, malic, shikimic and fumaric acids) in wild edible mushroom *Cantharellus cibarius* Fr., kept under four different conditions (dried, frozen, preserved in olive oil and in vinegar). The organic acids citric, ketoglutaric, malic, succinic, oxalic, ascorbic, quinic, shikimic and fumaric were also found in the edible mushrooms *viz.*, *Amanita caesarea* (Scop.) Pers., *Boletus edulis* Bull., *Gyroporus castaneus* (Bull.) Que'l., *Lactarius deliciosus* (L.) Gray, *Suillus collinitus* (Fr.) Kuntze and *Xerocomus chrysenteron* (Bull.) Que'l. (Valentao *et al.*, 2005b).

Kashmir being the temperate region with suitable climatic conditions which favours luxuriant growth of different mushroom species including different species of *Morchella*. The aim of present work is to analyse the anti-oxidant capacity of one of the dominantly found species *Morchella esculenta* var. as little or no work has been done so far, to check its antioxidant property to the best of our knowledge is mostly used by the tribals of the region to treat different diseases particularly for chronic arthritis, general weakness and feed *Morchella esculenta* to women along with milk during and after pregnancy and claims that it provides quick recovery and resistence to the women after birth.

Material and Methods

Preparation of Mushroom Extract

Morchella esculenta fruiting bodies were collected in March–May 2009 from coniferous forests of Kashmir (J and K). The fruiting bodies were dried in an oven at 40 °C for 4 hours. The specimens were taken to Mushroom Culture Collection Centre–Sherie Kashmir Agriculture University of Science and Technology (SKAUST) Srinagar (Kashmir) for identification. The dried fruiting bodies were crushed to powder by using electronic blender. About 50g of powder were taken in 500ml of methanol in soxhlet extraction unit for extraction at 30°C for 16-18 hours and filtered through Whatman No. 4 filter paper. The residue was then, extracted with two additional 500 mL of methanol as described above. The combined methanolic extract was then rotary evaporated at 40°C to dryness, redissolved in methanol to a concentration of 10 mg/ml and stored at 4°C for further use.

Antioxidant Activity

Chemicals

1,1 Diphenyl -2- picrylhydroxyl (DPPH), butylated hydroxytoluene (BHT), L-ascorbic acid, Trolox (6-hydroxy-2-5-8-tetramethyl chroman-2-carboxylic acid), Gallic acid, Tween-20, Folin ciocalteu's phenol reagent (FCR), Sodium carbonate, Sodium nitroprusside, methanol, chloroform and the other chemicals and reagents purchased from Biochem Pharmaceutical Industries (Mumbay). All other unlabeled chemicals and reagents were of analytical grade.

Scavenging Effect on 1,1-Diphenyl-2-Picrylhydroxyl (DPPH)

The hydrogen atom or electron donating ability of the methanolic mushroom extract was measured from the bleaching of the purple-coloured methanol solution of 1,1-Diphenyl-2-picrylhydroxyl (DPPH). This spectrophotometric assay uses the stable radical DPPH as a reagent (Burits M and Bucar F., 2000). 1000µl of various concentrations (20-200µg/ml) of the extract were added to 4 ml of 0.004 per cent methanol solution of DPPH. After 20-30 min incubation period at room temperature, the absorbance was read against a blank at $\lambda = 517$ nm. Inhibition of free radical by DPPH in per cent (per cent I) was calculated by the following formula.

$$\% \text{ inhibition} = (A_{blank} - A_{sample}/A_{blank}) \times 100$$

where, A_{blank} is the absorbance of the control (Solvent), and A_{sample} is the absorbance of the test compound. Extract concentration providing 50 per cent inhibition (IC_{50}) was calculated from the graph plotted inhibition percentage against extract concentration. Tests were carried out in triplicate.

Total Phenolic Compounds Determination

Total soluble phenolics in the mushroom methanolic extract was determined with Folin-Ciocalteu reagent according to the method of Slinkard and Singleton (1977) by using gallic acid as a standard. 1.0 ml mushroom extract solution was taken in a volumetric flask and was diluted with 45ml of distilled water. 1ml Folin-Ciocalteu reagent was added and mixed thoroughly. After 5 min, 2ml of Na_2CO_3 (2 per cent) was added and the mixture was allowed to stand for 2½ hours with intermittent shaking. The absorbance of developed blue colour was measured at 760 nm. The concentration of total phenols was expressed as mg/g of the dry extract (Kim *et al.*, 2003). The concentration of total phenolic compounds in the mushroom methanolic extract was determined as µg of gallic acid equivalent by using an equation that was obtained from standard gallic acid graph.

$$\text{Absorbance} = 0.0009 \times \text{gallic acid } (\mu g)$$

Nitric Oxide Scavenging Activity Assay

Sodium nitroprusside in aqueous solution at physiological pH spontaneously generates nitric oxide, which interacts with oxygen to produce nitrite ions.This can be determined by the use of the Griess Illosvoy reaction. 2 ml of 10 mM sodium nitroprusside in 0.5 ml phosphate buffer saline (pH 7.4) was mixed with 0.5 ml of extract at various concentrations and the mixture was incubated at 25°C for 2½ hours. From the incubated mixture 0.5 ml was taken out and added into 1.0 ml sulfanilic acid reagent (33 per cent in 20 per cent glacial acetic acid) and incubated at room temperature for 5 min. Finally, 1.0 ml naphthyl ethylenediamine dihydrochloride (0.1 per cent w/v) was mixed and incubated at room temperature for 30 min. The absorbance at 546 nm was measured by UV-Vis spectrophotometer (Figure 36.11). The nitric oxide radicals scavenging activity was calculated according to the following equation:

$$\text{Per cent Inhibition} = (A_0 - A_1)/A_0 \times 100$$

where,

A_0 is the absorbance of the control and A_1 is the absorbance of test sample.

Superoxide Radical Scavenging Activity Assay

This activity was measured using NBT (nitroblue tetrazolium reagent) method as described by Sabu and Ramadasan (2002). The method is based on generation of superoxide radical (O^-_2) by auto-oxidation of hydroxylamine hydrochloride in presence of NBT, which gets reduced to nitrite. Nitrite in presence of EDTA gives a color that was measured at 560 nm. Test solutions of extract (20–200 µg/ml) were taken in a test tube. To this, reaction mixture consisting of 1 ml of (50 mM) sodium carbonate, 0.4 ml of (24 mM) NBT and 0.2 ml of 0.1 mM EDTA solutions were added to the test tube and immediate reading was taken at 560 nm. About 0.4 ml of (1 mM) of hydroxylamine hydrochloride was added to initiate the reaction then reaction mixture was incubated at 25°C for 15 min and reduction of NBT was measured at 560 nm. Ascorbic acid was used as the reference compound. Decreased absorbance of the reaction mixture indicates increased superoxide anion scavenging activity. All the extracts of mushroom extract were treated in the similar manner, absorbance was recorded and the percentage of inhibition was calculated according to the following equation:

$$\% \text{ Inhibition} = (A_0 - A_1)/A_0 \times 100$$

where,

A_0 is the absorbance of the control (blank) and A_1 is the absorbance of test samples. All the tests were performed in triplicate and the graph was plotted with the mean values.

Statistical Analysis

Data are expressed as mean ± SD. Means of triplicate analyses were calculated. A difference was considered to be statistically significant when $p < 0.05$.

Results and Discussion

Antioxidant Activity of Methanolic Mushroom Extract

Inhibition of DPPH Radical

DPPH is a stable free radical at room temperature and accepts an electron or hydrogen radical to become a stable diamagnetic molecule (Soares *et al.*, 1997). The reduction capability of DPPH was determined by the decrease in its absorbance at λ=517 nm, which is induced by antioxidants. Positive

DPPH test suggests that the methanolic extract of the mushroom was free radical scavenger. The scavenging effect of mushroom extract and ascorbic acid on DPPH radical was compared. On the DPPH radical, mushroom extract had significant scavenging effects with increasing concentrations in the range of 20–100 μg/ml when compared with that of ascorbic acid (Figure 36.1). 100 μg/ml of mushroom extract and ascorbic acid exhibited 79.8 per cent and 99.8 per cent inhibition respectively (Table 36.1). The IC50 values were found to be 67.12 and 28.42 μg/ml for mushroom and ascorbic acid, respectively (Table 36.2). The different concentrations of mushroom extract (20, 40, 60, 80 and 100 μg/ml) showed antioxidant activities in a dose dependent manner on DPPH radical.

Table 36.1: Antioxidant Activity of *Morchella esculenta* of Different Concentrations of the Extract by Per cent Inhibition on Different Free Radical Formation and Ascorbic acid (Standard)

Group	*Concentration (μg/ml)*	*Per cent Inhibition*		
		Nitric -oxide	*DPPH*	*Super-oxide*
Methanolic extract of mushroom	20	37.2±0.45	39.7±0.87	36.12±0.77
	40	40.01±0.36	49.8±0.81	40.10±0.87
	60	42.04±0.53	58.9±0.96	44.9±0.34
	80	46.02±0.65	67.9±0.94	48.10±0.65
	100	49.04±0.23	70.8±0.89	52.9±0.76
Ascorbic acid (Standard)	20	48.3±0.56	64.2±0.65	46.10±0.98
	40	50.02±0.76	74.2±0.77	50.9±0.88
	60	52.04±0.87	84.2±0.98	54.10±0.79
	80	57.03±0.74	94.2±0.86	60.8±0.87
	100	63.02±0.84	104.3±0.87	64.9±0.86

Values are: Mean ± Standard Deviation (n = 3). $p < 0.05$.

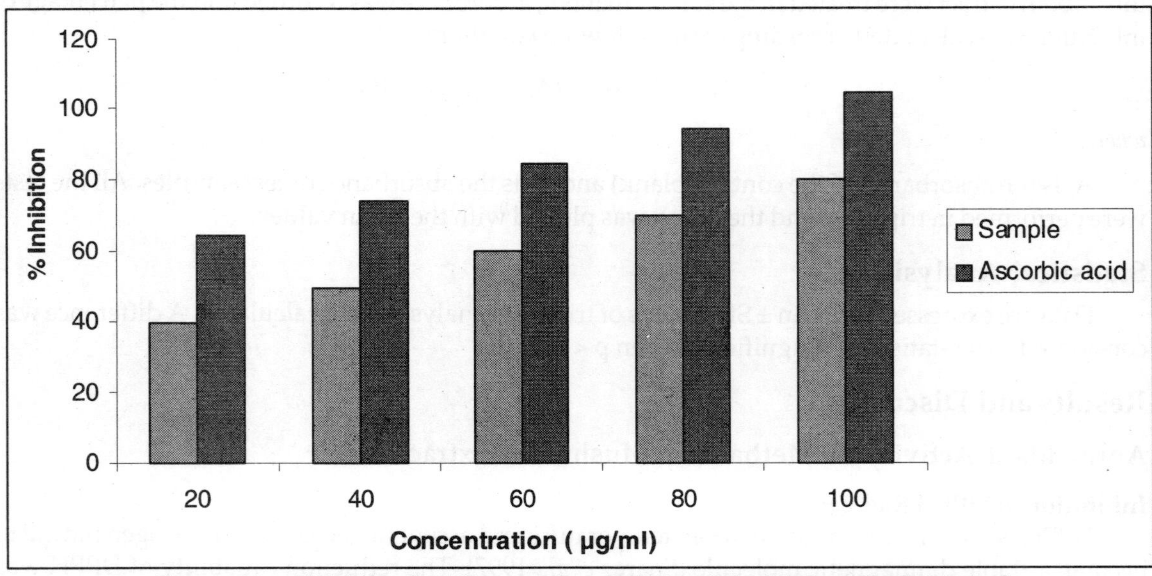

Figure 36.1: DPPH Radical Scavenging Activity of the Methanolic Extract of *Morchella esculenta* at Different Concentrations

Table 36.2: Total Phenolic Content (µg GAEs/mg extract) and IC50 (µg/ml) Values of DPPH, Super-oxide and Nitric-oxide of Methanolic Extract of *Morchella esculenta* and Ascorbic Acid (Standard)

Morchella esculenta	*Total Phenolic Compounds (µg GAEs/mg extract)*	*IC50 Values (µg/ml)*	*Mushroom methanolic Extract*	*Ascorbic Acid*
Methanolic extract	23.42±0.89	DPPH	67.12	28.42
		Super-oxide	102.14	36.23
		Nitric-oxide	114.34	67.13

Values: Mean ± Standard Deviaton (n = 3). $p < 0.05$.

Determination of Total Phenolic Content

The total amount of phenolic content present in the mushroom extract is shown in Figure 36.1, which was detected to be 47.01 ± 0.29 µg/mg gallic acid equivalent of phenols. These results suggest that the higher levels of antioxidant activity is due to the presence of phenolic components. Phenols are very important plant constituents because of their scavenging ability due to their hydroxyl groups (Hatano *et al.*, 1989). The phenolic compounds may contribute directly to antioxidative action (Duh *et al.*, 1999). It is known that polyphenolic compounds have inhibitory effects on mutagenesis and carcinogenesis in humans when ingested up to 1 g daily from a diet rich in fruits and vegitables (Tanaka *et al.*, 1998). Phenolic compounds from mushrooms are known to be good natural antioxidants. However, the activity of synthetic antioxidants was often observed to be higher than that of natural antioxidants (Ningappa *et al.*, 2007). Phenolic compounds, at certain concentrations, markedly slowed down the rate of conjugated diene formation. The interests of phenolics are increasing in the food industry because they retard oxidative degradation of lipids and thereby improve the quality and nutritional value of foods (Aneta *et al.*, 2007).

Nitric-oxide Radical Scavenging Assay

Nitric oxide plays an important role in various types of inflammatory processes in the animal body. In this study, the methanolic mushroom extract of *M. esculenta* was checked for its inhibitory effect on nitric oxide production. Nitric oxide radical generated from sodium nitroprusside at physiological pH was found to be inhibited by the mushroom extract. The various concentrations of the extract (20–100 µg/ml) showed 37.2 per cent, 40.01 per cent, 42.04 per cent, 46.02 per cent and 49.04 per cent inhibition, respectively. Results showed the percentage of inhibition in a dose dependent manner (Figure 36.2). A 100 µg/ml of the extract and ascorbic acid exhibited 49.04 per cent and 63.02 per cent inhibition, respectively. The concentration of the extract needed for 50 per cent inhibition (IC50) was found to be 114.34 µg/ml, whereas 67.13 µg/ml was needed for ascorbic acid (Table 36.2). These results were found to be statistically significant ($P < 0.05$).

Superoxide Radical Scavenging Assay

Superoxide is a reactive oxygen species, which can cause damage to the cells and DNA leading to various diseases. It was therefore proposed to measure the comparative interceptive ability of the antioxidant extracts to scavenge the superoxide radical. Several in vitro methods are available for generation of superoxide radicals (Vani *et al.*, 1997). In our study, superoxide radicals were generated by auto-oxidation of hydroxylamine in presence of NBT (nitroblue tetrazolium). The reduction of NBT in presence of antioxidants was measured. The decrease of absorbance at 560 nm with antioxidants

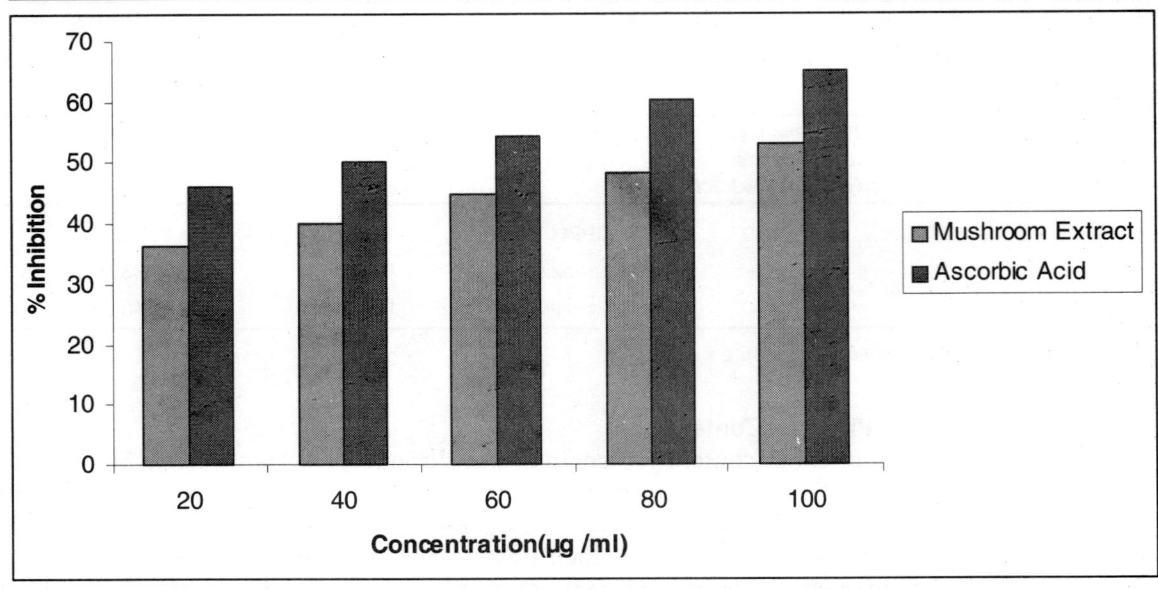

Figure 36.2: Nitric-oxide Radical Scavenging Activity of the Methanolic Extract of *Morchella esculenta*

thus indicates the consumption of superoxide anion in the reaction mixture. Different concentrations of methanolic mushroom extract (20–100 µg/ml) had strong superoxide scavenging activity (36.12 per cent,40.10 per cent, 44.9 per cent, 48.10 per cent and 52.9 per cent inhibition, respectively). A 100 µg/ml of methanolic mushroom extract and ascorbic acid exhibited 52.9 per cent and 64.9 per cent inhibition, respectively (Figure 36.3). IC50 value of methanolic mushroom extract on superoxide radical scavenging activity was found to be 102.14 µg/ml, whereas the IC50 value of ascorbic acid was found

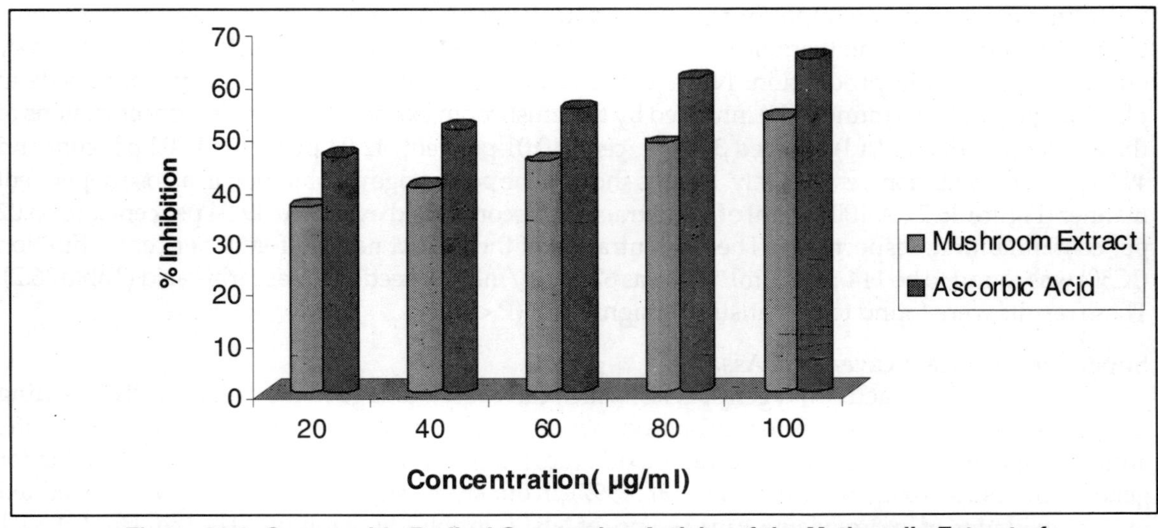

Figure 36.3: Super-oxide Radical Scavenging Activity of the Methanolic Extract of *Morchella esculenta* at Different Concentrations

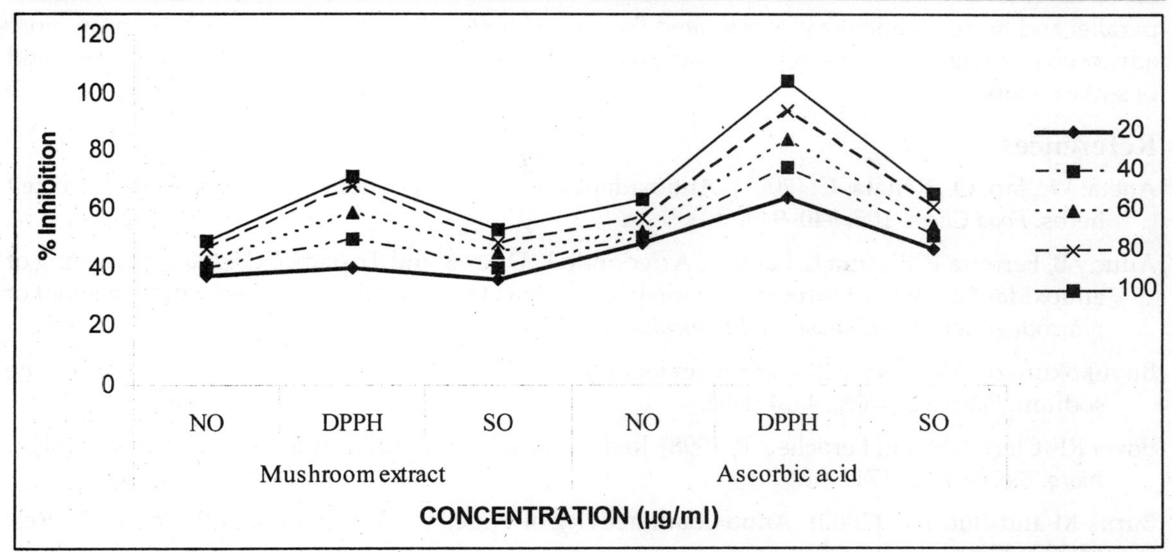

Figure 36.4: The Graph Represents Comparative Study of Per cent Inhibition of Different Free Radical Formation by Different Mushroom Concentrations along with Standard (Ascorbic acid)

Values are: NO = Nitric oxide, DPPH = 1,1-Diphenyl-2-picrylhydroxyl, SO = Superoxide

to be 36.69 μg/ml (Table 36.2). All of the extracts had a scavenging activity on the superoxide radicals in a dose dependent manner (20–100 μg/ml in the reaction mixture). Nonetheless, when compared to ascorbic acid, the superoxide scavenging activity of the extract was found to be low. This could be due to the presence of reactive concentration of bioactive constituents and mixture of other nutrients in the extract. Results were found statistically significant ($P < 0.05$).

Oxidative stress has been implicated in the pathology of many diseases such as Parkinson disease, Alzheimer, diabetes, cardiovascular disoders, aging and inflammatory conditions etc. The results obtained in the present studies may be attributed to several reasons *i.e.*, scavenging of superoxide radicals, nitric oxide radicals and DPPH radicals generated in the mammalian cells, involved in the regulation of various physiological processes. However, excess production of these radicals are associated with several diseases (Ialenti, 1993). In the present study the nitrite produced by the incubation of solutions of sodium nitroprusside in standard phosphate buffer at 25 °C was reduced by the methanolic extract of the investigated mushroom. This may be due to the antioxidant principles in the extract which compete with oxygen to react with nitric oxide thereby inhibiting the generation of these free radicals. Superoxide dismutase catalyses the dismutation of the highly reactive superoxide anion to oxygen and hydrogen peroxide (Kamalakkannan, 2003). Superoxide anion is the first reduction product of oxygen (Ray, 2002), which is measured in terms of inhibition of generation of O_2.

According to the several references which reported antiinflammatory,antibacterial and antitumoral activities of this mushroom have previously been investigated (Mau *et al.*, 2004; Elmasta *et al.*, 2006; Nitha *et al.*, 2007; Ramirez-Anguiano *et al.*, 2007). Based on a detailed report on the antioxidant activity of *M. esculenta*, it has exhibited excellent activity patterns in beta-carotene/linoleic acid, reducing power, and metal chelating effect systems (Mau *et al.*, 2004). In the light of these reports, our results are parallel and more excellent as investigated the antioxidant activity of the test mushrooms in more advanced scavenging test systems *viz.*, nitric oxide, super oxide and DPPH systems and find best and positive results.

References

Aneta, W., Jan, O., Renata, C. (2007). Antioxidant activity and phenolic compounds in 32 selected herbs. *Food Chem.* 105, 940–949.

Auudy B, Ferreira F, Blasina L, Lafon F, Arredondo F, Dajas R and Tripathi PC. (2003). Screening of antioxidant activity of three Indian medicinal plants traditionally used for the management of neurodegenerative diseases. *J. Ethanopharmacol.*, 84: 131-138.

Buyukokuroglu ME, Oktay M and Kufrevioglu (2001). *In vitro* antioxidant properties of dantrolene sodium. *Pharmacol. Res.*, 44: 491-95.

Boyer RF, Clark HM and Leroche AP (1998). Reduction and release of ferritin iron by plant phenols, *J. Inorq. Biochem.* 32: 171-181.

Burits M and Bucar F. (2000). Antioxidant activity of Nigella sativa essential oil. Phytother Res. 14:323–328.

Cuendet M, Hostettmann K and Potterat O. (1997). Iridoid glucosides with free radical scavenging properties from Fagraea blumei. *Helv Chim Ac.* 80: 1144-1152.

Duh, P.D., Tu, Y.Y., Yen, G.C. (1999). Antioxidative activity of water extracts of Hamgjyur (Chrysanthemum morifolium). Lebensm.-Wiss. *Technol.* 32: 269–277.

Dapkevicius, A., Venskutonis, R., Van Beek, T.A., Linssen, P.H. (1998). Antioxidant activity of extracts obtained by different isolation procedures from some aromatic herbs grown in Lithuania. *Journal of the Science of Food Agriculture.* 77: 140–146.

Hatano, T., Edamatsu, R., Mori, A. (1989). Effects of interaction of tannins with coexisting substances. *Chem. Pharm. Bull.* 37, 2016–2021.

Joyce DA. (1987). Oxygen radicals in disease. *Adv. Drug Reac. Bull.*, 127: 476-479.

Kim, D., Jeong, S., Lee, C.H. (2003). Antioxidant capacity of phenolic phytochemicals from various cultivars of plums. *Food Chem.* 81, 321–326.

Mau, J. L., Chang, C.-N., Huang, S.-J., and Chen, C.-C. (2004). Antioxidant properties of methanolic extracts from *Grifola frondosa*, *Morchella esculenta* and *Termitomyces albuminosus mycelia*. *Food Chemistry*, 87, 111–118.

Miller AL (1996). Antioxidant flavonoids: structure, function and clinical. *Alt. Med. Rev* 1: 103-111.

Ningappa, M.B., Dinesha, R., Srinivas, L. (2007). Antioxidant and free radical scavenging activities of polyphenol-enriched curry leaf extract (*Murraya koenigii* L.). *Food Chem.*. doi:10.1016/j.foodchem.2007.06.057.

Oyaizu, M. (1986). Studies on products of browning reactions: Antioxidative activities of products of browning reaction prepared from glucosamine. *Jpn. J. Nut.*, 44: 307-315.

Slinkard K and Singleton V L (1977) Total phenol analyses: automation and comparison with manual methods. *American J. Enolo. Viticul.* 28: 49–55.

Tiwari A. (2001). Imbalance in antioxidant defense and human diseases: Multiple approach of natural antioxidants therapy. *Curr. Sci.*, 81: 1179-1187.

Tanaka, M., Kuei, C.W., Nagashima, Y. (1998). Application of antioxidative maillrad reaction products from histidine and glucose to sardine products. *Nippon Suisan Gakkaishi* 47: 1409–1414.

Tiwari A. (2001). Imbalance in antioxidant defense and human diseases: Multiple approach of natural antioxidants therapy. *Curr. Sci.,* 81: 1179-1187.

Sabu, M.C., Ramadasan, K. (2002). Anti-diabetic activity of medicinal plants and its relationship with their antioxidant property. *J. Ethanopharmacol.* 81: 155–160.

Valentao, P., Lopes, G., Valente, M., Barbosa, P., Andrade, P. B., Silva, B. M., Baptista, P., and Seabra, R.M. (2005b). Quantitation of nine organic acids in wild mushrooms. *Journal of Agricultural and Food Chemistry*, 53: 3626–3630.

Microbial Biotechnology and Ecology (2011) *Pages* **616–623**
Editors: **Deepak Vyas, G.S. Paliwal, P.K.Khare and R.K Gupta**
Published by: **DAYA PUBLISHING HOUSE, NEW DELHI**

Chapter 37

Antibacterial Potential of *Morchella esculenta* Against Some Human Pathogenic Bacteria

Javed Ahmad Wagay*, Poonam Dehariya, Anjali C. and Deepak Vyas

Lab of Microbial Technology and Plant Pathology, Department of Botany, Dr. H.S. Gour Central University, Sagar – 470 03, M.P.

ABSTRACT

Methanolic extract of *Morchella esculenta* was investigated for its *in vitro* antibacterial activity.The antibacterial activity of this mushroom was evaluated against eight human pathogenic bacteria on the basis of inhibition zones by using disc diffusion and well diffusion methods.The minimum inhibitory concentration (MIC) and minimum bacterial concentration (MBC) of the extract (µg/ml)were also determined. The lowest value of MIC and MBC were obtained for *Vibrio cholariae* (MIC-78.52µg/ml) and *E. coli* (MBC-88.76 µg/ml) and maximum value of MIC and MBC were found against *Streptococcus* sp. (MIC-97.66 µg/ml) and *Vibrio* sp. (MBC-151.05 µg/ml). The mushroom was found to have no antagonistic effect against *Enterococcus* sp.

Introduction

Morchella esculenta (Guchi or sponge mushroom) belongs to family Helvellaceae is the most therapeutic and highly priced mushroom found in Himalayan ranges of extreme north western extremity of Indian subcontinent–Kashmir (J and K). The state is located between 32°-17 and 37°-5 north latitude and 73°-26 and 80°-30 east longitude and its average height from the mean sea level

* E-mail: ufaq07@rediffmail.com/javediqbal49@gmail.com

varies from 30 to 7200 meters. The average rain fall is 150cm and the temperature remains moderate from 20 to 30°C through out the year. Due to suitable environmental conditions the region is rich in mushroom diversity especially different species of *Morchella*. The mature ascocarp of *Morchella* consists of a stalk like portion–the stipe surrounded by hollow, conical cap. The cap is 3-6 cm in diameter, 4-8 cm long, pale brownish cream, globose to ovoid. Surface covered with irregularly interwoven pits of various shapes, framed by irregular ridges following the pits, edges of the ridges usually not darker than the pits. The stem (stipe) is 2-8 cm long, 2-4 cm in diameter, glabrous, round, much larger at the base, wrinkled, grooved longitudinally, covered with small scurfy tufts, fragile and hollow. The Asci long, cylindrical, hyaline, 280-320 × 18-22 μm in diameter. Flesh is waxy, thin, whitish and produce spores. Each spore is 18-25 × 115 μm in diameter, and ellipsoid in shape with smooth surface. The honey combed surface of pileus gives it the appearance of a sponge. It is pitted and ridged by and is about the same length as the stipe. It mostly grows in soil rich in organic matter usually in dense deciduous forest litler and fruits in the spring. Its growing season is usually from 15 April to July and is mostly used as food and ethenomedicine after sun dried by the tribals of Kashmir.

The usage of this mushroom as medicine has a long history dates back 3000 BC in the Roman and Greek civilisation (Singh, 2000). They produce a series of biologically active compounds to prevent themselves from being victimised to different microorganisms such as bacteria and pathogenic fungi. They provide a rich and varied source of terpenoids that have antibiotic and antifungal activities (Ayer and Browne, 1981). Benedict and Brady (1972) tested the potential of some mushrooms on some bacteria and reported that the best inhibitory responses were seen against some gram +ve organisms including acid fast bacterium (*M. smegnatis*) and pathogenic strains of yeast (*C. albicans*). *Morchella esculenta* is being used in traditional Chinese medicine to treat indigestion, phlegm, croup, and shortness of breath (Ying *et al.*, 1987). The anti-tumour activity of ethanolic extract of *Morchella esculenta* mycelium grown in submerged culture was determined by the mouse solid tumour model induced by Daltons Lymphoma ascite cells. Oral administration of the morel extract resulted in a 74.1 per cent inhibition in tumor volume and 79.1 per cent decrease in tumor weight 30 days after tumor cell implantation (Nitha and Janardhanan, 2005). Later research further confirmed the antitumor activity of the extract against both ascites and solid tumours (Nitha *et al.*, 2007). Methanolic extracts prepared from the mycelia of *M. esculenta* showed high antioxidant activity as compared to some antioxidants such as ascorbic acid, and α-tocopherol respectively (Mau *et al.*, 2004).

Although bioactive polysaccharides are wide spread among mushrooms, different species can produce different types of polysaccharides having different antimicrobial properties. Antimicrobial drugs have long been used for prophylactic and therapeutic purposes, but the recent increase in the drug resistant bacterial strians is creating serious problems. Consequently the antimicrobial activities of various antibacterial polysaccharides from different mushrooms are being evaluated in terms of their clinical efficacy. A lot of review is available which proved that research has been going the different aspects of *Morchella esculenta* especially its anticancerous and antidiabetic properties but little work has been reported on its antibacterial activity in Indian sub continent. So the present research was therefore designed to investigate antibacterial potiential of methanolic extract from whole ascocarp including stipe of *Morchella esculenta* against different human pathagenic bacteria.

Materials and Methods

Extraction

Morchella esculenta fruiting bodies were collected in March–April, 2009 from coniferous forests of Kashmir. The fruiting bodies were dried in an oven at 40°C for 4 hour. The specimens were taken to

Mushroom Culture Collection Centre–Sher-e-Kashmir Agriculture University of Science and Technology (SKAUST), Srinagar (Kashmir) for identification.The dried fruiting bodies were crushed to powder by using electronic blender. About 20g of powder were taken in 200ml of 95 per cent methanol in soxhlet extraction unit for extraction at 30°C for 12-18 hours. The extraction was filtered through Whatman no.4 filter paper. The methanolic extract was then vacuum rotary evaporated at 30°C to dryness. The extract was redissolved in 95 per cent methanol to a concentration of 10mg/ml and stored at 4°C for further use.

Test Microorganisms

Th antibacterial investigation of *M. esculenta* was measured against eight bacterial cultures namely *Klebsiella pneumoniae,Vibrio cholariae* (MTCC.1168), *E. coli* (MTCC.1581), *Pseudomonas auroginosa* (MTCC.1568), *Vibrio* sp., *Streptococcus* sp., *Bacilus* subtilis (MTCC.1789) and *Enterococcus* sp. Bacterial cultures were obtianed from Microbial type culture collection (MTCC) Chandigarh (Haryana) and Chandraka Pathological Laboratory, Jabalpur (M.P).The disc diffusion method outlined by the Natural committee for clinical laboratory standards (NCCLS) was used with 40µg/ml chloramphenical disc as reference antibiotic. The size of inhibitory zones were measured in millimeters after incubation period of 24 hours at 37±1°C in thermostate incubator.

Screening of Antibacterial Activity of Mushroom Crude Extract

Antibacterial property of *Morchella esculenta* methanol extract was determined by disc diffusion method (Brown *et al.*, 2005). All the bacterial strains mentioned were incubated at 37±0.1°C for 24-48 hours in Nutrient broth (NB). The culture suspension were prepared and adjusted by comparing against 0.4-0.5 MC Farland standard turbidity tubes. Nutrient agar was poured in to each sterilised Petri dish (10×100 mm) and allow it to solidify for overnight in refrigerator. The bacterial cultures (100µl of each) were inoculated on sterilized agar surface of each plate. The bacterial culture was being spread evenly on the surface by using a glass swab to and fro by rotating the plates at 60°C to ensure homogeneously distribution of inoculam. After allowing the inoculam to dry at room temperature, the disc loaded with the extract of desired concentrations and placed on the agar plates. The positive control was maintained using chloramphenicol (Antibiotic) solution of 0.40µg/ml concentration. The plates were then inoculated at 37±0.1°C for about 16-24 hours. Subsequently the plates were examined for bacterial growth inhibition and the radius of zones of inhibition around each disc was measured in millimeters respectively. The plates were made in trilicates to get the accurate antibacterial results.

Minimum Inhibitory Concentration (MIC) and Minimum Bacterial Concentration (MBC)

MIC and MBC were determined by varying the concentration of mushroom extract followed by Agar well diffusion assay (Prescottet, 2000). For MBC, the concentration ranging from 1-1000µg/ml were prepared that showed antibacterial activity during the preliminary screening. Four different concentrations were 100 µg/ml, 250 µg/ml, 500 µg/ml and 750 µg/ml respectively. A drop of each concentration of each extract was dispensed in to each well using calibrated dropper.The plates were incubated at 37±0.1°C for 18-24 hours. The minimum concentration that showed inhibition was taken as MIC (Table 37.2). Similarly the solution for MBC determination was prepared by 2 times serial decrease dilution from 290 to 100µg/ml. Wells of 6mm diameter were bored in each agar plate and each well was loaded with different concentrations to determine its MBC after incubation period of 24-

48 hours at 37±0.1ºC The lowest dilution yielding no growth at all was taken to be its MBC.The MIC and MBC assay were performed thrice to make accurate results.The different values of MIC and MBC are given in Table 37.2.

Results and Discussion

The *M. esculenta* used in the present investigation has been found to have broad antibacterial potential against different tested human pathogenic bacteria.This has been proved by clear zones of inhibition. Produced by methanol extract impregnated discs of different concentrations (Figure 37.1). The results proved that the mushroom extract was highly effective against all investigated test bacteria. The best *in vitro* antibacterial activity of extract was found against *Streptococcus* sp. in which zone of inhibition was measured to be 28.33 mm at an concentration of 100 µg/ml (Figure 37.1 and Table 37.1). The second bacteria which found to be highly susceptible against extract was *Klebsiella pneumoniae* in which zone of inhibition was measured to be 25.99 mm which is followed by *Bacllus subtilis, E. coli, Vibrio* sp., *Pseudomonas aeruginosa* and *V. cholariae* with zone diameters 25.83mm, 22.3mm, 22.30mm, 18.65mm and 16.66mm respectively (Table 37.1). The results clearly shows that extract has highest antigonastic activity against *Streptococcus* sp. and lowest against *Vibrio cholariae* respectively shown by graphical representation in Figure 37.2.

Table 37.1: Antibacterial Activity of Methanolic Extract (100µg/ml) of *Morchella esculenta* Against Different Human Pathogenic Bacteria

Name of Bacteria	*Zones of Inhibition (mm)*		
	Mushroom Extract	*Positive Control*	*Negative Control*
Streptococcus sp.	28.33±0.22	36.66±0.71	12.33±0.80
K. pneumoniae	25.99±0.5	33.83±1.82	9.16±0.88
Bacillus subtilis	25.83±0.33	32.0±0.16	9.83±0.5
E. coli	22.33±0.33	30.33±0.25	12.99±0.32
Vibrio sp.	22.30±0.43	31.83±0.5	0
P. auroginosa	18.65±0.67	28.8±1.67	0
V. cholariae	16.66±0.65	24.3±1.25	6.33±0.93
Enterococcus sp.	0	28.2±0	0

Values: Mean ±Standard deviation (SD).

Positive control = Chloramphenicol (Antibiotic).

Negative control = 95 per cent methanol.

The antibacterial activity of the extract was quantitively assessed by determining the minimum inhibitory concentration (MIC) and minimum bacterial concentration (MBC) shown in Table 37.2. It had been considered that if the MIC of the extract was less than 100µg/ml, the antibacterial property was best, if MIC value is ranging from 100-500 µg/ml was value found to better and if the MIC value was found to be ranging from 500-750µg/ml was considered weak and similarly if MIC was found to be ranging between 750-1000µg/ml was considered inactive respectively (Khan *et al.*, 2009).The present study on antibacterial activity of *M. esculenta* has been found to have broad antibacterial activities as its MIC against each test bacteria was below 100µg/ml respectively. However, the highest MIC value was found against *Streptococcus* sp. (97.66µg/ml) and least against *Vibrio cholariae* (78.52µg/ml).

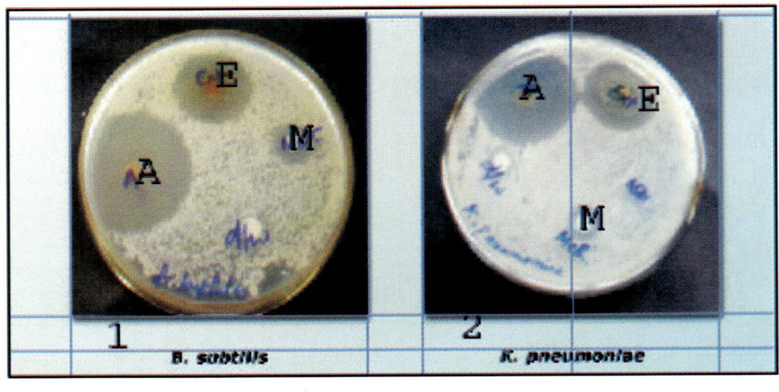

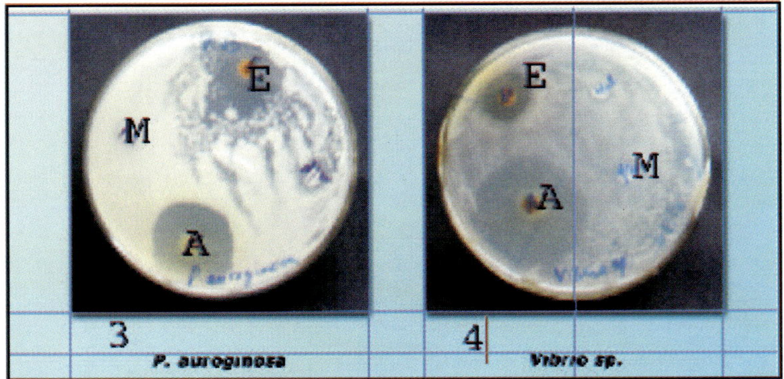

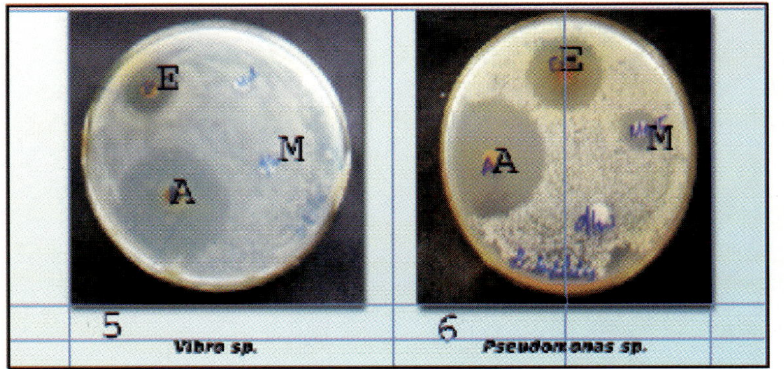

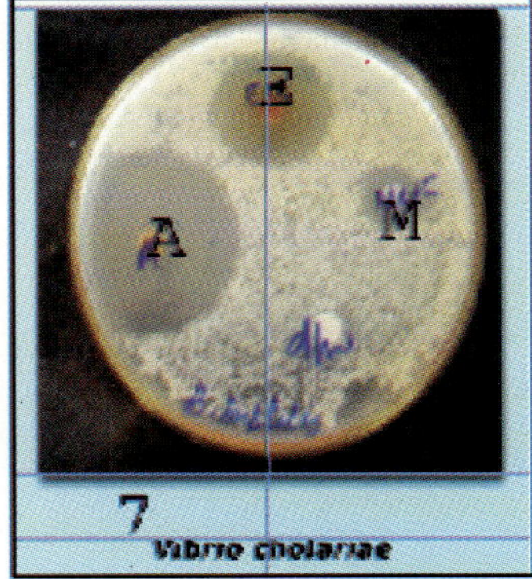

Figure 37.1: Plates Showing Zones of Inhibition by Mushroom Extract (mm), Positive and Negative Control Against Different Bacteria

Values: A = Positive control, E= Extract, M = Negative control

1: *Streptococcus* sp., 2: *K. pneumoniae*, 3: *B. subtilis*, 4: *E. coli*, 5: *Vibrio* sp, 6: *P. auroginosal* 7: *V. cholariae*

Similarly the minimum concentration at which no bacterial growth was observed was considered to be its MBC, the minimum value of MBC was found against *E. coli* (88.76µg/ml) and maximum value of MBC was found against *V. cholariae* (133.09 µg/ml). Table 37.2 also shows MIC and MBC values of mushroom extract against other bacteria as well. This clearly proved that the extract highly suppressed

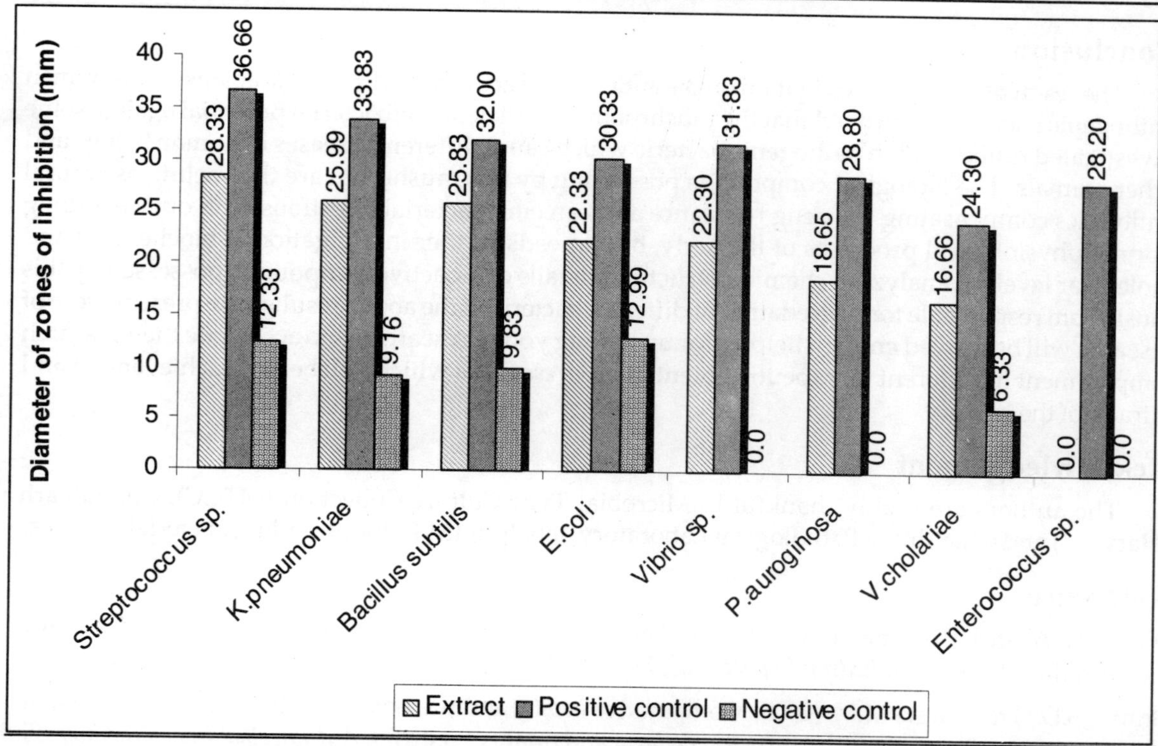

Figure 37.2: Graphical Representation of Extract Showing Different Values Against Each Bacteria

the growth and may not allow bacterial genome either to undergo normal processes of transcription and translation or may not allow for the synthesis of its cell wall which resulted the death of its strains simultaneously at very low concentrations which clearly proved beyond any doubt that *M. esculenta* is a valuable mushroom having sufficient therapeutic potential especially antibacterial activity. It also proved that most of the bio active compounds of this mushroom are highly soluble in methanol, hence methanol is a best solvent for extraction. The result also depicts that disc diffusion method is a satisfactory and result oriented method for the detection of antibacterial properties of mushrooms.

Table 37.2: Mushroom Extract of *M. esculenta* Shows Minimum Inhibitory Concentration (MIC in µg/ml) and Minimum Bacterial Concentration (MBC in µg/ml)

Bacteria	*MIC µg/ml*	*MBC µg/ml*
Streptococcus sp.	97.66	99.43
K. pneumoniae	95.87	101.12
B. subtilis	89.92	112.07
E. coli	89.68	88.76
Vibrio sp.	87.86	151.05
P. auroginosa	78.66	106.85
V. cholariae	78.52	133.09

Conclusion

The result of present investigation on the antibacterial activity of *M. esculenta* against some human pathogenic bacteria has proved that the mushroom has efficient antibacterial potential against some investigated tested human pathogenic bacteria which cause different diseases in human beings and other animals. The biological compounds possessing by this mushroom are thus acting as natural antibiotics compensating the drug resistance and can cure bacterial infections with out disturbing normal physiological processes of the body, but it needs further investigation at biochemical and molecular level for analyzing chemical structural details of bioactive compounds possessed by this mushroom responsible for degredation of different bacteria in the above results. The present piece of research will be proved enough helpful for upcoming young researchers to accelerate their research temperament in different therapeutic potential of *M. esculenta* which will be a big achievement and miracle of the century.

Acknowledgement

The authors are highly thankful to Microbial Type Culture Collection (MTCC), Chandigarh (Haryana) and Chandraka Pathological Laboratory, Jabalpur (M.P) for providing bacterial cultures.

References

Ayer, W.A and Browne, L.M. (1981). Terpenoid metabolites of mushrooms and related Basidomycetes.*Tetrahedron Report* 110(37): 2199-2248.

Brown, S.D., Traczewski M.M. (2005). Comparative *in vitro* antimicrobial activity of a new carbepenem, doripenem: Tentative disc diffusion criteria and quality control.*J. Antimicobial Chemotherapy*. 55: 944-949.

Benedict, R.C. and Brady, L.R. (1972). Antimicrobial activity of mushroom metabolites. *J. Pharm. Sci.* 61: 180-182.

Bon Chang, S.T. and Mshigeni, K.E. (2001). *Mushroom and human health: their growing significance as potent dietary supplements*. University of Namibia, Windhoek, Namibia, 79.

Bose, S.R. (1946). Antibiotics in a Polypours (*Polystictus sanguineus*). *Nature* 158: 292-296.

Ikekawa, T. (2001). Beneficial effects of edible and medicinal mushrooms on health care. *Int. J. Med. Mush*. 3: 291-298.

Kan, N.A, Qureshi, S, Pandey, A.K and Ashutosh, S. (2009). Antibacterial activity of some medicinal mushrooms of central India. *Tur. J. Biol*. 33: 1-5.

National Committee for Clinical Laboratory Standards (NCCLS). Performance Standards for antimicrobial susceptibility tests, Approved standard NCCLS Publication M2-A5, Villanova, PA, USA, 1993.

Prescott, L.M, Harley, J.P. and Klein, D.A. (2002). *Microbiology* 5th edn; MC Graw-Hill. New York, N.Y. 10020: pp. 809-811.

Singsh, S.K., Upadhyay, R.C. and Verona, R.N. (2000). Physico-Chemical preferences for efficient mycelial colonization in edible mushrooms. *Mush. Res*. 9(2): 85-89.

Nitha, B., Janardhanan, K.K. (2005). Antioxidant, anti-inflammatory and antitumor activities of cultured mycelia of morel mushroom, *Morchella esculenta*. *Ind J. Med. Res*. 121: 133.

Nitha, B., Meera, C.R, Janardhanan, K.K. (2007). Anti-inflammatory and antitumor activities of cultured mycelium of morel mushroom, *Morchella esculenta*. *Curr. Sci.* 92(2): 235-239.

Mau, J.L, Chang, C.N, Huang, S.J, Chen, C.C. (2004). Antioxidant properties of methanolic extracts from *Grifola frondosa, Morchella esculenta* and *Termitomyces albuminossus* mycelia. *Food Chem.* 87(1): 11-18.

Ying J, Mao X, Ma Q, Zong Y, Wen H. (1987). *Icones of Medicinal Fungi from China*. Science Press, Beijing. 14: pp. 38-45.

Microbial Biotechnology and Ecology (2011)
Editors: **Deepak Vyas, G.S. Paliwal, P.K.Khare and R.K Gupta**
Published by: **DAYA PUBLISHING HOUSE, NEW DELHI**

Pages **624–665**

Chapter 38

Production and Partial Characterization of Fungal and Bacterial Cellulases on CMC and Cellulose Powder

☆ ***Deepak Vyas*[1] *and Ashish Vyas*[2]**

[1]*Lab of Microbial Technology, Department of Botany, Dr. H.S.G. University, Sagar*
[2]*Department of Biotechnology, Lovely University, Jalandhar, Punjab*

ABSTRACT

The endoglucanases, exoglucanases and β-glucosidases (cellulases complex) of fungi and bacteria were determined and presented in chapter 5. It was observed that fungal spp. have much more potential to produce cellulase enzymes than bacterial spp. Among fungi, *Aspergillus terreus, Aspergillus nidulans, Aspergillus flavus, Fusarium oxysporum, Penicillium rubrum, Phoma* sp., *Trichoderma viride* were found to be effective producer of all the three enzymes tested. Among bacterial genera, *Bacillus marinus, Bacillus* sp. (V2) and *Bacillus subtilis* were promising candidate for cellulolytic activity. *Aspergillus terreus, Aspergillus nidulans, Fusarium oxysporum, Bacillus marinus, Bacillus* sp. (V2) and *Bacillus subtilis* were selected for detailed study for their enzymatic potential. All the three enzymes (endoglucanases, exoglucanases and β-glucosidases) were found optimally active at acidic pH range in selected three fungi and bacterial spp. However, *Fusarium oxysporum* was found to show stable endoglucanase activity at alkaline pH range too. 60°C was found optimum for the maximum activity of endoglucanase and β-glucosidase and 50°C temperature for exoglucanases by *Aspergillus nidulans. Aspergillus terreus* was optimally active at pH 4 and 40°C for all the three enzymes tested. The increasing importance of endoglucanase enzyme in different industrial applications has placed this enzyme to be more important among other cellulases enzymes. Therefore to know the functioning of endoglucanase enzyme an attempt has been made to know the effect of some chemical reagent (EDTA, 2, 4 DNP, $HgCl_2$, $SnCl_2$). EDTA was found to be moderately affecting the endoglucanase activity in all the test organisms. 2, 4 DNP and $HgCl_2$ were found to inhibit almost complete endoglucanase activity (more than 90 per cent) at 5mM in all the test organisms. $SnCl_2$ showed moderate inhibitory effect on endoglucanase activity at 5mM concentration in the test organism.

Introduction

Cellulases refer to a group of enzymes which acting together, hydrolyze cellulose. Cellulose, is a homopolymer of about 8,000-12,000 glucose unit linked linearly by β-1,4-gycosidic linkages forming a crystalline unit held together by hydrogen bonding (Brown, 1982). Based on this structure, Reese *et al.* (1950) proposed a hypothesis that enzymatic hydrolysis of cellulose requires at least two enzymes C_1 and Cx. According to this hypothesis, C_1 enzymes render the crystalline cellulose accessible for hydrolytic attack and a Cx enzyme then hydrolyze the modified cellulose interaction of the original model of the C_1–Cx cellulolytic systems, as proposed by Reese *et al.*, 1950.

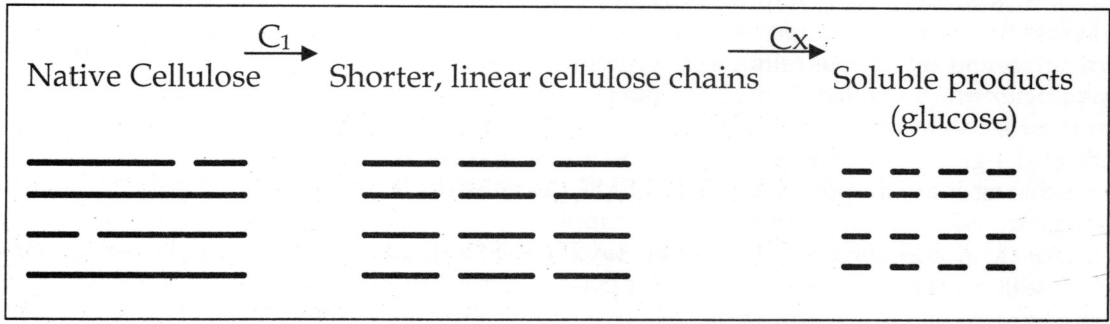

However, the original model of the C_1–Cx cellulolytic system as proposed by Reese *et al.* (1950). However, the precise action of C_1 was not made clear. Subsequently, Reese's suggestion was misinterpreted Cx was an endoglucanase that acted before C_1, a cellobiohydrolase (Wood *et al.*, 1989). The C_1 factor in 60s and 70s year of decade was not isolated and purified isolated and this model of cellulose degradation is now regarded as antiquated (Din *et al.*, 1994) and existence of C_1 enzyme is still obscure. However, furthermore considerable progress has been made in the understanding of the nature and function of cellulolytic enzymes therefore, the definition was modified. There are atleast three major types of hydrolytic enzymes involved in the degradation of native cellulose to glucose (Bhat and Bhat, 1997).

1. The endo-(1,4)-β-D-glucanase (synonyms: endoglucanase, endocellulase, carboxymethyl cellulase [EC 3.2.1.4]), which cleaves β-linkages at random, commonly in the amorphous parts of cellulose.
2. The exo-(1,4)-β-D glucanase (synonyms: cellobiohydrolases, exocellulase, microcrystalline cellulase, avicelase [EC 3.2.1.91]), which releases cellobiose from either the nonreducing or the reducing end, generally from crystalline part of cellulose.
3. The β-glucosidase (synonym: cellobiase [EC 3.2.1.21]), which releases glucose from cellobiose and short chain oligosaccharides.

Cellulases are distributed throughout the biosphere; they are most manifest in fungi and bacterial sources (Enari, 1983). In microbial sources these cellulolytic enzymes are either cell bound or extracellular. The ability to produce extracellular cellulolytic enzymes is widespread in fungi and bacteria and these systems have been extensively studied (Enari, 1983; Wood, 1985), however fungi are the most studied organisms with respect to cellulose degradation. Generally fungi hydrolyse cellulose to simple soluble sugar and utilize them as a carbon source in their metabolism. Cellulase biosynthesis is generally assumed to be subject to genetic and biochemical regulation. Cellulases are extracellular, inducible enzymes, the best inducer being cellulose, cellobiose, lactose and sophorose

(2-O-β-D-glycopyranosyl-D-glucose). Synthetic compounds as palmitate and acetate esters of disaccharides and thiocellobiose have also been shown to function as inducers of cellulases (Reese *et al.*, 1969). In virtually all microorganisms examined the synthesis of cellulases is induced by presence of cellulose and repressed in the presence of glucose. The most generally accepted view of the induction process is that the organism produced a basic level or a constitutive amount of cellulase thus giving rise to soluble hydrolysis product of cellulose, which enter the microbial cells and functions as inducer (Eriksson *et al.*, 1990). Cellulases catalyze the breakdown of the β-1,4 glucosidic linkages. It has been proposed that cellulase hydrolysis occurs by an acid catalysis mechanism at the active site (Reese *et al.*, 1950; Knowles *et al.*, 1987) proposed a two step mechanism that for a cellulase to attack crystalline cellulose two factors were required. Cx factor or carboxymethylcellulase is able to attack soluble derivatives and amorphous cellulose, but without activity against crystalline cellulose (*e.g.* cotton). C_1 was a factor which enabled Cx to act on cotton or native cellulose mechanism being by disrupting the structure of cellulose by breaking H-bonds. It is now well established fact that the C_1 fraction is an exo-acting β-1,4-glucanase (often referred as exocellulase or cellobiohydrolase) removing cellobiose from non reducing end of the polymer. It is now widely accepted that C_1 and cellobiohydrolase are identical (Gong *et al.*, 1979). The third member of the complex is β-1,4 glucosidase (cellobiase) which hydrolyze cellobiose to glucose. According to mechanism proposed by Eriksson (1969), amorphous region in the cellulose fibre are first attacked by endoglucanases, thereby exposing free chain ends. Exo-glucanases then come into action by hydrolytically removing cellobiose from the chain ends. The free cellobiose is hydrolyzed further to glucose through action of β-glucosidases. In general, cellulases are bimodular proteins with large catalytic and small cellulose binding module linked by short highly glycosylated protein sequence rich in Serine and Proline (Gilkes *et al.*, 1991). Most of the fungal cellulases are glycoproteins and exist in multiple forms (Coughlan and Ljunghdahl, 1988). These multicomponent enzymes are required to effectively participate in enzymatic reactions and physical homogeneity of the substrate. Proteolytic cleavage of cellulase separates the cellulose binding and catalytic fragments demonstrated the presence of a two-domain organisation in these enzymes (Gilkes *et al.*, 1988; Tomme *et al.*, 1988). The genes encoding cellulases are chromosomal in both fungi and bacteria. In fungi, cellulase genes are randomly distributed over the genome, with each gene having its own transcriptionally regulatory elements (Tomme *et al.*, 1995). In bacteria, the cellulase genes are either randomly distributed in *Clostridium thermocellum* (Guglielmi and Beguin, 1998) or clustered on the genome in *C. cellulolyticum, C. cellulovorans, C. acetobutylicum* (Belaich *et al.*, 1997; 1999). Cellulases enzymes are extracellular enzyme systems, strictly defined as those enzymes that have passed through the cytoplasmic membranes of the cell originally responsible for synthesis (Priest, 1984). Current theory indicates that these enzymes pass through the cell membranes in linear form and assume their tertiary structure outside the cell known as cotranslational secretion (Davis and Tai, 1980).

The best known fungal forms producing complete cellulase system is *Trichoderma reesei* (Mandel and Reese, 1964; Fagerstam and Pettersson, 1980) *Trichoderma koningi* (Wood and McCrae, 1972, 1975, 1986a; Fan *et al.*, 1987), *Penicillium funiculosum* (Wood *et al.*, 1980; Wood and McCrae, 1982; Wood and McCrae, 1986b), *Fusarium solani* (Wood, 1969, 1975; Wood and McCrae, 1977), *Fusarium oxysporum* (Christakopoulas *et al.*, 1989; Christakopoulas *et al.*, 1995a,b) and *Aspergillus niger* (Singh *et al.*, 1990, 1991) are other well known cellulolytic fungi. Anaerobic rumen inhabiting fungi also have the capability to degrade cellulose. The cellulolytic enzyme system is one of the rumen anaerobic fungi, *Neocalimastix frontalis*, has been studied by Wood *et al.* (1986).

Cellulose degradation in nature by bacterial system occur aerobically and anerobically. Bacterial degradation of cellulose seems to take by cluster of enzymes rather than by individual endo and exoglucanases as in the case of fungi (Ljungdahl and Eriksson, 1985). Cellulases of aerobic bacteria such as the *Cellulomonas* sp., appears to be tightly bound to their cellulose substrate and appear in the culture medium only in stationary phase (Langsford *et al.*, 1984). Various cellulolytic spp. of *Bacillus* such as *B. subtilis, B. polymyxa, B. brevis, B. licheniformis* and *B. cereus* have been described by number of workers (Knosel, 1971; Priest, 1977; Thayer, 1978; Robson and Chambliss, 1984, 1987).

Endoglucanase (CMCase) hydrolyze Carboxy Methyl Cellulose (CMC) or swollen cellulose in random fashion resulting in rapid decrease in chain length (Wood, 1985). Endoglucanases are thought to be primarily responsible for decreasing degree of polymerization by internally cleaving cellulose chain at relatively amorphous regions, thereby generating new cellulose chains ends susceptible to the action of cello biohydrolases (Teeri *et al.*, 1998). *Trichoderma reesei* produced three different endoglucanases *i.e.* EGI, EGII and EGIII, which also occur in multiple forms (Labudova and Farkas, 1983).

Exoglucanases act in a processive manner on the reducing or non-reducing ends of cellulose polysaccharides chains, liberating either glucose (glucanohydrolases) or cellobiose (cellobiohydrolases) as major products. Exoglucanases acts on microcrystalline cellulose, presumably peeling cellulose chain from the microcrystalline structure (Teeri, 1997). Cellobiohydrolases or exoglucanases degrade cellulose by hydrolyzing cellobiose units from non reducing end of the chain and have very limited action on substituted celluloses such as CMC and hydroxy ethyl cellulose (Bisaria and Mishra, 1989). Exoglucanases exhibit highly cooperative synergistic action in the presence of endoglucanases (Enari and Niku-Paavola, 1987; Bisharia and Mishra, 1989). Heterogeneity of cellobiohydrolases components from *T.reesei* and *Penicillium pinophillum* has been studied in detail (Wood and McCrae, 1986a; Wood *et al.*, 1988). A general feature of most cellulases is a modular structure of including both catalytic and carbohydrate modules (CBMs). The presence of CBMs is particularly important for the initiation and processivity of exoglucanases (Teeri *et al.*, 1998). Cellobiohydrolases activity is essential for the hydrolysis of microcrystalline cellulose. CBH I and CBH II are the principle components of the *T. reesei* cellulase systems representing 60 per cent and 20 per cent respectively, of the total cellulase protein produced by the fungus on the mass basis (Wood, 1992).

β-glucosidases or cellobiase (EC 3.2.1.21), one of the component of cellulase complex represent very small portion of the total extracellular protein secreted by *T. reesei.* β-glucosidase hydrolyzes degradation products of cellulose to glucose. β-glucosidases are characterized by their transferase activity, retention of the β-configration of glucose on hydrolysis, inhibition by low concentration of glucanolactone, and high activity toward cellotriose and less activity toward larger cellodextrins (Bisaria and Mishra, 1989). The purification of β-glucosidases from extracellular culture filtrates, intracellular extracts, and plasma membranes of organisms has reported by several groups (Bergem and Pettersson, 1973; Singh *et al.*, 1990). However, the exact genetic and biochemical relationship among these different β-glucosidases is not yet clear. Glycosides such as salicin (Mandel and Reese, 1964) are commercially available and have been used as substrate for determining β-glucosidase activity.

Cellulase activity in fungi and bacteria were greatly dependent upon factors like pH and temperature, and incubation period. In order to obtain economic hydrolysis of cellulose with maximum saccharification in short span of time it is essential to determine the optimum conditions. Enzymes being proteins contain ionizable groups and consequently the pH of the culture medium affects their structures and function.

In view of the above, an attempt has been made to investigate the cellulolytic capabilities of selected fungal and bacterial cultures. The present chapter is planned as follows:

- ☆ Determination of endoglucanase (CMCase), exoglucanase (FPase) and β-glucosidase enzyme activity in some fungal and bacterial cultures.
- ☆ Partial characterization of selected fungal and bacterial cultures *i.e.* determining its optimum pH and temperature range.
- ☆ Effect of some chemical reagents on endoglucanase (CMCase) activity of fungal and bacterial cultures.

Materials and Methods

Collection of Samples

The samples were collected from previously decomposing organic cellulosic and lignocellulosic waste subjected for degradation. For this different cellulosic substrates *viz.* Sugarcane bagasse waste, Sagaun saw dust, Mushroom wheat compost, Mushroom soyabean compost, decomposing *Polyalthia pendula* leaves manure, decomposing organic cellulosic waste, decomposing cellulosic laboratories waste, like cotton pieces, potato pith, paper waste etc were taken. For the above mentioned substrates (5 kg. each) were degraded in the pits of size 2ft. × 2ft. × 2ft. in the Botanic Garden of Department of Botany, Dr. Hari Singh Gour University, Sagar. These substrates were environmentally degraded for the period of 5 months from 28.09.01 to 28.02.02. After the appropriate time interval, 100 gm of decomposing residue is collected in the sterilized polythene bags and brought in the laboratory. The fungi were also isolated from Farmyard dung manure, nadib manure, chicken manure, decomposing newspaper, decomposing logs of wood, bark of *Magnifera indica* and garden soil and deseased portion of Lemon fruits (*Citrus* sp.), *Cicer arietinum, Saccharum officinarum.*

Isolation of Fungal and Bacterial Cultures

The decomposing residue brought in the laboratory was kept at 4°C±1. Isolation of fungi from the samples of different substrates was carried out using Czapek Dox Agar Medium (Dox, 1910).

Czapek Dox Agar Medium (gm/lt.)

☆ Sodium nitrate $NaNO_3$	3.00
☆ Dipotassium hydrogen phosphate K_2HPO_4	1.00
☆ Magnesium sulphate $MgSO_4.7H_2O$	0.50
☆ Potassium chloride KCl	0.50
☆ Ferrous sulphate $FeSO_4.7H_2O$	0.01
☆ Sucrose	30.00
☆ Agar	15.00
☆ Distilled Water	1000.00 ml
☆ pH	5.5

Fungi are isolated by direct agar plate method as per the method of Warcup (1955). A small amount of the sample (0.005-0.015 g) was taken from the sample with the help of sterile flattered tip needle and was dispersed in a drop of sterile water in the bottom of petridish. The sterilized Czapek

Dox Agar medium was then poured into the petri dish. The plated sample was dispersed in the plate by rotating the medium before its solidification. After this plates were kept in incubator at 28±1°C for their growth.

Isolation of cellulolytic bacteria was performed by enrichment techniques suggested by Hans and Srinivasan (1968). About 1 gm mixture of rotting cellulosic substrates was inoculated into the isolation media. Isolation media consisted of mineral salts solution supplemented with 0.1 per cent yeast extract and strip of filter paper. The mineral salt solution contain : NaCl, 6.0 gm; $(NH_4)_2SO_4$, 1.0 gm; KH_2PO_4, 0.5 gm; K_2HPO_4, 0.5 gm; $MgSO_4$, 0.1 gm; $CaCl_2$, 0.1 gm; and 1 lt. of water.

After 3 to 7 days of incubation at 30°C on reciprocal shaker, a patch of a yellow pigmented material appeared at the liquid air interface on the filter paper. As soon as the pigmented material appeared, a portion of filter paper was transferred with sterile wire and inoculated into fresh medium. The process was repeated several times to enrich aerobic and mesophilic cellulose utilizing organisms. The filter paper from the enriched culture was removed, macerated in a small amount of sterile water, and streaked on the plates containing carboxy methyl cellulose agar plates.

Representatives of the various colonies which developed on each of this media were further purified by pure culture techniques.

Purification of Fungal and Bacterial Isolates

The contaminated cultures of fungal isolates were purified and derived through single spores, using dilution plating. To ensure purity, cultures were derived from single spore in each case. The bacterial contamination was prevented by using antibiotic streptomycin in the medium during isolation and purification of fungi. After ensuring purity, the cultures were maintained in PDA slants at 4°C.

Purification of bacterial cultures was done by pour plate method. In these method four test tubes, each containing 10 ml of distilled water was taken. Test tubes were labelled from 1-4. Inoculate 1 ml. of mixed bacterial suspension into test tube no. 1 with the help of sterile pipette. Test tubes were shaked slowly to obtain uniform suspension from test tube no. 1 to test tube no. 2 and further 1ml. of bacterial suspension each from test tube no. 2 to test tube no. 4 each time by repeating the step. Prepare sterilized petri plates from no. 1-4. Transfer 1 ml of bacterial suspension each from test tube no. 1-4 to petri plates no. 1-4. Prepare nutrient agar medium and pour into petri plates and rotate the plates gently to ensure uniform distribution in plates. Invert the Petri plates after solidification and incubate at 37°C±1 for 24 hrs.

Congo Red (CR) Test

Cellulase (endoglucanase) activity is determined by method of Teather and Wood (1982) with slight modification. In this method, Mandels and Reese medium is prepared with following constituents:-

Mandels and Reese medium (gm/lt.)

☆ Proteose peptone	1.0
☆ Ammonium sulphate $(NH_4)_2SO_4$	1.4
☆ Potassium dihydrogen phosphate KH_2PO_4	2.0
☆ Urea NH_2-CO-NH_2	0.3
☆ Magnesium sulphate $MgSO_4.7H_2O$	0.3
☆ Calcium chloride $CaCl_2$	0.002

- ☆ Ferrous sulphate $FeSO_4.7H_2O$ 0.005
- ☆ Mangnese sulphate $MnSO_4.H_2O$ 0.001
- ☆ Zinc chloride $ZnCl_2$ 0.017
- ☆ Carboxy Methyl Cellulose (CMC) 10
- ☆ Distilled water 1000 ml
- ☆ pH 5.3

Mix all the constituent in flask and autoclave the medium at 15 psi for 15 min., 25 ml of Mandel and Reese medium was poured in 150 ml of sterilized flask. The flask was than inoculated with a spore/mycelial suspension by adding 2 ml. of sterile distilled water to freshly grown fungal agar slants (Reddy *et al.*, 1998) and incubated at 28±°C for 6 days. After appropriate incubation period, sample was withdrawn and centrifuged at 9500 rpm for 20 min in Centrifuge. The cell free supernatant is used as crude enzyme source. Cellulase activity is then revealed by pouring Mandel and Reese agar plates medium supplemented with CMC (1.2w/v). After solidification of medium, cylindrical probes were made in the centre of Petri plates of 6 mm diameter with the help of cork borer. These wells are then filled with crude enzyme of test organisms. Petri plates were then incubated at 28°C±1 for 2 days. After incubation the Petri plates are flooded with 10 ml of 0.1 per cent aqueous solution of Congo Red. The colouration is terminated after 20 min by pouring off the dye and flooding the plates with 10 ml of a 5 M NaCl solution. After an additional 20 min, the salt solution is discarded and endoglucanase activity is revealed by pale reddish zone around the well. In case of bacterial cultures, petri plates of Mandels and Reese agar medium supplemented with CMC (1.2 w/v) was streaked by bacterial test organism and incubated at 37±2°C for 48 hrs. After incubation period, the same process as followed in fungi were followed but instead of 0.1 per cent, 0.5 per cent Congo red is taken to reveal pale reddish zone around the bacterial colony. The zone around the well (in fungi) and bacterial colony were measured in mm. A control consisting of Mandels and Reese agar medium without CMC was also run simultaneously with the test.

Viscometric Method

CMCase (β-1, 4 glucanase) activity of the test organism was evaluated using Fenske Ostwald Viscometer (efflux time for water = 15 sec). The preparation of crude enzyme for fungi is mentioned under congo red test. In bacterial cultures, Mandel and Reese broth medium supplemented with CMC (1.2 w/v) is prepared and 25ml. of medium is dispensed in 150 ml. of flask and autoclaved at 15 psi for 15 min. The flask was then inoculated with 2 ml. of test bacterial suspension in nutrient broth which gave the absorbance of 1.2 at 660 nm in spectrophotometer. The flasks were then incubated in BOD incubator at 37±2°C for 2 days. After incubation, aliquot (5 ml.) is taken and centrifuged at 9500 rpm for 20 min. The supernatant obtained after centrifugation is used for viscometric analysis.

Reaction mixture consists of CMC solution (1.2 per cent w/v), citrate buffer (pH 4.8) and crude enzyme of test organism in the ratio of 4:1:2. The mixture is poured into the small arm and efflux time (ET_O) is immediately determined. Viscometer is then kept at water bath at 50°C. The efflux time is then determined after 60 min of incubation. A control consisting of enzyme boiled at 100°C is also run simultaneously with the test. Efflux time of reaction mixture is taken after 60 min and percent loss in viscosity of CMC is calculated using the formula of Capelline (1966):

$$V = \frac{ETo - ETt}{ETo - ETw} \times 100$$

where,

V: Percent loss in viscosity

ETo: Flow time of reaction mixture at zero time (*i.e.* before start of reaction)

ETt: Flow time of reaction mixture at time T intervals

ETw: Flow time of distilled water

Growth on Mandel and Reese agar Medium Containing Carboxy Methyl Cellulose (CMC) and Cellulose Powder

The growth of fungal and bacterial cultures is observed on Mandel and Reese medium agar medium containing CMC (1.2w/v) and cellulose powder (1 per cent w/v) as the sole source of carbon. The growth of fungal colonies (in mm) were measured on 3rd, 6th and 9th day at 28±1°C and growth of bacterial colony were measured on 2nd, 4th, and 6th day at 37±2°C. The test organisms showing growth on these polysaccharide was assumed to be positive for cellulolytic activity.

Thermophilic Property of Fungi and Bacteria

Cellulase positive fungi and bacteria were also screened for there thermophilic property. In each case fungal and bacterial cultures were grown on PDA medium and Nutrient Agar Medium plate at 45±1°C respectively.

Identification of Fungal and Bacterial Cultures

The fungal forms found to be positive for cellulolytic activity identified with the help of available literature (Thom and Raper, 1945; Subramanian, 1971; Barnett and Hunter, 1987; Gilman, 2001) and also with the help of online photographs and identification service from internet websites:

(www.mycologyonline.adelaide.ac.edu), (www.aspergillusman.ac.uk).

The bacteria positive for cellulolytic activity were identified on the basis of morphological and epigenetic characters *i.e.* biochemical test with the help of following keys:- Bergey's Manual of Systematic Bacteriology (Kreig and Holt, 1984; Sneath *et al.*, 1986), Bergey's Manual of Determinative Bacteriology (Holt *et al.*, 1994) and one species was further identified and confirmed from Microbial Type and Culture Collection and Gene Bank (MTCC) at Institute of Microbial Technology (IMTECH), Chandigarh, India.

Cellulase Enzyme Assay

Extracellular cellulases complex *viz.* endoglucanase, exoglucanase and β-glucosidase activity of test organisms *i.e.* fungal and bacterial cultures were determined by following methods:

Production Medium

Each test organism for endoglucanase activity was grown on Carboxy Methyl Cellulose (CMC), exoglucanase and β-glucosidase activity on cellulose powder as sole source of carbon in Mandel and Reese medium (Mandels and Reese, 1957).

Inoculum Preparation

Fungal cultures were grown on Potato Dextrose Agar (PDA) medium and the spores were harvested aseptically from 5 day old PDA slants. 2 ml of sterile distilled water is added to the fungal agar slants and shaked vigorously for preparing uniform suspension was used as inoculum (Reddy *et al.*, 1998). The bacterial inoculum consists of 2 ml of 24 hour old bacterial culture grown on nutrient broth giving absorbance of 1.2 at 660 nm.

Preparation of Buffer Solution

Citrate Buffer

Stock Solution

0.1 M solution of Citric Acid = 21.01 gm in 1 lt. of distilled water

0.1 M solution of Sodium Citrate = 29.4 gm in 1 lt. of distilled water

Table 38.1

pH	*0.1 M Citric Acid (in ml.)*	*0.1 M Sodium Citrate (in ml.)*
3.0	16.4	3.6
3.4	14.6	5.4
3.8	12.7	7.3
4.2	10.8	9.2
4.6	8.9	11.1
5.0	7.0	13.0
5.4	5.1	14.9

Potassium Phosphate Buffer

Stock Solution

0.2 M solution of KOH = 11.22 gm. in 1 lt. of water

0.2 M solution of KH_2PO_4 = 27.22 gm. in 1 lt. of water

Table 38.2

pH	*0.2 M KOH (in ml.)*	*0.2 M KH_2PO_4 (in ml.)*
5.8	3.5	50
6.0	5.8	"
6.2	9.1	"
6.4	13.0	"
6.6	18.0	"
6.8	24.0	"
7.0	30.0	"
7.2	35.0	"
7.4	40.0	"
7.6	43.0	"
7.8	45.0	"
8.0	47.0	"

Borax–NaOH Buffer (0.05 M Borate)

Stock Solution

0.05 M solution of Borax

0.2 N solution of NaOH

Mix stock solution and dilute to 200 ml. with water.

Table 38.3

pH	*0.05 M Borax (in ml.)*	*0.2 N NaOH (in ml.)*
8.3	50	0
9.3	"	11
9.6	"	23
9.8	"	34
10.0	"	43
10.1	"	46

Preparation of Enzyme Sample

Twenty five ml of Mandels and Reese medium was dispensed in each 150 ml of flask. All the flasks were then sterilized at 15 psi for 15 minutes. Fungal and bacterial inoculum is inoculated in Mandels and Reese medium containing CMC and cellulose powder separately. The experiment was done in duplicates and inoculated flasks were incubated at 28±1°C for fungi and 37±1°C for bacteria in an incubator under stationary condition. Aliquots (5ml.) were removed periodically from flasks under aseptic condition after 4th, 8th, 12th day in fungi and 2nd, 4th, 6th day of incubation in bacteria. The fungal mycelium was removed by filtering through whatmann filter paper nc. 1 and supernatant obtained was centrifuged at 9500 rpm for 20 minutes. The supernatant obtained was used for enzymatic activity.

Preparation of Di-Nitro Salicyclic Acid (DNS) Reagent

3, 5 di-nitro salicyclic acid reagent was prepared for determining the reducing sugar as per the method of Miller (1959).

☆ Distilled water	1416 ml
☆ 3, 5 di-nitro salicyclic reagent	10.6 gm
☆ Sodium hydroxide	19.8 gm

Dissolve the above chemicals, and then add

☆ Sodium Potassium Tartarate (Rochelle salt)	306 gm
☆ Phenol (melted at 50°C)	7.6 ml
☆ Sodium metabisulfite	8.3 gm

This reagent should be stored at 4°C in stoppered bottle untill used for enzymatic activity.

Assay of Endoglucanase Activity (CMCase)

Endo glucanase activity was measured as per the method described by Mandels (1974). Reaction mixture consist of 0.5 ml. of 1 per cent carboxy methyl cellulose (CMC) in citrate buffer (pH 4.8), 0.5 ml.

of enzyme sample, diluted with citrate buffer (pH 4.8). Several dilutions is made of enzyme such that one dilution will release from CMC substrate, slightly more than 0.5 mg. of glucose in the reducing sugar assay and other slightly less. The reaction mixture is incubated at 50°C for 30 minutes. After appropriate period of incubation, the reaction is stopped by adding 3 ml. of DNS reagent and the reaction mixture is boiled for exactly 5 minutes in vigorously boiling water bath. The tubes are cooled at room temperature and the absorbance is then measured at 540nm. A control consisting of substrate blank is also run simultaneously with the test so as to correct any amount of sugar present in the crude enzyme. The amount of reducing sugar or glucose formed after substraction from control is translated using linear glucose standard prepared by plotting glucose used against absorbance at 540nm, into microgram (μg) of glucose produced during enzymatic reaction. Enzyme activity is presented in term of International Units (IU), which is micromole (μm) of glucose release/min./ml.

$$\text{IU/ml.} = \text{mg. glucose} \times 0.37 \times \text{dilution factor}$$

or

$$\text{IU/ml.} = \frac{0.185}{\text{Enzyme dilution to give 0.5 mg. glucose}}$$

Assay of Exo Glucanase (FPU) Activity (FPase)

Exoglucanase activity determined as per the method of Mandels (1974). In this method, 1 ml. of citrate buffer (pH 4.8) is added to a test tube, followed by 0.5 ml of enzyme suitably diluted in the same buffer and 1 × 6 cm. strips of whatmann no. 1 filter paper (50 mg). At least two dilution of enzyme must be used. One dilution should be capable of releasing more than 2 mg. of glucose; the other should release slightly less. The reaction mixture is incubated at 50° C for 60 min., after the incubation period, reaction is stopped by adding 3 ml. of DNS reagent. The suspension is mixed well and the tubes are transferred to a boiling water bath for exactly 5 min. Tubes are immediately cooled in the cold water and absorbance is then measured at 540nm. A control consisting of substrate blank is also run simultaneously with test so as to correct any amount of sugar present in the crude enzyme. The amount of reducing sugar or glucose formed after subtraction from control is translated using linear glucose standard prepared by plotting glucose used against absorbance at 540 nm, into microgram (μg) of glucose produced during enzyme reaction. Enzyme activity is presented in term of International Units known as Filter Paper Units (FPU) which is micromoles (μm) of glucose released/min./ml.

$$\text{IU/ml.} = \text{mg. glucose} \times 0.185 \times \text{dilution factor}$$

or

$$\text{FPU/ml.} = \frac{0.37}{\text{Enzyme dilution to give 0.5 mg. glucose}}$$

Assay of β-glucosidase Activity

β-glucosidase activity is measured as per the method described by Mandels (1974). In this method, 0.5 ml of 1 per cent salicin prepared in citrate buffer (pH 4.8), 0.5 ml of enzyme sample, diluted with citrate buffer (pH 4.8) several dilutions are made of enzyme such that one dilution will release from salicin substrate, slightly more than 0.5 mg of glucose in the reducing sugar assay and other slightly less. The reaction mixture is incubated at 50°C for 30 min. After appropriate period of incubation, the reaction is stopped by adding 3 ml. of DNS reagent and the reaction mixture is boiled for exactly 5 min. in vigorously boiling water bath. The tubes are cooled immediately in cold water and the absorbance is then measured at 540 nm. A control consisting of substrate blank is also run simultaneously with test so as to correct any amount of sugar present in the crude enzyme. The amount of reducing sugar glucose formed after subtraction from control is translated using linear glucose standard prepared by plotting glucose used against absorbance at 540nm into microgram (µg) of glucose produced during enzyme reaction. Enzyme activity is presented in term of International Units (IU) which is micromole (µm) of glucose released/min/ml.

$$\text{IU/ml.} = \text{mg. glucose} \times 0.37 \times \text{dilution factor}$$

or

$$\text{IU/ml.} = \frac{0.185}{\text{Enzyme dilution to give 0.5 mg. glucose}}$$

Effect of pH on Activity of Cellulase Enzymes

The effect of pH was determined by measuring activity at standard assay over a pH range 3-10. Substrates CMC (1 per cent) for endoglucanase and salicin (1 per cent) for β-glucosidase activity was prepared in three buffer *viz.* citrate buffer (pH 3-5), Potassium Phosphate buffer (6-8), and Borax-NaOH buffer (9-10). Exoglucanase activity is assayed in buffers of different pH 3-10. Enzyme of test organism was mixed with substrate and cellulase assay was performed. Cellulase activity was determined in IU/ml.

Effect of Temperature on Activity of Cellulase Enzymes

The activity was determined by carrying out the standard assay at various temperatures between 30-90°C at optimum pH obtained for test organism. Enzyme mixed with substrate CMC for endoglucanase activity and salicin for β-glucosidase activity prepared at buffer of optimum pH activity obtained, exoglucanase activity was also performed in buffer of optimum pH. Endoglucanase, exoglucanase and β-glucosidase activity was carried out at different temperature range of 30-90°C. Cellulase activity was determined in IU/ml.

Effect of Chemical Reagents on Endoglucanase Activity

The effect of chemical reagents was evaluated on the endoglucanase activity of fungal and bacterial cultures as per the method of Ozaki and Ito (1991) with slight modification. EDTA, 2,4 DNP, $HgCl_2$ and $SnCl_2$ were prepared of three concentration *viz.* 0.1mM, 1mM and 5mM. The crude enzyme (1ml.) of test organism and each chemical reagents (1 ml.) were mixed and incubated at 30°C for 30 min. and an aliquot (0.5 ml.) was used for the assay. The endoglucanase activity was measured in IU/ml. A control was run consist of enzyme without reagent.

Chemicals

All chemicals which are used in the present investigation were of analytical grade. The majority of chemicals were of Ranbaxy, India followed by Himedia (CDH, Chemical India).

(Merck company, Darmstcidt, Germany), (Fluka Chemical Ltd. Gillingham, Dorset, UK)

Results

Cellulase Enzymes of Fungal Cultures

The endoglucanase (CMCase), exoglucanase (FPase), and β-glucosidase activity was determined on 4th, 8th and 12th day of incubation.

The data depicted in the Table 38.4 shows the activities of endoglucanase, exoglucanase and β-glucosidase activity in forty fungal cultures. In Zygomycotina class, two spp. of *Mucor* (AV69, AV62) shows best endoglucanase, exoglucanase and β-glucosidase activity on 8th day of incubation. *Rhizopus* sp. (AV 15) shows highest endoglucanase, exoglucanase and β-glucosidase activity on 12th day of incubation. In Ascomycotina class, among the spp. of *Chaetomium*, the endoglucanase, exoglucanase and β-glucosidase activity differs. In case of *Chaetomium cochliodes*, endoglucanase, activity was higher on 4th day but decreases gradually as the incubation period increased upto 12th day, whereas, exoglucanase activity was not observed on 4th day, it appeared on 8th day and show little increase on 12th day. No β-glucosidase activity was found. In case of *Chaetomium globosum*, the endoglucanase activity increased gradually upto 12th day of incubation. This result was total opposite of *Chaetomium cochloides*. Exoglucanase activity was found to increase gradually as the incubation period increases upto 12th day, for β-glucosidase, the activity increases upto 8th day and then reduces. In case of *Chaetomium* sp. (AV56), endoglucanase activity increases upto 8th day and become almost more than two fold of 4th day activity, but on 12th day significant reduction *i.e.* almost half of the 8th day of activity was observed. Exoglucanase activity was found increases upto 8th day and then became stable and no further increase in activity was observed. In β-glucosidase activity initially there was no change in the activity upto the 8th day a little higher activity was obtained in 12th day of incubation.

Table 38.4: Cellulases Enzymes of Fungal Cultures

Fungal Cultures	*Isolate Number*	*Incubation Time (in days)*	*Endoglucanase Activity (CMCase) (IU/ml)*	*Exoglucanase Activity (FPase) (FPU/ml)*	*β-glucosidase Activity (IU/ml)*
		ZYGOMYCOTINA			
Mucor sp.	AV62	4	0.515	0.010	0.084
		8	0.982	0.014	0.150
		12	0.881	0.013	0.148
Mucor sp.	AV69	4	0.440	0.030	0.199
		8	1.169	0.049	0.401
		12	0.924	0.040	0.180
Rhizophus sp.	AV15	4	0.201	0.011	0.029
		8	0.347	0.038	0.033
		12	0.593	0.066	0.090
		ASCOMYCOTINA			
Chaetomium cochliodes	AV6	4	0.210	ANO	ANO
		8	0.192	0.012	ANO
		12	0.186	0.018	ANO
Chaetomium globosum	AV17	4	0.919	0.013	0.053
		8	1.396	0.020	0.064
		12	1.515	0.021	0.054

Contd...

Table 38.4–Contd...

Fungal Cultures	Isolate Number	Incubation Time (in days)	Endoglucanase Activity (CMCase) (IU/ml)	Exoglucanase Activity (FPase) (FPU/ml)	β-glucosidase Activity (IU/ml)
Cheatomium sp.	AV56	4	0.510	0.015	0.088
		8	1.212	0.019	0.088
		12	0.688	0.019	0.093
		DEUTEROMYCOTINA			
Aspergillus flavus	AV23	4	0.380	0.010	0.202
		8	0.528	0.010	0.279
		12	1.065	0.010	0.217
Aspergillus nidulans	AV14	4	0.353	0.058	0.083
		8	0.636	0.102	0.189
		12	0.516	0.074	0.055
Aspergillus fumigatus	AV4	4	0.370	0.025	0.090
		8	0.485	0.029	0.103
		12	0.502	0.037	0.115
Aspergillus niger	AV8	4	0.102	0.024	0.112
		8	0.220	0.026	0.186
		12	0.362	0.030	0.203
Aspergillus sp.	AV36	4	0.056	0.019	0.059
		8	0.081	0.022	0.070
		12	0.082	0.025	0.070
Aspergillus sp.	AV51	4	0.179	0.010	0.134
		8	0.331	0.028	0.282
		12	0.567	0.029	0.483
Aspergillus terreus	AV49	4	0.444	0.069	0.062
		8	1.167	0.140	0.080
		12	0.833	0.097	0.067
Aspergillus ochraceous	AV65	4	0.251	ANO	0.009
		8	0.503	ANO	0.014
		12	0.455	ANO	0.015
Aspergillus sp.	AV70	4	0.515	0.092	0.045
		8	1.207	0.109	0.062
		12	1.118	0.078	0.060
Alternaria alternata	AV32	4	0.116	0.001	0.006
		8	0.214	0.024	0.005
		12	0.352	0.002	0.006
Curvularia sp.	AV39	4	0.156	0.007	0.037
		8	0.148	0.007	0.042
		12	0.147	0.007	0.046

Contd...

Table 38.4–Contd...

Fungal Cultures	Isolate Number	Incubation Time (in days)	Endoglucanase Activity (CMCase) (IU/ml)	Exoglucanase Activity (FPase) (FPU/ml)	β-glucosidase Activity (IU/ml)
Colletotrichum sp.	AV46	4	0.226	0.061	0.055
		8	1.063	0.089	0.065
		12	0.817	0.088	0.123
Drechslera sp.	AV31	4	0.556	0.070	ANO
		8	1.011	0.096	ANO
		12	0.897	0.091	ANO
Fusarium sp.	AV40	4	0.134	0.010	0.018
		8	0.703	0.013	0.087
		12	0.737	0.022	0.106
Fusarium oxysporum	AV43	4	0.425	0.010	0.022
		8	0.742	0.034	0.038
		12	0.541	0.022	0.034
Fusarium sp.	AV45	4	0.420	0.013	0.070
		8	0.823	0.016	0.103
		12	0.866	0.016	0.097
Geotrichum candidum	AV28	4	0.073	0.011	0.052
		8	0.148	0.013	0.058
		12	0.366	0.014	0.059
Helminthosporium sp.	AV59	4	0.083	0.042	ANO
		8	0.331	0.065	ANO
		12	0.320	0.062	ANO
Penicillium rubrum	AV18	4	0.493	0.018	0.062
		8	1.030	0.026	0.127
		12	0.752	0.045	0.193
Penicillium nigricans	AV1	4	0.181	0.009	0.031
		8	0.415	0.011	0.034
		12	0.714	0.029	0.055
Penicillium chrysogenum	AV10	4	0.182	0.011	0.026
		8	0.375	0.028	0.064
		12	0.614	0.031	0.092
Penicillium sp.	AV57	4	0.243	0.034	0.058
		8	0.553	0.068	0.120
		12	0.565	0.081	0.123
Penicillium sp.	AV41	4	0.390	0.007	0.120
		8	0.756	0.010	0.127
		12	0.679	0.008	0.119

Contd...

Table 38.4–Contd...

Fungal Cultures	*Isolate Number*	*Incubation Time (in days)*	*Endoglucanase Activity (CMCase) (IU/ml)*	*Exoglucanase Activity (FPase) (FPU/ml)*	*β-glucosidase Activity (IU/ml)*
Phoma sp.	AV50	4	0.821	0.013	0.023
		8	1.187	0.015	0.032
		12	1.110	0.025	0.045
Rhizoctonia sp.	AV67	4	0.275	ANO	0.011
		8	0.344	ANO	0.014
		12	0.361	ANO	0.011
Trichoderma viride	AV13	4	0.657	0.089	0.031
		8	1.267	0.152	0.810
		12	1.058	0.155	0.729
Trichoderma sp.	AV21	4	0.826	0.022	0.187
		8	2.168	0.084	0.509
		12	1.947	0.117	0.399
Trichoderma koningi	AV34	4	0.490	0.018	0.125
		8	0.589	0.032	0.159
		12	0.596	0.034	0.151
Trichothecium roseum	AV54	4	0.301	0.006	ANO
		8	0.704	0.009	ANO
		12	1.810	0.013	ANO
Mycelia sterlia (Black)	AV5	4	0.599	0.011	0.123
		8	1.079	0.011	0.157
		12	0.479	0.012	0.157
Mycelia sterlia (Yellow)	AV29	4	0.173	0.012	0.070
		8	0.617	0.021	0.081
		12	0.316	0.021	0.078
Unidentified 1	AV55	4	0.144	0.003	0.009
		8	0.189	0.004	0.023
		12	0.217	0.004	0.023
Unidentified 2	AV48	4	1.695	0.015	0.076
		8	1.295	0.016	0.106
		12	0.906	0.022	0.116
Unidentified 3	AV53	4	0.271	0.055	ANO
		8	0.542	0.089	ANO
		12	0.452	0.069	ANO

ANO: Activity Not Observed

All data given are the mean value of the two independent experiments.

In Deuteromycotina, twenty nine cultures were evaluated for cellulase complex. Among nine spp. of *Aspergillus*, three spp. of *Aspergillus viz. A.terreus, Aspergillus* sp. (AV70) and *A.nidulans* shows good activity of endoglucanase, exoglucanase and β-glucosidase on 8th day of incubation, whereas in *Aspergillus* sp. (AV51), *A. flavus, A. fumigatus, A. niger* and *Aspergillus* sp. (AV36) shows good endoglucanase, exoglucanase and β-glucosidase activity on 12th day of incubation. Interestingly, in *A.ochraceous* maximum endoglucanase and β-glucosidase activities was obtained on 8th day, however no exoglucanase activity was found in it. Out of five spp. of *Penicillium*, except *Penicillium rubrum* and isolate no. AV41, all the three *Penicillium* spp. *i.e. P. nigricans, P. chrysogenum* and *Penicillium* sp. (AV57) shows higher activity of endoglucanase on 12th day whereas, in case of *P. rubrum* and *Penicillium* sp. (AV41) higher activity of endoglucanase was observed on 8th day. Higher activity of exoglucanase and β-glucosidase was observed on 12th day of incubation in *P.rubrum, P.nigricans, P.chrysogenum* and *Penicillium* sp. (AV57), whereas in *Penicillium* sp. (AV41) best activity of exoglucanase and β-glucosidase was observed on 8th day. In three spp. of *Trichoderma, Trichoderma* sp. (AV21) shows maximum endoglucanase and β-glucosidase activity on 8th day of incubation, whereas, activity of exoglucanase was found maximum on 12th day of incubation. Almost similar trend in activity of endoglucanase, exoglucanase and β-glucosidase was observed in *Trichoderma viride* and *Trichoderma koningi*.

During the present investigation, it was found that three spp. of *Fusarium* shows good amount of endoglucanase, exoglucanase and β-glucosidase activity. Among the three species of *Fusarium, Fusarium oxysporum* shows best endoglucanase, exoglucanase and β-glucosidase activity on 8th day of incubation whereas, best endo- and exoglucanase activity in *Fusarium* spp. (AV45, AV40) was observed on 12th day of incubation. However, β-glucosidase activity in *Fusarium* sp. (AV 45 and AV 40) was observed maximum on 8th and 12th day of incubation respectively. *Alterneria alternata* was found to show maximum activity of endoglucanase and β-glucosidase on 12th day and exoglucanase activity on 8th day of incubation. *Curvularia* sp. showed maximum endoglucanase and exoglucanase activity on 4th day, however endoglucanase activity decreased upon with the increase in incubation period whereas exoglucanase activity was found to be static. β-glucosidase activity was found to be maximum on 12th day of incubation. In *Colletotrichum* sp. maximum endoglucanase and exoglucanase activity was found on 8th day and β-glucosidase activity on 12th day of incubation. In *Drechslera* sp., maximum endo- and exoglucanase activity was observed on 8th day of incubation. β-glucosidase activity was found to be absent. In *Geotrichum candidum* maximum endoglucanase activity was observed on 12th day, whereas exoglucanase and β-glucosidase activity was almost similar on 8th and 12th day of incubation. In *Helminthosporium* sp. maximum endoglucanase and exoglucanase activity was observed on 8th day of incubation and β-glucosidase activity was found absent. *Phoma* sp. shows maximum endoglucanase activity on 8th day of incubation. Exoglucanase and β-glucosidase activity was found to be maximum on 12th day of incubation. *Rhizoctonia* sp. shows maximum endoglucanase activity on 12th day of incubation. β-glucosidase activity was found to be best on 8th day of incubation. Exoglucanase activity was found to be absent. *Trichothecium roseum* shows maximum endoglucanase and exoglucanase activity on 12th day of incubation, while β-glucosidase activity was found to absent. Mycelia sterlia (AV5) and (AV29) showed maximum endoglucanase, exoglucanase and β-glucosidase activity on 8th day of incubation respectively.

In case of Unidentified 1 (AV55) endoglucanase activity was highest was 12th day. Interestingly no change in exoglucanase and β-glucosidase activity was recorded after 8th day of incubation. In case of Unidentified 2 (AV48) endoglucanase activity was highest on 4th day and then decreased after further period of incubation, whereas exoglucanase and β-glucosidase activity were observed maximum in 12th day of incubation. Unidentified 3 (AV53) showed optimum endoglucanase and exoglucanase activity on 8th day of incubation. β-glucosidase activity was found to be absent.

Effect of pH on Activity of Cellulase Enzymes in Three Fungal Cultures

Two *Aspergillus* spp. *viz. A.nidulans* and *A.terreus* and one sp. of *Fusarium oxysporum* was selected for their endoglucanase, exoglucanase and β-glucosidase activity for their optimum pH range. In *A.nidulans* it was found in range of pH 5-9, 4-6, 4-6 for endoglucanase, exoglucanase and β-glucosidase activities respectively. For endoglucanase optimum pH was 6, and for exoglucanase and β-glucosidase optimum pH was 5. Above and below this optimum range, the endoglucanase, exoglucanase and β-glucosidase activity declines rapidly.

Aspergillus terreus showed very broad pH range from 3-6. For endoglucanase and exoglucanase activities, optimum pH was 4. β-glucosidase activity was found optimum at pH 5. *Fusarium oxysporum* also showed a very broad range of tolerance for pH from 4-9 and pH 5 was optimum for endo- and exoglucanase activities and for β-glucosidase activity optimum pH was 4 (Table 38.2 and Figure 38.1).

Effect of Temperature on Activity of Cellulase Enzymes in Three Fungal Cultures

In the present investigation, fungal cultures were taken to evaluate the optimum and active temperature ranges. The data were depicted in Table 38.3 and Figure 38.2. It is clearly evident from results that *A.nidulans* shows a very broad stable temperature range for endoglucanase, exoglucanase and β-glucosidase activity ranging from 30-80°C, 30-60°C and 40-80°C respectively with maximum 60°C for endoglucanase and β-glucosidase activities, 50°C for exoglucanase activity. In *A.terreus,* endoglucanase activity was found to be active from 30-70°C with optimum at 40°C. The exoglucanase and β-glucosidase activities range 30-50°C and 40-50°C respectively. *Fusarium oxysporum* shows temperature range 30-60°C for endoglucanase, 30-50°C for exoglucanase and β-glucosidase activities. However, optimum temperature 60°C, 50°C and 50°C respectively for endo-, exoglucanase and β-glucosidase activity was observed.

Effect of Chemical Reagents on Endoglucanase Activity of Three Fungal Cultures

Figures 38.3 and 38.4 shows the effect of chemical reagent on endoglucanase activity of *Aspergillus nidulans*. It is clearly evident from the result that EDTA and $SnCl_2$ did not affect much, whereas 2, 4 DNP and $HgCl_2$ were found to reduce endoglucanase activity more severely. The lower concentration (0.1 mM) of 2, 4 DNP reduces the endoglucanase activity more than 50 per cent and higher concentration (5 mM) was found to inhibit activity more then 90 per cent. Lower concentration (0.1 mM) of $HgCl_2$ was more inhibitory and found to inhibit endoglucanase activity more than 80 per cent and its higher concentration causes 93 per cent inhibition in the activity.

Figures 38.5 and 38.6 depicts the effect of chemical reagents on endoglucanase activity of *Aspergillus terreus*. The result shows that EDTA and $SnCl_2$ did not affect much as 5 mM concentration of EDTA causes 37 per cent and same concentration of $SnCl_2$ inhibits only 22 per cent activity. 2, 4 DNP and $HgCl_2$ were found to reduce endoglucanase activity more severely. The lower concentration (0.1 mM) of 2, 4 DNP reduce the endoglucanase activity upto 70 per cent and higher concentration (5 mM) was found to inhibit 94 per cent activity. Concentration of 0.1 mM of $HgCl_2$ inhibited 87 per cent of endoglucanase activity and higher concentration (5 mM) of $HgCl_2$ causes 97 per cent inhibition in activity.

The results of effect of chemical reagents on endoglucanase activity of *Fusarium oxysporum* are shown in Figures 38.7 and 38.8. It is evident from the result that unlike *Aspergillus nidulans* and *Aspergillus terreus*, EDTA inhibit (48 per cent) of endoglucanase activity at (0.1 mM) and 63 per cent inhibition at 5 mM. $SnCl_2$ also shows effect on endoglucanase activity as 5 mM concentration causes

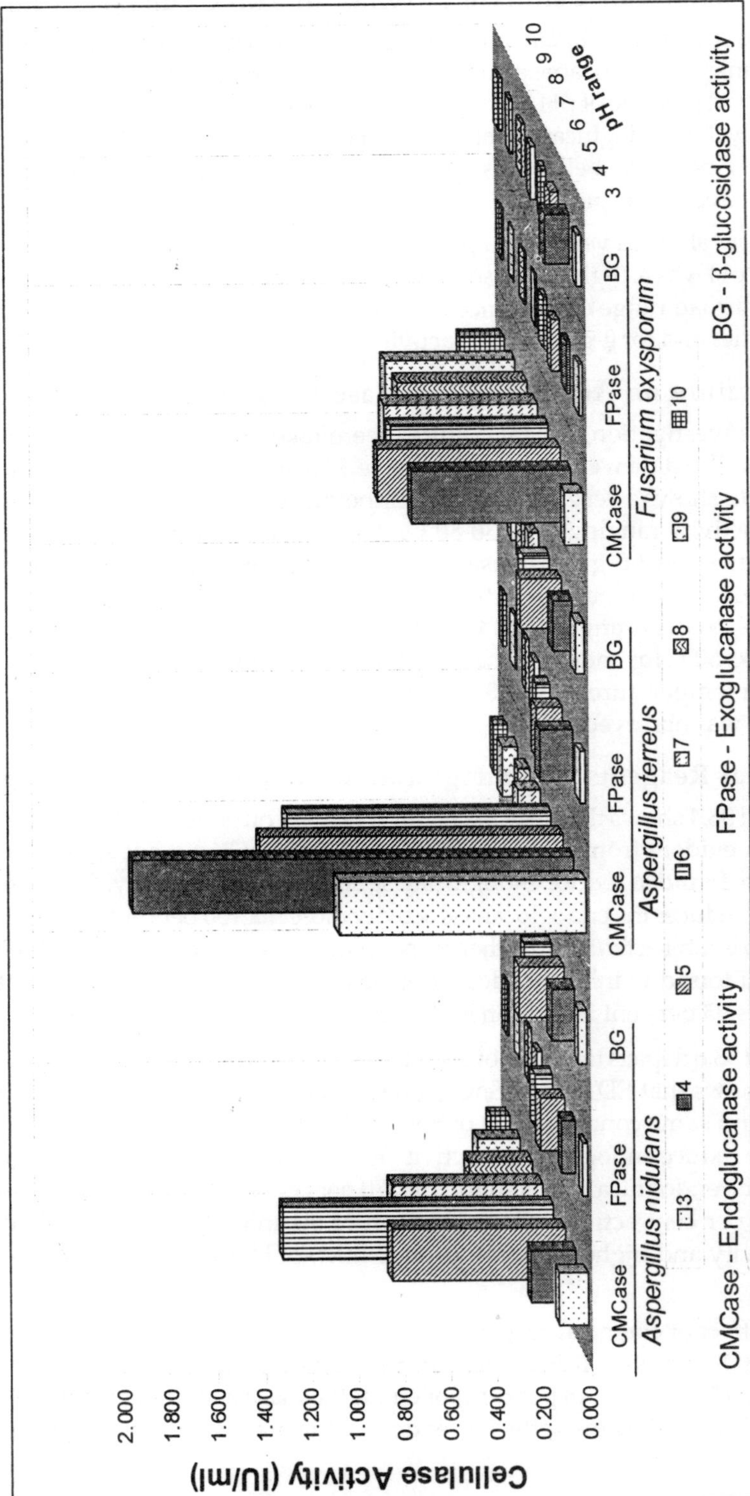

Figure 38.1: Effect of pH Range on the Activity of Cellulase Enzymes in Three Fungal Cultures

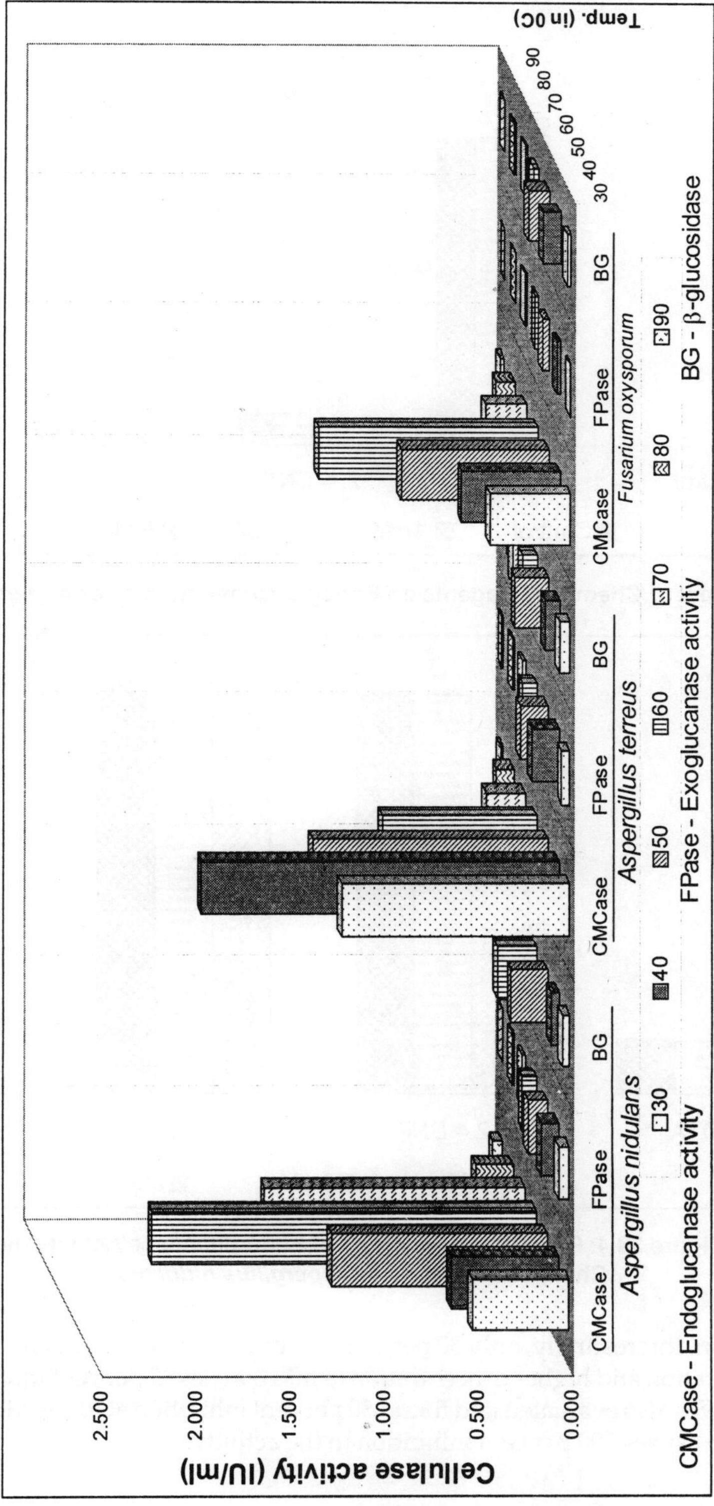

Figure 38.2: Effect of Temperature Range on the Activity of Cellulase Enzymes in Three Fungal Cultures

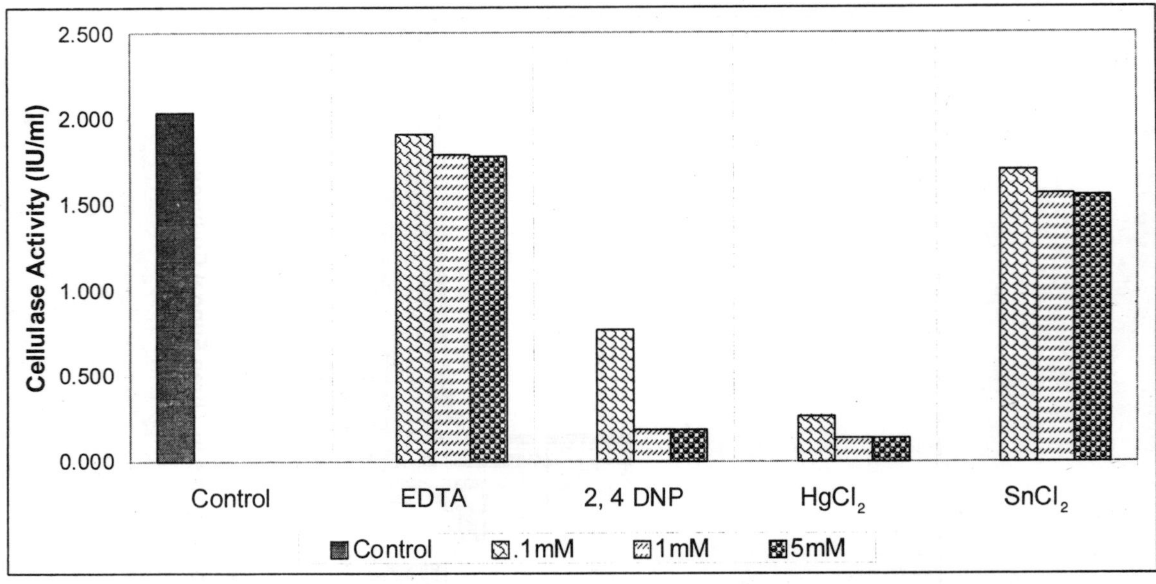

Figure 38.3: Effect of Chemical Reagents on Endoglucanase Activity of *Aspergillus nidulans*

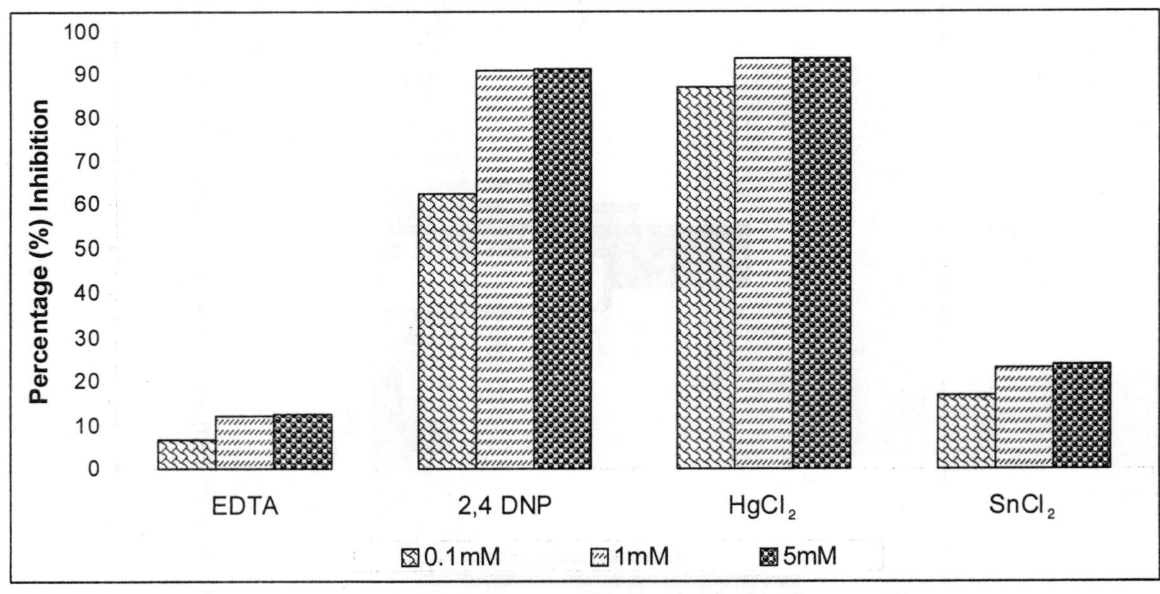

Figure 38.4: Percentage Inhibition of Endoglucanase Activity by Chemical Reagents in *Aspergillus nidulans*

35 per cent inhibition. Interestingly, only 38 per cent inhibition in endoglucanase activity was found at (0.1 mM) concentration and higher concentration (5 mM) causes 83 per cent inhibition by 2, 4 DNP. The effect of $HgCl_2$ was also evaluated and found 80 per cent inhibition at (0.1 mM) concentration and 5 mM concentration causes 100 per cent inhibition in the activity.

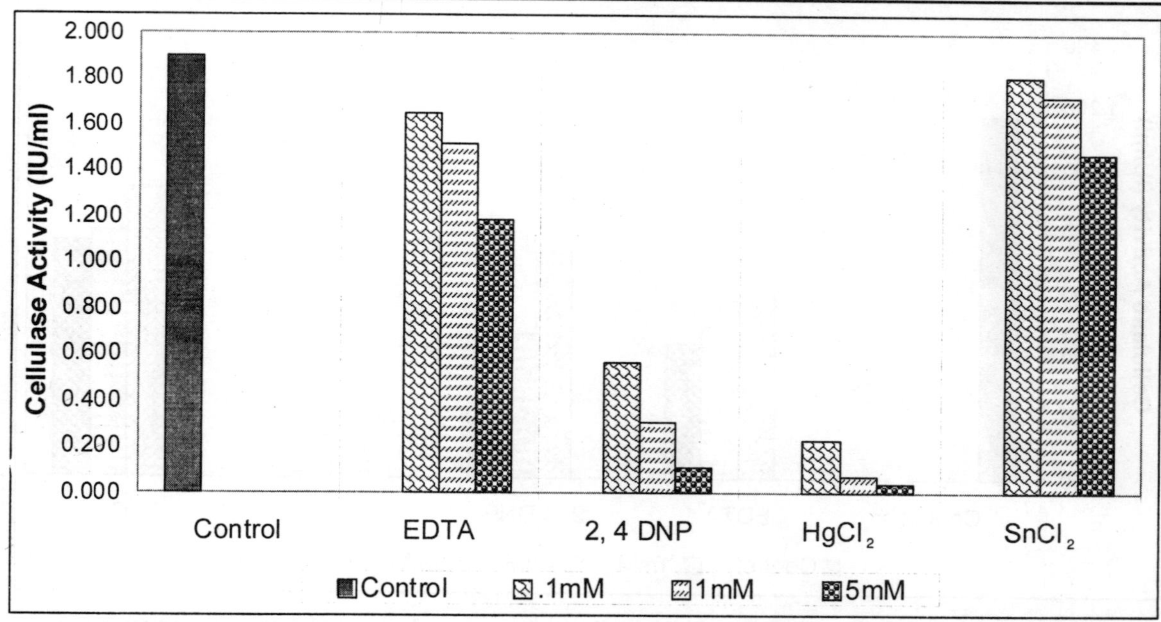

Figure 38.5: Effect of Chemical Reagents on Endoglucanase Activity of *Aspergillus terreus*

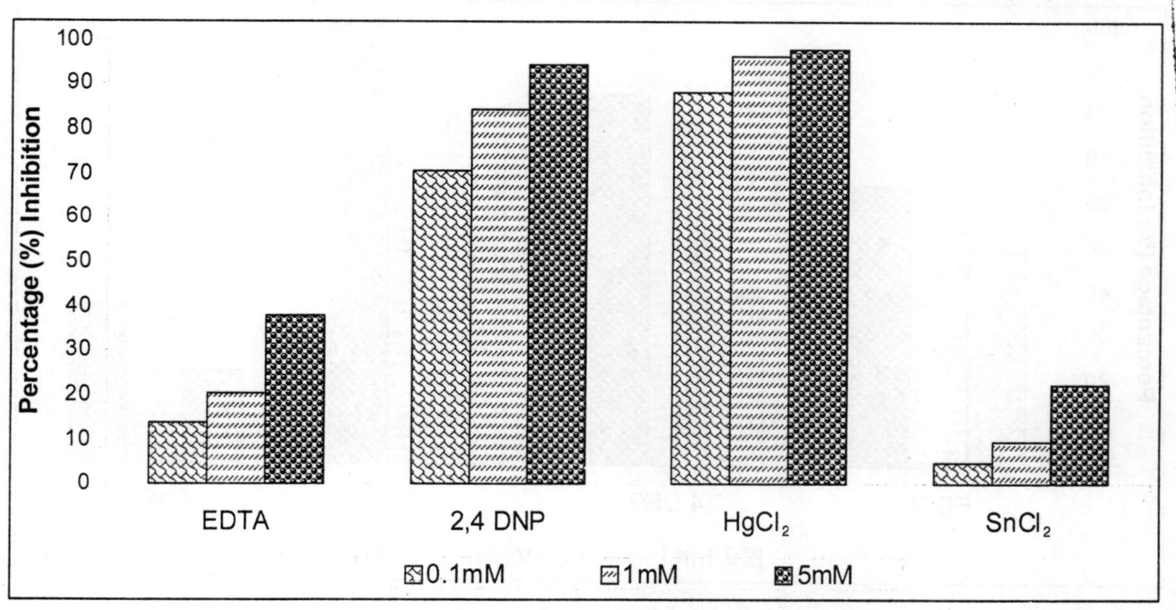

Figure 38.6: Percentage Inhibition of Endoglucanase Activity by Chemical Reagents in *Aspergillus terreus*

Cellulase Enzymes of Bacterial Cultures

The results of cellulase activity of bacterial cultures were presented in Table 38.4. The cellulolytic activity was measured as endoglucanase, exoglucanase and β-glucosidase. Out of the five bacterial

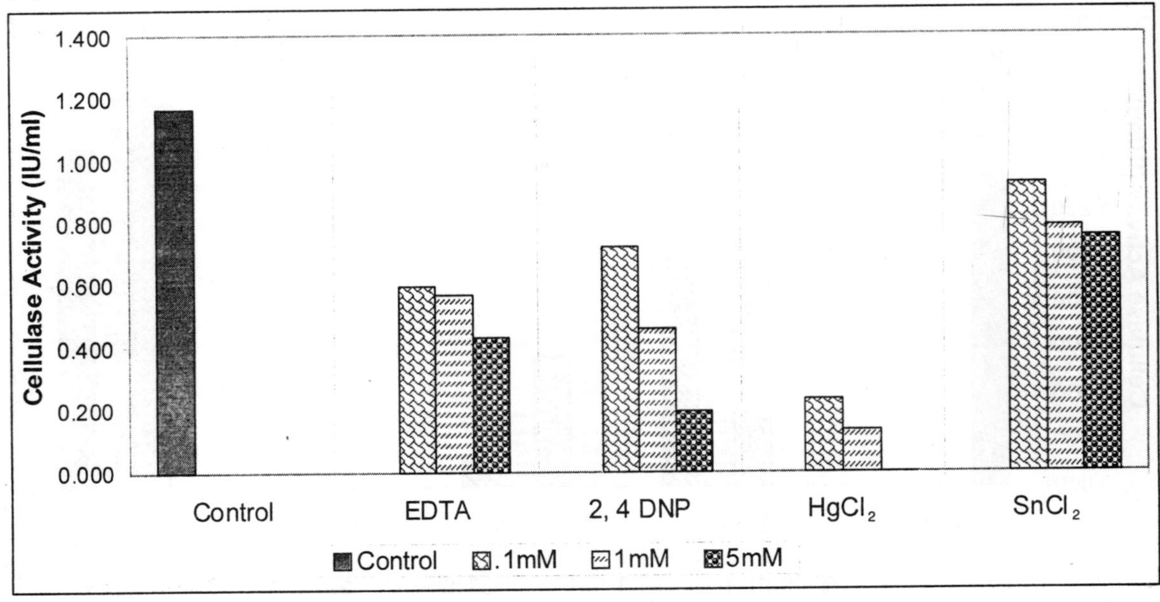

Figure 38.7: Effect of Chemical Reagents on Endoglucanase Activity of *Fusarium oxysporum*

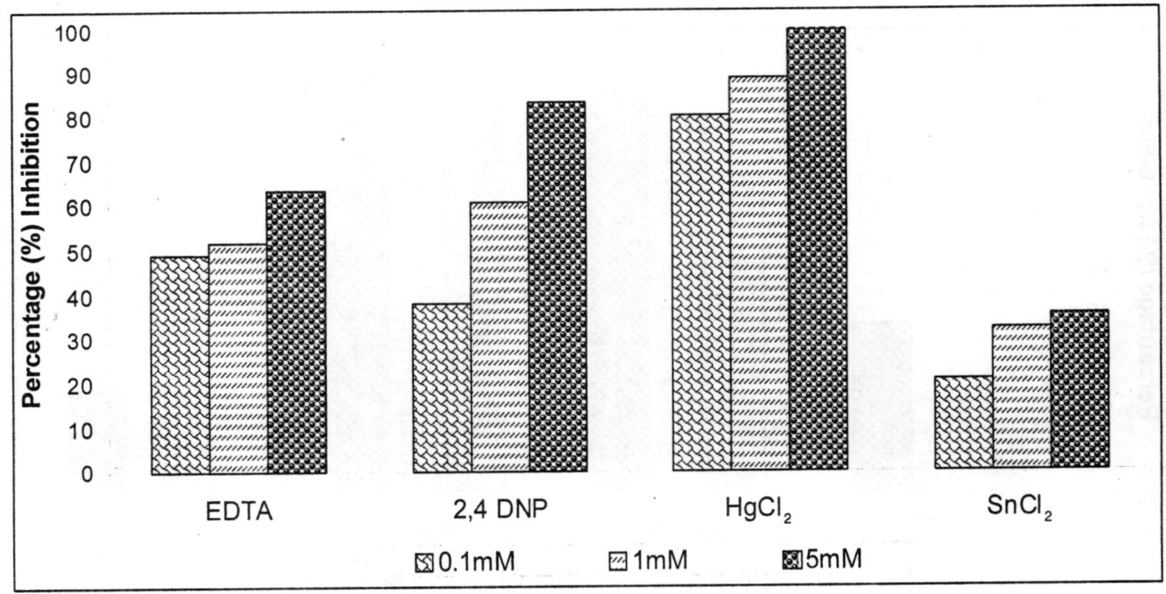

Figure 38.8: Percentage Inhibition of Endoglucanase Activity by Chemical Reagents in *Fusarium oxysporum*

cultures, four belongs to genus *Bacillus*. All the test *Bacillus* species shows endoglucanase, exoglucanase and β-glucosidase activities. In *Bacillus marinus*, *Bacillus* sp. (V2), *Bacillus subtilis* and *Bacillus* sp. (J2) best endo-, exoglucanase and β-glucasidase activity was observed on 6th day of incubation. *Bacillus marinus* was found best because it shows maximum endo- and exoglucanase activity on 6th day of incubation. Interestingly, β-glucosidase activity was recorded higher in *Bacillus* sp. (J3). *Aeromonas hydrophila* shows best endoglucanase, exoglucanase and β-glucosidase activity on 4th day of incubation.

Effect of pH on Activity of Cellulase Enzymes in Three Bacterial Cultures

The data presented in Table 38.5 and Figure 385.9 shows the active pH range for cellulase complex of three selected bacterial cultures. In *Bacillus marinus*, endoglucanase activity was observed at broader pH range *i.e.* 4-9 with optimum at pH 6, whereas, exoglucanase and β-glucosidase activity was found to show pH range 4-8 and 3-8 respectively, with optimum at pH 5 and 6 respectively. *Bacillus* sp. (V2) shows pH range from pH 3-8, for endoglucanase activity with optimum at pH 6. For exoglucanase activity pH range 4-7 with optimum was observed at pH 6 whereas, for β-glucosidase activity pH range was 3-7 with optimum at pH 5. In *B.subtilis*, for endoglucanase activity range of pH lies between 4-8 and optimum was observed at pH 5. For exoglucanase activity pH range was 3-8 and optimum was observed at pH 5.

Table 38.5: Effect of pH Range on the Activity of Cellulase Enzymes in Three Fungal Cultures

Sl.No.	*Fungal Culture*	*pH Range*	*Endoglucanase Activity (CMCase) (IU/ml)*	*Exoglucanase Activity (FPase) (FPU/ml)*	*β-glucosidase Activity (BG) (IU/ml)*
1.	*Aspergillus nidulans*	3	0.122	0.018	0.032
		4	0.191	0.060	0.101
		5	0.742	0.105	0.192
		6	1.165	0.078	0.118
		7	0.649	0.022	0.071
		8	0.270	0.009	0.020
		9	0.186	0.004	0.018
		10	0.082	0.005	0.017
2.	*Aspergillus terreus*	3	1.060	0.022	0.034
		4	1.892	0.145	0.083
		5	1.300	0.111	0.175
		6	1.138	0.059	0.115
		7	0.099	0.023	0.041
		8	0.046	0.008	0.029
		9	0.070	0.009	0.020
		10	0.055	0.009	0.022
3.	*Fusarium oxysporum*	3	0.076	0.013	0.019
		4	0.683	0.016	0.108
		5	0.786	0.035	0.036
		6	0.683	0.018	0.022
		7	0.665	0.005	0.020
		8	0.559	0.004	0.011
		9	0.563	0.004	0.013
		10	0.186	0.004	0.014

All data given are the mean value of the two independent experiments.

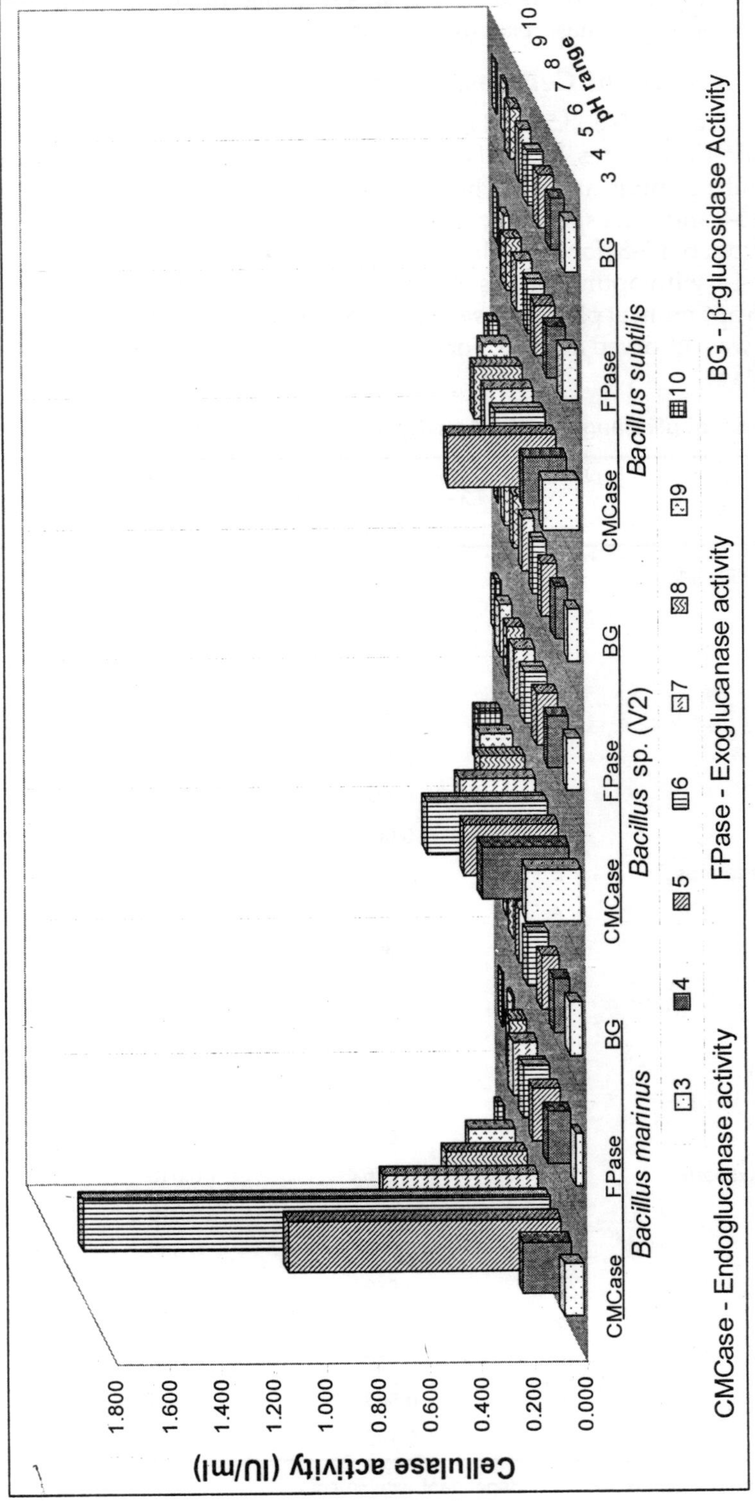

Figure 38.9: Effect of pH Range on the Activity of Cellulase Enzymes in Three Bacterial Cultures

Effect of Temperature on Activity of Cellulase Enzymes in Three Bacterial Cultures

The cellulase enzymes of selected bacterial cultures were subjected to different temperature range to evaluate optimum temperature for cellulolytic activities. The data obtained from the experiment are depicted in Table 38.6 and Figure 38.10. It is evident from the results that *Bacillus marinus* has very narrow range of temperature tolerance for endoglucanase, exoglucanase and β-glucosidase activity *i.e.* from 30-50°C. The maximum activity of all the three enzymes complex was best at 50°C. Any further increase in the temperature was found detrimental for the cellulases activity. The *Bacillus* sp. (V2) shows much broader range of temperature tolerance ranging from 30-80°C for endoglucanase activity whereas 30-70°C was found good for exoglucanase and β-glucosidase activities, 60°C was found best and optimum for all the three enzymes. *B.subtilis* shows broader range of temperature tolerance *i.e.* 30–70°C temperature for endoglucanase, exoglucanase and β-glucosidase activities. 50°C temperature was found best for all the three enzymes.

Table 31.6: Effect of Temperature Range on Activity of Cellulase Enzymes in Three Fungal Cultures

Sl.No.	*Fungal Culture*	*Temperature Range (°C)*	*Endoglucanase Activity (CMCase) (IU/ml)*	*Exoglucanase Activity (FPase) (FPU/ml)*	*β-glucosidase Activity (BG) (IU/ml)*
1.	*Aspergillus nidulans*	30	0.518	0.057	0.040
		40	0.567	0.090	0.039
		50	1.144	0.105	0.193
		60	2.040	0.074	0.210
		70	1.386	0.018	0.100
		80	0.202	0.009	0.087
		90	0.050	0.007	0.019
2.	*Aspergillus terreus*	30	1.210	0.045	0.055
		40	1.900	0.145	0.073
		50	1.250	0.146	0.177
		60	0.818	0.074	0.078
		70	0.211	0.018	0.071
		80	0.093	0.009	0.021
		90	0.013	0.009	0.015
3.	*Fusarium oxysporum*	30	0.430	0.007	0.025
		40	0.520	0.015	0.092
		50	0.788	0.035	0.110
		60	1.165	0.014	0.024
		70	0.218	0.009	0.012
		80	0.101	0.002	0.010
		90	0.022	0.001	0.003

All data given are the mean value of the two independent experiments.

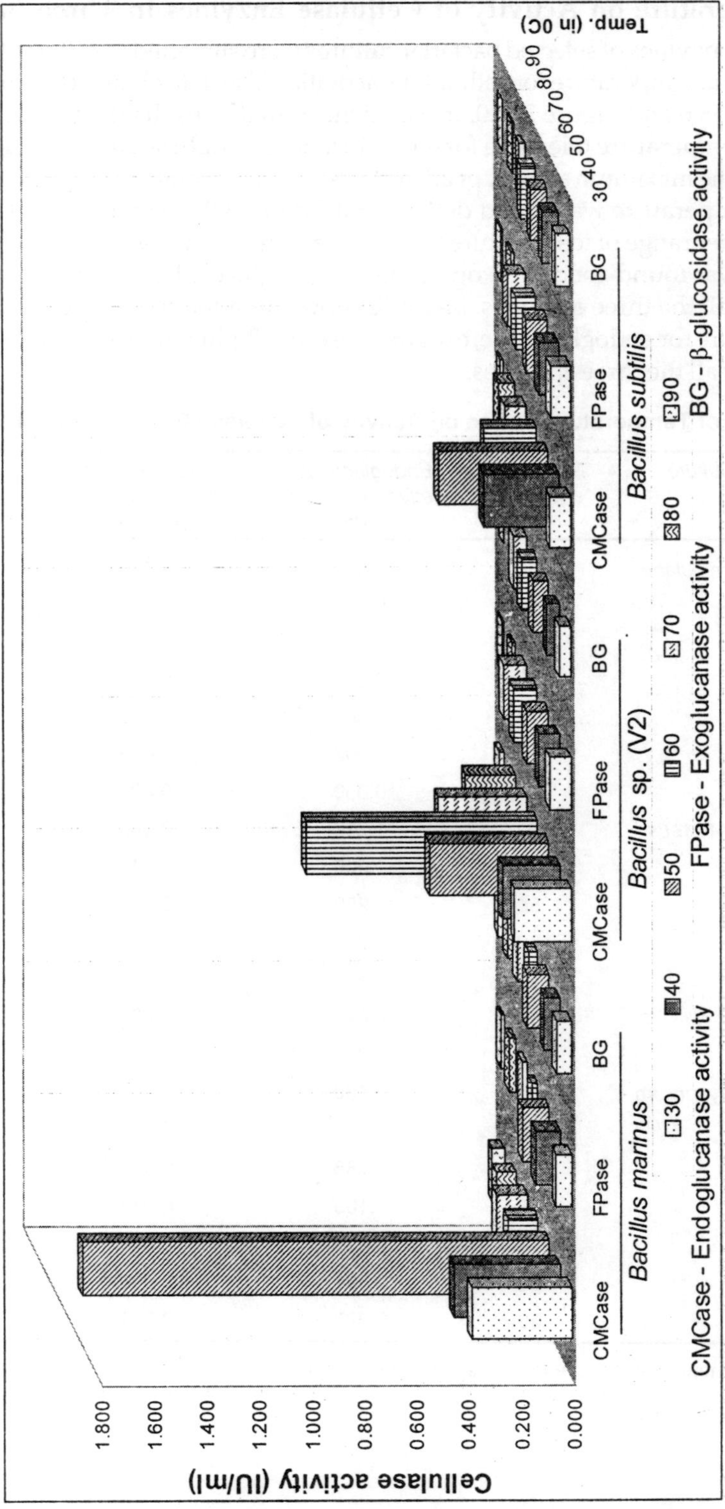

Figure 38.10: Effect of Temperature Range on the Activity of Cellulase Enzymes in Three Bacterial Cultures

Table 38.6: Cellulase Enzymes of Bacterial Cultures

Bacterial Cultures	*Isolate Number*	*Incubation Time (in days)*	*Endoglucanase Activity (CMCase) (IU/ml)*	*Exoglucanase Activity (FPase) (FPU/ml)*	*β-glucosidase Activity (IU/ml)*
Aeromonas hydrophila	J2	2	0.116	0.025	0.046
		4	0.238	0.069	0.057
		6	0.192	0.058	0.051
Bacillus marinus	O1	2	0.190	0.044	0.048
		4	0.404	0.086	0.065
		6	0.606	0.101	0.067
Bacillus subtilis	M1	2	0.204	0.030	0.044
		4	0.307	0.073	0.042
		6	0.393	0.074	0.056
Bacillus sp.	V2	2	0.189	0.042	0.036
		4	0.191	0.068	0.049
		6	0.425	0.081	0.057
Bacillus sp.	J3	2	0.102	0.024	0.112
		4	0.220	0.026	0.186
		6	0.362	0.030	0.203

All data given are the mean value of the two independent experiments.

Table 38.7: Effect of pH Range on the Activity of Cellulase Enzymes in Three Bacterial Cultures

Sl.No.	*Bacterial Culture*	*pH Range*	*Endoglucanase Activity (CMCase) (IU/ml)*	*Exoglucanase Activity (FPase) (FPU/ml)*	*β-glucosidase Activity (BG) (IU/ml)*
1.	*Bacillus marinus*	3	0.073	0.028	0.049
		4	0.187	0.09	0.065
		5	1.046	0.103	0.069
		6	1.783	0.100	0.077
		7	0.594	0.095	0.066
		8	0.311	0.063	0.044
		9	0.178	0.009	0.028
		10	0.022	0.004	0.025
2.	*Bacillus* sp. (V2)	3	0.208	0.051	0.045
		4	0.334	0.081	0.050
		5	0.362	0.081	0.057
		6	0.463	0.085	0.049
		7	0.294	0.081	0.044
		8	0.173	0.062	0.035
		9	0.128	0.048	0.028
		10	0.094	0.020	0.009

Contd...

Table 38.7–Contd...

Sl.No.	Bacterial Culture	pH Range	Endoglucanase Activity (CMCase) (IU/ml)	Exoglucanase Activity (FPase) (FPU/ml)	β-glucosidase Activity (BG) (IU/ml)
3.	*Bacillus subtilis*	3	0.136	0.061	0.049
		4	0.168	0.074	0.056
		5	0.415	0.077	0.061
		6	0.190	0.063	0.059
		7	0.185	0.061	0.044
		8	0.182	0.060	0.037
		9	0.109	0.022	0.009
		10	0.040	0.002	0.004

All data given are the mean value of the two independent experiments.

Table 38.8: Effect of Temperature range on Activity of Cellulase Enzymes in Three Bacterial Cultures

Sl.No.	Bacterial Culture	Temperature Range (°C)	Endoglucanase Activity (CMCase) (IU/ml)	Exoglucanase Activity (FPase) (FPU/ml)	β-glucosidase Activity (BG) (IU/ml)
1.	*Bacillus marinus*	30	0.379	0.059	0.058
		40	0.407	0.096	0.060
		50	1.776	0.100	0.083
		60	0.116	0.020	0.033
		70	0.114	0.019	0.033
		80	0.074	0.021	0.031
		90	0.046	0.012	0.021
2.	*Bacillus* sp.(V2)	30	0.215	0.080	0.046
		40	0.220	0.080	0.048
		50	0.456	0.085	0.057
		60	0.885	0.090	0.058
		70	0.336	0.084	0.046
		80	0.188	0.010	0.003
		90	0.020	0.004	0.001
3.	*Bacillus subtilis*	30	0.078	0.077	0.054
		40	0.288	0.077	0.061
		50	0.418	0.080	0.062
		60	0.199	0.078	0.056
		70	0.080	0.068	0.020
		80	0.061	0.009	0.005
		90	0.009	0.003	0.002

All data given are the mean value of the two independent experiments.

Effect of Chemicals Reagents on Endoglucanase Activity of Three Bacterial Cultures

Figures 38.11 and 38.12 shows the effect of chemical reagents *viz.* EDTA, 2, 4 DNP, $HgCl_2$ and $SnCl_2$ on *Bacillus marinus*. It is clearly evident from the results that EDTA and $SnCl_2$ did not much affected the endoglucanase activity. On the other hand, 2, 4 DNP and $HgCl_2$ were found to inhibit severely. The lower concentration (0.1 mM) of 2, 4 DNP reduces the endoglucanase activity upto 67 per

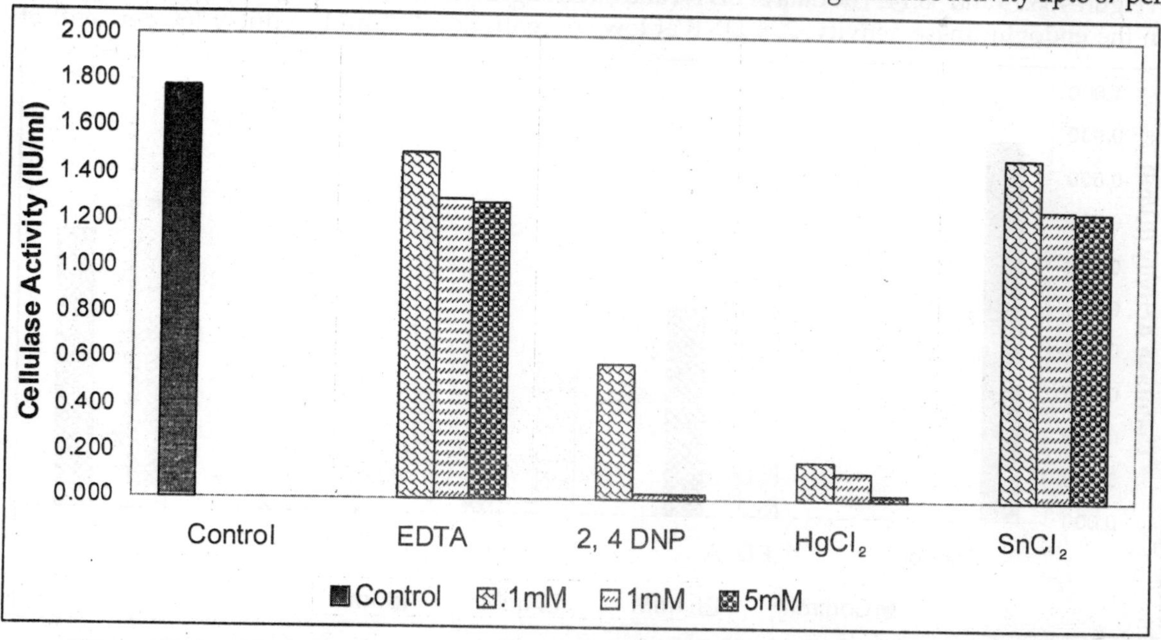

Figure 38.11: Effect of Chemical Reagents on Endoglucanase Activity of *Bacillus marinus*

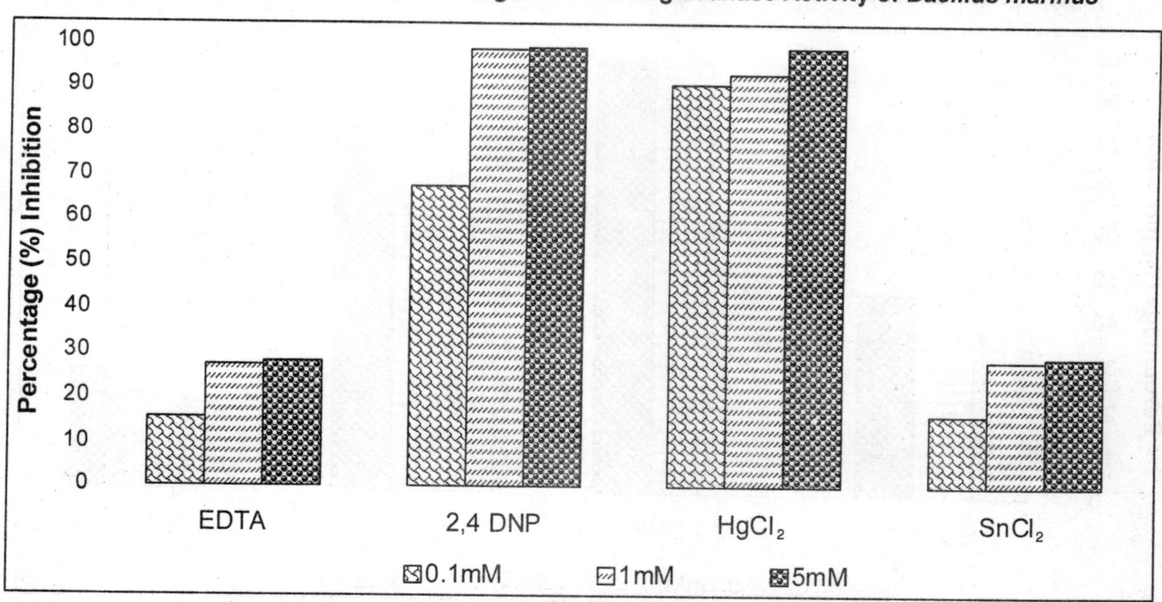

Figure 38.12: Percentage Inhibition of Endoglucanase Activity by Chemical Reagents in *Bacillus marinus*

cent and higher concentration (5 mM) were found to inhibit activity more than 95 per cent, and 0.1 mM concentration of $HgCl_2$ causes 95 per cent inhibition and higher concentration (5 mM) inhibited 100 per cent activity.

The results of effect of chemical reagent on endoglucanase activity of *Bacillus* sp. (V2) were presented in Figures 38.13 and 38.14. The data of EDTA and $SnCl_2$ suggest that they have lesser negative influence on the endoglucanase activity. 2, 4 DNP at low concentration (0.1 mM) reduces (60 per cent) of

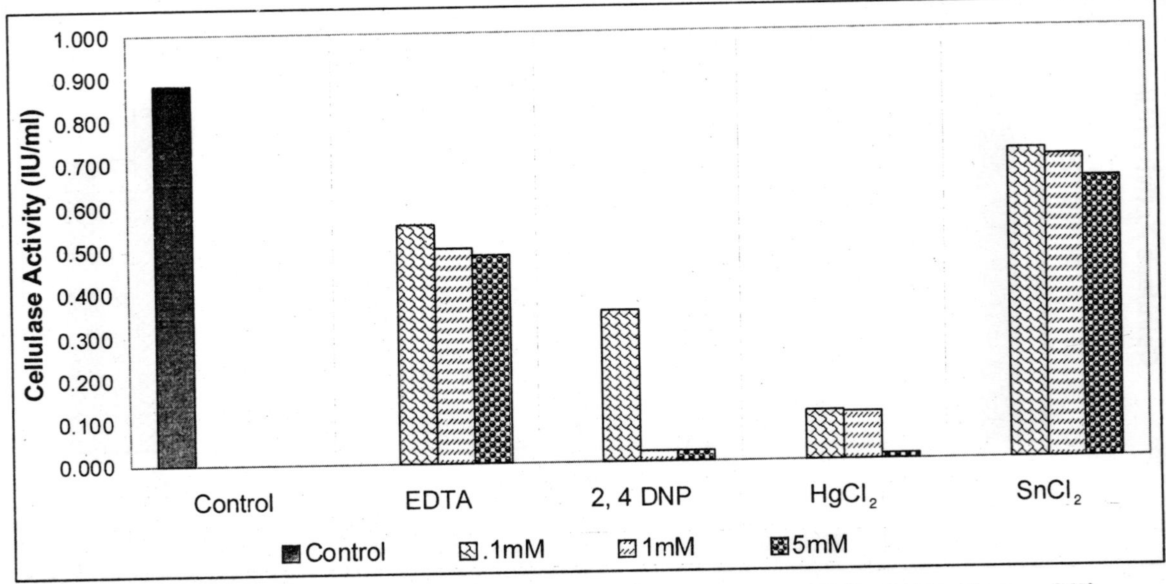

Figure 38.13: Effect of Chemical Reagents on Endoglucanase Activity of *Bacillus* sp. (V2)

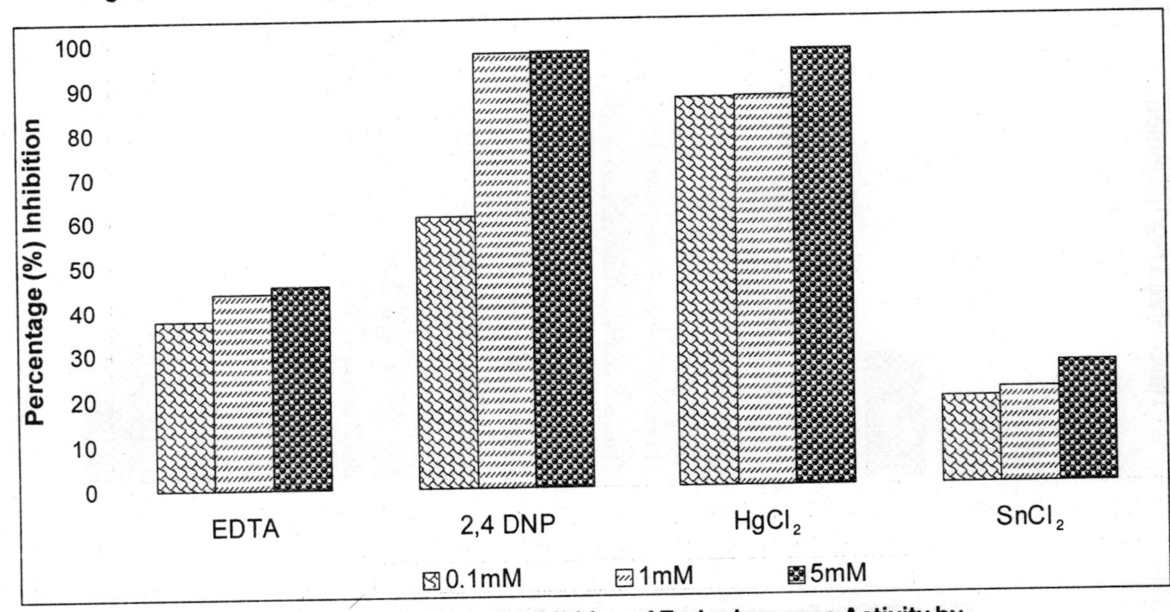

Figure 38.14: Percentage Inhibition of Endoglucanase Activity by Chemical Reagents in *Bacillus* sp. (V2)

endoglucanase activity and at higher concentration (5 mM) causes 97 per cent inhibition. Lower concentration (0.1 mM) of $HgCl_2$ causes 87 per cent inhibition and inhibited 98 per cent at 5 mM concentration.

Figures 38.15 and 38.16 shows the effect of chemical reagent on endoglucanase activity of *Bacillus subtilis*. The results clearly reveal that EDTA moderately inhibited the activity (40 per cent) at 0.1 mM and at 5 mM concentration causes 58 per cent inhibition. $SnCl_2$ made no significant adverse affect on

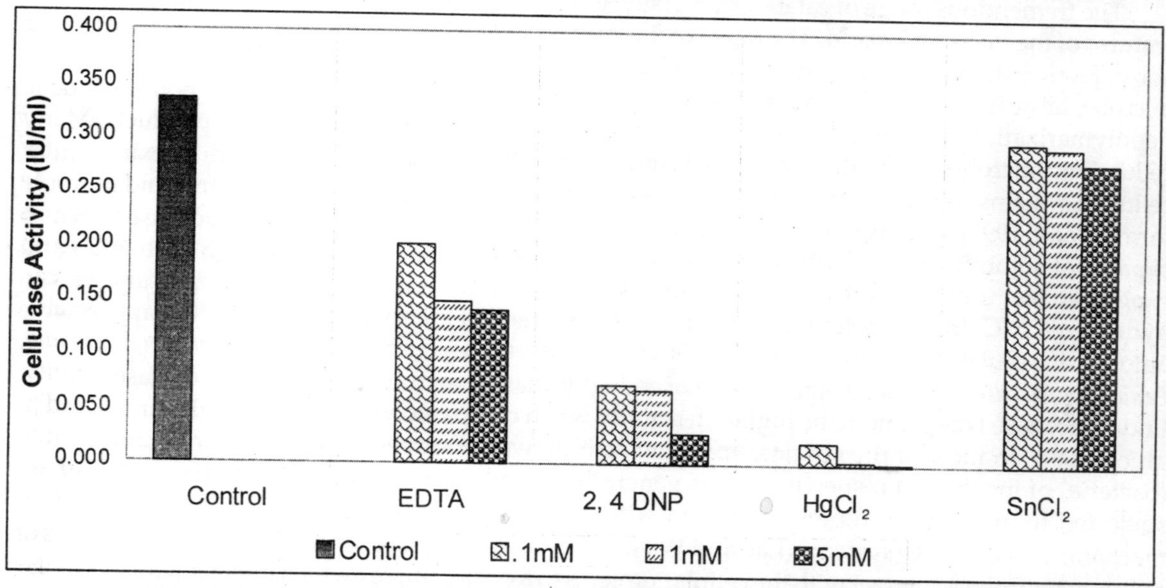

Figure 38.15: Effect of Chemical Reagents on Endoglucanase Activity of *Bacillus subtilis*

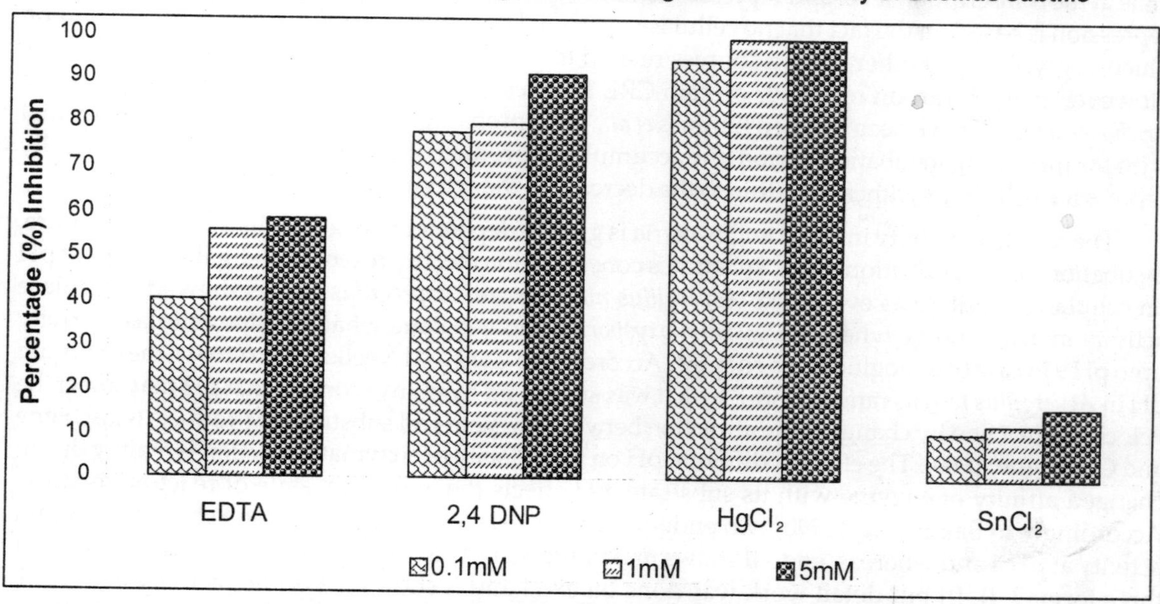

Figure 38.16: Percentage Inhibition of Endoglucanase Activity by Chemical Reagents in *Bacillus subtilis*

the activity. 2,4 DNP inhibited 77 per cent endoglucanase activity at 0.1 mM concentration and 5 mM concentration causes 90 per cent inhibition. $HgCl_2$ was found to the potent inhibitor as 94 per cent inhibition of endoglucanase activity at 0.1 mM concentration and 5 mM concentration causes 100 per cent inhibition of the activity.

Discussion

The tremendous range of catabolic diversity among microorganisms is one of the distinguishing features of the microbial world. The range of this diversity also differs widely among species utilizing one or few substrates to number of compounds as sole carbon and energy sources; however cellulolytic microbes lie near the specialist end of this continuum. The cellulose catabolism involves both enzymatic depolymerization of insoluble cellulose and cellular utilization of the hydrolytic products. Many cellulolytic microbes especially fungi when cultured on cellulosic carbon source produce extracellular cellulase systems consisting of endoglucanases, exoglucanases and β-glucosidase in free and multiple form (Wood, 1992). In comparison with fungi, most bacteria produce mainly endoglucanase enzymes capable of solubilizing amorphous and swollen cellulose (Wood, 1985). Although both endo and exoglucanases show very high activity toward amorphous cellulose, only endoglucanases can hydrolyze CMC. In the present investigation all the screened microbial forms secreted appreciable amount of cellulases in culture filterates. Species of *Aspergillus, Trichoderma, Chaetomium, Fusarium, Penicillum, Bacillus* produced high amount of endoglucanase, exoglucanase and β-glucosidase activity. Endoglucanase was found to be higher in activity when compared with that of exoglucanase and β-glucosidase. In most of the species, optimum activity was observed on 8th day (fungi) and 6th day (bacteria) of incubation respectively. It is generally accepted view that both bacteria and fungi are subjected to an inducer–repressor system with catabolite repression involved in the regulation mechanism of cellulase systems (Lao and Wilson, 1994). In catabolite repression the end products of cellulose hydrolysis interact with the cellular proteins to form a complex which interact with particular gene at the transcription level and represses cellulase synthesis (Lewin, 1987). The proof for catabolite repression is based on the fact that no cellulase in formed during the growth of a microorganisms on glucose, glycerol and other carbon sources related to glycolytic metabolism (Bhat and Bhat, 1997). However, general carbon repressor protein CRE 1 represses the transcription of cellulase genes in *Trichoderma reesei* have been isolated (Strauss *et al.*, 1995) probably support our finding indirectly that with the increasing incubation period, the accumulated product of cellulose hydrolysis catabolically repress the cellulase synthesis leading to the decrease in the enzyme activity.

The cellulase activity in fungi and bacteria is greatly dependent on factors like pH, temperature, incubation period, nutritional salt, substrates concentration etc. In present investigation effect of pH on cellulase activity was evaluated. *Aspergillus nidulans* and *Aspergillus terreus* showed a cellulase activity in acidic range whereas *Fusarium oxysporum* showed somewhat alkaline cellulase activity upto pH 9 in case of endoglucanase enzyme. According to Garg and Neelkanthan (1981), the optimum pH in *Aspergillus terreus* ranges from 3 to 6. It was suggested by many workers that pH may affect the velocity of reaction by changing the attraction between enzyme and substrate or products (Gascoigne and Gascoigne, 1960). The effect of different pH on the velocity of enzymatic reaction is mainly due to changed affinity of enzyme with its substrate, pH effects the ionization state of reaction mixture. Accordingly to Bagga *et al.* (1990) two endoglucanases exist endo I and II. Endo I shows maximum activity at pH 4 and whereas, endo II shows maximum activity at pH 5. Exoglucanases also occurs in three forms I, II, III but detail work was done on exo I and it shows maximum activity at pH 5.5. Similarly, β-glucosidase also exist in two forms I and II. β-glucosidase I shows maximum activity at pH 6 and pH 5 was enough for maximum activity of β-glucasidase II in *Aspergillus nidulans*. Tavolibov *et al.* (1988), Buachidze *et al.* (1987), Rodinova *et al.* (1987) have reported optimum pH of 4.5 for β-glucosidase in *Aspergillus terreus.* Cellulase activity has previously been reported in number of *Aspergillus* spp. (Rodionova *et al.*, 1987; Murao *et al.*, 1988; Tabolibov *et al.*, 1988; Bagga *et al.*, 1990; Himmel *et al.*, 1993; Galas and Romanowska, 1997; Chikamatsu *et al.*, 1999), *Fusarium oxysporum* (Christakopoulos, 1995 a,b), *Penicillium* sp. (Wood and McCrae, 1982; Bhat *et al.*, 1989; Reddy *et al.*, 1998).

Temperature is another important parameter for enzyme activity as lower temperature retard and higher temperature often inactivates the enzyme proteins by denaturing. The optimum temperature of an enzyme varies with factors such as enzyme purity, substrate, presence of activator or inhibitors, its usefulness for the purpose of characterizing enzyme is limited. *Aspergillus nidulans* showing temperature stability from 30-70°C indicate this fungi to exhibit thermophilic properties. *Aspergillus terreus* and *Fusarium oxysporum* was found to show mesophilic properties. Bagga *et al.* (1990) has reported maximum endoglucanases activity at 65°C, exoglucanase activity at 50°C and β-glucosidase activity at 65°C. However, in our finding maximum endoglucanase activity is observed at 60°C, exoglucanase and β-glucosidase activities are found at 50°C. Buachidze *et al.* (1987), Rodionova *et al.* (1987), Tavbolibov *et al.* (1988) reported the temperature optima of 55-60°C for β-glucosidase activity in *Aspergillus terreus. Fusarium oxysporum* showed optimum temperature 60°C (endoglucanase), 50°C (exoglucanase and β-glucasidase activities). Christakopoulos *et al.* (1995a) reported 55°C as optimum for endoglucanase activity in *Fusarium oxysporum.*

The number of bacterial genera was reported to produce cellulase enzymes. Among these *Bacillus* spp. were found to be dominant spp. in decomposing cellulosic waste. In nature *Bacillus* spp. are ubiquitous. There is a great diversity in physiology among member of the genus *Bacillus,* whose collective features include degradation most of all substrates derived from plant and animal sources including cellulose, starch, pectin, protein, agar, hydrocarbons and other antibiotic production, nitrification, denitrification, nitrogen fixation facultative lithotrophy, autotrophy, acidophily, alkaliophily, psychrophily, thermophily. Member of *Aeromonas* sp. were reported to produce cellulases (Ohya *et al.*, 1977; Nihlani and Satanarayana, 1992; Joshi and Bal, 1993). In the present finding, *Bacillus marinus* has broad pH and narrow temperature range for endoglucanase, exoglucanase and β-glucosidase activities, maximum enzymatic activities, at pH 6 and 50°C temperature were observed and therefore safely can be designated as mesophilic. This is the first ever report about the cellulolytic property of *Bacillus marinus. Bacillus subtilis* showed pH 5 and temperature optima 50°C for the three enzymes tested. *Bacillus* sp. (V2) showed optimum pH 6 for endo and exoglucanase activities and 5 pH for β-glucosidase activity. Temperature 60°C for endoglucanase, exoglucanase and β-glucosidase activities was observed optimum in *Bacillus* sp. (V2). However, Ozaki and Ito (1991) have reported the optimum pH 5.2 and 45°C temperature for cellulase activity in *Bacillus* sp. KSM-330. Robson and Chambliss (1984) observed optimum pH 4.8 and temperature 58°C for cellulase activity in *Bacillus* isolate. The capacity of selected *Bacillus* strains to produce and secrete large quantities of extracellular enzymes has placed them among the most important industrial enzyme producers. The ability of different *Bacillus* spp. to ferment in the acid, neutral and alkaline pH ranges, combined with the presence of thermophily in the genus, has lead to the development of variety of new commercial product with the desired temperature, pH activity and stability properties to address a variety of specific applications like deinking of pulp and paper industry and biostoning in textile industry. The endoglucanases enzyme system of bacteria seem to be quite complex. Yamne *et al.* (1970) identified two extra cellular (A and B) and one cell bound (c) endoglucanase components of bacteria *Pseudomonas fluorescens* var. *cellulosa,* which were purified and characterized. There are relatively few reports

(Sashihara *et al.*, 1984) of *Bacillus* spp. producing endoglucanases. Endoglucanases act synergistically with cellobiohydrolases and β-glucosidase during solubilization of crystalline cellulose (Nidetzky *et al.*, 1994; Bhat and Bhat, 1997). The best characterized example is *Bacillus subtilis* DLG (Robson and Chambliss, 1987). A number of *Bacillus* spp. were studied for their cellulase activity (Tewari and Chahal, 1977; Dhillon *et al.*, 1985; Robson and Chambliss, 1987; Nihlani and Satanarayana, 1992; Joshi and Bal, 1993; Gorska *et al.*, 2001).

Previously, there has been attempt to identify the active sites of endoglucanases, as these enzymes of cellulases complex have been widely used in the industrial processes. Active sites of cellulases have been carried out by chemical modification and inhibition studies (Dinur *et al.*, 1986). Chelator EDTA was found to effect endoglucanase activity in all fungi and bacterial cultures moderately at 5 mM concentration (not more than 45 per cent inhibition) accept *Fusarium oxysporum* and *Bacillus subtilis* in which 63 per cent and 53.86 per cent inhibition in endoglucanase activity was observed at 5 mM. The results probably suggest that EDTA is a metal chelator and probably might not chelate a possible divallent(s) required for endoglucanase activity. However, Robson and Chambliss (1984) reported that EDTA at concentration 50 mM inhibited only 10 to 20 per cent of TNP-CMC degrading activity in *Bacillus* sp. DLG and concluded that these compounds were not chelating cations required TNP-CMC degrading activity. Kotchoni *et al.* (2003) also reported 20 per cent inhibition in endoglucanase activity at 1 mM of EDTA in wild strain of *Bacillus pumillus* BPCRI. However in our finding 27.08 per cent of endoglucanase activity was inhibited in *Bacillus marinus*, 43 per cent and 55.65 per cent in *Bacillus* sp. (V2) and *Bacillus subtilis* respectively. The most notable inhibition was caused by 2,4 DNP and $HgCl_2$ in all the microbial form tested and inhibited almost complete endoglucanase activity at 5 mM concentration. 2,4 DNP, however has been reported as an uncoupler for oxidative phosphorylation (Ali and Sayed, 1992) indicating that a series of phosphorylation steps may play a crucial role in signaling transduction leading to cellulase synthesis. 2,4 DNP is a phenolic compound and phenol compound are well known repressor of cellulases enzymes (Varadi, 1972). Kotchoni *et al.* (2003) reported 100 per cent inhibition of endoglucanase activity in *Bacillus pumillus*. Metal shows both stimulatory as well as inhibitory effect on microorganisms while, iron ions are essential for growth of microorganisms. Although desired in minute concentration, some ions like mercury and silver are toxic even at small concentration. In our results $HgCl_2$ was found to inhibit almost complete endoglucanase activity in all the test organisms. The sensitivity toward $HgCl_2$ may be results of the interaction with a trypthophan residues(s) at the active site of endoglucanase as earlier suggested by Eriksson and Pettersson (1968) and Ozaki and Ito (1991). $SnCl_2$ also moderately inhibit the endoglucanase activity at high concentration. $SnCl_2$ is the member of p block, IV group metals (De, 1999). Lead, is also the member of same block and was found to be inhibiting cellulase activity in *Trichoderma reesei* (Kim *et al.*, 2001). $SnCl_2$ is also heavy metal like lead and probably might be inhibiting cellulase activity due to non-specific salt formation. Generally speaking cellulases enzymes are inhibited by Hg^+, Ag^{++}, Co^{++}, Cr^{++}, Pb^{++}, Zn^{++} salts at 10^{-3} M (Mandels and Reese, 1963). Similarly, Okada (1977) also reported the complete inhibition of endoglucanase (3.2.1.4) activity at 1 mM by Hg^{++} in *Trichoderma viride*.

Acknowledgement

Authors are thankful to Head, Department of Botany, Dr. H.S.G. Uinversity, Sagar, M.P. for providing laboratory facilities. AV greatfully acknowleged Head, Department of Biotechnology, Lovely University, Jalandhar, Punjab.

References

Ali, S., and A. Sayed. (1992). Regulation of cellulase biosynthesis in *Aspergillus terreus*. *World J. Microbiol. Biotechnol.* 8: 73-75.

Bagga, P.S., D.K. Sandhu, and S. Sharma. (1990). Purification and characterization of cellulolytic enzyme produced by *Aspergillus nidulans*. *J. Appl. Bacteriol.* 68: 61-68.

Belaich, J.P., A. Belaich, H.P. Fierobe, L. Gal, C. Gaudin, S. Pages, C. Reverbel-Leroy, and C. Tordif. (1999). The cellulolytic system of *Clostridium cellulolyticum*. p. 479-487. In: K. Ohmiya, K. Hayashi, K. Sakka, Y. Kobayashi, S. Karita, and T. Kimura ed., *Genetics, biochemistry and ecology of cellulose degradation*. Uni. Publishers, Tokyo, Japan.

Belaich, J.P., C. Tordif, A. Belaich, and C. Gaudin. (1997). The cellulolytic system of *Clostridium cellulolyticum*. *J. Biotechnol.* 57: 3-14.

Bergem, L.E.R., and L.G. Pettersson. (1973). The mechanism of enzymatic cellulose degradation, purification of a cellulolytic enzyme from *Trichoderma viride* active on highly ordered cellulose. *Eur. J. Biochem.* 37: 21-30.

Bhat, M.K. (2000). Cellulases and related enzymes in biotechnology. *Biotechnol. Adv.* 18: 355-383.

Bhat, M.K., and Bhat, S. (1997). Cellulose degrading enzymes and their potential industrial application *Biotechnol. Adv.* 15: 583-620.

Bhat, M.K., Gaikwad, J.S. and Maheswari, R. (1993). Purification and characterization of an extracellular β-glucosidase from thermophilic fungus *Sporotrichum thermophile* and its influence on cellulase activity. *J. Gen. Microbiol.* 139: 2825-2832.

Bhat, M.K., S.I. McCrae, and T.M. Wood. (1989). The endo-(1-4)-α-D-glucanase system of *Penicillium pinophillum* cellulase: isolation, purification and characterization of five major endoglucanase components. *Carbohyd. Res.* (190: 279-297.

Bisaria, V.S., and Mishra, S. (1989). Regulatory aspects of cellulase biosynthesis and secretion. *CRC Crit. Rev. Biotechnol.* 9: 61-103.

Brown, R.M. (1982). *Cellulose and Natural Polymer Systems: Biogenesis, Structure and Degradation*. Plennum. New York.

Buachidze, T.S., I.M. Tavabilov, N.A. Rodinova, and G.I. Kvesitadze. (1987). Isolation and purification of β-D-glucosidase from the thermophilic mutant *Aspergillus terreus*. *Appl. Biochem. Microbiol.* 23: 187-196.

Chikamatsu, G., K. Shirai, M. Kato, T. Kobayashi, and N. Tsukagoshi. (1999). Structure and expression properties of the endo-β-1, 4-glucanase A gene from the filamentous fungus *Aspergillus nidulans*. *FEMS Microbiol. Lett.*, 175: 239-245.

Christakopoulos, P., B.J. Macris, and D. Kekos. (1989). Direct fermentation of cellulose to ethanol by *Fusarium oxysporum*. *Enzyme Microb. Technol.*, 11: 236-239.

Christakopoulos, P., D. Kekos, B.J. Macris, M. Claeyssens, and M.K. Bhat. (1995a). Purification and characterization of a less randomly acting endo-1, 4-β-D-glucanase from culture filterates of *Fusarium culmorum*. *Arch. Biochem. Biophys.* 316 (1): 428-433.

Christakopoulos, P., D. Kekos, B.J. Macris, M. Claeyssens, and M.K. Bhat. (1995b). Purification and mode of action of low molecular mass endo-1, 4-α-D-glucanase from *Fusarium oxysporum*. *J. Biotechnol.* 39: 85-93.

Coughlan, M.P., and L.G. Ljungdahl. (1988). Comparative biochemistry of fungal and bacterial cellulolytic enzyme systems. p. 11-30. *In* J.P. Aubert, P. Beguin, and J. Millet ed. *Biochemistry and genetics of cellulose degradation*. FEMS Sym. 43. Academic Press, London.

Davis, B.D., and P.C. Tai. (1980). The mechanism of protein secretion across membranes. *Nature* (London). 283: 433-438.

De, A.K. (1999). *A text book of inorganic chemistry* Eighth edition. New Age Intel.

Dhillon, N., S. Chhibber, M. Saxena, S. Pajni, and D.V. Vadehera. (1985). A constitutive endoglucanase (CMCase) from *Bacillus licheniformis*-1. *Biotechnol. Lett.* 7: 695-697.

Din, N., H.G. Damude, N.R. Gilkes, R.C. Miller, R.A.J. Warren, and D.G. Kilburn. (1994). C_1-Cx revisited: intramolecular synergism in a cellulase. *Proc. Natl. Acad. Sci. USA*. 91: 11383-11387.

Dinur, T., K.M. Osiecki, G. Legler, S. Gatt, R.J. Desnick, and G.A. Grabourki. (1986). *Proc. Natl. Acad. Sci. U.S.A.* 83: 1660-1664.

Eggins, H.O.W., and G.J.F. Pugh. (1962). Isolation of cellulose decomposing fungi from the soil. *Nature* London 193: 94-95.

Ehrlich, P.R., and E.O. Wilson. (1991). Biodiversity studies. Science and Policy. *Science*. 253: 758-762.

Eidsa, G. (1972). Cellulase from *Coniophora cerebella* (Pers.) Duby. *Thesis*. University of Bergen.

Elberson, M.A., F. Malekzadeh, M.T. Yazdi, N. Kameranpour, M.R. Noori-Dioii, M.H. Matt, M. Shahamat, R.R. Colwell, and K.R. Sowers. (2000). *Cellulomonas persica* sp. nov. and *Cellulomonas iranensis* sp. nov. mesophilic cellulose degrading bacteria isolated from forest soil. *Int. J. Syst. Evol. Microbiol.* 50: 993-996.

Enari, T.M. (1983). Microbial cellulases, p. 83-223. *In* W.F. Forgaty (ed.) *Microbial enzymes and biotechnology*. Applied Sciences Publishers, London.

Enari, T.M., and M.L. Niku-Paavola. (1987). Enzymatic hydrolysis of cellulose: is the current theory of the mechanisms of hydrolysis valid? *CRC Crit. Rev. Biotechnol.* 53: 67-87.

Eriksson, K.E. (1969). New methods for the investigation of cellulases. *Adv. Chem. Ser.* 95: 88-104.

Eriksson, K.E. (1975). Enzymatic mechanism involves in the degradation of wood component. 12-14 *March. Symposium on enzymatic hydrolysis of cellulose.* Aulan Ko. Finland.

Eriksson, K.E. (1978). Enzyme mechanism involved in cellulose hydrolysis by rot fungus *Sporotrichum pulverulentum*. *Biotechnol. Bioeng.* 70: 317-332.

Eriksson, K.E., and G. Pettersson. (1968. Studies on the cellulolytic enzymes V. some structural properties of the cellulase from *Penicillium notatum*. *Arch. Biochem. Biophys.* 124: 160-166.

Eriksson, K.E., R.A. Blanchette, and P. Ander. (1990). "*Microbial and Enzymatic Degradation of Wood and Wood Components*". Springer Verlag, Berlin. Heidelberg. Germany.

Fagerstam, L.G., and L.G. Pettersson. (1980). The 1, 4-β-Glucan cellobiohydrolases of *Trichoderma reesei* QM 9414. A new type of cellulolytic synergism. *FEBS Lett.* 119: 97-100.

Fan, L.T., M.M. Gharpuray, and Y.H. Lee. (1987). *Cellulose Hydrolysis*. Berlin, Germany: Springer–Verlag 3: 1-68.

Fan, L.T., Y.H. Lee, and D.H. Beardmore. (1981). The influence of major structural features of cellulose on rate of enzymatic hydrolysis. *Biotechnol. Bioeng.* 23: 419-424.

Galas, E., and I. Romanowska. (1997). Purification and some properties of β-glucosidase from *Aspergillus niger* IBT-90. *Acta Microbiol. Pol.* 46: 241-252.

Garcia-Martinetz, D.V., A. Shinmyo, A. Madia, and A.L. Demain. (1980). Studies on cellulase production by *Clostridium thermocellum*. *Eur. J. Appl. Microbiol. Biotechnol.* 9: 189-197.

Gardner, R.M., K.C. Doerner, and B.A. White. (1987). Purification and characterization of exo-β-1, 4 glucanase from *Ruminococcus flavifaciens* FD-1. *J. Bacteriol.* 169: 4581-4588.

Garg, S.K., and S. Neelkanthan. (1981. Effect of cultural factors on cellulase activity and production by *Aspergillus terreus*. *Biotechnol. Bioeng.* 23: 1653-1659.

Gascoigne, J.A., and M.M. Gascoigne. (1960). *Biological degradation of cellulose*. Butterworths and Co. (Publ.) Limited. London. 264.

Ghose, T.K. (1969). Continuous enzymatic saccharification of cellulose with culture filterate of *Trichoderma viride* QM6a. *Biotechnol. Bioeng.* 11: 239.

Ghosh, M., and B. Nandi. (1995). p. 53 A.K. Roy, and K.K. Sinha ed. In: *Recently Advances in Phytopathology*. MD Publication, New Delhi.

Ghosh, S., B.P. Kapadnis, and N.B. Singh. (2000). Composting of cellulosic hospital waste: A potentially novel approach. *Int. Biodeter. Biodegrad.* 45: 89-92.

Ghosh, T.K., T. Panda, and V.S. Visaria. (1984). In: *VII*th *Int. Biotechnol. Sym.* IIT, New Delhi. 620.

Gilkes, N.R., B. Henrissat, D.G. Kilburn, R.C. Miller Jr., and R.A.J. Warren. (1991). Domains in microbial β-1, 4-glycanases: sequence conservation function and enzyme families. *Microbiol. Rev.* 55: 303-315.

Gilkes, N.R., R.A.J. Warren, R.C. Miller Jr., and D.G. Kilburn. (1988). Precise excision of the cellulose binding domains from two *Cellulomonas fimi* cellulases by a homologous protease and effect on catalysis. *J. Biol. Chem.* 263: 10401-10407.

Gilman, J.C. (2001). *A manual of soil fungi*. Biotech Book, New Delhi.

Gong, C.S., M.R. Ladisch, and T.G. Tsao. (1979). Biosynthesis, purification and mode of action cellulases of *Trichoderma reesei*. *Adv. Chem. Ser.* 181: 261-287.

Gorska, E., B. Tudek, and S. Russel. (2001). Degradation of cellulose by nitrogen-fixing strain of *Bacillus polymyxa*. *Acta Microbiol. Pol.* 50: 129-137.

Guglielmi, G., and P. Beguin. (1998). Cellulase and hemicellulase genes of *Clostridium thermocellum* from five independent collections contain few overlap and are widely scattered across the chromosome. *FEMS Microbiol. Lett.* 161: 209-215.

Hans, Y.W., and V.R. Srinivasan. (1968). Isolation and characterization of cellulose utilizing bacterium. *Appl. Microbiol.* 16: 1140-1145.

Hawksworth, D.L., and R.R. Colwell. (1992). Biodiversity amongst microorganisms at its relevance. *Biodiv. Conserv.* 1: 221-345.

Hawksworth, D.L., P.M. Kirk, B.C. Sutton, and D.N. Peglar. (1995). *Dictionary of Fungi*. CAB Intl.

Himmel, M.E., W.S. Adney, J.W. Fox, D.J. Mitchell, and J.O. Baker. (1993). Isolation and characterization of two forms of β-D-glucosidase from *Aspergillus niger*. *Appl. Biochem. Biotechnol.* 39/40: 213-225.

Joshi, A., and B. Ball. (1993). Extracellular alkaline enzymes of facultative bacteria of $CaCO_3$ kilns near Jabalpur. *Ind. J. Microbiol.* 33: 179-183.

Kim, D.W., Y.H. Jang, C.S. Kim, and N.S. Lee. (2001). Effect of metals ions on the degradation and adsorption of two cellobiohydrolases on microcrystalline cellulose. *Bull.*

Knosel, D. (1971). Continued investigation for pectolytic and cellulolytic activity of different *Bacillus* species. Zentralblatt. fur. *Bacteriologie* 126: 604-609.

Knowles, J.K.C., P. Lehtovaara, T.T. Teeri, M. Penttila, I. Salovuori, and L. Andre. (1987). *Philos. Trans. R. Soc.* London. 321: 449-454.

Kotchoni, O.S., O.O. Shonukan, and W.E. Gachomo. (2003). *Bacillus pumilus* BpCRI 6, a promising candidate for cellulase production under condition of catabolite repression. *Afr. J. Biotechnol.* 2: 140-146.

Labudova, I., and V. Farkas. (1983). Multiple enzyme forms in the cellulase system of *Trichoderma reesei* during its growth on cellulose. *Biochem. Biophys. Acta.* 744: 135-140.

Langford, M.L., N.R. Gialkes, W.W. Wakarchuk, D.G. Kilburn, R.C. Miller, and R.A.J. Warren. (1984). The cellulase system of *Cellulomonas fimi. J. Gen. Microbiol.* 130: 1367-1376.

Lewin, B. (1987). *Genes III, An up-to-date treatment of the molecular genetics of both eukaryotes and prokaryotes, along with related cell and molecular biology.* John Wiley, New York.

Ljungdahl, L.G., and K.E. Eriksson. (1985). Ecology of microbial cellulose degradation. *Adv. Microb. Ecol.* 8: 237-299.

Mandels, M., and E.T. Reese. (1963). Inhibition of cellulase and β-glucosidase. p. 115-158. *In* E.T. Reese, ed. *Advances in Enzymatic Hydrolysis of Cellulose and Related Materials.* Pergamon Press, London.

Mandels, M., and E.T. Reese. (1964). *Fungal cellulases and the microbial decomposition of cellulosic fabric. Development in Industrial* (Amer. Inst. Biol. Sci.) Washington D.C. Microbiol. 5: 5-20.

Murao, S., S. Sakamoto, and M. Arai. (1988). Cellulases of *Aspergillus aculeatus. Methods Enzymol.* 160: 275-299.

Nidetzky, B., W. Steiner, M. Hayn, and M. Claeyssens. (1994). Cellulose hydrolysis by the cellulases from *Trichoderma reesei::* a new model for synergistic interactions. *Biochem. J.* 298: 705-710.

Nihlani, D., and T. Satanarayana. (1992). Isolation and characterization of extracellular enzyme producing bacteria. *Ind. J. Microbiol.* 32 : 434-449.

Ohya, T., N. Yokoi, and T. Mase. (1977). "Process for preparation of enzymes". *UK Patent.* 1465307.

Okada, G. (1977). Enzymatic studies on a cellulase systems of *Trichoderma viride* II Purification and properties of two cellulases. *J. Biochem.* 77: 33-42.

Ozaki, K., and S. Ito. (1991). Purification and properties of an acid endo-1, 4-β-glucanase from *Bacillus* sp. KSM–330. *J. Gen. Microbiol.* 137: 41-48.

Priest, F.G. (1984). *Extracellular enzymes.* American Soc. Microbiol, Washinghton, D.C.

Reddy, B.R., G. Narsimha, and G.V.A.K. Babu. (1998). Cellulolytic activity of fungal culture. *J. Scient. Ind. Res.* 57: 617-620.

Reese, E.T., J.E. Lola, and F.W. Parrish. (1969). Modified substrates and modofied products as inducers of carbohydrolases. *J. Bacteriol.* 100: 1151-1154.

Reese, E.T., R.G.H. Siu, and H.S. Levinson. (1950). The biological degradation of soluble cellulose derivatives and relationship to the mechanism of cellulose hydrolysis. *J. Bacteriol.* 59: 485-497.

Robson, L.M., and G.H. Chambliss. (1984). Characterization of the cellulolytic activity of *Bacillus* isolate. *Appl. Environ. Microbiol.* 47: 1039-1046.

Robson, L.M., and G.H. Chambliss. (1987). Endo-β-1, 4 glucanase gene of *Bacillus subtilis* DLG. *J. Bacteriol.* 169: 2017-2025.

Rodionova, N.A., I.M. Tavobilov, L.I. Martinovich, T.S. Buachidze, G.I. Kvesitadze, and A.M. Bezborodov. (1987). β-Glucosidases from cellulolytic fungi *Aspergillus terreus, Geotrichum candidum* and *Trichoderma longibrachiatum* as typical glycosidases. *Biotechnol. Appl. Biochem.* 9: 239-250.

Sashihara, N., T. Kudo, and K. Horikoshi. (1984). Molecular cloning and expression of cellulase genes of alkaliphilic *Bacillus* sp. strain N-4 in *Escherchia coli. J. Bacteriol.* 158: 503-506.

Singh, A., A.B. Abidi, N.S. Darmwal, and A.K. Agrawal. (1991). Single cell protein production by *Aspergillus niger* and its evaluation. *Zentbl. Mikrobiol.* 146: 181-184.

Singh, A., A.K. Agrawal, A.B. Abidi, and N.S. Darmwal. (1990). Properties of cellobiose from *Aspergillus niger. Appl. Microbiol. Biotechnol.* 34: 356-358.

Singh, J.S., and E. Khurana. (2002). Paradigms of Biodiversity: An overview. *Proc. Ind. Natn. Sci. Acad. (PINSA).* B68 (3): 273-296.

Strauss, J., R.L. Mach, S. Zeilinger, G. Hartler, G. Stoffler, M. Wolschek, and C.P. Kubichek. (1995). Cre1, the carbon catabolite repressor protein from *Trichoderma reesei. FEBS. Lett.* 376: 103-107.

Subramanian, C.V. (1971). *Hyphomycetes: An account of Indian species except Cercosporae.* Indian Council of Agricultural Research. New Delhi. India.

Tavolibov, I.M., T.S. Buachidze, N.A. Rodionova, G.I. Kvesitadze, and A.M. Bezborodov. (1988). Substrate specificity and certain catalytic characteristic of β-glucosidase from *Aspergillus terreus. Biochemistry* 49: 847-853.

Teeri, T.T. (1997). Crystalline cellulose degradation: new insight into function of cellobiohydrolases. *Trends Biotechnol.* 15: 160-167.

Teeri, T.T., A. Koivula, M. Linder, G. Wohlfahrt, C. Devine, and T.A. Jones. (1998). *Trichoderma reesei* cellobiohydrolases: why so efficient on crystalline cellulose? *Biochem. Soc. Trans.* 26: 173-178.

Tewari, H.K., and D.S. Chahal. (1977). Growth and cellulase formation by *Bacillus* sps. *Ind. J. Microbiol.* 17: 23.

Tewari, H.K., S.S. Marwaha, and L. Singh. (1988). Studies on cellulase production from groundnut shell. *J. Res. (PAU)* 25: 424-432.

Thayer, D.W. (1978). Carboxymethylcellulase produced by facultative bacteria from the hind gut of the termite *Reticulitermes hesperus. J. Gen. Microbiol.* 106: 13-18.

Tomme, P., R.A.J. Warren, and N.R. Gilkes. (1995). Cellulose hydrolysis by bacteria and fungi. *Adv. Microbiol. Physiol.* 37: 1-81.

Varadi, J. (1972). In "*Biodetorioration of materials*". pp. 129-135 *In.* A.H. Walters and E.H. Hueck van der plas (eds). Applied Science, London.

Vyas, A., and D. Vyas. (2002). Cellulolytic activity of fungal cultures isolated from cellulosic laboratory waste. *J. Basic Appl. Micol.* 1: 183-185.

Vyas, A., D. Vyas, and K.M. Vyas. (2003a). Screening of Extracellular cellulases producing fungi from different lignocellulosic waste. *J. Basic Appl. Mycol.* 2: 41-43.

Vyas, A., D. Vyas, and K.M. Vyas. (2003b). Cellulolytic strains of *Aspergillus* and *Penicillium. J. Bot. Soc. University of Saugor. (Formerly Bull. Bot. Soc.)* 39: 61-77.

Warcup, J.H. (1955). The soil plate method for isolation of fungi from soil. *Nature* (London): 116-117.

Wood, P.J. (1980). Specificity in the interaction of direct of direct dyes with polysaccharides. *Carbohydr. Res.* 85: 271-287.

Wood, T.M. (1969). The cellulase of *Fusarium solani*. Resolution of the enzyme complex. *Biochem. J.* 115: 457-464.

Wood, T.M. (1975). Properties and mode of action of cellulase. pp. 111-137 *In* G.R. Wilki ed. *Cellulose as chemical, energy source,* N. York. John Wiley. New York.

Wood, T.M. (1985). Properties of cellulolytic enzyme system. *Biochem. Soc. Trans.* 13: 407-410.

Wood, T.M. (1992). Microbial enzymes involved in the degradation of cellulose components of plant cell walls. pp. 10-24. *In*: Rowett Research Institute Annual Report.

Wood, T.M., and S.I. McCrae. (1972). The purification and properties of the C_1 component of *Trichoderma koningii* cellulases. *Biochem. J.* 128: 1183-1192.

Wood, T.M., and S.I. McCrae. (1975). pp. 231-254. *In* M.J. Bailey, T.M. Enari, and M. Linko (ed.). *"Enzymatic hydrolysis of cellulose"* SITRA Helsinki.

Wood, T.M., and S.I. McCrae. (1977). Cellulase from *Fusarium solani*: Purification and properties of the C_1 components. *Carbohydr. Res.* 53: 117-133.

Wood, T.M., and S.I. McCrae. (1982). Purification and some properties of (1, 4)-β-D-glucan glucanohydrolase associated with the cellulase from the fungus *Penicillium funiculosum. Carbohydr. Res.* 110: 291-303.

Wood, T.M., and S.I. McCrae. (1986a). The cellulase of *Penicillium pinophilum*: synergism between enzyme components in solubilizing cellulosic with special reference to the involvement of two immunologically distinct cellobiohydrolases. *Biochem. J.* 234: 93-94.

Wood, T.M., and S.I. McCrae. (1986b). Purification and properties of a cellobiohydrolases from *Penicillium pinophillum. Carbohydr. Res.* 148: 331-344.

Wood, T.M., C.A. Wilson, S.I. McCrae, and A.L. Joblin. (1986). A highly active extracellular cellulase from anaerobic rumen fungus *Neocallimastix frontalis FEMS Microbiol. Lett.* 34: 37-40.

Wood, T.M., S.I. McCrae, and C.C. MacFarlane. (1980). The isolation purification and properties of the cellobiohydrolase components of *Penicillium funiculosum* cellulase. *Biochem. J.* 169: 51-65.

Wood, T.M., S.I. McCrae, and M.K. Bhat. (1989). The mechanism of fungal cellulase action. Synergism between enzyme components of *Penicillium pinophillum* cellulase in solubilizing hydrogen bond ordered cellulose. *Biochem. J.* 260: 37-43.

Wood, T.M., S.I. McCrae, C. Wilson, M.K. Bhat, and L. Gow. (1988). Aerobic and anaerobic fungal cellulases with special reference to their mode of attack on crystalline cellulose. pp. 31-53. *In* J.P. Aubert, P. Beguin, and J. Millet (ed.). "*Biochemistry and genetics of cellulose degradation*. FEMS Symp. 43 Academic Press London.

www.aspergillus.man.ac.uk

www.mycologyonline.adelaide.ac.edu

www.textbookofbacteriology.net/Bacillus.html

Yamane, K., H. Suzuki, and K. Nisizawa. (1970). Purification and properties of extracellular and cell bound cellulase components of *Pseudomonas fluorescens* var. *cellulosa*. *J. Biochem*. 67: 19-35.

Wood, M., S.J. McCormack, [illegible] and [illegible] with [illegible] In: [illegible] Academic Press, London.

www.aspergillus.man.ac.uk

www.[illegible]

www.textbookofbacteriology.net/Bacillus.html

Yamane, K., [illegible] and K. Nakazawa [illegible] components of [illegible]

Ecology

Microbial Biotechnology and Ecology (2011) *Pages* **669–682**
Editors: **Deepak Vyas, G.S. Paliwal, P.K.Khare and R.K Gupta**
Published by: **DAYA PUBLISHING HOUSE, NEW DELHI**

Chapter 39

Lichen Bioindicator Communities in Achanakmar: Amarkantak Biosphere Reserve, Madhya Pradesh and Chhattisgarh

☆ ***Satya and D.K. Upreti****

Lichenology Laboratory, National Botanical Research Institute (CSIR)
Rana Pratap Marg, Lucknow – 226 001, U.P.

ABSTRACT

Achanakmar-Amarkantak area, an interstate Biosphere Reserve falling in Madhya Pradesh and Chhattisgarh state, has been designated as 14th Biosphere Reserve by Government of India in the year 2005. Based on the habitat together with some morphological and anatomical characters the lichen taxa of the Achanakmar–Amarkantak Biosphere Reserve, categorized into 11 lichen communities. The biosphere reserve exhibit maximum cover of Physcioid lichen communities represented by 18 per cent followed by 16 per cent Pertusarioid, 13 per cent of Lecanoroid and 12 per cent of Lecideoid communities. On the basis of different lichen communities the study area can be clearly demarcated into undisturbed, moderately disturbed and disturbed areas. The Attaria, Kurkhuredader and near to Kabirchabutra area falls under the undisturbed area. The Kapildhara, Mai ki bagia, 7 km before Karanjia from Gorakhpur, Chauradader, Khurkhuridader VALCO mining site vergin forest area are moderately disturbed while 5 km before Chaparwa from Amarkantak, Pataleshwar, Durgadhara, Dindori forest rest house, 13 km before Kabirchabutra from Chauradader, are the disturbed area of the biosphere.

Keywords: *Bioindicator, Lichen Communities, Achanakmar-Amarkantak Biosphere Reserve.*

---

* E-mail: upretidk@rediffmail.com

Introduction

Conservation agencies are interested in promoting and maintaining biodiversity, based on rapidly measurable forest characteristics for effective implementation of protective measures (Neitlich and McCune, 1997). The lichens are one of the important components of biodiversity as they are well known as bioindicators. Lichens are vital components of the ecosystem serving as substrates, shelter, food, nutrient cycles and succession (Gradstein, 1992). Lichens are sensitive and widely accepted as indicators of air quality, biodiversity and climate change. Large scale data on lichens and environmental variables that determine their distribution are an integral component of many global conservation programmes.

Plants and allies can serve as bioindicators of environmental conditions and ecosystem health. Lichens communities are currently used as indicators of forest ecosystem function in several contexts. Region wide studies have goals of monitoring the relation of major factors such as climatic, air quality and forest tree species composition to variation in lichen communities, and how these relations interact and change over time. Studies of lichens of particular forest type often have goals of monitoring effects of forest management practices and landscape context, including a variety of indirect human impacts on forest environment. The presence of some particular communities of lichens in a forest indicates the status of the habitat. In the recent years lichen community are included in the forest health monitoring programs because they help to answer several key assessment questions. Repeated sampling of lichen communities in permanent plots can be utilized to document the changes in the condition of lichen communities overtime which also reflects the environmental condition of the area.

Owing to the vast natural resources, diverse and rich flora and fauna, unique topography and geographical situation, the Achanakmar–Amarkantak area an interstate Biosphere Reserve has been designated as 14th Biosphere Reserve by Government of India in the year 2005. Though, a number of information regarding the higher group of plants are available from the Biosphere Reserve, however, the studies on most of cryptogamic plants are quite neglected. Recently, Satya (2006), enumerated 130 species belonging to 44 genera and 25 families of lichens from the Biosphere Reserve. In the present paper an attempt has been made to provide the detailed account of Bioindicator lichen communities in the Biosphere Reserve. The available account of bioindicator communities and their distribution pattern can be used as an useful tool for defining and presenting the disturbed and undisturbed areas of the Biosphere Reserve. The bioindicators communities also used in indicating areas of conservation interest.

Materials and Methods

Study Area

The Achanakmar-Amarkantak Biosphere Reserve (AABR) lies between 22º15' to 22º58' N and 81º25' to 82º5' E, having an area of 3835.51 sq km (Figure 39.1 and Table 39.1). It comprises part of Bilaspur district of Chhattisgarh, Dindori and Anuppur districts of Madhya Pradesh falling in agro-climatic zone. Out of 3835.51 sq km area, 1224.98 sq km falls in Madhya Pradesh and remaining area of 2610.53 sq km in Chhattisgarh state. The AABR area includes one core zone *i.e.* Achanakmar Wildlife Sanctuary lying in Bilaspur district with a total geographical area of 551.15 sq km.

The AABR has a varied topography, the districts of Bilaspur and Anuppur has plane rice fields. The Dindori has undulating hillocks, while Maikal range of Satpuras culminating in the Amarkantak plateau of bauxite rocks. Numerous streams and "nallas", many of which are perennial, cut up the whole area. Thus variety of landforms is one of the major attributes of AABR. The Biosphere Reserve is one of the major watershed of the peninsula and it is the source of three major river systems namely

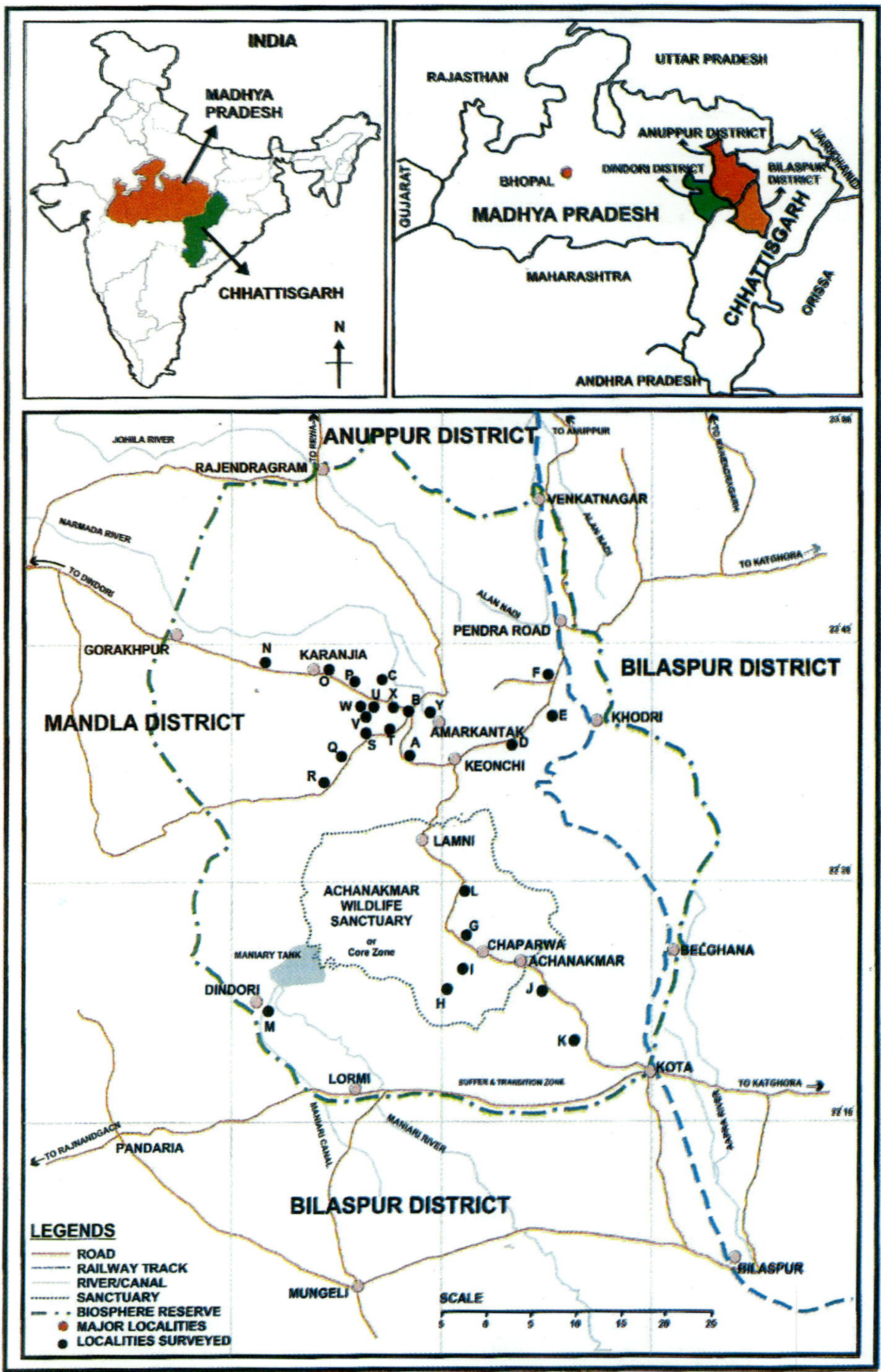

Figure 39.1: Map Showing the Localities Surveyed for Lichen Study, for Legends Please see Table 39.1

Narmada, Johilla and Sone (Ganga basin) and Ama nallah stream that join Arpa river (Mahanadi basin).

Table 39.1: The Sites Selected for Collection of Lichens, their Altitude and Major Phorophytes

Locality Codes	*Localities*	*Altitudes (m)*	*Phorophytes*
A	Attaria	680	*Shorea robusta*
B	Kabirchabutra	808	*Shorea robusta, Mangifera indica, Syzygium cuminii, Ficus* sp.
C	Kapildhara	808	*Shorea robusta, Syzygium cuminii, Mallotus philippensis*
D	Mai ki Bagia	804	*Shorea robusta*
E	Jwaleshwar	804	*Shorea robusta, Emblica officinalis, Ficus* sp, *Terminalia arjuna, Mallotus philippensis*
F	Durgadhara	784	*Mangifera indica,* Unidentified tree, *Syzygium cuminii*
G	5 km before Chaparwa from Amarkantak	476	*Mallotus philippensis, Shorea robusta,* Unidentified tree
H	Gabhighat	488	*Mallotus philippensis, Ficus racemosa, Terminalia arjuna, Mangifera indica, Syzygium cuminii,* Unidentified tree
I	Chaparwa naala	457	*Mallotus philippensis, Shorea robusta, Ficus racemosa*
J	5 km away from Chaparwa towards Kota	439	*Mallotus philippensis, Syzygium cuminii, Shorea robusta*
K	Border of Achanakmar Wildlife Sanctuary	448	*Mallotus philippensis, Shorea robusta, Bauhinia* sp., *Syzygium cuminii,* Unidentified tree
L	22 km before Keonchi from Chaparwa	488	*Mallotus philippensis, Syzygium cuminii, Shorea robusta, Mangifera indica, Emblica officinalis,* Unidentified
M	Dindori forest rest house	303	*Acacia nilotica*
N	7 km. before Karanjia from Gorakhpur	400	*Mangifera indica, Pongamia Pinnata, Grewia* sp., *Azadirachta indica, Acacia nilotica*
O	Karanjia forest rest house	400	*Shorea robusta, Mangifera indica*
P	Jagatpur forest rest house	393	*Shorea robusta*
Q	Chauradader	454	*Shorea robusta*
R	Tarwartola	448	*Shorea robusta*
S	13 km. before Kabirchabutra from Chauradader	454	*Grewia* sp., *Pongamia pinnata* sp.
T	8 km. before Kabirchabutra from Chauradader	448	*Shorea robusta, Emblica officinalis*
U	Khurkhuridader VALCO mining site plantation area	448	*Shorea robusta*
V	Khurkhuridader VALCO mining site vergin forest	448	*Shorea robusta, Mangifera indica, Eucalyptus* sp., *Grewia* sp.,
W	Khurkhuridader	454	*Shorea robusta.*
X	Near to Kabirchabutra	424	*Shorea robusta.*
Y	Patalashwar temple	808	Lime plaster of monuments.

Sampling Method

The lichen samples were collected from rocks and trees from 25 localities of AABR Madhya Pradesh and Chhattisghar. The lichen specimens were identified by studying their morphology, apothecial anatomy, chemistry and following the literature of Awasthi (1988, 1991) and Upreti (1991). The chemical investigations of the specimens were performed according to Walker and James (1980).

Results and Discussion

Bioindicator Lichen Communities

The presence of some particular communities of lichens in a forest indicate the status of the habitat. In the recent years lichen communities are included in the forest health monitoring programs because they help to answer several key assessment questions. Repeated sampling of lichen communities in permanent plots can be utilized to document the changes in the condition of lichen communities overtime which also reflects the environmental condition of the area.

Lichens respond to the environmental changes in the forest, including changes in forest structure, air quality and climate. The disappearance of lichens in a forest may indicate environmental stress, such as high level of sulphur dioxide based pollutants and nitrogen.

The lichen taxa so far known from the biosphere reserve represents eleven lichen community types, based on the habitat together with some morphological and anatomical characters of the lichens (Figure 39.2).

Pyrenocarpous Lichen Community

The lichen community is represented by the perithecia bearing lichen taxa and growing mostly on the smooth barked trees in moist evergreen phorophytes. *Dermatocarpon miniatum* a single saxicolous

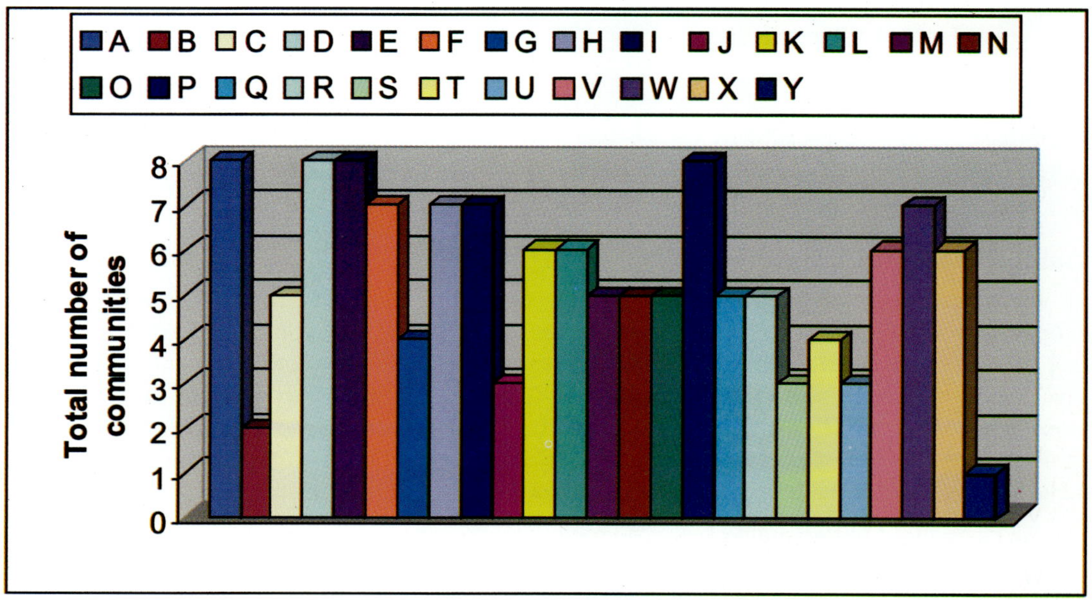

Figure 39.2: Bioindicator Lichen Communities in Different Localities of AABR

species of pyrenocarpous lichens is known from the Kapildhara falls area found growing on moist boulders under shade. The Chaparwa area, 5 km before Chaparwa from Amarkantak, 22 km before Keonchi from Chaparwa are the sites exhibit occurrence of *Pyrenula fuscoolivacea* and *P. subglobriscula*, dence forest patches with evergreen phorophytes (Plate 39.1).

Graphidaceous Lichen Community

The fruiting bodies (apothecia) in Graphidaceous lichen taxa are modified into elongate, simple to branched structures called lirellae, represented by the lichen genera *Graphis*, *Phaeographis* and *Arthonia*. The graphidaceous lichens grow both on dry and moist places. In dry well lit areas of the forest they grow in association with Lecanoroid communities while in moist habitats, pyrenocarpous lichens are their companions.

The Jagatpur forest rest house, Khurkhuridader, Near to Kabirchabutra, Attaria, Kapildhara, Mai ki Bagia, Jwaleshwar, Durgadhara and Gabhighat area clearly indicates the moist evergreen forest patches with in the dry deciduous forest, and hence represent excellent growth of graphidaceous lichen communities (Plate 39.1B).

Cynophycean Lichen Community

Collema, *Leptogium* and *Peltula* are the major blue-green alga containing lichen taxa of the biosphere reserve. Both *Collema* and *Leptogium* have ability to grow on soil, rocks and barks of the trees while *Peltula* species only grows on rocks. The cynophycean lichen indicates the nutrient poor, moist and shady locations of the biosphere reserve (Plates 39.1C). The Kapildhara, Gabhighat, Chaparwa nala, 5 km away from Chaparwa towards kota, Border of AWLS, Tarwartola, Khurkhuridader VALCO mining site plantation area, Khurkhuridader VALCO mining site vergin forest, near to Kabirchabutra area are with perennial streams and have shallow vallies which provides a moist and shady habitat for cynophycean lichen communities to colonize. The rocks both exposed and under forest, bear luxuriant growth of *Peltula*.

Lecanoroid Lichen Community

The Lecanoroid community is characterized by the apothecia bearing crustose lichens. Presence of Lecanoroid communities indicates the well lit habitats of the Biosphere Reserve. Twelve species of the Lecanoroid lichen communities comprising *Lecanora*, *Lecidella* and *Vainoria* sp., are found growing on both thick, thin, dry and moist bark of trees. The Chaperwa nala area exhibit the maximum diversity of the Lecanoroid communities (Plate 39.1D).

Parmelioid Lichen Community

The Parmelioid lichen communities are characterized by the leafy growth formed lichens, best developed in well lit, moderately acidic substrates (Plate 39.1E). The rough-barked trees of *Shorea robusta* both in more open and closed canopy forest area provide a suitable habitat for Parmelioid lichens. *Shorea robusta* tree is a suitable phorophyte for the luxuriant growth and development of crustose lichen. Out of 64 lichen, species recorded from *Shorea robusta* trees in various forests sites of India, 42 species fall under the crustose lichens (Satya *et al.*, 2005). The Tarwartola and Jagatpur Forest Rest House area exhibit the best habitat for colonization of this community.

Some Parmelioid member also grows on rocks both in exposed and on rocks covered under thick forest canopy. Such rocks in Kapildhara, Jwaleshwar forest and Kurkhuridader area exhibit the growth of saxicolous Parmelioid lichens in association with *Caloplaca*, *Peltula*, *Buellia*, *Staurothele* and *Diploschistes* species.

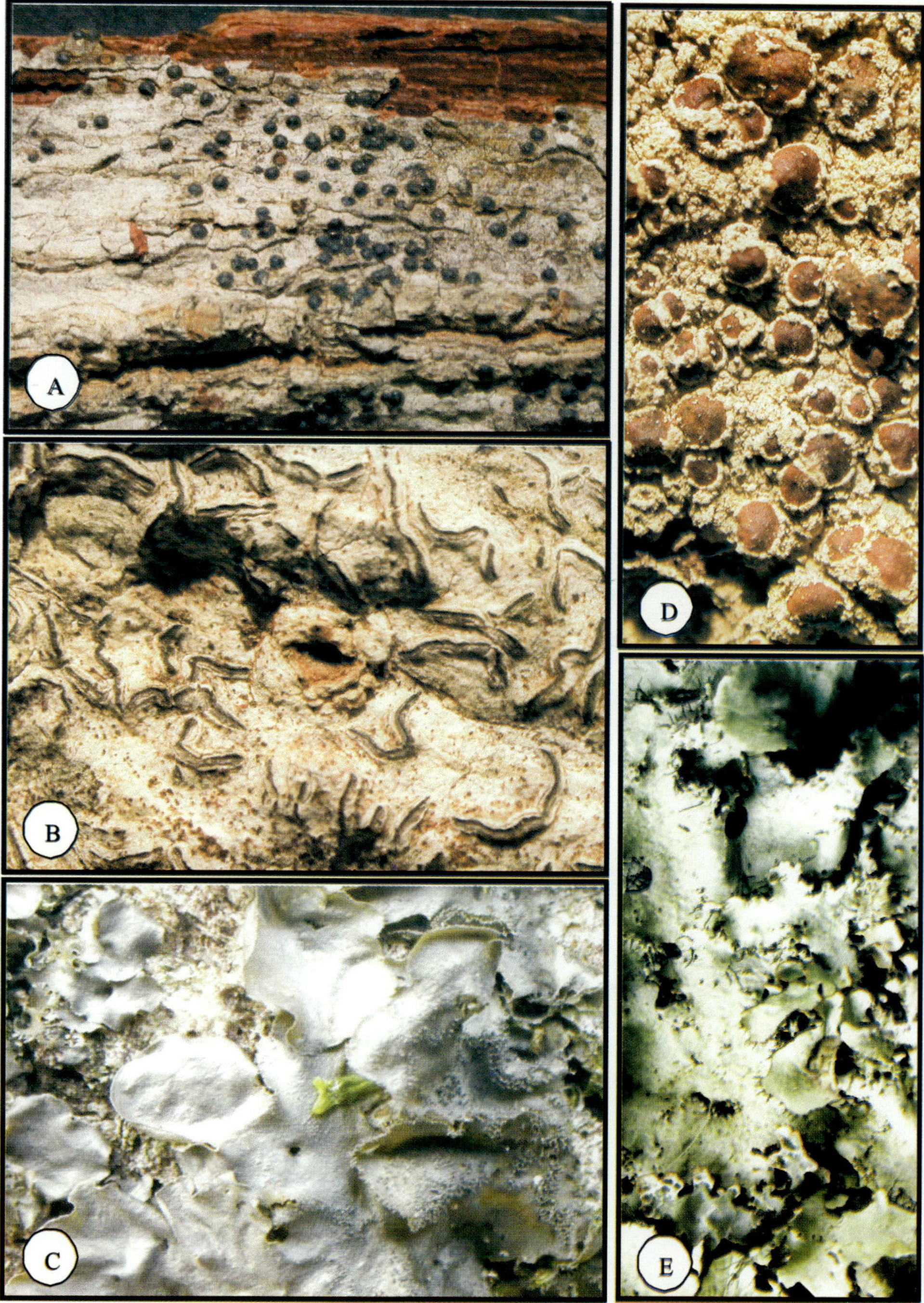

Plate 39.1 A–E: Bioindicator Lichen Communities

A: Pyrenocarpous lichen *Pyrenula* sp.; B: Graphidaceous lichen, *Graphis* sp.; C: Cynophycean lichen, *Leptogium* sp.; D: Lecanoroid lichen, *Lecanora* sp.; E: Parmelioid lichen, *Parmotrema* sp.

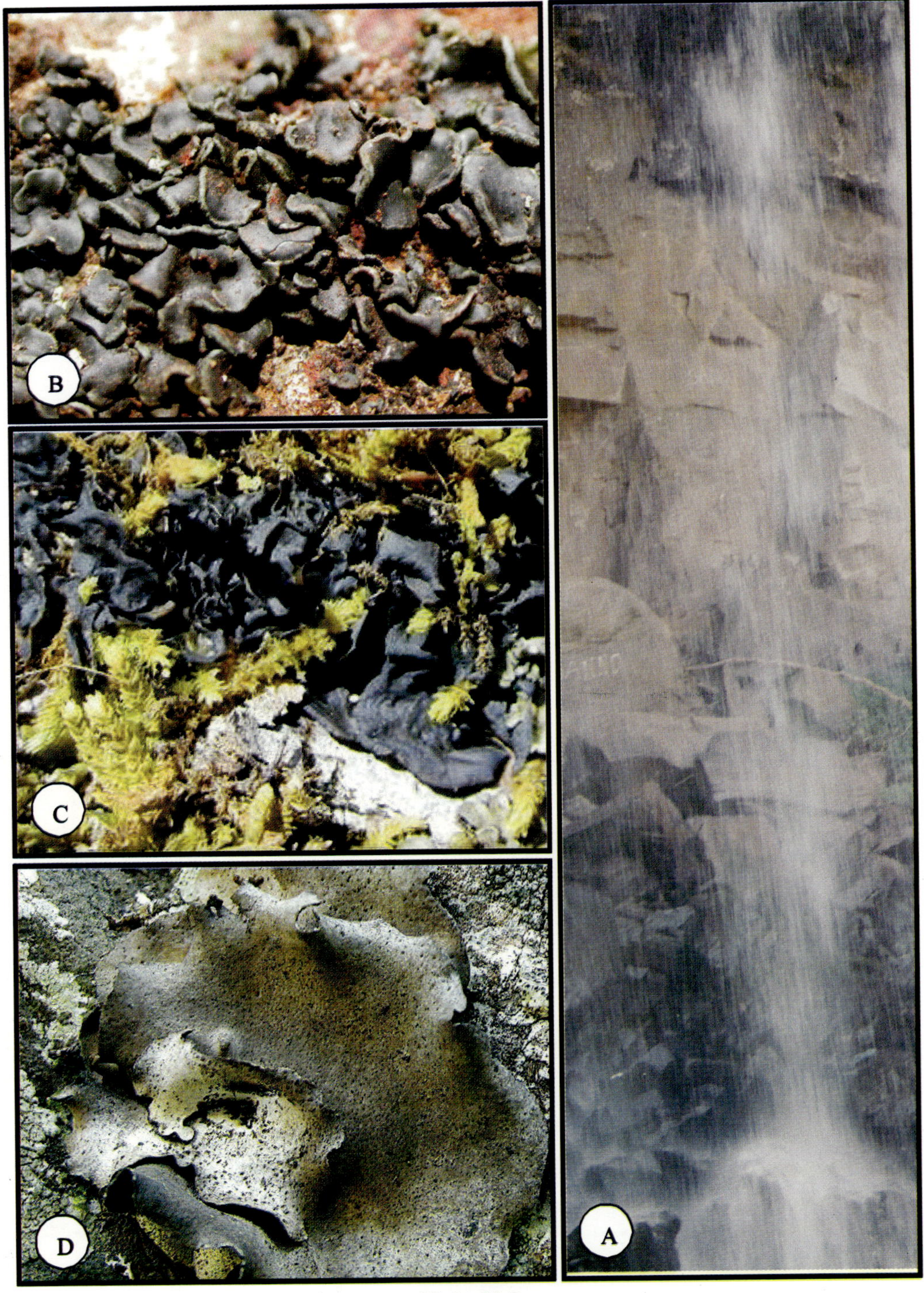

Plate 39.2

A: Water Fall in Kapildhra Area; B: *Peltula* sp.; C: *Collema* sp.; D: *Dermatocarpon miniatum*

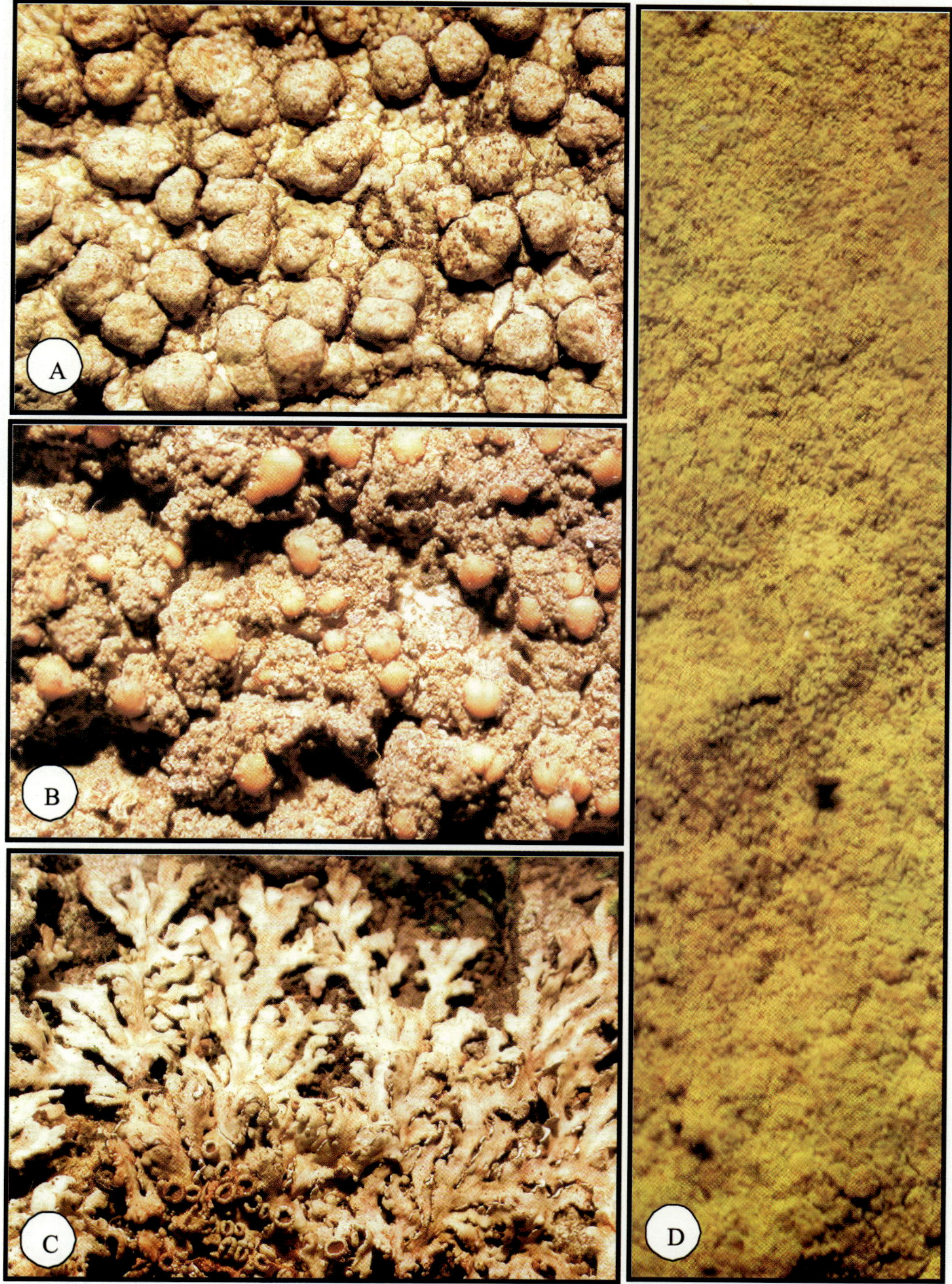

Plate 39.3 A–D: Bioindicator Lichen Communities

A: Pertusarioid lichen, *Pertusaria* sp.; B: Lecideoid lichen, *Bacidia* sp.; C: Physcioid lichen, *Hetetodermia* sp.; D: Leprarioid lichen, *Chrysothrix* sp.

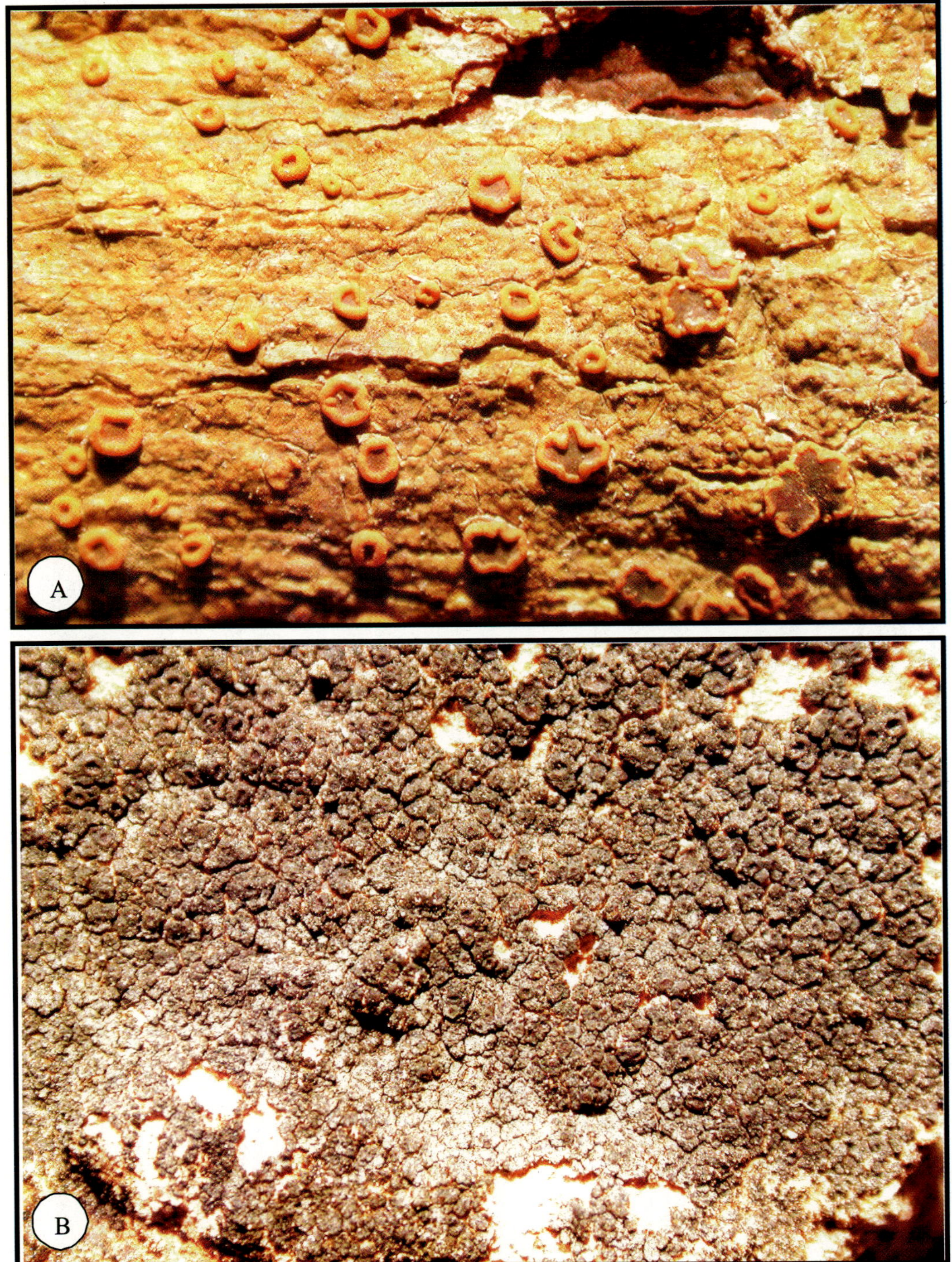

Plate 39.4 A–B: Bioindicator Lichen Communities

A: Teloschistaceous lichen, *Letrouitia* sp.; B: Lichinioid lichen, *Phylliscum* sp.

Pertusarioid Lichen Community

The community is characterized by crustose, verrucose-fertile and verrucose-sorediate thallus. The community indicates old tree forest. The thick, rough-barked trees of *Shorea robusta* in the dry deciduous forest appears exellent host for the Pertusarioid communities with verrucose-fertile taxa as 19 such species are reported on the *Shorea robusta* trees, while the *Pertusaria amara* (a verrucose-sorediate) taxon often colonize on rather more smooth-bark trees of *Grewia*. The community member grows on exposed roots of *Shorea* on trunk at base, on branches and twigs in association with the members of both foliose and crustose lichens. The common foliose taxa are the species of *Dirinaria* while *Buellia*, *Lecanora* and lirelliforem species of Graphidaceous lichen are the common crustose lichens (Plate 39.2A).

Lecideoid Lichen Community

The community is characterized by crustose to squamulose thalloid lichens bearing apothecia without thalline cover. The members of the community colonized on the bark of deciduous trees in sheltered and well lit sites. The genera *Bacidia*, *Phyllopsora* and *Schadonia* have similar morphology of thallus which grow on thick, rough-barked trees at their basal parts in moist, shady places while *Haematomma* and *Protoblastenia* prefers smooth barked trees in open area. The rock inhabiting lecideoid community belongs to a single genus *Trapeliopsis* sp., which grows on moist rocks in Kabirchabutra area. The members of Graphidaceous lichens, *Buellia*, *Lecanora* are the common associates of this community (Plate 39.2B).

Leprarioid Lichen Community

The community has the members of lichens having powdery thallus of varnish like crust over substrates. *Chrysothrix*, *Cryptothecia* and *Lepraria* are the common genera of the Leprose lichen in the Biosphere Reserve. The member of this community grows both on rocks and trees. The rocks in vertical moist places exhibit luxuriant growth of Lepraria while *Chrysothrix* and *Cryptothecia* mostly colonized on dry, rough-barked trees in moist and dry places in association with Lecanoroid and Teloschistaceous lichens. After forest fire, the *Chrysothrix* grows mostly on mature *Shorea robusta* trees at basal parts and trunks as the pioneer colonizer (Plate 39.2D).

Physcioid Lichen Community

The members of the family Physciaceae belongs to this community. Comprising of both to the crustose and foliose form of lichens, growing on a varied range of substrates. The foliose genera *Dirinaria*, *Pyxine*, *Physcia*, *Heterodermia* and *Phaeophyscia* under this community exhibit the maximum host diversity. The saxicolous taxa of the community mostly grows on rocks in moist places. The crustose taxa of the community such as *Buellia* and *Rinodina* are mostly grows in moist places. Mature *Shorea robusta* trees in moist places exhibit luxuriant growth of *Dirinaria* in association with *Heterodermia* in the Khurkhuridader area while Kabirchabutra and Kapildhara area has luxuriant growth of *Heterodermia diademata* on soil, rocks and barks of different trees (Plate 39.2C).

Teloschistaceous Lichen Community

The community is characterized by anthraquinone containing yellow crustose thallus and lichen genera *Caloplaca* and *Letrouitia* belongs to this community. *Letrouitia* is a corticolous genus while *Caloplaca* grows both on rocks and bark of trees. The members of *Caloplaca* indicate the moist as well as well lit area of the biosphere reserve. The members grow both on rough and smooth surfaced rocks in exposed and mostly on the semi shaded rocks. The Kapildhara area with semi shaded moist rocks are the excellent habitat for *Caloplaca* to colonize. *Letrouitia* species exhibit their luxuriant growth on smooth, hard barked trunks of *Mallotus* trees (Plate 39.3A).

Lichinioid Lichen Community

The lichen genus *Phylliscum* is the only member of this community known from the biosphere reserve and found growing on man-made substrate in Amarkantak area. This genus has dark brown black crustose to squamulose thallus, which forms large black patches on the lime plaster of buildings and monuments. The member of the community also indicates the presence of calcareous rocks in the Biosphere Reserve. The member of Pyrenocarpous lichens such as *Endocarpon* and *Staurothele* also grow in association of this community.

The biosphere reserve exhibit the maximum 18 per cent cover of Physcioid lichen communities followed by 16 per cent Pertusarioid, 13 per cent Lecanoroid and 12 per cent of Lecideoid communities. The members of Physciaceae family are more tolerant to extreme environment (Backor *et al.*, 2003).

The Cynophycean, Graphidaceous and Pyrenocarpous lichen communities are represented each by 7 per cent, while the Lichinioid lichen community has the minimum cover of 1 per cent (Figure 39.3).

Based on the occurrence of the different lichen communities the study area can be clearly demarcated into undisturbed, moderately disturbed and disturbed areas (Figure 39.3). The Attaria, Kurkhuredader and near to Kabirchabutra area falls under the undisturbed area. The Kapildhara, Mai ki bagia, Border of AWLS, Jwaleshar, 7 km before Karanjia from Gorakhpur, Karanjia forest rest house, Jagatpur forest rest house, Chauradader, Khurkhuridader VALCO mining site plantation area, Khurkhuridader VALCO mining site vergin forest area are moderately disturbed while 5 km before Chaparwa from Amarkantak, Pataleshwar, Durgadhara, Dindori forest rest house, 13 km before Kabirchabutra from Chauradader, 8 km before Kabirchabutra from Chauradader falls under the disturbed category.

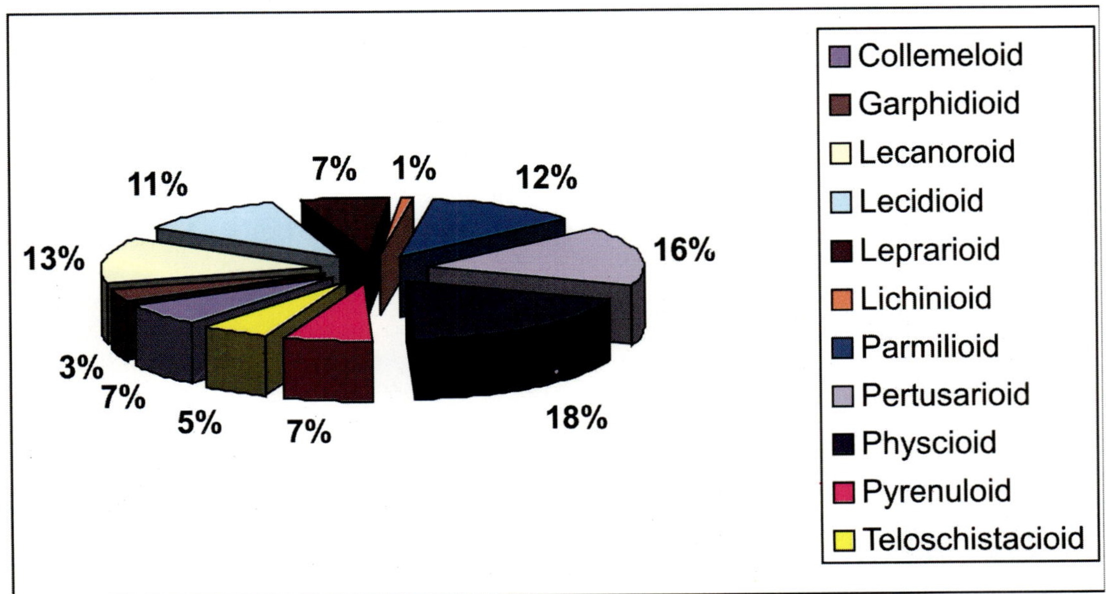

Figure 39.3: Frequency of Bioindicator Lichen Communities in AABR

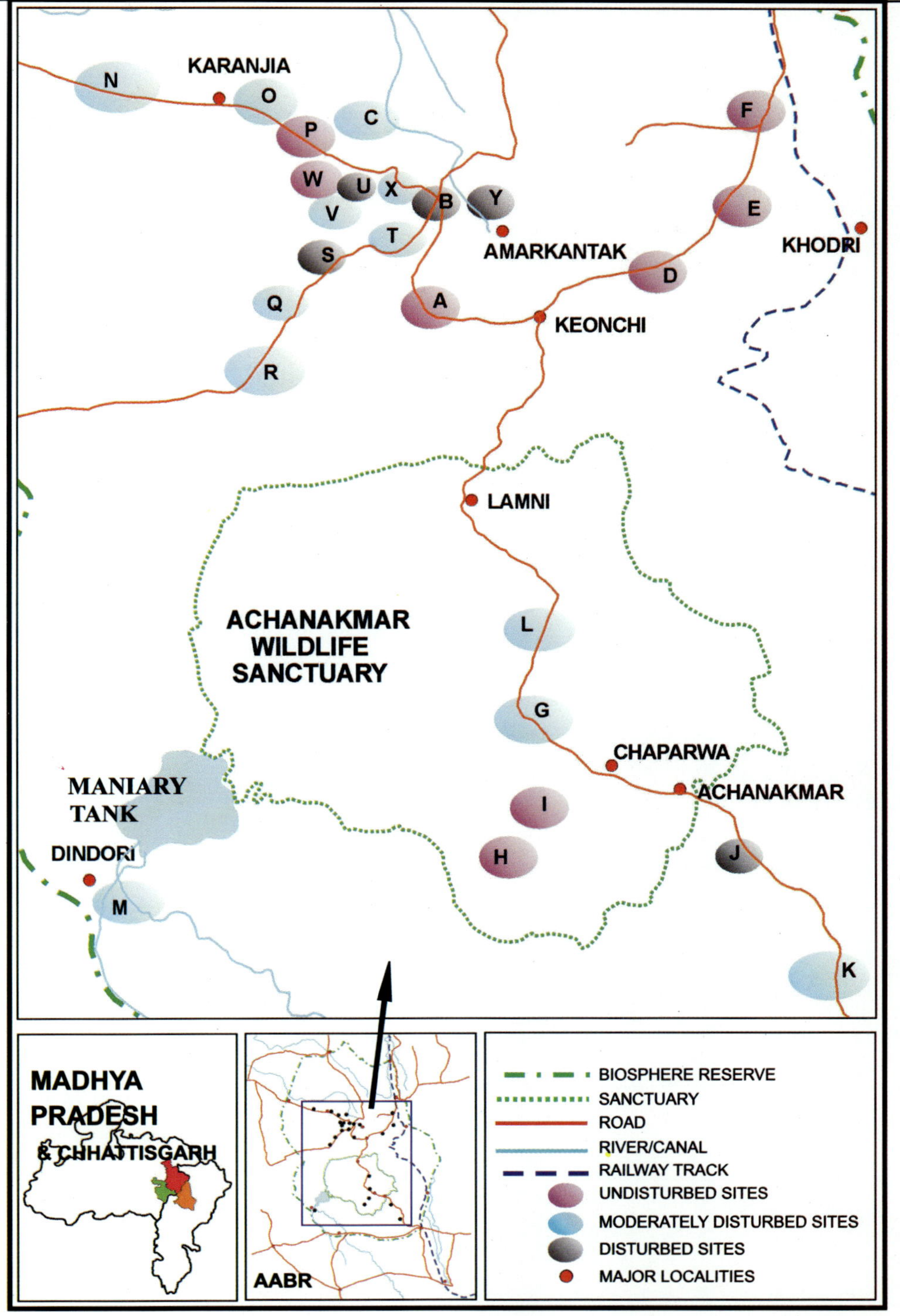

Figure 39.4: Lichen Exploration Sites Showing Different Level of Disturbance in AABR

Conclusion

In future to conduct studies, for the forest health monitoring progrmmes the available account of the lichen communities will help to answer several key assessment questions. The periodical monitoring of lichen communities in the are can be utilized to document the changes in the condition of the lichen communities overtime which also reflect the change in environmental condition of the area.

Acknowledgements

We are thankful to Director, National Botanical Research Institute for providing necessary laboratory facilities to work, to Ministry of Environment and Forests for financial support, to forest officers of Achanakmar-Amarkantak Biosphere Reserve for their cooperation.

References

Awasthi, D. D. (1988). A key to the macro lichens of India and Nepal. *Journal of Hattori Botanical Laboratory* 65: 207-302.

Awasthi, D.D. (1991). A key to the microlichens of India, Nepal and Sri Lanka. *Bibliotheca Lichenologica*. 40: 1-337.

Backor, M., Fahselt, D., Davidson, R.D. and Wu, C.T. (2003). Effect of copper on wild and tolerant strains of the lichen photobiont *Trebouxia erici* (Chlorophyta). and possible tolerant mechanisms. *Archives of Environmental Contamination and Toxicology* (45): 159-167.

Gradstein, S. R. (1992). The vanishing tropical rain as an environment for bryophytes and lichens. In *Bryphytes and Lichen in Changing Environment*, (Eds. J. W. Bates and A. M. Farmer). pp. 234-253. Clarendon, Oxford.

Neitlich, P. N. and B. McCune (1997). Hot spot of Epiphytic Lichen diversity in Two Young Managed Forests. *Conservation Biology* (11): 172-182.

Satya, Upreti, D.K. and Nayaka, S. (2005). *Shorea robusta*, an excellent host tree for lichen growth. *Current Science* 89 (4): 594-595.

Satya (2006). Ecological Studies of lichens in Amarkantak Biosphere Reserve. *Ph.D. Thesis*. University of Lucknow.

Upreti, D.K. (1991). Lichen genus *Pyrenula* from India: The species with spores of *Pyrenula brunnea* type. Bull. Soc. Bot. Fr. 138. *Letters Bot*. 3: 241-247.

Walker, F.J. and James, P.W. (1980). A revised guide to microchemical technique for the identification of lichen products. *Bulletin of British Lichen Society*. 46: 13-29.

Microbial Biotechnology and Ecology (2011) *Pages* **683–707**
Editors: **Deepak Vyas, G.S. Paliwal, P.K.Khare and R.K Gupta**
Published by: **DAYA PUBLISHING HOUSE, NEW DELHI**

Chapter 40

Silvipastoral Systems: The Solution for the Sustainable Production in Semi Arid Tropics

☆ ***R.K. Bhatt, A.K. Mishra and H.S. Tiwari***

Indian Grassland and Fodder Research Institute, Jhansi – 284 003, U.P.

Introduction

The traditional land use system in India have become fragile and unproductive due to over exploitation of natural resources, resulting in large scale degradation and consequent occurrence of wastelands. In India land degradation is a continuous process primarily due to increase in human and animal population pressure on a limited land resource. According to the estimates given by NBSSLUP (Sehgal and Abrol, 1994), 57 per cent of land (187.7 million ha) in the country is potentially exposed to various degradation forces; of which a dominant fraction is under water erosion 45 per cent (149.9 million ha), wind erosion 4.1 per cent (13.5 million ha), chemical deterioration 4.2 per cent (13.8 million ha) and physical deterioration 3.6 per cent (11 million ha). As per record of Ministry of Agriculture (1994), 37 per cent of total geographical area of the country (107.43 million ha) is degraded due to various causes of land degradation.

The problem of overgrazing is faced and presently the grazing pressure is 3.34 ACU/ha against the normal carrying capacity of 1 ACU/ha for a productive grassland. The over grazing resulted replacement of suitable grass cover by poor quality grasses and weeds (UNESCO, 1979). The grazing pressure on the rangelands under some semi arid region particularly in Bundelkhand region is still higher nearly 5 ACU/ha. It is higher than the national is (2.5 ACU/ha) average (Singh and Singh, 1994). The carrying capacity of a well managed rangeland in the region does not exceed 1 ACU/ha (Shanker *et al.*, 1988). Increasing demand of fuel wood, fodder, timber and lack of cash and infrastructure in many developing countries are some most relevant arguments for tree integration into farming and pastoral areas. It is aims at sustained productivity and conservation, rather than destructive exploitation of natural resources. The consequences of deforestation and desertification call for immediate action. Agro forestry systems have a great potential to solve a number of such problems. The semi-arid and arid lands with mostly marginal soil cover the largest area of land in the tropics and subtropics. The use of trees and shrubs to enhance organic matter production to maintain soil fertility, and to reduce erosion and to create more even microclimate has been found very effective. Thus, for sustainable production, the best alternative is to promote appropriate integrated agroforestry systems in the arid and semi-arid areas.

Silvipastoral land use has been identified as a holistic approach to rehabilitate the degraded lands and rangelands for meeting the needs of fodder and fire wood by rural masses and conservation of natural resources (Paroda 1990). Silvipastoral system is a suitable technology for the management of degraded and rangelands as this have been described as a low input technology (Deb Roy and Pathak, 1974, 1984). The establishment of silvipastoral system on wastelands/degraded and rangelands is not only to improve the soil health and microclimate but also facilitate the needs of human and livestock. The basic concepts of silvopastoral system based on sound ecological principles (productivity + conservation of resources) and are very much similar to natural approach.

Silvipastoral System

The term silvipasture essentially refers to an integrated system of growing and managing the tress/shrubs in association with grass or grasses and/or grass–legume mixture simultaneously on the same piece of land, where animals may or may not become a part of the system. Thus the system will include tree + pasture and/or animals. Tejwani (1987) used two different terms "Silvopasture" and "Pastoral Silviculture" for this type of integrated system of land use. It has been suggested that a combination of tree and grasses is referred to as "Silvipasture". If the grazing land is in a forest; where as the system is referred to as "pastoral silviculture" if tree are scattered in a pasture or wasteland.

A multi tired silvopasture systems will be near natural comparatively stable and what is more important is that it will also ensure better solar energy flow through the food chain. A Silvopasture structured on the functional pattern of natural ecosystem will, therefore, be a viable proposition (Paroda and Jatasra, 1985). Trees and shrubs are used as forage either through browsing or lopping and other forage like grasses and legumes as under story seasonal crops. The tree species also provide timber and other minor products to the inhabitants as well as shade and shelter to the grazing animals. The tree and shrubs grow luxuriantly even during the drought years as their deep tap root system enables them to grow independently of moisture. Trees improve soil through leaves and other litter and in addition to decomposition of old roots besides its capacity to fix its atmosphere nitrogen. They act as a nutrient and moisture pumping machine by drawing nutrients and moisture from deeper layers of soil. The presence of trees acts as a protective barrier against soil erosion or as wind breaks. Tree reduces the soil moisture evaporation by lowering the soil surface temperature. Grasses while conserving soil and water also utilize off season precipitation. The legumes enrich soil by nitrogen fixation and in the mixture they help growth of the grasses and trees besides improving the forage quality. Compared with other land uses, in marginal and sub marginal lands the silvopastoral system provides forage/grazing availability and quality for a longer period of the year.

Silvopastoral system is a mixed community composed of trees and crops, which form entirely different pattern for the utilization of light, water and nutrients. The growth and productivity of component crops in such system depends upon the use of available resources. The available soil moisture, mineral nutrients and light are the main resources governing plant productivity. The infiltered light affect the growth and other biological phenomenon of the crops and as well as the physical parameters under the canopy and to the surroundings. The solar radiation transmission a tree crop system is the major basis for understanding the principle of yield patterns and construction of a model for optimum yield and sustainability.

A suitable tree species to be planted for silvopastoral system should be of extreme economic, social and ecological significance because these systems maintain the socio-economic and environmental balances of ecosystem. For these programmes there is a need to focus research attention on identifying the potential tree species which are required to be grown along with the crops. It has been recommended that the tree species should be multipurpose, easy availability and wider distribution, fast growing, nitrogen fixing capacity, deep root system, good coppicing ability, higher rate of leaf fall during deciduous period with rapid decomposition of leaf, water stress tolerant, pest resistant, capacity to withstand in intensive frequent lopping and promising better under canopy growth.

Silvipastoral Development

Realising the importance of silvipasture systems for meeting the biomass requirements, the research work was initiated during the sixties at several institute in the country. The result obtained during past decades indicate that fodder and fuel wood production could be increased several folds from the existing levels through proper management of wasteland. In India, silvipasture research was initiated during the early sixties at the Central Arid Zone Research Institute (CAZRI), Jodhpur. This institute worked out the technologies for establishment of shelterbelts, stabilization of sand dunes and development of agri-silviculture systems. Later on comprehensive studies on such system were taken up around 1970s at Indian Grassland and Fodder Research Institute (IGFRI), Jhansi. The studies included on designing and development of silvopastoral system on degraded lands with special emphasis on fodder production one hand and the conservation on the other hand. Gradually the other institutes *viz.*, Central Soil and Water Conservation Research and Training Institute (CSWCRTI), Dehra Dun and Central Institute for Dry Land Agriculture (CRIDA), Hyderabad initiated work on such systems to develop appropriate land use system in their respective region. Besides these, an All India Coordinated Research Project on Agroforestry (AICRPAF) with 20 centers was initiated by ICAR during the year 1983. Agroforestry research in India was further strengthened during the seventh plan (1985-90) by adding 11 more centers to the AICRPAF and by creating a National Research Center for Agroforestry (NRCAF) at Jhansi during the year 1988. Now studies on various aspects of Agroforestry are also under taken by most of the state Agricultural Universities (SAUs) and some traditional universities as well.

Land Development

In the wasteland, fellow lands, sloppy and uneven topography the rain water harvesting techniques with a watershed management approach is the pre-requisite for providing the conservation of water, soil and soil moisture and checking erosion and loss of nutrients. The small staggered contour bunds, trenches and intermittent pitting is essential to provide this effect and channelize the water on one side for slow disposal and storage. The trenches of 3 × 0.5 × 0.3 m size (length adjusted depending upon the slope) are the requirement for soil moisture conservation. Their number per hectare was determined based upon the rainfall intensity and storms and plan to check maximum of the peak storm intensity erosion.

The cattle proof trench (CPT) of 1.2 × 1 × 0.7 m size depositing the earth on one side and sowing seeds of non palatable woody species *viz., Prosopis juliflora, Euphorbia* sp. etc. mixed with *Acacias, Dichrostachys cineria* and *Stylos* make a very effective green impenetrable wall to keep off the animals. Besides it produces desirable biomass in time.

Planting Technique

Multiple purpose trees were planted in the existing pastures/grazing lands or on wastelands or denuded lands followed by sowing/planting grasses, legumes or cereals in between the lines of trees. The 45 cm^3 pits were dug at a spacing 3 × 3 or 3 × 4 or 4 × 5 m. With the onset of monsoon, the tree seedlings were planted in these pits after applying 100 g mixture of urea, single super phosphate and potash in a ratio of 1:4:1 with 10 g BHC around the seedling to protect it from termites. The intermittent space between these seedlings was sown with the seeds of adaptable grasses and legumes in alternate lines. The small seeds were either pelleted with soil and fertilizers mixture or with a small dose of super phosphate and urea were sown. The grass and legume lines were at a distance of 0.5 m. The grass seedlings/root slips were intermittently planted in line providing good establishment.

Where the grass seeds are not available, Pathak (1983) advanced the simple technique for larger area of wastelands. The technique involves surface seeding of legumes *viz., Stylosanthes hamata* and *Macroptilium atropurpureum* at a line spacing of 1 m. On the trench mounds, contours, around the pits and earth deposits of cattle proof trenches its early colonization, growth and formation of a compact mat saves the soil from erosion and provides a good association with native grasses suppressing most of the seasonal weeds. While sowing, the seeds are mixed with single super phosphate @ 40 kg phosphorus/ha. This method gave better success on very poor undulating sites and even in ravenous areas.

In the first year the area was given a top dress of 25-30 kg/ha of nitrogen during early August. The grasses and legumes were harvested during November in the first year when the legumes have shed their seeds. In the subsequent years the harvesting could be done twice depending upon the area. The trees when form good canopy after 5-7 years they were lopped seasonally to provide additional forage and also light canopy cover to provide optimum light at the grass growth level.

Afterwards the area was maintained either as seasonal hay plot followed by aftermath grazing by animals or grazing the animals as per the carrying capacity of the land in a rotational or deferred rotational grazing system.

Choice of Woody Species

The species are selected based on tolerance to high incidence of pruning, multiple purpose *viz.,* forage, firewood, nitrogen fixing, low crown diameter to bole diameter ratio, tolerant to side shade, phyllotaxis to permit penetration of light to the ground, the phenology specially leaf flushing and fall to be advantageous to the growth of annual crops, litter fall and decomposition to be advantageous to ground flora and soil. They should be compatible to, other species with ideal root growth habit and should be efficient nutrient pumps most of these have been desired for agroforestry species also (King 1979). Most of the native grasses have been found to associate well with trees (Deb Roy and Pathak 1974; Wilson 1951 and Krishnaswamy 1942).

Micro-environmental Changes in Silvipastoral System

Although much work has been done on the production aspects of grasses in the experimental field trials, in the grassland system and also in silvopastoral system but little work is available on tree-crop interaction with respect to micro-environmental changes and physiological processes of the grasses under tree canopies in the silvopasture systems in the semi arid tropics. Therefore, the work on tree–crop interaction with respect to the micro-environmental changes in the system, growth behavior, productivity, assimilatory processes and quality of the under storey grasses and also to find out relationships between these factors with the productivity was started by Bhatt (1988) at IGFRI, Jhansi.

The extent and amount of effect of trees on productivity and adaptation of under growing grasses in silvipastoral system can be explained by the physical and physiological influences in the system and/or on the surrounding environment. In such systems the components and environmental parameters influences one another by which the environment causes a response in plant functions and growth, and the plant then show the effect on environment. Researches on tree-crop system will, therefore, primarily concern on the interaction of components and influences on the surroundings. The law of temporal and spatial distribution of the tree shading and variation in light intensity may help in improving the farming technique in order to bring in to full play the productive potential of tree-crop inter cropping system (Liu, 1991). The radiation distribution pattern is variable in different plantation with spacing. The solar radiation received by crop varied with the shading effect of trees. To see the effect of the light it is best account the daily sum of shady area and shade light intensity. The vertical and horizontal distribution of radiation is also important for crop productivity. Radiation intensity of a point varies greatly from place to place, depending on the sun elevation angle, which leads to corresponding changes in the horizontal distribution in the daily course. The physical parameters such as temperature of the canopy and to its surroundings, relative humidity, wind velocity, light transmission, soil temperature, soil moisture and energy balance such as net radiation, latent heat flux, soil heat flux etc. are the important parameters, which interact in the system. It is very important to study the seasonal and diurnal light transmission and distribution in silvipastoral system throughout the growth of under canopy crop. The spatial and temporal distributions of available light under tree canopies may help in improving the productivity in the tree-crop inter cropping system.

Light Transmission Under Different Tree Canopies

Mishra and Bhatt (1994) studied light transmission under different silvopastoral systems in semi arid tropics. *Acacia tortilis* and *Hardwickia binata* allowed 60 per cent and 55 per cent Photosynthetically Active Radiation (PAR) infiltration of the total PAR whereas *Leucaena leucocephala* infiltered least amount of PAR (33 per cent). The diurnal photosynthetically active radiation (PAR) distribution patterns varied under tree canopies. Figure 40.1 showed diurnal variation in the PAR transmission under full grown tree canopies of *L. Leucocephala* and in open and revealed that PAR transmission increased from 6 AM and reached at peak during 12 to 14 hours and then decreased gradually (Bhatt *et al.*, 2003). On an average, *Leucaena* canopies allowed only 28-32 per cent PAR at the tree spacing 4 × 4m at full canopy growth. The amount and intensity of PAR infiltered by the *Leucaena* tree canopy reduced to a great extent. The seasonal variation in light transmission under tree canopies during different months depends on the canopy growth and different phenological phases (Figure 40.2). The PAR transmission increased gradually from January to July because of leaf senescence and reached maximum is May–June when the canopy was leaf less.

Studies on microclimate variations around the tree cover by Ramakrishna (1984) revealed under 13 year old *Acacia tortilis* based Silvopastoral system, the total incident radiation just beneath the tree canopy was only 14 to 30 per cent of that received in open area. It was insufficient for good growth and productivity of pasture grasses like *Cenchrus ciliaris*. Similarly micro metrological parameters reported

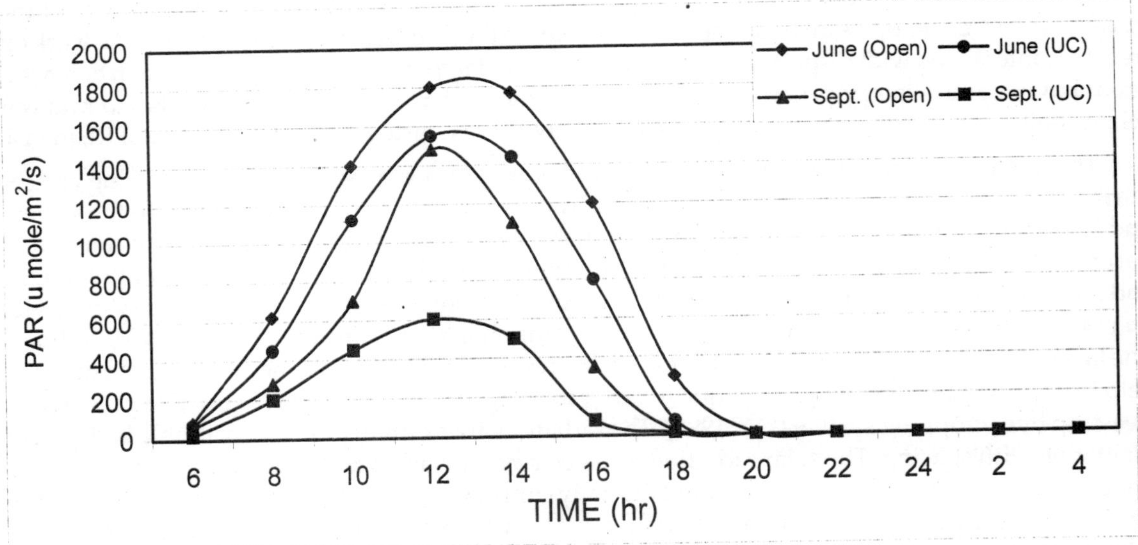

Figure 40.1: Diurnal Variation in Light Transmission Under *Leucaena leucocephala* Tree Canopies

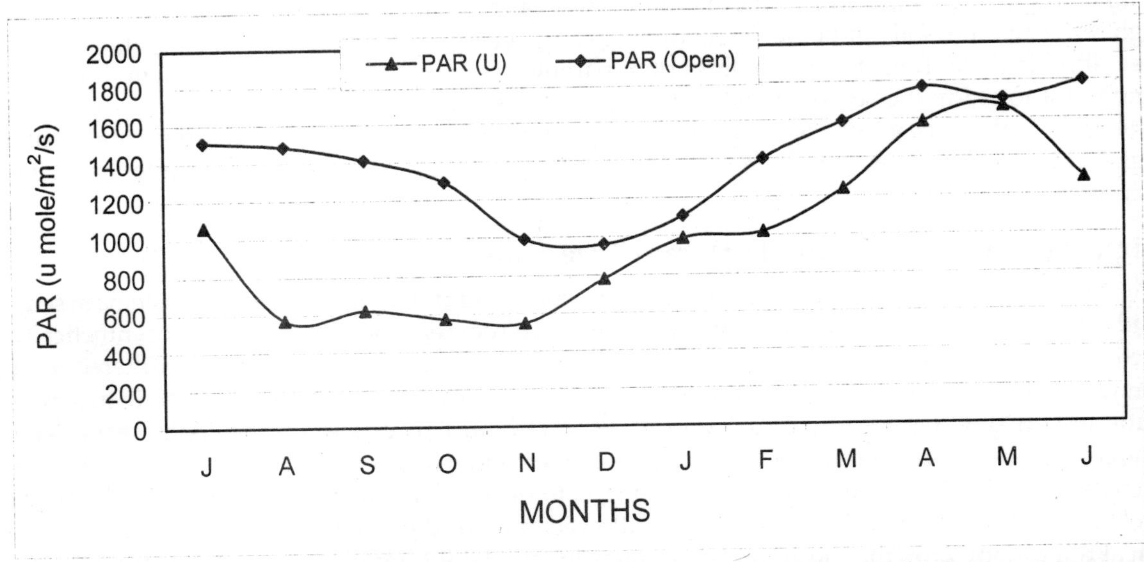

Figure 40.2: Monthly Variation in Light Transmission Under *Leucaena leucocephala* Tree Canopies

by Hazra (1994) in different silvopastoral systems revealed that under the *A. nilotica* canopies, the light infiltration was minimum of 59.2 per cent of PAR while it was maximum in association with *H. binata* (83.1 per cent). Studies on micro metrological parameters by Hazra and Patil (1986) in 4 tree species (*A. lebbek, A. procera, L. leucocephala* and *A. tortilis*) at the age of 4-5 years under silvopastoral condition revealed that the light filtration under different tree canopies varied from 74 to 93 per cent of photosynthetic active radiation (PAR). The tree cover maintained higher relative humidity (62-70 per cent) as compared to open filed (56 per cent).

Temperature Variations Under Different Tree Canopies

Leucaena trees have major influence on temperature pattern (Figure 40.3). The shading of the canopy and reduction in radiation led to decreased under canopy air temperature. The under canopy temperature was lower to air temperature of open field during June–July whereas in winter months it was higher to air temperature (Figure 40.4). Higher canopy–air temperature difference was recorded under *Leucaena leucocephala*. In Open field at the grass canopy the temperature was significantly higher whereas in the silvipasture system the canopy temperature was lower to air temperature. The under canopy temperature was lower to air temperature in *Leucaena leucocephala–Panicum maximum* silvipasture system in all the months except in December. *Acacia tortilis–Cenchrus* based silvipasture system maintains relatively higher canopy temperature as compared to *L. leucocephala–Panicum* based silvipasture system. The canopy temperature during the full canopy growth was 32 °C and 33.5 °C as recorded in the month of Sept.–Oct. in *L. leucocephala* and *Acacia tortilis* based silvipasture systems respectively. On average of two years data the canopy–air temperature difference was highest (–4.5°C) under *L. leucocephala* canopies where as under *A. tortilis* canopies the canopy temperature difference was about –1.7 °C (Table 40.1). In open the temperature of grass canopy was 35.8 °C with canopy air temperature difference of –1.2 °C.

Table 40.1: Average Value of Canopy Temperature (CT), CT–AT, and PAR Transmission in the Silvopastoral Systems

Parameters	*Canopy*	*1999*	*2000*	*Average*
CT (°C)	*A. tortilis*	30.2	29.8	30.0
	L. leucocephala	28.8	28.4	28.6
CT–AT	*A. tortilis*	-1.6	-1.8	-1.7
	L. leucocephala	-4.6	-4.4	-4.5
PAR µmole/m²/s	*A. tortilis*	845	825	835
	L. leucocephala	520	475	498

The change is soil temperature under tree canopies at different soil depth was gentle and following the same trends during different months and day time. The soil temperature decreases with decreasing in soil depth. The maximum soil temperature (41°C) was recorded in June and minimum (18 °C) in January. The night soil temperature was higher in *Leucaena* field than in the control and under canopy air temperature. During the day time variation in soil temperature was due to shading under *Leucaena* trees canopies. The light transmission under tree canopies was low because of shading of tree canopies and grass canopies which caused decrease in soil temperature during full canopy growth of trees and grasses, whereas it increases in summer months.

The mean daily maximum soil temperature beneath the tree canopy of *Acacia tortilis* and grass was lower by as much as 10 °C to 16 °C in the top soil zone (0.5 cm) and 4 °C to 5 °C at 30 cm depth than recorded in the open which indicates a better soil thermal region under the tree plantation (Ramakrishna and Sastri 1977 b). Studies carried in a 7 year old *Acacia tortilis* plantation during the monsoon season at Jodhpur showed that during the morning hours air temperature beneath the tree canopy was lower by 0.1 °C to 0.7 °C than these recorded in the open, while during the afternoon period the temperatures underneath the tree canopy remained lower by as much as 0.6 °C to 2.0 °C than those recorded in the open (Rama Krishna and Sastri, 1977 a).

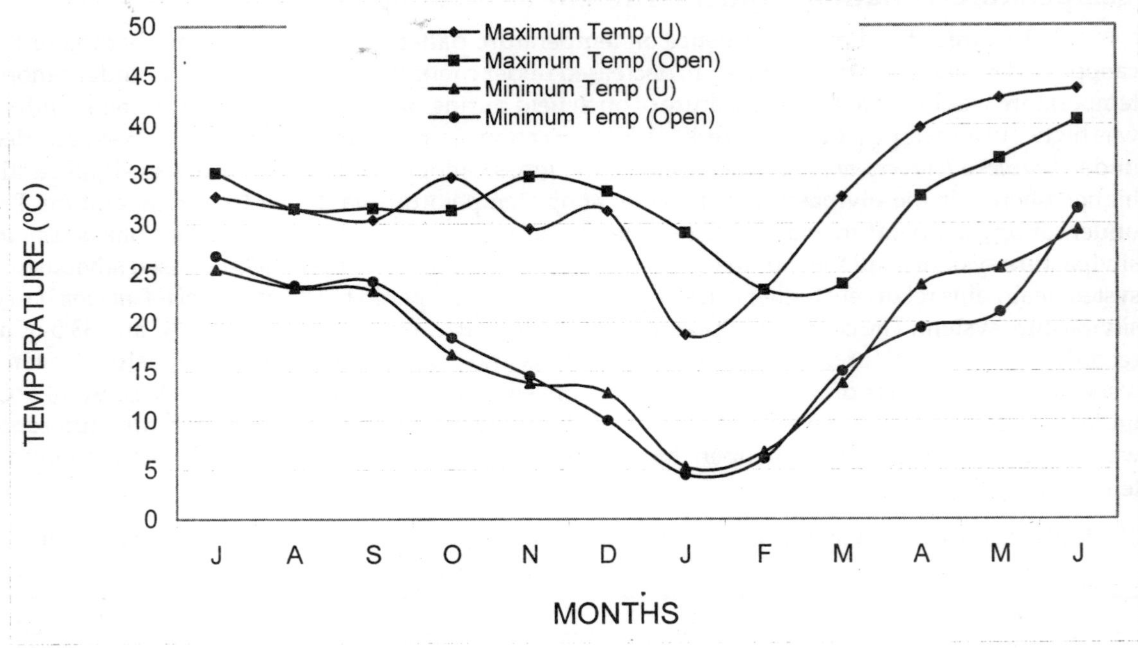

Figure 40.3: Seasonal Variation in Canopy Temperature Under the Trees of *L. leucocephala*

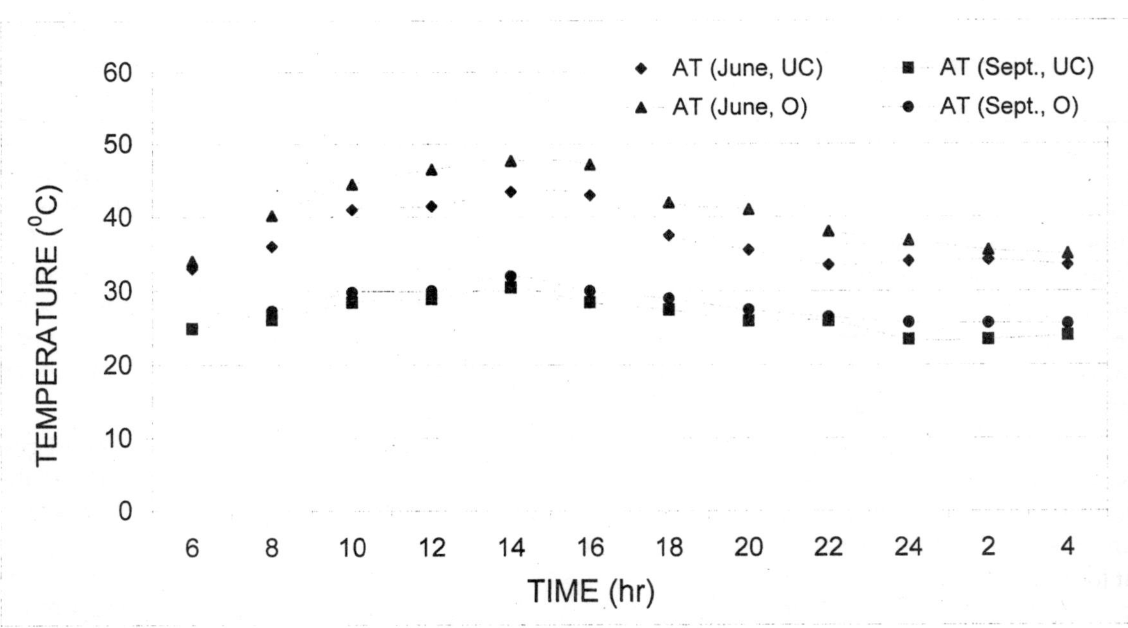

Figure 40.4: Diurnal Variation in Canopy Temperature Under the Trees of *L. leucocephala*

Photosynthetic Pigments

Bhatt *et al.* (1994) studied the accumulation of photosynthetic pigments in various grasses under the canopies of ten year old tree of *Hardwickia binata, Acacia tortilis, Albizia lebbeck, A. amara* and in open field condition and they found that (Chl-a and Chl-b) in *Sehima nervosum* and *Heteropogon contortus* was higher under the tree canopies than in open field. Higher synthesis of Chl b in these grasses under canopies indicates their shade adaptation ability. *S. nervosum* accumulated higher amount of Chl-b as compared to *H. contortus.* The high chlorophyll content (Chl a and Chl b) of the *Cenchrus ciliaris* and *Panicum maximum* under tree canopies of *L. leucocephala* also estimated by Bhatt *et al.* (1994) and reported that maximum chlorophyll a:b was observed in *C. ciliaris* indicating its fast adaptation to light intensity. The accumulations of photosynthetic pigments in grasses were higher under shading of tree canopies. The more accumulation of chlorophyll b under tree canopies indicates shade adaptation efficiency of these grasses (Table 40.2).

Table 40.2: Photosynthetic Pigments in Grasses Under Different Tree Canopies

Canopy	*Grasses*	*Photosynthetic Pigments (mg/g f.wt.)*			
		Chl-a	*Chl-b*	*Chl a+b*	*Chl a:b*
Open	*S. nervosum*	0.34	0.29	0.63	1.17
	H. contortus	0.33	0.12	0.45	2.75
A. tortilis	*S. nervosum*	0.49	0.36	0.85	1.36
	H. contortus	0.43	0.37	0.8	1.16
H. binata	*S. nervosum*	0.69	0.55	1.24	1.25
	H. contortus	0.3	0.29	1.54	1.03
L. Leucocephala	*S. nervosum*	0.38	0.39	0.77	0.97
	H. contortus	0.25	0.27	0.52	0.93
A. amara	*S. nervosum*	0.35	0.29	0.64	1.21
	H. contortus	0.32	0.38	0.7	0.84
A. lebbeck	*S. nervosum*	0.31	0.32	0.63	0.97
	H. contortus	0.18	0.18	0.55	0.49

Total chlorophyll and carotenoid content were more in the shade grown plant on the other hand the chl a/b ratio was lower in shade grown plants as compared to sum plants (Naidu and Swamy, 1993). Shade plants have a higher relative content of chl b than chl a (Egle 1960, Goodchild *et al.*, 1972). The decrease in chl a/b ratio was usually accompanied by an increase in chl b and specific leaf weight, which shows the shade adaptive feature in the grass species as observed by Bhatt and Shinha (1990). On the basis of high chl a:b *Chrysopogon fulvus, Paspalum notatum, Cenchrus ciliaris* and *Setaria sphacelate* were identified for higher productivity. Some shade tolerance grasses (*Chloris gyana* and *Brachiaria*) were selected on the basis of their chlorophyll accumulation (Bhatt and Sinha, 1990). Chlorophyll content (a + b) was maximum under 50-75 per cent shading in most of the grass species (Bhatt, *et al.*, 2006).

Physiological Processes of Grasses Under Tree Canopies

The production potentiality of the system components can be determined by physiological phenomenon, *viz.* Pigment adaptation, photosynthesis, transpiration, carboxylation efficiency, water use efficiency, and biomass accumulation, partitioning of biomass and mineral accumulation. These physiological processes in the silvipastoral systems are controlled by under-canopy micro-environmental parameters. Therefore, this research was concentrated on the interface between tree and crops, the micro-environmental changes and resultant physiological processes to understand the adaptation behavior, sustainability, productivity and feasibility of a tree-crop system.

Physiological Processes of *Cenchrus ciliaris* and *Panicum maximum* Under Leucaena Tree Canopies

The rate of photosynthesis, transpiration, stomatal conductance and accumulation of photosynthetic pigments was evaluated in grasses (*Panicum maximum* and *Cenchrus ciliaris*) in open and under *Leucaena leucocephala* tree canopies. Rate of photosynthesis, transpiration, stomatal conductance and leaf temperature of grass species decreased significantly under *Leucaena* tree canopies due to high degree of shading. In *C. ciliaris* maximum rate of photosynthesis was 39.28 µmole/m^2/s at 1806 µmole/m^2/s PAR and 10.27 µmole/m^2/s at 408 µmole/m^2/s PAR in open field and under tree canopies respectively. Whereas in *P. maximum* higher rate of assimilation (37.44 µmole/m^2/s) was recorded at 1800 µmole/m^2/s PAR and 16.51 µmole/m^2/s at 350 µmole/m^2/s PAR (Tables 40.3 and 40.4). Variation in the rate of photosynthesis in grass species was observed at different places under the tree canopies which were due to changing in PAR intensity. The rate of photosynthesis is linearly related to the available PAR (r=0.91) (Figures 40.5 and 40.6).

Table 40.3: Physiological Parameters in *Cenchrus ciliaris* in Open and Under *Leucaena* Canopies

Months	*PN (µ mole/m²/s)*		*LT (°C)*		*CINT (ppm)*		*CS (cm/s)*		*PN/CINT*		*PN/TR (µ mole CO_2/ µmole H_2O)*		*TR (µmole H_2O)*	
	Open	*Shade*	*Open*	*Shade*	*Open*	*Shade*	*Open*	*Shade*	*Open*	*Shade*	*Open*	*Shade*	*Open*	*Shade*
July	38.25	10.09	39.66	34.69	153	206	1.02	0.56	0.25	0.049	3.64	1.72	10.50	5.86
Aug	39.28	10.27	39.11	34.71	135	239	1.05	0.55	0.291	0.043	3.63	1.71	10.82	6.00
Sept	39.28	10.80	39.13	35.25	135	225	1.21	0.57	0.291	0.048	3.62	1.79	10.85	6.03
Oct	29.24	5.12	37.31	34.62	170	233	0.976	0.235	0.172	0.022	2.14	1.29	13.66	3.96
Nov	15.74	7.67	28.82	25.84	254	294	0.579	0.474	0.062	0.023	2.69	1.77	5.85	4.33
Dec	5.59	5.08	28.53	24.63	245	254	0.364	0.278	0.031	0.02	1.86	1.99	4.08	2.55

Table 40.4: Physiological Parameters in *Panicum maximum* in Open and Under *Leucaena* Canopies

Months	*PN (µ mole/m²/s)*		*LT (°C)*		*CINT (ppm)*		*CS (cm/s)*		*PN/CINT*		*PN/TR (µ mole CO_2/ µ mole H_2O)*		*TR (µ mole H_2O)*	
	Open	*Shade*	*Open*	*Shade*	*Open*	*Shade*	*Open*	*Shade*	*Open*	*Shade*	*Open*	*Shade*	*Open*	*Shade*
July	34.34	14.36	37.55	35.61	162	266	1.194	0.768	0.212	0.054	2.89	1.83	11.88	7.84
Aug	36.19	16.63	37.41	35.69	154	264	1.26	0.768	0.235	0.063	3.02	1.97	11.98	8.44
Sept	37.44	16.51	37.41	35.66	144	254	1.28	0.796	0.26	0.065	3.07	1.95	12.19	8.46
Oct	31.05	9.93	35.74	32.55	115	191	0.829	0.344	0.27	0.052	4.12	2.15	7.53	4.61
Nov	13.55	11.04	27.49	26.4	154	181	0.294	0.271	0.088	0.061	3.15	4.14	4.30	2.66
Dec	10.16	9.28	28.69	25.20	242	211	0.177	0.319	0.042	0.044	3.70	3.33	2.74	2.78

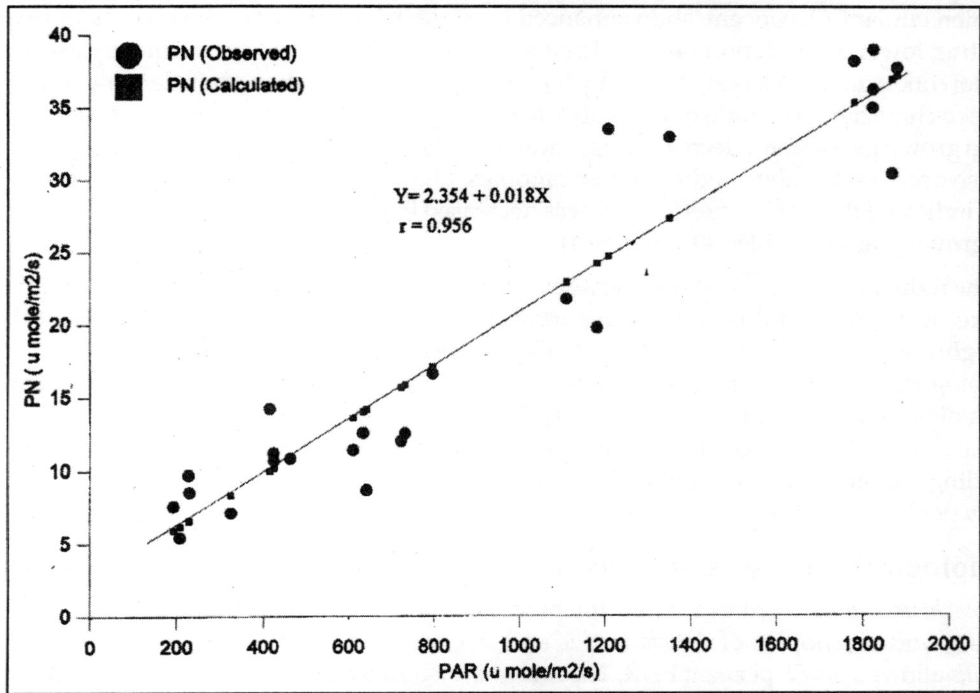

Figure 40.5: Rate of Photosynthesis (PN) in *P. maximum* at Various Levels of PAR in Open and Under *Leucaena* Species

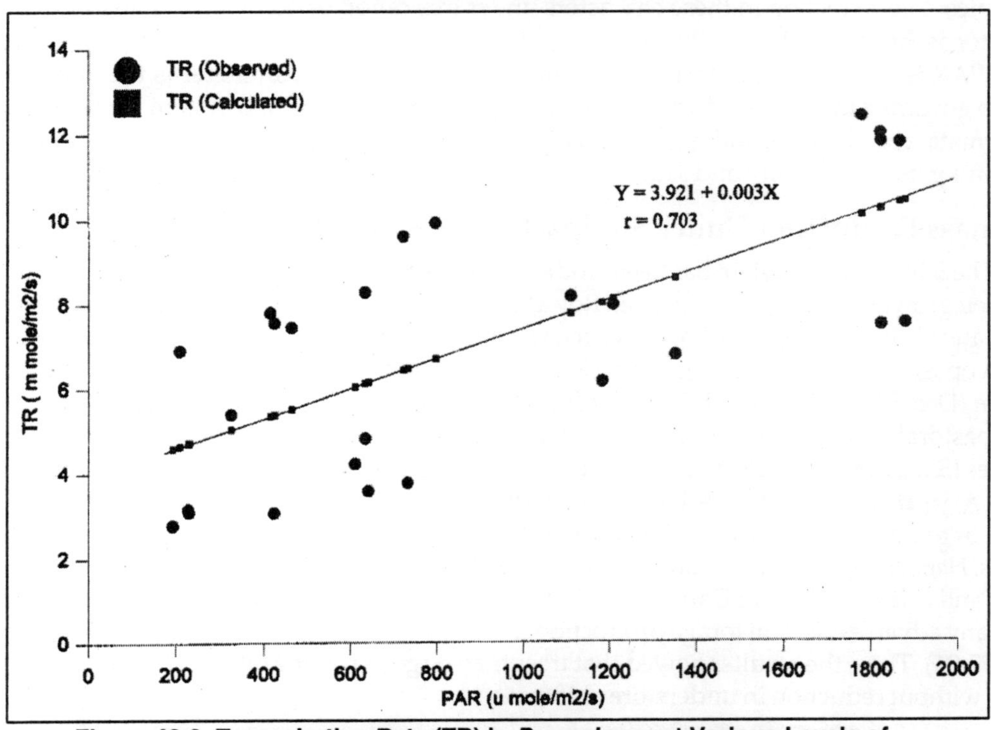

Figure 40.6: Transpiration Rate (TR) in *P. maximum* at Various Levels of PAR in Open and Under *Leucaena* Species

Intercellular CO_2 concentration enhanced two fold in both the grass species under tree canopies exhibiting lower assimilation of CO_2. The rate of CO_2 assimilation was intimately associated with stomatal conductance as it is evidenced by highly significant correlation coefficient ($r = 0.8796$) between these two characters. The ratio of PN/CINT which represents the carboxylation efficiency was higher in open grown grasses and decreased significantly under high shading of tree canopies. Transpiration rate also decreased under shading of tree canopies. Photosynthesis and transpiration ratio (PN/TR) which indicated the water use efficiency was decreased in grasses under tree canopies as compared to open grown grasses (Tables 40.3 and 40.4).

The reduction in these physiological activities under tree canopies of *L. leucocephala* might be due to decrease in PAR and through which partial closure of stomatal pore occurred (Bhatt *et al.*, 1994). The highly significant correlation of these parameters with PAR is suggestive of the fact that these physiological processes are mainly influenced by these micro-environmental parameters. For maintaining the optimum functioning of all physiological parameters and sustaining the productivity under *L. leucocephala* based silvopastoral system it is essential to manage the canopy size either by pollarding, lopping and maintaining the ideal spacing between the trees or to workout threshold trees density per hectare for optimum PAR distribution in the system.

Physiological Processes of *Cenchrus ciliaris* Under *Acacia* Based Silvipastoral

Cenchrus ciliaris were evaluated for productivity, adaptational behaviour and physiological activities under canopies of *Acacia tortilis* and in open field condition. The full grown canopy of *A. tortilis* allowed 50–55 per cent PAR. The rate of transpiration, photosynthesis, leaf temperature and stomatal conductance of *C. ciliaris* decreased under tree canopies as compared to open field. Similar to these attributes PN/TR, PN/CI and PN/COND also decreased under the shade environment of tree canopies. The reduction in these characters under tree canopies occurred due to low availability of PAR for assimilation of CO_2. The highly significant correlation of physiological characters and DMY with PAR is suggestive the fact that this micro-environmental parameter is the only major factor which governed the yield and adaptation of grasses under silvipastoral system. The lowest reduction in stomatal conductance and higher specific leaf mass, chl b and chl a:b in *C. ciliaris* under *A. tortilis* exhibiting its associability and sustainability in this system under semi-arid region.

Biomass Production Under Silvipastoral Systems

The Silvipastoral system has been studied for their advantage over existing agricultural practices for their growth and productivity (Deb Roy and Pathak 1983, Pathak and Roy 1994, Pathak *et al.*, 1995, Grewal *et al.*, 1996). Also there have been a few attempts to monitor productivity (In ecosystem context) of Silvopasture system based on *Albizia lebbeck. Albizia procera* and *Hardweckia binata* in Bundelkhand region (Deb Roy 1986, Roy 1995). The information's available on forage production under different silvopastoral systems in different agroclimatic conditions were generally on the basis of 4 to 6 years studies (Singh and Puri, 1975; Deb Roy *et al.*, 1980 Singh and Roy, 1991; Hazra *et al.*, 1994; Dogra *et al.*, 1997, Arya *et al.*, 1998, etc.). A long term studies conducted on silvipastoral systems at Jhansi and Datia in red gravelly soils with five tree species at each location (*Albizia amara, Albizia lebbek, Acacia tortilis, Hardwickia binata* and *Leucaena leucocephala*) at Jhansi and (*A. amara, A. lebbek, A. tortilis, Dalbergia sissoo* and *L. leucocephala*) at Datia under 3 spacing (4×3, 4×4 and 4×6 m) revealed that trees did not have any adverse effect on forage production up to 11-12 years at any spacing (IDRC Reports, 1982-83 to 1993-94). Thus, the results showed that trees may be grown at the rate of 825 plants/ha up to 11-12 years without reduction in understorey biomass.

In arid condition, it has been observed that in addition to indigenous species like *Prosopis cineraria* and *Zizyphus numularia*, the introduced species such as *A. tortilis, D. cinerea, Colophospermum mopane* showed very good performance in silvopastoral systems (Ahuja, 1980). Forage production from lower storey crops under 14-18 years old plantation of 4 desert trees (*P. cineraria, Tecomella undulata, A. lebbek* and *Acacia senegal*) ranged from 0.6 to 1.5 t/ha/year (Ahuja, 1980).

The relative forage yield under *A. procera* was minimum (70.7 per cent) while relative dry forage production of 94.6 per cent was recorded higher in association with *A. lebbeck*. It was also observed that reduction in forage yield of understory crop, light transmission through canopy is not only responsible factor but moisture contents seems to be another factor as relative humidity under *A. nilotica* was maximum (70 per cent) although lowest relative yield of 70.7 per cent was recorded in association with *A. procera*. (Hazra 1994)

On the basis of more than 20 years studies in shallow red gravelly soils under semi arid condition at Jhansi, Pathak *et al.* (1996) reported that the degraded lands producing hardly up to 1 t/ha/year biomass which can be improved up to 10 t/ha/year at a 10 years rotation through silvopastroal systems. Besides yield improvement by 8 to 10 times, the quality of mixed forage has also improved by 6 to 7 times.

A fifteen years studies in Yamuna ravine near Agra, revealed that a silvipastoral system consisting of *A. nilotica* + *C. ciliaris* and *A. tortilis* + *C. ciliaris* planted at 3 × 3 m spacing produced on an average the total biomass yield of 5.0 t/ha/year (2.5 t fuel + 2.5 t forage) and 6.9 t/ha/year (4.2 t fuel + 2.7 t forage), respectively (Prajapati *et al.*, 1993). Studies on the production potential of pasture alone (*C. ciliaris*), fodder trees alone (*H. binata* + *C. mopane*) and silvopastoral systems (*C. ciliaris* + *H. binata* + *C. mopane*) were done at CAZRI, Jodhpur for nine years. On the basis of nine years results, it was observed that silvopastoral systems was better for higher average forage production (1.73 t/ha/yr) and livestock maintenance (4.1 Acu/ha) followed by pure pasture and pure trees block (Harsh *et al.*, 1992).

Grass production in 14–18 year old plantation of four desert trees was monitored by Ahuja *et al.*, 1978 in arid situation. The peak forage yield was reported under *Prosopis cineraria* (1.54 t DM/ha) and the least production was under *Acacia Senegal* (0.69 t DM/ha). The increase in grass yield was attributed to increased availability of nutrients under *P. cineraria*. Deb Roy *et al.* (1978) studied the forage production of *Cenchrus ciliaris* and a mixture of *Chrysopogon fulvus*, + *Sehima nervosum*, under different tree spacing of *Hardweckia binata* and *Albizia amara* from a typical degraded site in Bundelkhand. Forge production from the mixture of *C. fulvus* + *S. nervosum* (4.23 t DM/ha) was higher than *C. ciliaris* (3.74 t DM/ha). Deb Roy (1989) studied average forage production (5 year) of *Cenchrus ciliaris* and *Cenchrus setigerus* in association with *Acacia tortilis* gave an average forage production of 3.5 t DM/ha while in association with *Leucaena leucocephala* it gave higher production (4.1 t DM/ha). In contrast, *Cenchrus setigerus* gave higher production (3.1 t DM/ha) in association with *Acacia tortilis* when compared to *Leucaena Leucocephala* (3.0 t DM/ha).

In the silvopastoral systems under semi arid tropics crop growth rate (CGR) and dry matter yield (DMY) of grasses (*Sehima nervosum* and *Heteropogon contortus*) were higher under the canopies of *A. tortilis* and *H. binata* while the maximum reduction in yield of these grasses were recorded under *L. leucocephala* trees. The DMY was closely associated with available PAR (r= 0.71) under the tree canopies indicating that for the optimum production of these grasses about 55-60 per cent PAR is required (Misra and Bhatt, 1994). Thus on the basis of physiological adaptation and biomass production it is indicative that *A. tortilis* and *H. binata* are suitable tree species with *H. contortus* and *S. nervosum* under silvipastoral systems in the semi-arid region. About 98 per cent dry matter yield of grasses was obtained under *Hardwickia binata* and *Acacia tortilis* canopy when compared with the dry matter yield in open field Bhatt *et al.* (1994).

In one of the study *C. ciliaris* and *P. maximum* have produced 15.78 t. and 27.83 t/ha forage production under the tree canopies of *A. tortilis* and *L. leucocephala* respectively in the 5th year of growth (Bhatt *et al.*, 2006). The dry matter yield was 4.72 t/ha and 8.37 t/ha in *C. ciliaris* and *P. maximum* under the tree canopies (Figure 40.7). The biomass yield and leaf area index was increased continuously up to 5th year and then sustained up to 8th year in both the grass species in open and under the tree canopies (Table 40.5). Plant height and tiller production per plant varied from year to year depending on the environmental conditions but the new tiller production continued every year. On average of all the years, the biomass production was 5.29 t/ha and 4.20 t/ha in open and under tree canopies of *A. tortilis* in *C. ciliaris* whereas it was 7.56 t/ha and 6.84 t/ha in *P. maximum* in open and under *L. leucocephala* trees. Overall the biomass production was reduced by 21 per cent in *C. ciliaris* under the tree canopies of *A. tortilis* and 10 per cent in *P. maximum* under *L. leucocephala* canopies indicating that the productivity of these grasses sustained for longer time (Figure 40.7). The dry matter yield was significantly correlated (r = 0.931) with the available PAR under tree canopies exhibiting that for the optimum production of these grasses under the shading environment of trees, about 40–60 per cent PAR is required.

Table 40.5: Growth, Physiological and Quality Characters of Grasses Grown in Open and Under Tree Canopies (Figure in parenthesis indicates percent reduction and gain)

Characters	*C. ciliaris*		*P. maximum*	
	Open	*UC*	*Open*	*UC*
Photosynthetic rate (μmole/m²/s)	32.36	16.52(–49.0)	30.51	18.69 (–48.2)
Transpiration (μmole/m²/s)	10.33	4.8(–53.5)	9.57	5.82 (–39.2)
Stomatal conductance (cm/s)	0.96	0.48(–50.0)	0.97	0.58 (–40.2)
Canopy Photosynthesis (PN X LAI)	153.06	69.71(–54.4)	215.09	127.65(–40.6)
Chlorophyll a (mg/g f.wt.)	2.28	2.32(+1.7)	2.48	2.66 (+7.2)
Chlorophyll b (mg/g f.wt.)	1.02	1.22(+19.6)	1.10	1.32 (+20.0)
Sugar (per cent)	2.13	2.53(+18.8)	2.12	2.62(+23.8)
Starch (per cent)	6.22	6.38(+2.6)	6.12	6.56(+7.2)
Crude Protein (per cent)	6.39	7.12(+11.4)	10.12	10.48(+14.9)
Plant height (cm)	129	136(+5.4)	153	152(+6.5)
Tillers/plant	34	31(–8.8)	28	26(–7.1)
Leaf Area Index (LAI)	4.73	4.22(–10.8)	7.05	6.83(–3.1)
Forage yield (t/ha)	16.78	13.27(–20.9)	22.83	21.74(–4.8)
Crude Protein Yield (kg/ha)	333.65	268.6(–19.47)	683.1	716.83(+4.9)

UC: Under tree canopies.

Production of fuel wood at 8 years of growth under silvipasture produced 28t/ha in *A. tortilis* and 38t/ha/yr in *A. amara* (3.5 and 4.75 t/ha/year on an average). For most of the short rotation species on such lands on a cycle of 10 years one could expect from 4-6 t/ha/year fuel wood production at a tree density of 500/ha. In many trees annual lopping at 6-7 years has been found to give 2.3-3.5 t/ha

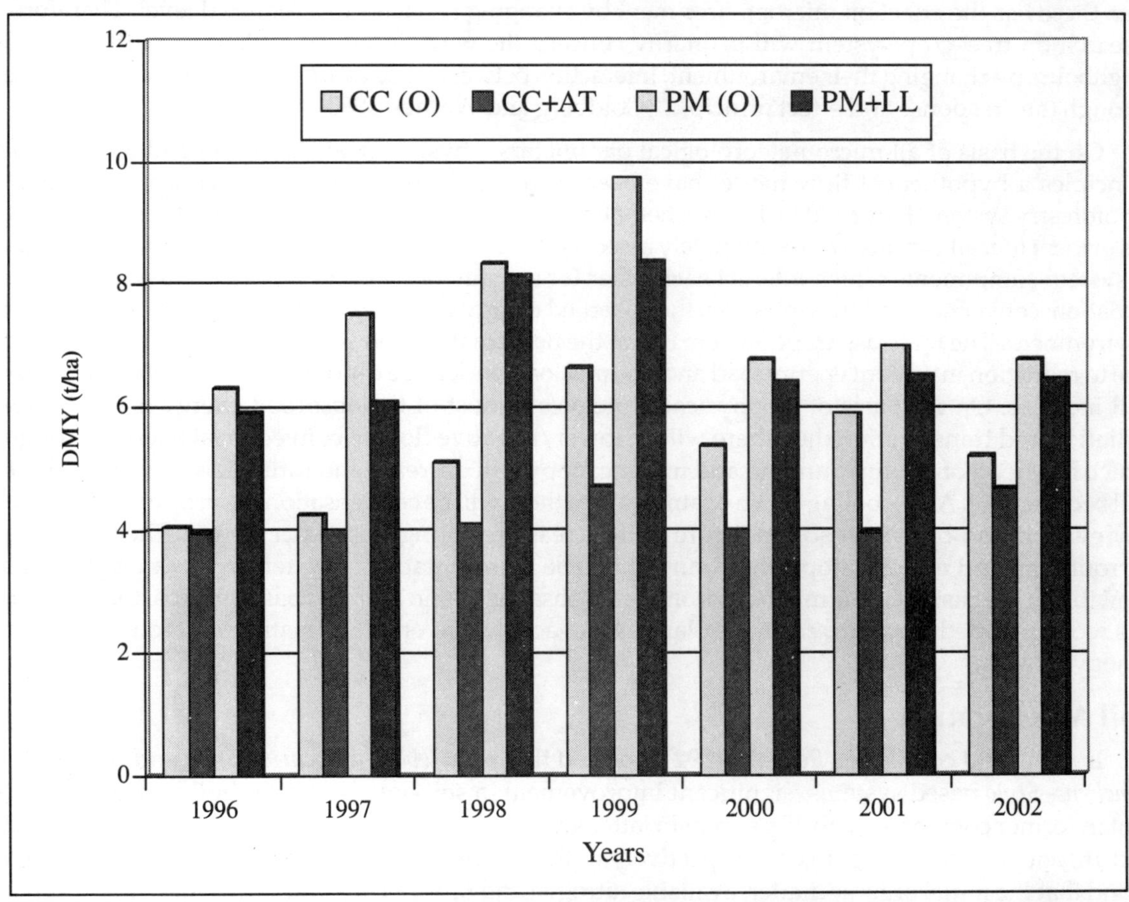

Figure 40.7: Dry Matter Yield in *C. ciliaris* (CC) and *P. maximum* (PM) in Open (O) and Under Tree Canopies of *A. tortilis* (AT) and *L. leucocephala* (LL)

fodder and 4.5-6.5 t/ha firewood. Thus, forage and top feed combined yield produced 5.3-9.5 t/ha forage and 5 t/ha firewood or 10-14.5 t/ha total harvestable biomass.

Biophysical Modelling of Tree-Crop Intercropping System

The adaptation and ability to survive of plants with in a given environment depends upon the extent of their interaction with the surroundings through phenomena such as transpiration, light absorption and energy exchange. PAR adversely affects the relative humidity, stomatal diffusion resistance and therefore, transfer of water vapour increased (Nobel, 1977). Transpiration is influenced by environmental factors such as temperature, light intensity, wind velocity, relative humidity, soil moisture and resistance to water movement. Transpiration increase with increase in temperature and decrease in relative humidity during the day time (Kaul, 1974). The rate of transpiration and the water content of leaves have an inverse relationship with each other and mainly governed by the relative humidity and temperature variation under tree canopies. The crop components interact with each other through the coupling with the environment and causing response on plant functioning and then these has the effect on microenvironment by changing its factor to a required level. Therefore, research on tree–crop system will primarily concern the ways in which a plant can influence its neighbours by changing their environment. Interaction between species are mediated by environment through the "response and effect principle"(Goldberg and Werner, 1983).

On the basis of all micrometeorological parameters, physiological characters and biophysical principles a hypothetical flow model have been developed for tree–crop intercropping system/ agroforestry system (Figure 40.8). From schematic diagram and flow chart and preceding discussion, it is evident that all parameters are intimately associated with the physiological economy and adaptation of system components which interact each other for sustainability of the system. By the process of radiation, convection and transpiration, the absorbed energy exchanges between canopy surface and environment. The main assumption here is that the net radiation and sensible heat flux will reduced due to reduction in radiant energy load and thermal load under tree canopies whereas latent heat flux will increase. On the basis of biophysical principles if most of the absorbed energy is lost by re-radiation and transpiration then there will be lower/negative flow of convectional energy through which heat load of the surrounding and under canopy will decrease and ultimately the atmosphere will become cool. After cooling down of atmosphere there will be condensation of surface water due to low evaporation by which soil moisture will increase resulting less water deficit. Therefore, the surrounding and under canopy environment will be more suitable for better under canopy crops's growth. On the basis of these micro environmental observations in *Leucaena* based silvipastoral system it is recommended that *Leucaena* trees planting can achieve favorable climatic conditions for under canopy growth.

Soil Amelioration

In semi-arid conditions Pathak (1992) reported that in *A. lebbek–Cenchrus–Stylo* and *A. procera–Cenchrus–Stylo* based systems, significant improvement in soil organic matter build up was 38 per cent in former compared with 25 per cent in latter system. Available phosphorus and potash were 22 and 16, and 9.5 and 11.0 per cent, respectively in the above systems. In another study, it has been found that the initial organic matter, available nitrogen and phosphorus and field capacity of 0.32 per cent, 131 kg/ha, 6.2 kg/ha and 11 per cent were enhanced to 0.78 per cent, 267 kg/ha, 15.5 kg/ha and 15.5 per cent, respectively over a period of 10 years of establishment of silvopastoral system (Pathak, 1994).

Yadava and Varsheny (1997) reported on the basis of five years that silvopastoral system reduced the run off and soil loss about 6 and 11 times, respectively against a bare land. Similarly loss of total soluble salts, dissolved nitrogen and potassium was reduced at the tune of 69, 67 and 43 per cent, respectively as compared to barren land. While improvement in organic carbon and available nitrogen and phosphorus in silvipastoral system was 53, 23 and 8 per cent, respectively against the initial status of the nutrients of this area. In case of potassium status in the system was almost maintained. However, in case of bare land all the nutrients were decreased after 4 years as compared to initial status.

In arid condition, Singh and Lal (1969) investigated profile characteristics and level of fertility under *P. cineraria* and *A. nilotica* canopies and concluded that silvopasture systems enhanced organic matter, total nitrogen, available phosphorus, soluble calcium and down the pH. Better mechanical composition of soil up to 120 cm depth due to silvopasture systems promoted the growth and yield of crops grown in the vicinity of *P. cineraria*. Aggarwal *et al.* (1975) concluded that status of available micronutrients generally improved under plantation especially under *P. cineraria*. Comparative study

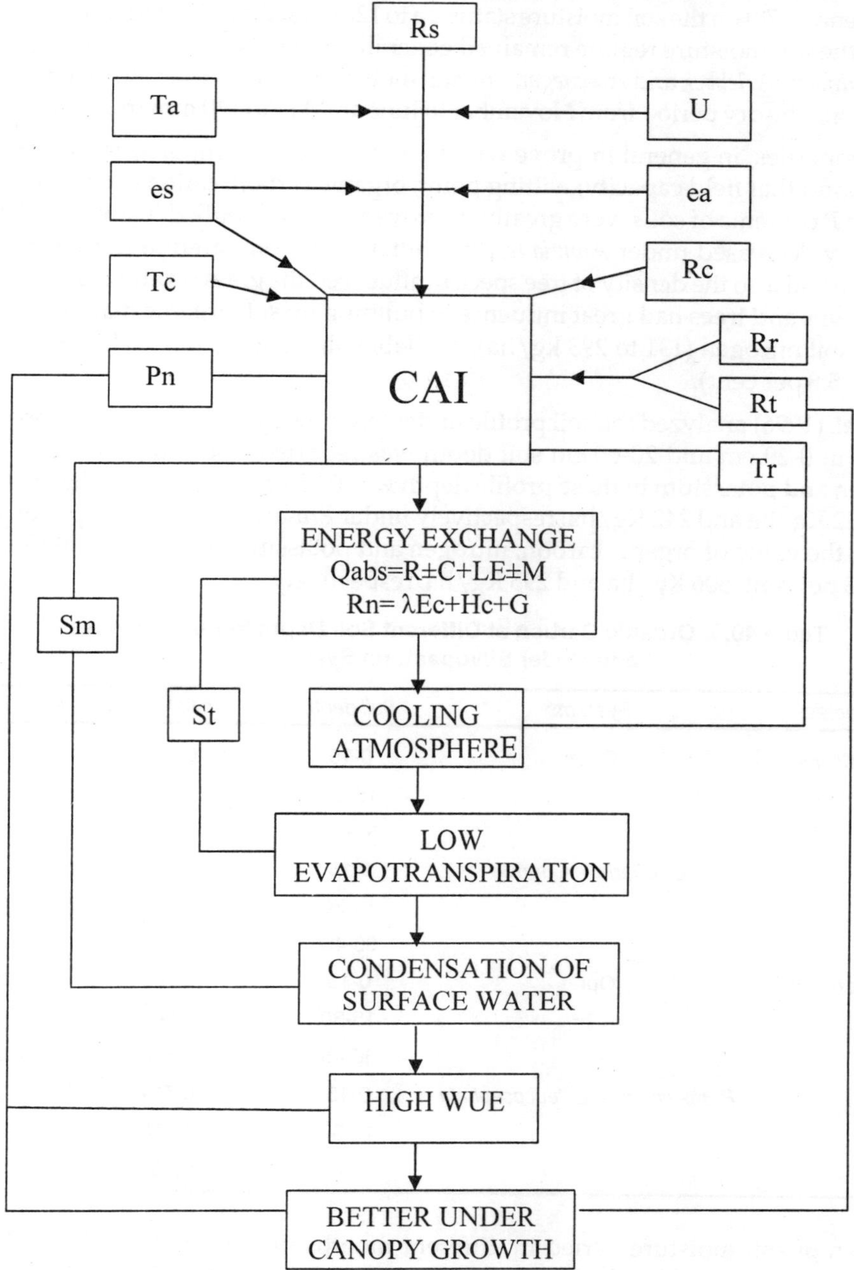

Figure 40.8: Energy Flow Chart for Agroforestry

Rs: Solar radiation; Ta: Air temperature; U: Wind velocity; es: Air humidity; ea: Boundary layer resistance; Tc: Canopy temperature; Rc: Canopy resistance; CAI: Canopy Area Index; Rr: Reflected light; Rt: Transmitted light; Pn: Photosynthesis; Tr: Transpiration; Sm: Soil moisture; St: Soil temperature; WUE: Water Use Efficiency; Qabs: Energy absorbed; R: Radiation energy; C: convection energy; LE: latent energy; M: Metabolic energy; Rn: Net radiation; λEc: Long wave radiation; Hc: Heat convection; G: Ground energy.

(Gupta and Saxena, 1978) on the soil moisture status up to 120 cm soil profile under five tree plantations suggested that the soil moisture regime remained generally higher below *P. cineraria* and *T. undulata* than that in *P. juliflora*, *A. lebbek* and *A. senegal*. The soil moisture under *P. cineraria* vicinity ranged from 27 to 50 mm during the dry period from November to June and 115 to 140 mm from July to September.

The soil properties, in general improve with tree cropping as compared to non-tree situation. Hazra (1990) found that field capacity; wilting point, organic carbon, cation exchange capacity and available N and P contents of soils were greatly improved, whereas bulk density, pH and EC values were appreciably decreased under *Albizia lebbek* plantation as compared to normal cropping. The canopy structure and also the density of tree species influenced the grass production underneath. The leguminous shrubs and trees had great influence in building up soil organic matter (0.32 to 0.91 per cent) available soil nitrogen (131 to 293 kg/ha), available phosphorus (6.2 to 18.5 kg/ha) and field capacity (11 to 15.8 per cent).

Sharma *et al.* (1996) analyzed the soil profile under tree canopy and open field conditions. Better nutrient status in 0-20 cm and 20-60 cm soil depth was reported under tree canopy. The organic carbon, nitrogen and potassium in these profile depth was 0.15 per cent, 512 Kg/ha, 309 Kg/ha and 0.13 per cent, 522 Kg/ha and 242 Kg/ha, respectively under *Prosopis cineraria* canopy respectively. In open situation, the value of organic carbon, nitrogen and potassium were 0.13, 449 Kg/ha and 290 Kg/ha and 0.13 per cent, 506 Kg/ha and 295 Kg/ha, respectively.

Table 40.6: Organic Carbon at Different Soil Depth in Pure Grasses and Under Silvopastoral Systems

Grass Species	*Systems*	*Soil depth*	*Initial Year*	*After Two Years*
Cenchrus ciliaris	Open	0-15	0.426	0.505
		15-30	0.406	0.44
		30-45	0.421	0.45
	C. ciliaris + A. tortilis	0-15	0.69	0.88
		15-30	0.499	0.64
		30-45	0.606	0.60
Panicum maximum	Open	0-15	0.600	0.63
		15-30	0.541	0.60
		30-45	0.556	0.59
	P. maximum + L. leucocephala	0-15	0.714	0.80
		15-30	0.556	0.65
		30-45	0.531	0.67

The pattern of soil moisture varied in different months under the A. *tortilis* + C. *ciliaris* and *L. leucocephala* + *P. maximum* based silvipastoral systems (Mishra, 2002). The moisture availability under the tree canopies was higher for longer time for sustainability of the system productivity. On average the soil moisture at 0–30 cm soil depth was 7.5 per cent and 8.57 per cent in open field of grasses and 8.87 and 9.73 per cent under the tree canopies of *A. tortilis* and *L. leucocephala* respectively during the active growth stage of the crop (July to November). The organic carbon content in the soil was 0.45 per cent in open field of *C. ciliaris* and 0.67 per cent in *A. tortilis* + *C. ciliaris* while it was 0.53 per cent under sole *P. maximum* in open field and 0.79 per cent in *L. leucocephala* + *P. maximum* based silvipastoral system. Higher relative humidity, soil moisture and organic carbon content under the tree canopies as compared to the open grown grasses (without trees) indicating that the system has improved the microclimate and soil health for the sustainable production of the system for longer period.

Mishra (2002) reported that organic carbon was maximum at the top layer (0-15 cm) followed by (30–45 cm) soil depths in pure grasses in open field as well as in the *C. ciliaris* + *A. tortilis* and *P. maximum* + *L. leucocephala* based silvipastoral systems. The increase in organic carbon by 10 to 40 per cent under the silvopasture system as compared to sole pastures may be because of more litter decomposition and available root biomass. The increase in organic carbon under the silvopasture systems has indicated the improvement in soil health, which intern higher system productivity and sustainability. *Leucaena leucocephala* + *Panicum maximum* based silvipasture system maintained higher organic carbon and therefore, the sustainability of system production were maintained over the years. Maximum increase was estimated in case of available nitrogen, phosphorus and potassium content under the tree pasture canopies than the sole pasture.

Maximum nutrients were estimated at the top layer of the soil than at different depths. Generally, higher level of nutrients under tree + pasture based silvopasture systems during two years may be due to decay of litter, root biomass and other organic carbon matter (Mishra, 2002). The availability of phosphorus and potassium significantly improved under the tree canopies exhibiting the more available nutrients for maintaining the sustainable production of the systems in the degraded land. Many workers have also reported the more availability of nutrients under tree cover (Sanchez *et al.*, 1985, 1987; Nair, 1989). Also symbiotic nitrogen fixations by trees often result in increase of soil nitrogen availability (Alpizar *et al.*, 1986; Dommer gues 1987). Root decay may be another source of adding organic carbon and nutrients in the soil (Young, 1991; George and Kumar, 1998).

The analysis of soils after 6 years of silvipasture establishment indicated increase in the nutrients like nitrogen, phosphorus, organic carbon and potash in time even when grasses were harvested and removed every year (Singh *et al.*, 1977). Misra *et al.* (1982) also observed improvement in soil physical properties, pH, nitrogen and organic carbon with 4 years silvipasture plantation on a calcareous soil. In another study it has been found that the initial organic matter, available nitrogen, available phosphorus and field capacity of 0.32 per cent, 131 kg/ha, 6.2 kg/ha and 11 per cent were changed to 0.78 per cent, 267 kg/ha, 15.5 kg/ha and 15.5 per cent respectively over a period of 10 years. From these studies it was amply indicated that poor soils on the wastelands could restore their fertility under such systems.

Carbon Sequestration

Effective carbon sequestration in wasteland can be achieved by means of silvopastoral, pastoral and watershed approach. R and D in the wasteland development programme may increase the carbon sequestration rate by considering all the ecological, social, and economic implications. There are two fundamental approaches to sequestering carbon in such ecosystems: (1) protection of ecosystems that store carbon so that sequestration can be maintained or increased; and (2) enhancement of the ability of ecosystems to increase carbon sequestration beyond current conditions. Restoration of degraded lands offers significant benefits and carbon sequestration potential in both below and above ground systems.

Early estimates of huge losses of carbon from soils due to degradation and erosion of soils gave the idea to develop wastelands as carbon storage. The major strategy for increasing carbon sequestration is to increase afforestation. Such increases in productivity will likely lead to greater amounts of carbon sequestration in both above- and below-ground plant parts, as well as in soils. Reclamation of wastelands increased the vegetation cover and biomass production along with the soil carbon. However, sequestration of carbon implies not only increasing the amount of carbon entering the soils but also a decrease with amount leaving either through decomposition or erosion (Johnson and Kern, 1991). The silvopastoral systems of *Leptochloa* along with *Acacia* and *Prosopis* in degraded lands in 4 to 7 years rotations have produced 20 Mg/ha/yr and 4 Mg/ha/yr biomass of tree and grass along with increase in soil carbon (Singh *et al.*, 1988). Growth of high nitrogen fixing tree species like *Sesbania* rapidly increased soil carbon even in moderate sites (Rao *et al.*, 1990).

The organic carbon content of rakar soils in degraded lands of Bundelkhand region was estimated only 0.155 per cent with bulk density of 1.5 Mg/m^3 at the soil depth of 0–15 cm. The initial organic carbon stock of such soils was calculated as 3.49 Mg C/ha. The initial productivity of such land was only 1 Mg/ha/yr with carbon content of 0.5 Mg/ha/yr (assuming that vegetation contain 50 per cent C out of the total biomass). After the establishment of silvopasture systems the organic carbon stock of the soils was estimated to 10.125 Mg C/ha after ten years of rotation. This land has produced 11mg/ha biomass at the 10th years of growth of the system. The carbon stock in vegetation was calculated as 5.5 Mg/ha/yr (Bhatt, 2008). Therefore, the total carbon sequestration in such lands was 11.60 Mg/ha which have improved the productivity of the such lands. This has suggested that integration of trees with naturally growing grasses could be a viable land use option for improving biological productivity and carbon sequestration of highly degraded soils.

Agroforestry has tremendous potential in carbon sequestration because of carbon storage potential in its multiple plant species and soil as well as its applicability in agricultural lands and in reforestation (Montagnini and Nair, 2004). Proper development of agroforestry systems can make them effective carbon sinks. In total the extent of C sequestered depends on the amounts of C in standing biomass, in roots, and C sequestered in wood products. Average carbon storage by agroforestry practices has been estimated as 9, 21, 50, and 63 Mg C ha^{-1} in semiarid, subhumid, humid, and temperate region. For smallholder agroforestry systems in the tropics, potential C sequestration rates range from 1.5 to 3.5 Mg C ha^{-1} yr^{-1}. Agroforestry can also have an indirect effect on C sequestration when it helps decrease pressure on natural forests, which are the largest sink of terrestrial C. Another indirect avenue of C sequestration is through the use of agroforestry technologies for soil conservation, which could enhance C storage in trees and soils. Agroforestry systems with perennial crops may be important carbon sinks. In order to exploit this vastly unrealized potential of C sequestration through agroforestry in both subsistence and commercial enterprises in the tropics and the temperate region, innovative policies, based on rigorous research results, have to be put in place.

References

Aggarwal, R.K., Gupta, J.P., Saxena, S.K. and Muthana, K.P. (1975). Studies on soil Physico–chemical and ecological changes under twelve year old five desert species of west Rajastha, *Indian For.*, 102; 863-872.

Ahuja, L.D. (1980). Grass production under Khejri. *In:* Khejri (*Prosopis cineraria*) in Indian Deserts its role in agroforestry (*Eds.* H.S. Mann and S.K. Saxena) *Monograph* No. 11, CAZRI, Jodhpur, pp. 28-30.

Ahuja, L.D., Verma, C.M, Sharma, S.I. and Lamba, T.R. (1978). Range management studies on the contribution of ground storey (grass) in afforested areas in arid region. *Ann. Arid Zone*, 17: 304-331.

Alpizer, L.H.W., Fassbender, Heuveldop, H.P. and Enriquez, G. (1986). Modelling agroforestry system of Coco (*Theobroma cocoa*) with Laurel (*Cordia alliodora*) and Poro (*Erythrina poeppigiana*) in Costa Rica. I. Inventory of organic matter and nutrients. *Agroforestry system*, 4: 175-189.

Arya, R.L., Singh, A., Yadav, R.B., Singh, S.P., Gangwar, M.K. and Lal, Banwari. (1998). Early performance of trees and grasses under silvipastoral systems in salt affected soil of Indo Gangetic plains of Uttar Pradesh. *Range Mgmt. and Agroforestry* 19: 53-57.

Bhatt, R. K. (2008). Climate change and mitigation options through silvipastoral systems. Paper presented in the National Seminar of National Institute of Ecology, New Delhi, 26-27 Aug.

Bhatt, R. K., H. S. Tiwari, Vandana and L.P. Misra. (2006). Photosynthesis and shade tolerance in tropical range grasses and legumes. *Indian J. Plant Physiol*, Vol. 11, No. 2, (N.S.) pp. 172-177.

Bhatt, R. K., Khan, T.A., Pathak, P.S. and Misra, A.K. (2006). Sustainable forage production under silvipastoral systems in semiarid tropics. *Indian J. of Agroforestry* Vol. 8 No.1:1, 22-25.

Bhatt, R. K., Suresh, G., and Ram Newaj (2003). Biophysical aspects of tree crop interactions in silvipastoral system. Pub. In Agroforestry potentials and Opportunities. (ed.) P. S. Pathak and Ram Newaj, Pub. By Agrobios, Jodhpur pp. 249-265.

Bhatt, R. K. (1988). IGFRI, Annual report.

Bhatt, R. K., Misra, L. P. and Pathak, P. S. (1994). Forage yield and related plant processes in *Cenchrus* and *Panicum* under silvipastoral system. In: *Agroforestry system for Degraded Lands.* (ed. Panjab Singh, P.S. Pathak and M.M. Roy), Oxford and IBH Publishing Co. Vol.2: 732-738.

Bhatt, R.K. and Sinha, N.C. (1990). Photosynthetic pigment–a pre-requisite of grass productivity. *Photosynthetica* 24(1): 147-150.

Deb Roy, R. (1986). Studies on some aspects of renewable energy (fuel) and pasture production in an ecosystem of *Albizia lebbek* (L.) Benth. With grass and legumes. *Ph.D.Thesis*, Jiwaji University Gwalior (India).

Deb Roy, R. (1989). Biomass production potential of fodder cum fuel tree under silvipastoral system. In: Promotion of Fodder and Fuelwood Tree (eds N.G. Hedge, L.L. Relwani and V.D. Kelkar). BAIF, Pune: 70-76.

Deb Roy, R. and Pathak, P. S. (1974). Silvipastoral management, *Indian Farming* 24:41-42.

Deb Roy, R. and Pathak, P. S. (1983). Silvipastoral research and development in India. *Indian Rev. of Life Science* 3:247-264.

Deb Roy, R. and Pathak, P. S. (1984). Silvipastoral research and development in India. *Indian Rev. of Life Science* 3: 247-64.

Deb Roy, R., Patil, B.D. and Pathak, P.S. (1978). Silvipastoral farming for amelioration and increased productivity for aird and semi arid region. In: Proceeding of the International symposium on Arid Zone Research and Development.CAZRI, Jodhpur, India: 531p.

Deb Roy, R., Patil, B.D. Pathak, P.S. and Gupta, S.K. (1980). Forage production of *Cenchrus ciliaris* and *Cenchrus setigerus* under silvipasture system. *Indian J. Range Mgmt.*, 1: 113-120.

Dogra, K., Katoch, B.S., Sood, B.R. and Singh, Gurudev (1997). Production potential and quality of silvi–herbage system vis-à-vis natural grasslands.

Dommergues, Y.R. (1987). The role of biological fixation in agroforestry. *In: Agroforestry: A Decade of Development* (eds. H.A. Skppler and P.K.R. Nair). ICRAF. Nairobi (Kenya): 245-271.

Egle, K. (1960). Menge and verhaltnis der pigment–In: Ruhland, W(*ed.*): *Handbuch der flanzen Physiologie.* Vol. VII pp. 444-496. Springer-Verlag, Berlin–Gottingen–Heidelberg.

George, S.J. and Kumar, B.M. (1998). Liter dynamics and soil fertility improvement in silvopastoral systems of the humid tropics of southern India. Intt. *Tree crops J.*, 9: 267-282.

Goldberg, D. E. and Werner, P. A. (1983). Equivalence of competitors in plant communities: a null hypothesis and a field experimental approach. *Am. J. Bot.* 70: 1098-1104.

Good Child, D. J., Bojorkman, D. and Pyliotis, N. A. (1972). Chloroplast ultrastructure, leaf anatomy and content of chlorophyll and soluble protein in rain forest species. In: *Carnegic Institute Year Book* 71:102-107.

Grewal, S.S., Singh, K., Juneja, M. L. And and Singh, Shivcharan (1996). Relative growth, fuel wood yield, litter accumulation and conservation potential of seven Acacia species and an under storey grass on a sloping bouldery soil. *Indian J. Forestry.* 19: 174-182.

Gupta, J.P. and Saxena, S.K. (1978). Studies on monitoring of the dynamics of moisture in the soil and the performance of ground flora under desertic communities of trees. *Indian J. Ecol.*, 5: 30-36.

Harsh, L.N., Tiwari, J.C., Berman, U. and Sharma, S.K. (1992). Agroforestry for arid region. *Indian Fmg.* 42: 32-37.

Hazra, C.R. (1990). Revitalization of degraded land resources through silvipastoral system for herbage production. In: *Silvipasture system in India* (eds. P.S. Pathak and Punjab Singh). RMSI, IGFRI, Jhansi: 81-86.

Hazra, C.R. (1994). Role of agroforestry for amelioration as edaphclimatic conditions for increased for productivity. *In:* Advances in Agroforestry and its Role for Sustainable Agriculture and Environment. (*Eds.* R. Deb Roy, A.K. Bisaria and P.Rai). NRCAF, Jhansi. pp. 105-118.

Hazra, C.R. and Patil, B.D. (1986). Forage production under silvipastural system–light and temperature interaction. *Indian J. Range Mgmt.*, 7: 33-36.

Hazra, C.R., Singh, D.P. and Kaul, R.N. (1994). Greening of Common Ilands in Jhansi through Village Resource Development–a case study. National Aforestation and Eco-development Board, New Delhi.

IDRC (1982-1994). Annual Report of Silvipasture Operational Research Project for the Bundelkhand Region, IGFRI, Jhansi.

Johnson, M. G. and Kern, J. S. (1991). Sequestering Carbon in Soil. In: *Proc. EPA Workshop.* p. 85 USPEAERL. Corvallis, USA.

Kaul, R. (1974). Study of the seasonal variation of the water content of the leaves and the rate of transpiration in *Hemigraphis dura. J. Indian Bot. Soc.* 53: 97-99.

King, K.F.S. (1979). Key note address: Some principles of agroforestry, Proc. *Agroforestry Seminar*, ICAR, 17–26.

Krishnaswamy, M.H. (1942). Revised working plan of Kurnool East forest division for the period 1940–51, Govt Press Madras, 181 P.

Liu Naizhaung. (1991). Light distribution in tree intercropping area and its agricultural value. In agroforestry system in China (ed. Zhu Zhaohua *et al.,*). *China Academy of Forestry and IDRC.* Publ. Pp. 14-20.

Mishra, A. K. (2005). Growth, productivity and physiological process of grasses under silvopastoral system in semi-arid region. *Ph. D. Thesis,* Bundelkhand University, Jhansi.

Misra, L.P. and Bhatt, R.K. (1994). Productivity and adaptation of grasses under silvipastoral system in semiarid region. In *Proc. Agroforestry systems for Degradedlands* (ed. Panjab Singh, P.S. Pathak and M.M. Roy), Oxford and IBH Publishing Col. Vol.2, PP.727-731.

Misra, L.P. and Bhatt, R.K. (1994). Productivity and adaptation of grasses under silvipastoral system in semi arid region. *In:* Agroforestry systems for Degraded Lands (*Eds.* P.Singh, P.S. Pathak and M.M. Roy). Oxford and IBM Publishing Co. Pvt. Ltd., New Delhi. pp. 727-731.

Misra, S.M., Patil, B.D. and Pathak, P.S. (1982). Comparative differences in soil properties as a result of growing different grass, legume and tree combinations. *Indian J. Range Mgmt.* 3(1 and 2) : 71–74.

Montagnini, F. and Nair, P. K. (2004). Carbon Sequestration: An under-exploited environmental benefit of agroforestry systems. *Agroforestry Systems* 61: 281-295.

Naidu, C.V. and Swamy, P.M. (1993). Effect of shade on growth, biomass production and associated physiological parameters in *Pongamia pinnata* (Linn.) Pierre. *Indian J. Plant Physiol.* XXXVI (4) : 212-214.

Nair, P.K.R. (1989). The role of trees in soil productivity and protection. *In: Agroforestry systems in the Tropics* (ed. P.K.R. Nair). ICRAF, Nairobi and Kluwer Academic Publishers, Dordoecht, (the Netherlads): 567-589.

Nobel, P.S. (1977). Water relations and photosynthesis of a barrel cactus, *Ferocactus acanthodes* in colorado desert, *Oecologia* 27: 117.

Paroda, R. S. (1990). Silvipastoral approach for wasteland development: present options and future strategy. In: *Silvipastoral systems in India* (eds. PS Pathak and Panjab Singh). Range Management Society of India, Indian grassland and Fodder research Institute, Jhansi, pp. 1-3.

Paroda, R.S. and Jatasra, D.S. (1985). Forages for arid lands. In: *Current Practices in Dryland Resources and Technology.* (eds. Alani Singh and G.R. Chowdhary). Scientific and Geo–environ Academia, Jodhpur, 256p.

Pathak, P. S. and Roy, M. M. (1994). *Silvipastoral System of Production.* IGFRI, Jhansi: 55 p.

Pathak, P.S. (1983). Silvipasture through natural vegetation manipulation- an ecological assessment, Nat. Seminar on Silvipastoral System, 8–10 Oct., IGFRI, Jhansi.

Pathak, P.S. (1992). Silvopastoral technology for wasteland development. NARP training program on agroforestry, forage production and animal nutrition. pp. 14-20.

Pathak, P.S. (1994). Silvipastoral system of production for degraded lands in India. *In:* Advances in Agroforestry and its Role for Sustainable Agriculture and Environment (*Eds.* R.Deb Roy, A.K. Bisaria and P. Rai). NRCAF, Jhansi. pp. 186-201.

Pathak, P.S., Gupta, S.K. and Singh Punjab (1995). Rehabilitation of degraded lands. IGFRI Jhansi : 23.

Pathak, P.S., Gupta, S.K. and Singh, P. (1996). IGFRI Approaches Rehabilitation of Degraded lands. IGFRI, Jhansi, pp. 1-23.

Prajapati, M.C. K., Nambiar, T.N., Puri, D.N., Singh, J.P. and Malhotra, B.M. (1993). *Acacia nilotica* and *Cenchrus ciliaris* silvipasture for sustainable productivity of fuel and fodder in ravines.*In* Agroforestry for 2000 AD for the semi arid and arid tropics. Extended abstract (Late arrivals) (*Eds.* A.S. Gill, R. Deb Roy and A.K. Bisaria). NRCAF, Jhansi. pp. 33-34.

Ramakrishana, Y.S. and Sastri, A.S.R.A.S. (1977b). Microclimate under *Acacia tortilis* plantations. *Annual Report*. CAZRI, Jodhpur: 69-70.

Ramakrishna, Y.S. (1984). Forest Microclimate and its importance in agroforestry. *In: Agroforestry in Arid and Semi-Arid Zones* (ed K.A. Shankarnarayan). CAZRI, Jodhpur : 9-14.

Ramakrishna, Y.S. and Sastri, A.S.R.A.S. (1977a). Climatological studies on rainfall interception, diurnal variation in the total and net radiant energy available under *Acaci tortilis* trees. *Annual Report*, CAZRI, Jodhpur: 69 p.

Rao, D.L.N., Gill, H.S. and Abrol, I.P. (1990). Regional experience with perennial Sesbania in India. In: *Perennial Sesbania Species in Agroforestry Systems* (Eds. Macklin, Bill and Evans, D.O.), NFTA, Hawail, USA pp. 189-98.

Roy, M.M. (1995). Productivity of *Hardwickia binata* based silvopastures in Bundelkhand region. *Ph.D. Thesis*, Bundelkhand University, Jhansi: 182 p.

Sanchez, P.A. (1987). Soil productivity and sustainability in agroforestry. In: *Agroforestry : A Decade of Development* (eds. H.A. Steppler and P.K.R. Nair) ICRAF, Nairobi (Kenya): 205-223.

Sanchez, P.A., Palm, C.A., Davey, C.B., Szott, L.T. and Russell, C.E. (1985). Tree crops as soil improvers in humid tropics. In : *Attributes of Tree as Crop Plants* (eds. M.G.R. Cannell and J.E. Jackson). Institute of Terrestrial Ecology, National Environmental Research Council, Abbets Ripton, Huntingdon, England: 327-350.

Sehgal, J.L. and Abrol, I.P. (1994). *Soil Degradation in India status and impact.* 80 Oxford and IBH Publishing Co., Pvt. Ltd. New Delhi, India.

Shankar, V., Kumar, Suresth and Tyagi, R.K. (1988). Grazing resources of semi arid and arid regions. In: *Pasture and Forage Crop Research–A state of knowledge* Report (ed. Punjab Singh). RMSI, Jhansi: 63-65.

Sharma, S.K. Datta, B.K. and Tiwari, J.C. (1996). *Prosopis cineraria* (L) Druce in silvipastoral system in arid regions of western Rajasthan. *Range Mgmt. and Agroforestry*, 17: 81-85.

Singh, D., Mannikar, N.D., Srivas, N.C. and Saxena, D.C. (1977). Changes in soil fertility under long term cultivation of fodder crops and grasses. *J.Indian Soc. Soil* 25: 28–32.

Singh, J.P. and Puri, D.N. (1975). Economic utilization of ravines for fuel cum fodder. Annual Report, CSWCR and TI, Dehra Dun. pp. 39-40.

Singh, K.S. and Lal, P. (1969). Effect of khejri (*Prosopis cineraria*) and Babul (*Acacia arabica*) trees and soil fertility and profile characteristics. *Ann. Arid Zone*, 8: 33-36.

Singh, P. and Roy, M.M. (1991). Forage production through agroforestry constraints and priorities. *Range Mgmt. And Agroforestry* 12: 169-178.

Singh, V.P., Dey, S.K. and Murthy, K.S. (1988). Effect of low light stress on growth and yield of rice. *Indian J. Plant Physiol. 31*: 84-91.

Tajwani, K.G. (1987). Agroforestry practices and research in India. In: *Agroforestry: Realities, Possibilities and Potentials* (ed. H.L. Gholz), Martinus Nijhoff Publisher, Dordrecgt, Netherlands, pp. 109-136.

UNESCO (1979). *Tropical Grassland Ecosystem- A state of Art Report.* United National Educational Scientific and Cultural Organization, Paris: 65p.

Wilson, J.A. (1951). Grazing management and improvement in Madras Province. Proc. 7th Silvicultural Conf. FRI, Dehradun.

Yadava, R.B. and Varshney, R.B. (1997). Multistorey silvipastoral approach for sustaining soil fertility in degraded rangelands of Bundelkhand. *Range Mgmt. and Agroforestry* 18: 195-200.

Young, A. (1991). Soil Fertility. In: *Biophysical Research for Asian Agroforestry* (eds M.E. Avery, M.G.R. Cannell and C. Ong). Winrock International, USA: 187-207.

Microbial Biotechnology and Ecology (2011) *Pages* 708–723
Editors: Deepak Vyas, G.S. Paliwal, P.K.Khare and R.K Gupta
Published by: DAYA PUBLISHING HOUSE, NEW DELHI

Chapter 41

Agroforestry: Conservation of Natural Resources, Biomass Production and Climate Moderations

☆ *Ashok Shukla* and V.D. Tripathi*

National Research Centre for Agroforestry, Jhansi – 284 003, U.P.

ABSTRACT

Agroforestry, a land use system/technology in which trees are deliberately planted on the same units of land with agricultural crops and/or animals, has been recognized as one of the most promising strategy for rehabilitating the already degraded areas. It has been a way of life in India ever since the evolution of human beings through the forests. Uses of trees for different purposes include, wood, shelter and, medicines have been the common feature. The benefits of agroforestry includes, it optimizes production, provide supplement food and fodder, increase farm income, amelioration of soil chemical and physical properties, reduction of soil erosion, utilization of waste and degraded lands, improve environment, minimize adverse effect of climatic factors etc. The present chapter enlighten the brief account on the importance of agroforestry systems *viz.*, system productivity and enhancement, amelioration of problematic soil, conservation of natural resources and climate moderation.

Introduction

Agroforestry is an intensive land use management system that integrates trees, shrubs, crops and livestock on a landscape level to achieve optimum benefits (Garret *et al.*, 1994). It has been a way of life in India ever since the evolution of human beings through the forests. Uses of trees for different

* E-mail: ashokshukla06@gmail.com

purposes include, wood, shelter and medicines have been the common feature. Agroforestry systems have several advantages and some of these advantages are optimizes production, gives supplement food and fodder, improve soil, utilize wasteland and degraded lands, provide employment opportunities, increase farm income, minimize adverse effect of climatic factors and aid industrial growth.

Agroforestry research is more than hundred years old in India beginning with introduction of shade trees in tea gardens, but organized research was initiated during fifties in few ICAR institutes. India has been at the forefront since organized research in agroforestry started worldwide. In 1979 first seminar on agroforestry was organized by the ICAR at Imphal to accumulate and compile the data on the R and D of agroforestry in India. The All India Coordinated Research Project (AICRP) on Agroforestry with 20 centers all over the country was launched in 1983. At present 36 centers are under AICRP on agroforestry. These centers represent almost all the agro-climatic zones of the country. In addition to ICAR, ICFRE, private organizations (WIMCO, ITC, BAIF, IFFDC, West Coast Paper Mills Ltd, Hindustan Paper Mills Ltd and National Tree Growers Cooperatives) and NGOs are also engage in research and promotion of the agroforestry in the country. Agroforestry research and education has been started in more than 15 State Agricultural Universities. The major thrust of agroforestry research in the beginning was as follows:

1. Diagnostic survey and appraisal of existing agroforestry practices.
2. Collection and evaluation of promising tree species/cultivars of fuel, fodder and small timber.
3. Studies on management practices of agroforestry systems.
4. Environment, wasteland and community land development through agroforestry interventions, and
5. Integration of livestock, fishery, apiculture, lac etc. as a component of agroforestry.

Table 41.1: Area Under Various Types of Tree Plantation in India

Plantation Type	*Area (M ha)*
Agroforestry and social forestry	23.00
Externally aided social forestry	
(a) Farm forestry/agroforestry	1.24
(b) Village woodlots	0.50
(c) Strip plantation	0.07
(d) Rehabilitation of degraded forests	0.24
Sub total	2.06
By NGOs/Vas	0.04
Tree growers co-operatives	0.04
Conservative forestry	0.19
Afforestation (windbreaks/shelterbelt), Under irrigation region development program of the Indira Gandhi Canal Project	0.40
Total	25.72

As per one of the estimate about 25.72 M ha area is under various types of tree plantations (Table 41.1), which include agroforestry, social forestry, farm forestry and others. According to FSI (2005) the total forest cover in India is 67.8 M ha. Of this 5.1 M ha is very dense forest, 33.9 M ha is moderately dense forest and 28.8 M ha is open forest. Recently Dhyani *et al.*, 2006 estimated that 7.45 M ha area is under agroforestry. There is scope for using modern tool and products like RS and GIS to ascertain the information. National Research Centre for Agroforestry, Jhansi has taken a lead in this regard recently.

Dhyani *et al.* (2007) has illustrated the potential of agroforestry contributions like fuel wood, timber, fodder, fruits, livestock and bio-energy. The scenario of timber for domestic and industrial purposes is given in Table 41.2. Currently the gap between supply and demand is met through imports. The deficit of 16 M cum as on date (2008) could be met by promoting fast growing exotics like *Eucalyptus*, Subabul, *Poplar*, *Acacia mangium* etc. The major contribution of agroforestry has been in the supply of small timber, where more than half of the demand is being met from agroforestry.

Table 41.2: Demand and Supply of Timber for Furniture, Agriculture and Industry (M cum)

Particulars	*2001*	*2006*	*2010[a]*	*2020[a]*	*2025[a]*
Demand	73	82	89	107	116
Supply from forest	12	12	12	12	12
Supply from plantation and agroforestry	47	53	61	90	100
Deficit	14	17	16	5	4

[a]Estimates; (Note: 2.2 cum = 1 tone); Ganpathy (1997) and Saxena (1990)

Table 41.3: Prominent Agroforestry Systems in Different Regions of Country

Agroclimatic Zone/Region	*Agroforestry Systems*					
	AS[a]	*AHS*	*AH*	*HP*	*SP*	*Specialized*
Western Himalayan	4	4	5	4	4	-
Eastern Himalayan	5	3	5	4	3	Jhum (shifting cultivation)
Lower gangetic plain	5	-	3	2	2	Energy plantation
Middel gangetic plain	4	-	2	-	-	Homestead
Upper gangetic plain	5	-	5	-	-	Agri-horticulture
Upper gangetic plain	5	-	5	-	-	Agrihorti-silviculture
Trans-gangetic plain	5	-	4	3	4	Block plantation
Eastern plateau and hills	4	-	5	4	4	Block plantation
Western plateau and hills	4	-	5	2	4	-
Southern plateau and hills	5	-	3	2	4	-
East coast plateau and hills	4	5	4	4	2	Home garden/shelterbelt
West coast plains and ghats	4	5	4	2	2	Home garden
Gujarat plains and hills	4	2	4	3	5	Block plantation
Western plains dry area	5	3	4	-	5	Shelterbelt
The islands	4	5	4	1	2	Home garden

AS: Agrisilviculture; AHS: Agrihortisilviculture; AH: Agrihorticulture; HP: Hortipastoral; SP: Silvipastoral (Solanki, 2006).

The research and development efforts undertaken during the last two decades have clearly demonstrated the potential of agroforestry for resource conservation, improvement of environmental quality, rehabilitation of degraded lands and providing multiple outputs to meet the day to day demand of the rural population. The diagnostic survey and appraisal of existing agroforestry practices in the country revealed that there are enumerable agroforestry practices prevalent in agroclimatic zones (Pathak *et al.*, 2000, Sharda *et al.*, 2001, Solanki, 2006). On the basis of the design (D and D) exercise, the prominent agroforestry systems from different regions of the country are given in Tables 41.3 and 41.4, respectively.

Table 41.4: Prominent Agri-horticulture Systems in India

State	*Based Agri-horti Systems*
J and K, Himachal Pradesh, Uttranchal	Apple
Punjab, Haryana	Citrus
Uttar Pradesh	Mango, Aonla
Bihar	Litchi
NEH region	Citrus
Maharashtra, Goa	Pomegranate, Mango, Coconut
Karnataka, Andhra Pradesh	Mango, Coconut
Kerala, Tamil Nadu	Coconut, Arecanut, Palmira
Rajasthan	Ber
Gujarat	Mango
Orissa, West Bengal	Coconut, Palmira

Present chapter enlighten the brief account on the importance of agroforestry systems *viz.*, system productivity and enhancement, amelioration of problematic soil, conservation of natural resources and climate moderation.

System Productivity and Enhancement

Solanki *et al.* (2000) assessed the biomass production of different trees after 7 years of plantation (Table 41.5). Highest biomass was recorded in *Casuarina equisetifolia* (171 t ha^{-1}), followed by *Leuceana leucocephala* (159 t ha^{-1}), *Eucalyptus* hybrid (152 t ha^{-1}) and *Dalbergia sissoo* (65 t ha^{-1}).

Table 41.5: Biomass Production of Different Tree Species

Species	*Productivity*
Casuarina equisetifolia	171
Leuceana leucocephala	159
Eucalyptus hybrid	152
Dalbergia sissoo	65

Comparative Biomass of Poplars in Different Localities

The performance of Poplar plantation with same and different ages in various locations is being presented in Table 41.6. Comparing the growth performance of Poplars in terms of productivity, it was higher in tropical countries compared to temperate countries. The growth greatly depends on edapho-climatic conditions of the particular region. For instance in India, the productivity varied from 3.2 Mg ha^{-1} yr^{-1} (North central) to 17.9 and 22.3 Mg ha^{-1} yr^{-1} (Alluvial plain and Tarai region, respectively).

Table 41.6: Comparative Account of Distribution of Above Ground Biomass of Poplar

Species	Location	Age (yrs)	Density (ha^{-1})	Biomass (Mg ha^{-1})	Reference
Populus deltoides	India (Tarai)	1-4	666	7.4-89.3	Lodhiyal and Lodhiyal, 1997
P. deltoides	India (Tarai)	5-8	400	67.4-134.3	Lodhiyal *et al.*, 1995
P. tremuloides	North Central	8	-	25.4	Ruark and Bokheim, 1988
P. tremuloides	Wiscosin Canada	5	-	8.3-34.8	Wang *et al.*, 1995
P. deltoides	Albana	8	-	89.7	Carker and Tandon, 1997
P. deltoides	India Dehra Dun	5	-	22.5	Negi and Tandon, 1997
P. deltoides (Clone IC)	India	10	500	105.4	Singh, 1989
P. deltoides	India	14	-	44.5	Raizada and Srivastava, 1989
P. deltoides	USA	16	-	133.7	Shelton *et al.*, 1982
P. deltoides	India (Hisar)	9	208-2250	715-251.5	Puri *et al.*, 1994
P. deltoides (Agrisilvi)	India (Raipur)	4	666	20.9-35.8	Puri and Swamy, 2005

The large variability in aboveground biomass among different clones is probably due to genetic make up of individual clones. Among different components, the proportion of biomass was highest in stem followed by branches, bark and leaves. The proportion of biomass stored in roots were found to be 15-20 per cent of the total biomass, which are higher than the value 10-12 per cent reported for eucalyptus (Feller 1980) and equal to 5 years old poplar plantations (Lodhiyal *et al.*, 1992).

Eucalyptus

Chaturvedi (1981) assessed the yield potential of *Eucalyptus* hybrids in different site qualities (I-V) on a 6-9 years rotation (Table 41.7). The air dry tonnage yield varied from 6.9 $ha^{-1}yr^{-1}$ (site quality I) to 0.7 $ha^{-1}yr^{-1}$ (site quality V).

Table 41.7: Yield Potential of *Eucalyptus hybrid* in Different Site Quality

Site Quality	Rotation (yrs)	No. of Stems ha^{-1}	ADT ($ha^{-1}yr^{-1}$)
I	6	964	7.9
II	6	1038	5.1
III	7	1105	3.0
IV	8	1202	1.6
V	9	1345	0.7

The productivity potential of seven years old *E. tereticornis* managed under short rotation high density system were studied in the mid hill zone of H.P. (Saralch, 2005). The productivity per plant in all plant components declined significantly with increase in plant densities where as results on one hectare basis for the same parameters were exactly opposite to it (Table 41.8).

Mixed plantations of *Acacia mearnsii* (black wattle) and *Eucalyptus globulus* (blue gum) made in alternative rows at different spacing resulted in increased yield of wood and leaves over pure plantation in a 10 years rotation (Table 41.9).

Table 41.8: Above Ground Biomass and Productivity of *E. tereticornis*

Parameters	Density		
	27,778 trees ha^{-1} (60 x 60 cm)	12,346 trees ha^{-1} (90 x 90 cm)	6,944 trees ha^{-1} (120 x 120 cm)
Biomass (kg $tree^{-1}$)	4.57	5.74	7.13
Biomass (t ha^{-1})	127.07	70.85	49.49
Productivity (kg $tree^{-1}$ yr^{-1})	0.65	0.82	1.02
Productivity (t ha^{-1} yr^{-1})	18.15	10.12	7.07

Table 41.9: Biomass of Black Wattle and Blue Gum in Mixed Plantation (Cu mha^{-1})

Tree Species	3.5 x 3.5 m	3.65 x 3.65 m	3.65 x 4.57 m	Mean
Eucalyptus globules	274	226	318 460	330
Acacia mearnsii	180	228	108 90	152

Source: Forest Department, Tamil Nadu.

Leucaena leucocephala

The yield of three different varieties of *L. leucocephala* at Jhansi was studied by Pathak and Patil (1980) over a period of 10 years. The total productivity of Salvador registered 82 per cent and 64 per cent over K-8 and K-28 respectively (Table 41.10).

Table 41.10: Biomass Production of *L. leucocephala* Varieties

Variety	Main Stem $ADTha^{-1}yr^{-1}$	Branchwood	Total
Salvador	31.6	11.8	43.4
K-8	21.8	3.0	23.8
K-28	22.7	3.7	26.4

In 1994, Pathak and Gupta assessed the growth and biomass production of *L. leucocephala* provenances and promising selection at IGFRI, Jhansi. They found that selection S24 was quite promising and better than K8 and it can be used in northern India (Table 41.11).

Table 41.11. Growth and Production of *L. leucocephala* Provenances and Selections

Provenance	DBH (cm)	Height (m)	Biomass (kg $tree^{-1}$)
K8	9.10	12.80	41.34
K 217	8.90	12.70	37.07
K 601	9.20	12.20	41.27
K 636	8.90	12.90	31.26
K 397	8.30	12.50	31.30
K 340	8.70	11.60	34.93

Contd...

Table 41.11–Contd...

Provenance	DBH (cm)	Height (m)	Biomass (kg tree^{-1})
K 29	8.90	11.70	41.98
IGFRI 123-1	9.30	11.40	40.19
SP 1	8.50	11.60	39.94
S 10	10.10	12.50	50.16
S 14	9.90	12.50	43.18
S 15	9.00	11.70	36.58
S 22	8.90	11.70	44.73
S 23	7.70	10.70	23.91
S 24	9.50	12.80	56.36

Dalbergia sissoo

Gupta (1993) evaluated the performance of *D. sissoo* in the site quality class of VII at two different spacing *viz.*, 3 × 3 m and 2 × 2m. He found that at 6th year the plantation with 2 × 2 m spacing yielded 60.22 m^3ha^{-1} but it was achieved only in 10th when spaced 3 × 3m (Table 41.12).

Table 41.12: Standing Volume of *D. sissoo* on Class VII Land

Age (yrs)	DBH (cm)	Height (m)	Volume ha^{-1} (m^3)
Spacing 3 x 3m			
4	4.80	5.36	4.29
5	6.88	6.02	9.88
6	8.58	6.82	17.40
7	9.81	7.22	24.05
8	11.47	7.77	35.69
9	12.20	8.40	44.29
10	13.90	9.00	60.16
11	15.14	9.82	77.32
Spacing 2 x 2m			
4	7.90	7.21	35.21
5	8.70	8.20	48.51
6	9.20	9.08	60.22
7	9.40	10.03	69.20

Amelioration of Problematic Soil

In addition to biomass production, mitigating climate change, the trees plays a vital role in ameliorating the problematic soil by improving physical, chemical and biological properties of the soil. Nitrogen fixing trees ameliorate alkali soils at much faster than non nitrogen fixing trees.

Soil salinity and alkalinity have degraded about 7.41 M ha of land in India (Sharma, 1998). A large acreage in the canal irrigated tracts of arid and semi arid regions of the country suffer from water logging and salinity and the resultant loss to crop production is increasing at an alarming rate. Establishment of tree plantations on salt affected soils sets in amelioration process by favorably affecting physical, chemical and biological properties of soil (Sing *et al.*, 1993). As per an estimate 45.3 per cent land degradation of the total degraded land of India is caused by water erosion (Table 41.13).

Table 41.13: Land Degradation in India

Type of Degradation	*Area (M ha)*	*Per cent of Total Area*
Water erosion	148.9	45.3
Wind erosion	13.5	4.1
Chemical deterioration (salinity etc.)	13.8	4.2
Water logging	11.6	3.5
Total	187.8	57.1

Some woody trees differ in their tolerance to alkali soil conditions at the genetic as well as species level. Under saline conditions, only those which can withstand high salt content and thrive under high water table conditions should be selected for planting. The promising tree species for plantation under salt affected soils are listed here according to their degree of tolerance (Table 41.14).

Table 41.14: Promising MPTs for Reclamation

Alkali Soils	*Saline Soils*	*Bio-drainage*
Prosopis juliflora	*Casuarina equisetifolia*	*Populus deltaidus*
Acacia nilotica	*Leucaena leucocephala*	*Terminalia arjuna*
Tamarix articulata	*Prosopis juliflora*	*Eucalyptus tereticornis*
Eucalyptus tereticornis	*Acacia nilotica*	*Acacia auriculiformis*
Pongamia pinnata	*Tamarix troubii*	*Syzigium cuminii*
Terminalia arjuna	*Tamarix articulata*	*Albizia lebbeck*
Dalbergia sissoo	*Acacia farnesiana*	*Pongamia pinnata*
	E. Camaldulensis	*Dalbergia sissoo*

Singh *et al.* (1997) evaluated agriculture, forestry and agroforestry practices in a moderately alkali soils in northwestern India over a period of six years at CSSRI, Karnal. The soil conditions were much improved in terms of the build up of soil organic matter, N, P and K when trees were associated with crops (Table 41.15).

The ameliorating effects of 20 years old plantations of *Prosopis juliflora, Acacia nilotica, Albizia lebbeck* and *Terminalia arjuna* were reported by Singh (2000). The ameliorating effect on the soil appeared to be in the order: *Prosopis>Acacia>Terminalia>Albizia* (Table 41.16).

An experiment conducted by Kumar and Warsi (2000) in salt affected soils of Daleep Nagar due to the presence of hand par (Kanpur pan) between 70 to 125 cm depth. The planted trees *viz., D. sissoo, L. leucocephala, A. indica* and *A. nilotica* were substantially improved the physico-chemical property over a period of 4 years due to extraction of salt by plants, addition of organic matter (Table 41.17).

Table 41.15: Role of Agroforestry for Changes in some Soil Properties

Land Use System	pH	EC (dSm^{-1})	OC (%)	Available Nutrients (Kg ha^{-1})		
				N	P	K
Initial soil properties						
Sole crops	9.26	0.56	0.22	65	14.3	238
Eucalyptus based system	9.32	0.61	0.25	65	13.8	224
Acacia based system	9.34	0.67	0.28	72	13.6	212
Poplar based system	9.27	0.60	0.26	68	14.4	237
After five years						
Sole crops	**8.81**	**0.45**	**0.29**	**75**	**13.6**	**20.8**
Eucalyptus based system	8.65	0.32	0.37	86	18.5	259
Acacia based system	8.71	0.41	0.48	103	31.9	286
Poplar based system	8.47	0.35	0.43	93	21.7	321

Table 41.16: Ameliorating Effect of Tree Plantation on an Alkali Soil

Species	Original		After 20 years	
	pH	Organic C (per cent)	pH	Organic C (per cent)
A. nilotica	10.3	0.12	9.03	0.55
A. lebbek	10.3	0.12	8.67	0.47
T. arjuna	10.3	0.12	8.15	0.58
P. juliflora	10.3	0.12	8.03	0.58

Table 41.17: Changes in Physico-chemical Properties of Sodic Soils

Parameters	Initial	After 4 yrs
pH	10.5	8.6
ESP	65.2	36.8
EC (dSm^{-1})	2.93	1.92
Org carbon (per cent)	0.48	0.52

Singh and Lal (1969) reported that there is an increase in nutrient content of soil under *Prosopis* species in arid environments (Table 41.18).

Conservation of Natural Resources

Agroforestry systems have the potential to contribute significantly to maintaining or improving soil and water quality. The degree to which these and other ecological functions can be provided will depend on plant species composition and their physical structure both above and below ground. Agroforestry systems are generally perceived to be sustainable and to enhance soil properties. Growing trees in conjunction with annual crops or pastures is believed to provide a more thorough plant cover to protect the soil from erosion and a deeper or more prolific root system to enhance nutrient cycling. Appropriate agroforestry systems improve soil physical properties, maintain soil organic matter and promote nutrient cycling. Narain *et al.* (1994) studied the soil and water conservation efficiency of the different agroforestry systems (Tables 41.19 and 41.20).

Table 41.18: Nutrient Content of Soil Under Two *Prosopis* Species in Arid Region

Tree	*Site*	*Org C (per cent)*	*Total N (per cent)*	*Total P*	*Total K*
P. juliflora	Under tree	0.73	0.075	37	296
	Open area	0.25	0.027	31	294
P. cineraria	0-30 cm				
	Under tree	0.37	0.045	3.82	12.2
	Open area	0.25	0.038	1.52	7.52
P. cineraria	31-60 cm				
	Under tree	0.11	0.02	1.95	9.31
	Open tree	0.04	0.01	1.23	6.36

Table 41.19: Soil and Water Conservation by Different Agroforestry Systems

Land use	*Runoff %*	*Soil Loss (t)*	*% Reduction in*	
			Runoff	*Soil Loss*
Maize alone	18.3	17.7	-	-
Maize + Subabul	8.9	5	51.9	71.8
Maize + Eucalyptus	3.6	0.91	80.3	94.9
Chrysopogon fulvus	1.6	0.33	91.3	98.1
Grass + Subabul	0.6	0.13	96.7	99.3
Subabul	0.4	0.04	97.8	99.8
Grass + Eucalyptus	0.1	0.02	99.5	99.9
Eucalyptus	0.1	0.01	99.5	99.9

Table 41.20: Runoff, Soil and Nutrient Loss from Different Land Use Systems in Shivalik Region

Land Use Systems	*No. of Years of Observations*	*Runoff*	*Soil Loss (t ha^{-1})*	*Nutrient loss (Kg ha^{-1})*	
				N	*K*
Eucalyptus-Bhabar grass	6	0.05	0.07	0.46	0.90
Acacia catechu-forage grass	3	2.0	0.24	6.97	0.52
Leucaena-Napier grass	3	4.4	0.28	6.60	1.20
Teak-Leucaena-Bhabar grass	3	3.3	0.43	2.08	0.55
Eucalyptus-*Leucaena*-Turmeric	5	2.6	0.59	2.47	0.73
Poplar-*Leucaena*-Bhabrar grass	5	4.8	1.54	5.90	1.10
Sesamum-rape seed	3	20.5	2.69	42.5	3.00
Cultivation fallow	3	23.0	5.65	51.3	5.00

Climate Moderation

Carbon Sequestration by Trees

Intergovernmental Panel on Climate Change (2000) defines carbon sequestration is an increase in carbon stocks in any non-atmospheric reservoir. Carbon sequestration by trees from the atmosphere is a function of the land use, time for growing and technological progress. By two ways, trees can be used to reduce carbon omissions. One is direct carbon sequestration by reforestation and afforestation that yields a stock of carbon in shading trees. The other is the use of forest products as substitutes for fossil fuel or fossil fuel intensive goods such as steel and concrete.

Direct carbon sequestration by trees has been proposed as an emergency stop-gap measure to stop or reverse the increase in atmospheric CO_2, while allowing time to develop and implement clean energy technologies. The use of tree biomass for fossil fuel substation can be a long-term measure because harvesting and replanting in a given piece of land can be carried out in perpetuity. Additionally, the use of biomass for energy production helps rural economics to grow and enhances energy security.

Mechanism

Trees take atmospheric CO_2 during photosynthesis and fix it in woody (branches, stems and woody roots) and non-woody (foliage and fine roots) parts. Woody and non-woody parts have different growth dynamics and decay characteristics (Dewar and Cannel, 1992). At the end of the each rotation, a portion of biomass transferred to wood product, or energy feedstocks. The energy feedstocks release carbon back to the atmosphere upon combustion. The wood products eventually decay to release the carbon either by aerobic or anaerobic decomposition (Figure 41.1).

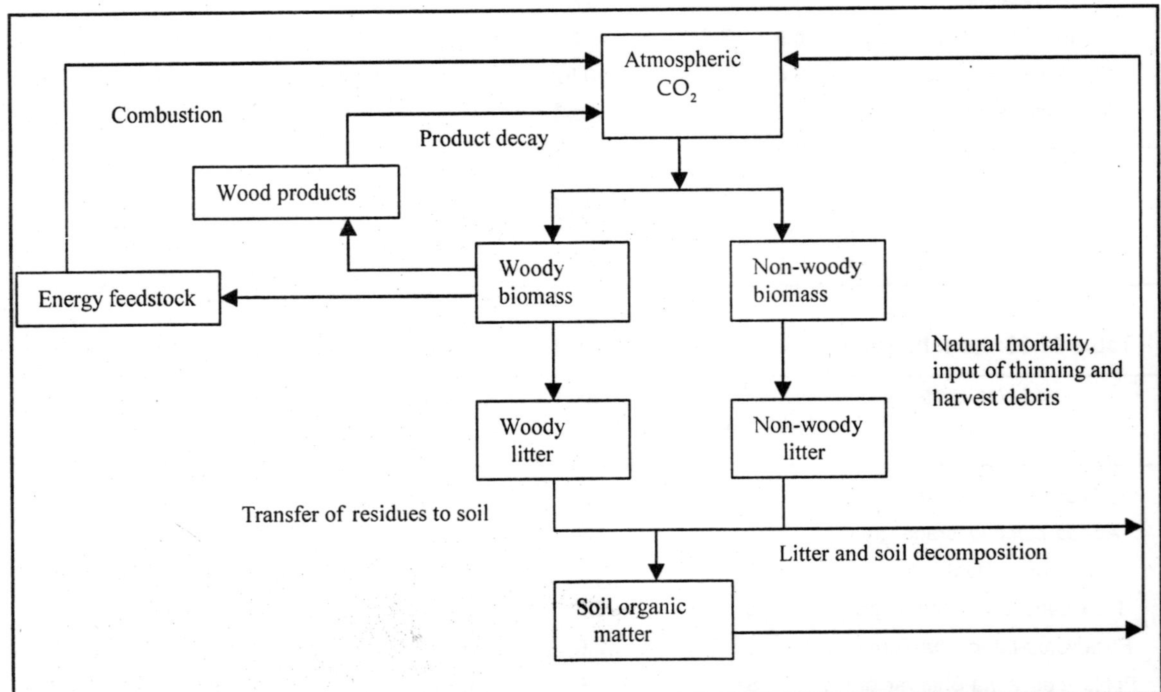

Figure 41.1: Carbon Mitigation by Trees, which are Regularly Harvested and Planted (*Source*: Dewar and Cannel, 1992)

The forest floor receives dead woods and non-woody litter continuously as tree components die because of natural mortality throughout each rotation and also at each thinning and harvest. A portion of litter is decomposed by microorganisms in to CO_2, which eventually returns to the atmosphere.

The amount of carbon that can be sequestered by trees depends on the biomass accumulation rate and rotation length. For long rotation forests, the present forest management can provide harvestable yields of about 4-8 dry metric tons/ha/yr in temperate and 10-12 metric tons/ha/yr in tropical areas (Hall *et al.*, 1991). For short rotation woody crops (SRWC), yields as harvestable woody biomass in range of 9-16 metric tons ha^{-1} yr^{-1} (Wright *et al.*, 1992). The yields of SRWC largely depend on genotype, cultural practices and site quality (Graham *et al.*, 1992).

Carbon Storage and Flows in India

The carbon emission and sequestration estimates for India are given in Table 41.21. The standing biomass (above and below ground) is estimated to be 8357 Mt for the year 1986. The corresponding carbon storage is 4179 Mt (assuming 50 per cent of woody biomass as carbon). The total carbon stored in forests, including soil, is estimate to be 9578 Mt. When the net annual carbon emission in forest ecosystem is considered (uptake-release) for India, the carbon emission is nearly offset by sequestration in forests under succession and in tree plantations.

Table 41.21: Carbon Storage and Flows in India (Mt of C) Estimated for the Year 1986

Carbon Flux	*1986*
Carbon storage#	
Forest vegetation	4179.0
Soil	5399.0
Total	9578.0
Carbon emissions$	
Shifting cultivation (Combustion and decomposition of woody litter)	1.5
Combustion of wood (from clear felling, forest degradation) during the year	31.9
From past long term use (as structural timber 30 years earlier)	1.4
From past short term use (as pulp, packaging etc. with a life of 3 years)	3.1
Current short term use (as pulp)	2.8
Release from soil in clear felled forests	3.9
Biomass decomposition of woody litter in forests	18.8
Total carbon emission	63.4
Carbon uptake in 64 million ha forests and plantations*	68.8
Total C uptake	68.8

#: Carbon storage is estimated for different forest types by taking area under forest types and standing biomass from literature. The tree crown cover and standing biomass relations are considered. C storage in soil is estimated using area under forest types and organic carbon content of different forest types; $: C emissions are estimated by considering various land conversions, end use of felled forest biomass and timing of C emissions. Combustion; same year, long term; structural timber with 30 year storage, short term; pulp, rayon, packing with C release over 3 years. C emissions from combustion of wood from non-forest sources (farm trees, homestead gardens, shrubs in commons) are not included, only the forest source is included; *C uptake: C sequestration in tree trunk and large branches in forest under succession and tree plantations in the range of 1.28 to 2.84 t of wood biomass/ha/year based on productivity values.

Source: Ravindranath *et al.* (1992).

Brown *et al.* (1996) estimated that by 2050, plantation in tropical countries have the potential to capture as much as 16.4 Gt C whereas agroforestry has the potential to capture 6.3 Gt C. The estimates of Trexler and Haugen (1994) are much lower than this, especially for agroforestry (Table 41.22), indicating that there is large degree of uncertainty regarding estimates of potential C sequestration at a global scale.

Table 41.22: Potential for C Sequestration in Tropical Countries in Gt C by 2050

Production System	*Texler and Haugen (1994)*	*Browen et al. (1996)*
Plantations	2.0–5.0	16.4
Agroforestry	0.7–1.6	6.3
Forest re-growth	9.0–23.0	11.5–28.7

Carbon Stocking in Different Agroforestry Systems

The amount of C sequestration largely depends on the agroforestry system being practiced. Factors influencing C storage in agroforestry systems include tree species, system management, environment and socio-economic aspects. The C storage potential of agroforestry system in different regions is presented in Table 41.23. Its varies from 12 to 228 Mg C ha^{-1}.

Table 41.23: Potential C Storage for Agroforestry Systems in Different Eco-regions of the World

Country	*Eco-region*	*System*	*Mg C ha^{-1}*	*References*
Africa	Humid tropic high	Agro-silvicultural	29-53	Dixon *et al.*, 1993
South America	Humid tropic low Dry low land	Agro-silvicultural	39-102[a] 39-195	
Southeast Asia	Humid tropical Dry low land	Agro-silvicultural	12-228 68-81	Krankina and Dixon 1994
Australia	Humid tropic low	Silvopastoral	28-51	
North America	Humid tropic high Humid tropic low Dry low land	Silvopastoral	133-154 104-198 90-175	Schroeder 1994
Northern Asia	Humid tropical low	Silvopastoral	13-18	Winjum *et al.*, 1992

a: Carbon storage value were standardize to 50 year rotation.

Many reports are available that the tree component in agroforestry has a higher capacity of biomass production than natural vegetation (Table 41.24). The table summarizing the prominent agroforestry practice for higher organic C content for the different regions. Das and Itnal (1994) reported that organic C content was about double in agri-horticultural and agroforestry systems as compared to sole cropping.

Total C Storage Under Agroforestry Systems in Different Regions of Country

C storage capacities of different agroforestry system under different agro-ecological regions have been given in Table 41.25. In semi arid region of U.P, C dynamics was studied by Ram Newaj *et al.* (2006) under agrisilviculture involving three pruning regimes and two crop sequences. C content in tree and crop was slightly higher in greengram-wheat (35.13) then blackgram-mustard (34.77) crop sequence.

Table 41.24: SOC Content in Some Agroforestry Systems

Region	*Agroforestry Practices*	*SOC (g Kg[1] soil)*	*References*
Semi-arid	Alley cropping		Kang *et al.* (1990)
Tropics	*Leucaena leucocephala* (pruning retained)	10.7	
	L. leucocephala (pruning removed)	6.5	
	L. leucocephala (pruning + 80 Kg N ha^{-1})	11.9	
Dry-land region	Sole cropping	3.9	Das and Itnal (1994)
	Agroforestry	7.2	
	Agri-horticulture	7.3	
	Agri-silviculture	4.7	
Bay Islands and	Monoculture systems (Coconut)	9.6	Liyange and Dessanayake
Kerala	Mixed farming with coconut and cacao/coffee/ pepper/clove/cinnamon	16.3 12-14.6	(1993)

Table 41.25: Total C Storage Under Agroforestry Systems in Different Regions of Country

Region	*Agroforestry System and Components*	*Total Storage (t C ha^{-1})*	*References*
Semi-arid	Silvipastoral (age 5 yrs)		Rai *et al.*, 2001
	A. nilotica + natural pasture	9.5-17.0	
	A. nilotica + established pasture	19.7	
	D. sissoo + natural pasture	12.4	
	D. sissoo + established pasture	17.2	
	H. binata + natural pasture	16.2	
	H. binata + established pasture	17.0	
North-western India	Silvipastoral (age 6 yrs)		Kaur *et al.*, 2002
	Acacia/Dalbergia/Prosopis + *Desmostacya*	6.8-18.55	
	Acacia/Dalbergia/Prosopis + *Sporobolus*	1.5-12.32	
Central India	Block plantations (age 6 yrs)		Swamy *et al.*, 2003
	Gmelina arborea	24.12-31.12	
Arid region (Rajasthan)	Agri-silvicultural (age 8 yrs)		
	E. officinalis + *V. radiata*		
Semi-arid region	Agri-silvicultural (age 11 yrs)		NRCAF 2005
	D. sissoo + crop	26.02	
Semi-arid region	Agri-silvicultural (age 5 yrs)		Ram Newaj *et al.*, 2006
	A. procera + black-gram-mustard	34.77	
	A. procera + green-gram-wheat	35.13	
North-western Himalaya	Silvipastoral system	2.17	AICRPAF 2006
	Agri-hortipastoral	1.15	
	Hortipastoral	1.08	

References

Brown, S., Sathaye, J, Cannell, M. and Kauppi, P. (1996). Management of forest for mitigating of greenhouse gas emissions. In: *Climate Change 1995* (Eds. Watson, R.T., Zinyovera, M.C. and Moss, R.H.), Impact Adaptation and Mitigation of Climate Change: Scientific-technical Analysis. Cambridge University Press, NY.

Chaturvedi, A.N. (1981). Yield tables for *E. hybrid* Forest Research Development Circle, U.P. Publ. No. 44.

Das, S.K. and Itnal, C.J. (1994). Capability based land use systems: role in diversifying dryland agriculture. In: *Soil Management for Sustainable Agriculture in dryland Area Bulletin*. Indian Society of Soil Science, 16:107-128.

Dewar R.C., Cannel, M.G.R. (1992). Carbon sequestration in the trees, products and soils of forest plantations: an analysis using UK examples. *Tree Physiology*, 11: 49-71.

Dhyani, S. K, Kareemulla, K. and Handa, A.K. (2006). *Agroforestry potential and returns across agroclimatic zones*. NRCAF, Jhansi.

Dhyani, S. K., Samra, J.S, Ajit, Handa, A.K. and Uma. (2007). Forestry to Support to Increase Agricultural Potential: Focus on Employment Generation and Rural Development. *Agricultural Economics Research Review*, 20: 179-202.

FSI 2005. State of Forest Report (2005). *Forest Survey of India*. Ministry of Environment and Forest, Dehradun, India.

Feller, M.C. (1980). Biomass and nutrient distribution in two eucalypt forest ecosystems. *Aust. J. Eco.* 51: 309-333.

Garret, H.E., Buck, L.E., Gold, M.A., Hardest, L.H., Kurt, W.B., Lassoie, J.P., Pearson, H.A. and Slusher, J.P. (1994). *Agroforestry: An integrated land-use management systems for production and farmland conservation*. USDA SCS 68-3A75-3-134. Washington, DC: US Department of Agriculture.

Graham, R.L., Wright, L.L. and Turhollow, A.F. (1992). The potential for short-rotation woody crops to reduce US CO_2 emissions. *Climatic Change*, 22: 223-38.

Gupta, R.K. (1993). *Multipurpose trees for agroforestry and wasteland utilization*. Oxford and IBH Publishing Co. Pvt. Ltd., New Delhi, pp. 562.

Hall, D.O., Mynic, H.E. and Williams, R.H. (1991). Alternative roles for biomass in coping with greenhouse warming. *Science and Global Security*, 2: 113-51.

Intergovernmental Panel on Climate Change (IPCC) (2000). *Land use, land-use change and forestry*. IPCC Special Report: Summery for Policymakers.

Kumar, M. and Warsi, A.S. (2000). Role of MPTs in management of wastelands with special reference to sodic soils. In: *MPTs: Research-Retrospect and Prospect*, (Eds.) K.R. Solanki, A.K. Bisaria and A.K. Handa) Agrobios (India), Jodhpur. (198-202 pp.

Lodhiyal, L.S., Singh, R.P. and Rana, B.S. (1992). Biomass and productivity in an age series of short rotation Populus deltoids plantation. *Tropical Ecol.* 33(2): 214-222.

Pathak, P.S. and Patil, B.D. (1980). Fuel wood and forage production from *L. leucocephala*. *Leucaena Newsletter*, 1: 11.

Pathak, P.S. and Gupta, V.K. (1997). In: *Agroforestry System Degraded Lands* (Eds. P. Singh, P.S. Pathak and M.M. Roy), Oxford and IBH Publishing Co. Pvt. Ltd., New Delhi, India

Pathak, P.S., Pateria, N.M. and Solanki, K.R. (2000). *Agroforestry Systems in India: A Diagnosis and Design Approach*. National Research Centre for Agroforestry. ICAR, Pp. 166.

Ram Newaj, Shanker, A.K. and Yadav, R.S. (2006). *Carbon and nitrogen dynamics in Albizia procera based agroforestry systems*. Annual report of ICAR ad-hoc scheme, NRCAF, Jhansi (Unpublished data).

Sharda, V.N., Dhyani, S. K. and Sharma, A.R. (2001). *Role of agroforestry in disaster management*. HPC (DM Plan) DOA and C, Govt of India, New Delhi, pp.37.

Sharma, R.C. (1998). Nature, extent and classification. In: *Agricultural Salinity Management in India*. CSSRI, Karnal.

Singh, G. (2000). Management of MPTs for salt affected soils in agroforestry system. In: *MPTs: Research-Retrospect and Prospect* (Eds.: K.R. Solanki, A.K. Bisaria and A.K. Handa) Agrobios (India), Jodhpur. 190-197 pp.

Singh, G. and Lal, P. (1969). *Ann. Arid Zone*, 8: 33-36.

Singh, G., Singh, N.T. and Tomar O.S. (1993). *Agroforestry in salt affected soils*. Bulletin No. 17, CSSRI, Karnal, 65.

Singh, G. Singh, N.T., Dagr, J.C., Singh, H. and Sharma, V.P. (1997). An evaluation of agriculture, forestry and agroforestry practices in a moderately alkali soil in northwestern India. *Agroforestry Systems*, 37: 219-295.

Solanki, K.R., Bisaria, A.K. and Handa, A.K. (2000). *Multipurpose tree species: Research Retrospect and Prospect*. Agrobios (India), Jodhpur, pp. 337.

Solanki, K.R. (2006). Agroforestry: Opportunity and challenges. In: *Production Technology and Management of Agroforestry Models* (Eds; S.K. Chauhan, S.S. Gill, H.N. Khajuria and R. Chauhan). Agrotech Publishing Agency, Udaipur, pp.14-15.

Trexler, M.C. and Haughen, C. (1994). Keeping it Green: Tropical Forestry: A Partial Literature Review. Report to GTZ for Enquette Commission, German.

Wright, L.L., Graham, R.L., Turhollow, A.F. and English, B.C. (1992). Opportunities to mitigate carbon dioxide build-up using short rotation woody crops. In: Sampson RN, Hair D, editors. *Forest and Global Change*, Washington, DC: American Forestry Association; 1: 123-156.

Microbial Biotechnology and Ecology (2011) *Pages* **724–728**
Editors: **Deepak Vyas, G.S. Paliwal, P.K.Khare and R.K Gupta**
Published by: **DAYA PUBLISHING HOUSE, NEW DELHI**

Chapter 42

Soil Mycoflora of Forest Field at Jagdalpur Region

☆ ***K.L. Tiwari, S.K. Jadhav and S. Kunjam***

School of Studies in Biotechnology
Pt. Ravishankar Shukla University, Raipur – 492 010, C.G.

ABSTRACT

Soil is a rich habitat for the growth of microorganisms, among these microorganisms, fungi are one of the dominant group present in soil. Soil samples are collected from different places of forest fields at Koprab and Kolawal forest area of Jagdalpur. From soil samples fungi are isolated with the help of serial dilution methods on Potato Dextrose Agar (PDA) medium. During present study 29 fungal species (251 fungal colonies) are recorded. Among them, the percentage contributions of different fungal groups are as follows, Zygomycotina (13.79 per cent), Anamorphic Fungi (68.96 per cent), Unknown groups (13.79 per cent) and sterile mycelia (3.44 per cent) are observed. Anamorphic fungi are dominated to the total fungal groups. During present study, the maximum percentage contribution of *Aspergillus awamori* (11.15 per cent) followed by *Penicillium* sp. IV (10.75 per cent), *Aspergillus niger* (9.96 per cent), *Aspergillus nidulans* (9.56 per cent) and *Penicillium* sp. V while minimum percentage contribution of *Drechslera* sp., *Aspergillus flavus*, *Cladosporium* sp., and *Penicillium purpurogenum* (0.79 per cent) similarly *Aspergillus versicolor*, *Cunninghamella* sp. and *Penicillium rugulosum* (0.39 per cent) are recorded.

Introduction

Soil forms a rich and dynamic medium for all microorganisms. Fungi occur in soil either in mycelial state or reproductive stage. Soil is a rich habitat for the growth of microorganisms. Among these microorganisms, fungi are one of the dominant groups present in soil.

An exhaustive work has been done on the taxonomy of forest soil fungi in India by the different scientist *i.e.* Madhusudan Rao and Manoharachary (1981), Manoharachary *et al.* (1990), Venugopal Rao (1984), Mohanty and Panda (1994) etc. have studied the soil fungi of different forests. Very little information is available regarding diversity of forest soil fungi of Jagdalpur region.

Materials and Methods

Soil samples are collected from different places of forest fields at Koprab and Kolawal forest area of Jagdalpur with the help of sterile plastic tubes. Fungi are isolated using serial dilution methods on Potato Dextrose Agar (PDA) medium and plates are incubated at 28±1º for incubation periods. After the incubation period fungal colonies are counted, isolated and maintained pure culture. The percentage contribution and percentage frequency are assessed by given formula. Fungi are identified with the help of available literatures (Nagmani *et al.*, 2006; Barnett, 1969; Ellis, 1971; Gilmans, 1959) and finally identified by authentic authority.

$$\text{Percentage Frequency} = \frac{\text{No. of observations in which a sp. observed}}{\text{Total no. of observations}} \times 100$$

$$\text{Percentage Contribution} = \frac{\text{No. of fungal colonies of individual sp. in all the observations}}{\text{Total no. of colonies of all sp.}} \times 100$$

Results and Discussion

29 fungal species of 251 fungal colonies are recorded during present investigation (Table 42.1). Among them, the percentage contributions of different fungal groups are as follows, Zygomycotina (13.79 per cent), Anamorphic Fungi (68.96 per cent), Unknown groups (13.79 per cent) and sterile mycelia (3.44 per cent) are observed (Figure 42.1). Anamorphic fungi are dominated to the total fungal groups.

During present study, the maximum percentage contribution of *Aspergillus awamori* (11.15 per cent) followed by *Penicillium* sp. IV (10.75 per cent), *Aspergillus niger* (9.96 per cent), *A. nidulans* (9.56

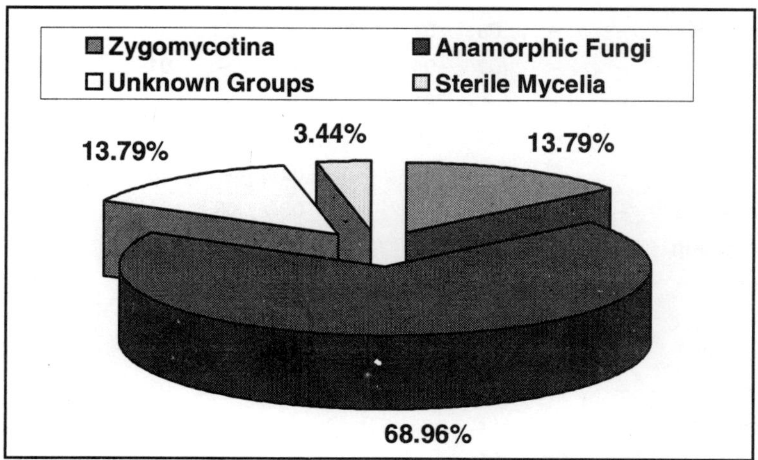

Figure 42.1: Percentage Contributions of Fungal Groups of Forest Soil Mycoflora

per cent) and *Penicillium* sp. V (7.56 per cent) (Figure 42.2) while *Mucor* sp. I (6.77 per cent), *Aspergillus* sp. (6.37 per cent) and *Pycnidial* sp. I (5.97 per cent) etc. are moderate contributions and *Cunninghamella* sp., *Aspergillus versicolor*, *Fusarium* sp. II, *Penicillium rugulosum* and *Penicillium* sp. VI (0.39 per cent) etc. are least contributions (Table 42.1).

Table 42.1: Fungal Distribution and Percentage Contributions of Soil Mycoflora of Forest Fields

S.N.	*Name of Fungi*	*Soil Sample*								*Total No. of Fungal Colonies*	*Percentage contributions*
		I	*II*	*III*	*IV*	*V*	*VI*	*VII*	*VIII*		
	Zygomycotina										
1.	*Absidia* sp.	–	–	–	–	03	–	–	–	03	1.19
2.	*Cunninghamella* sp.	–	–	–	–	–	–	01	–	01	0.39
3.	*Mucor* sp. I	–	–	01	01	14	–	–	01	17	6.77
4.	*Mucor* sp. II	–	–	01	01	–	–	–	–	02	0.79
	Anamorphic Fungi										
5.	*Aspergillus awamori*	–	10	02	08	01	05	02	–	28	11.15
6.	*A. flavus*	–	–	01	01	–	–	–	–	02	0.79
7.	*A. fumigatus*	–	–	01	–	–	01	–	–	02	0.79
8.	*A. nidulans*	–	02	–	17	05	–	–	–	24	9.56
9.	*A. niger*	–	03	10	10	01	–	01	–	25	9.96
10.	*A. versicolor*	–	01	–	–	–	–	–	–	01	0.39
11.	*Aspergillus* sp.	–	–	07	–	–	07	02	–	16	6.37
12.	*Cladosporium* sp.	–	–	–	–	–	01	01	–	02	0.79
13.	*Drechslera* sp.	–	02	–	–	–	–	–	–	02	0.79
14.	*Fusarium* sp. I	–	01	–	01	01	–	01	02	06	2.39
15.	*Fusarium* sp. II	–	–	01	–	–	–	–	–	01	0.39
16.	*Penicillium lilacinum*	–	–	–	–	–	02	–	04	06	2.39
17.	*P. purpurogenum*	–	–	–	–	–	–	02	–	02	0.79
18.	*P. rugulosum*	–	–	–	–	–	–	–	01	01	0.39
19.	*Penicillium* sp. IV	–	–	08	04	12	–	03	–	27	10.75
20.	*Penicillium* sp. V	–	–	02	04	12	–	–	01	19	7.56
21.	*Penicillium* sp. VI	–	–	–	01	–	–	–	–	01	0.39
22.	*Pycnidial* sp. I	–	–	03	06	–	06	–	–	15	5.97
23.	*Pycnidial* sp. II	–	–	–	04	–	04	–	06	14	5.57
24.	*Trichoderma viridae*	–	–	04	–	–	03	03	01	11	4.38
	Unidentified group										
25.	Unknown sp. I	03	–	–	–	–	–	–	–	03	1.19
26.	Unknown sp. II	01	–	01	02	–	–	–	11	14	5.57
27.	Unknown sp. III	–	–	01	–	–	–	–	–	01	0.39
28.	Unknown sp. IV	–	–	–	–	–	–	–	01	01	0.39
	Sterile mycelia										
29.	Sterile mycelia	–	03	01	–	–	–	–	–	04	1.59

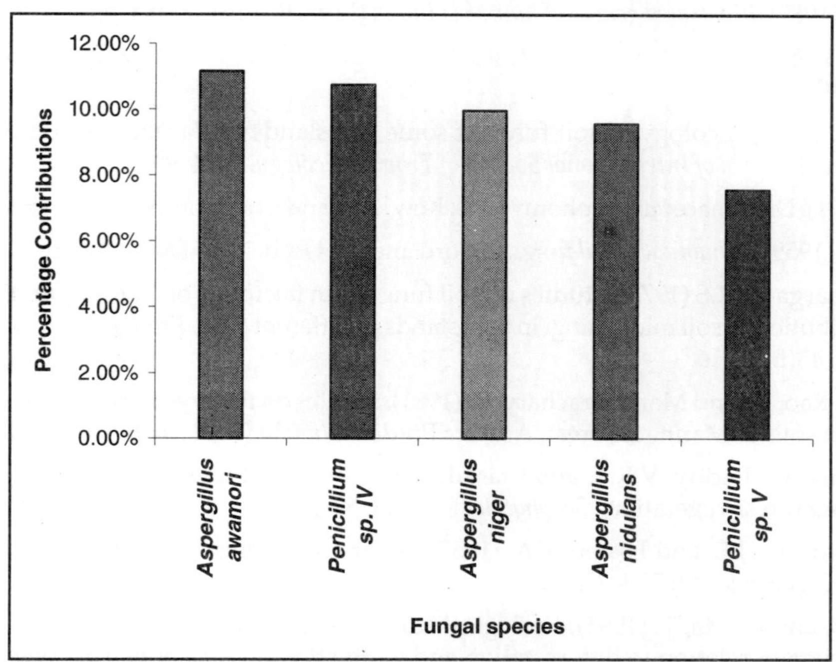

Figure 42.2: Maximum Percentage Contribution Fungal Species from Forest Soil Mycoflora

It is also observed that *Aspergillus awamori, A. niger, Fusarium* sp. I are most frequent fungi while *Cunninghamella* sp., *Aspergillus versicolor, Drechslera* sp., *Fusarium* sp. II etc are showing least frequent fungi.

Chaudhary and Sachar (1934), Saksena (1955), Miller *et al.* (1957) studied seasonal variation in forest soil fungi and pointed out seasonal changes in soil mycoflora and fungal population, which drastically differ from season to season. Tresner *et al.* (1954), Persiani *et al.* (1998) also observed seasonal variations in forest soil mycoflora. Dwivedi (1966) discussed seasonal variations of fungal population in some soil types.

Among all isolated fungal species, the Anamorphic fungi are dominated in forest soil. *Aspergillus* and *Penicillium* sp. are the most dominated genus to the total fungal flora. These observations in the present investigation are similar to Manoharachary *et al.* (1990), Kamal and Bhargava (1973), Rane and Gandhe (2006), who have reported that the *Aspergillus* occur more frequent in soil mycoflora, similar results are also reported by Amin and Abdalla (2004) and observed that *Aspergillus niger, A. fumigatus* and *A. nidulans* are most dominant fungi. Most frequent genera are *Aspergillus* and *Penicillium* is also recorded by Abdel Hafez (2004) at Saudi Arabia.

References

Abdel Hafez, S.I.I (2004). Survey of the mycoflora of desert soils in Saudia Arabia. *Mycopathologia*. 80 (1): 3–6.

Amin, E.N.E and Abdalla, M.H. (2004). Survey of soil fungi from the Sudan Gezira. *Mycopathologia*. 71 (3): 131–136.

Barnett, H.L. (1969). *Illustrated genera of Imperfect fungi.* (Mins Burgess Pub. Co.).

Chaudhary, H. and Sachar, G.S. (1934). A study of fungus flora of Punjab soils. *Annales of Mycology.* 32: 90--110.

Dwivedi, R.S. (1966). Ecology of soil fungi of some grasslands of Varanasi–II, distribution of soil mycoflora. *Bulletin of International Society of Tropical Ecology.* 7: 84–99.

Ellis, M.B. (1971). Diatomaceous Hyphomycetes. Kew, England Common Wealth Mycological Institute.

Gilmans, J.C. (1959). *A manual of soil fungi.* Oxford and IBH Pub. New Delhi, India.

Kamal and Bhargava, K.S (1973). Studies on soil fungi from tak forest of Gorakhpur. Edaphic factors and distribution of soil micro fungi in teak stands of different ages. *Proceedings of National Academy of Science.* 43(B): 9–16.

Madhusudan Rao, M. and Manoharachary, C. (1981). Studies on the myco-ecology of two pond muds and forest soils of Mannaur forest, Andhra Pradesh. *Indian Journal of Botany.* 4(2): 137-148.

Manoharachary, C., Reddy, V.R.T. and Prasad, U. (1990). Distribution and phenology of soil fungi supporting forest vegetation. *Geophytology.* 20 (2): 58–70.

Miller, J.H, Giddins, J.E. and Foster, A.A. (1957). A survey of fungi of forest and cultivated soils of Georgia. *Mycologia.* 49: 779–808.

Mohanty, R.B. and Panda, T. (1994). Ecological studies of the soil micro fungi in a tropical forest of South Orissa in relation to deforestation and cultivation. *Journal of Indian Botanical Society.* 73: 213–215.

Nagmani, A, Kunwar, I.K. and Manoharachary, C. (2006). *Handbook of Soil fungi.* I. K. International Pvt. Ltd. New Delhi.

Persiani, A.G., Maggi, M.A. and Pineda, F.D.C. (1988). Diversity and variability in soil fungi from a distributed tropical rain forest. *Mycologia.* 90 (2): 206–214.

Rane, G. and Gandhe, R.V. (2006). Seasonal distribution of soil fungi from forest soils of Jalgaon district, Maharashtra. *Zoos Print Journal.* 21 (9): 2407–2409.

Saksena, S.B. (1955). Ecological factors governing the distribution of soil micro fungi in some forest soils of Sagar. *Journal of Indian Botanical Society.* 34: 262–298.

Tresner, H.D., Bakus, M.P. and Curtis, J.T. (1954). Soil micro fungi in relation to hardwood forest continuum in Southern Wiskinson. *Mycologia.* 46: 314–333.

Venugopal Rao, K., Rao, N.K. and Manoharachary, C. (1984). Thermophilic fungi from forest soils of Andhra Pradesh. *Indian Botanical Report.* 3 (2): 158-161.

Microbial Biotechnology and Ecology (2011) Pages 729–740
Editors: Deepak Vyas, G.S. Paliwal, P.K.Khare and R.K Gupta
Published by: DAYA PUBLISHING HOUSE, NEW DELHI

Chapter 43

Study of Life-Forms and Biological Spectrum of Forest of Sagar District, Madhya Pradesh

☆ *A.S. Thakur*[1] *and P.K. Khare*[2]*

[1]*Department of Botany, Govt College, Khurai, Sagar – 470 117, M.P.*
[2]*Department of Botany, Dr. H.S. Gour Vishwavidyalaya, Sagar – 470 003, M.P.*

ABSTRACT

Present study was carried out in tropical dry deciduous vegetation of Sagar district selecting ten study sites having uniform composition. Vegetation was studied taking samples of three different sizes for trees, shrubs and herbs. Life forms occurring in the vegetation were recorded and biological spectrum of the entire district was constructed. Life forms of the angiosperms belonging to 54 families, 130 genera and 160 species have been studied. Life forms in order of importance were phanerophytes (55 per cent), therophytes (31.87 per cent), geophytes (6.25 per cent), chamaephytes (5 per cent), epiphytes (1.25 per cent) and hemicrytophyte (0.62 per cent). The dominance of phanerophytes and therophytes reveals that phytoclimate of the area as Phanero-therophytic.

***Keywords**: Biological spectrum, Phanero-therophytic phytoclimate, Dry deciduous forest.*

Introduction

Life form is an important character in describing vegetation which represents a preliminary picture of the ecological character of the vegetation (Cain, 1950). Life forms also help in ecological

* E-mail: pramodpkk@rediffmail.com; p.k.khare@gmail.com

interpretation of the vegetation of a region (Sharma and Singh, 1995). Raunkiaer (1934) defined the life forms as the sum of adaptation of plants to the climate. Adaptation of plants to the survival of unfavorable seasons, especially with regard to the position of perennating buds on plants and degree of their protection during adverse condition. The life form classes reflects the stratification of different layers above and further indicate how a plant passes the unfavorable seasons for growth (Rao, 1968).

The concept of life forms in the study of vegetation proposed for the first time by Humboldt (1806) who suggested groupings of vegetational types on the physiognomic basis. Later, several workers like Kerner (1890), Grisebach (1873) and Drude (1890) have emphasized the dependence of life forms on climate and assessed the role of species in vegetation, with special reference to duration of protection to the perennating organs and mode of propagation. Raunkiaer's system (1934) of classification of life forms is the most widely accepted one and has been universally followed. Raunkiaer's life form spectrum was modified by Braun-Blanquet (1951) and Ellenberg and Muller-Dombois (1967).

The ratio of life forms of different species in terms of number or percentage in any floristic community is called "Biological spectrum" or "the spectrum of life forms" (Milne and Milne, 1971) which can be used to calculate numerical results quickly (Lemon, 1962) to indicate the stratification and layering pattern of community (Rao, 1968; Krebs, 1994), to indicate the prevailing environment (Kotiwar *et al.*, 1996), its aridity or humidity (Meher-Homji, 1964), to monitor the impact of ambient stress factors on climate (Palit *et al.*, 2002) and to determine the nature of bioclimate or phytoclimate (Malik *et al.*, 2006).

Geographically, widely separated plant communities can be usefully compared with one another on the basis of their biological spectrum. Since life forms are related to the environment, biological spectrum is also an indicator of the prevailing environment (Meher-Homji, 1981). The occurrence of similar biological spectra in different regions indicate similar climatic conditions. The bioclimate of the regions according to Raunkiaer is characterized by life form(s) whose percentage value is much higher than the normal spectrum. This indicates the predominance of a particular type of climate and other condition that favour the development of the life form(s) in higher proportions; however due to biotic disturbance, life form may change.

The present chapter describes the biological spectrum of tropical dry deciduous forests in Sagar district of Madhya Pradesh which can be regarded as well as for the Central Indian region.

Study Area

Sagar district is located in the north of Narmada valley. Total geographical area of the district is 10,252 sq. km. The general elevation of the district varies from *Ca*. 400m to 580m above mean sea level (MSL). It is situated between 23°10' and 24°27' latitude North and from 78°04' to 79°22' longitude East. The climate of Sagar district is monsoonal. The whole year can be divisible into three well marked seasons; *i.e.* rainy (mid June to September), winter (October to February) and summer (March to mid June). Average annual rainfall is *Ca* 1200 mm, almost 90 per cent of the rainfall is received in rainy season and winter rains are of common occurrence. The maximum temperature is recorded during summer (45°C) and mean minimum temperature during winter (12.5°C).

Natural vegetation of the district comprises of tropical dry deciduous type after Champion (1936) and Champion and Seth (1968). Forests envelope 26.95 per cent of geographical area. In general, vegetation of the district is teak dominating. Mainly two major rock formation *viz.* Basalt or deccan trap and Vindhyan sandstone are found in the district. Black soil derived from weathering of basalt rock covers a wide area in district. This soil supports good vegetation with dominance of teak (*Tectona grandis*) (Thakur and Khare, 2006). Red soil occur in the area covered by Vindhyan sandstone, it generally support poor vegetation.

Material and Methods

Floristic analysis of all the study sites was carried out after sampling of vegetation by taking 100 random quadrats of 10 × 10 m, 5 × 5 m and 1 × 1 m for trees shrubs and herbs species, respectively. A list of all angiospermic species including climbers and epiphytes encountered in sampling area was prepared. For the construction the biological spectrum life forms of all plant species were determined on the basis of the position of perennating buds following Raunkiaer (1934) and Muller-Dombois and Ellenberg (1974). The number of species in each life form class were calculated. The percentage of species belonging to each life forms was determined by the following formula.

$$\text{Percentage of species in life form} = \frac{\text{Number of species in the life form}}{\text{Total number of species of all life forms}} \times 100$$

Biological spectrum for the district was prepared on the basis of percentage species composition in each life form and taking all the study sites.

Results and Discussion

Floristic composition of vegetation showed that a total number of 160 species of angiospermic plants were encountered during the sampling of vegetation. Out of these, 73 species were of trees, 14 of shrubs, 65 of herbs, 11 of climbers and 2 of epiphytes. They belong to 54 families out of which 47 were dicotyledons and 07 were monocotyledons. Depending upon the number of inclusion of species, family wise top position upheld by Fabaceae (22 species). Other dominating families are Euphorbiaceae, Asteraceae and Rubiaceae (Table 43.1).

The vegetation of Sagar district showed highest percentage of phanerophytes (55 per cent), other groups of life forms are in the order of importance were therophytes (31.87 per cent), geophytes (6.25 per cent), chamaephytes (5 per cent), epiphytes (1.25 per cent) and hemi-cryptophytes (0.62 per cent) (Table 43.2 and Figure 43.1). Similar proportions were found at different study sites of the district. Results showed dominace of phanerophytes and therophytes having contributions of 47.05-59.59 and 30.30-42.18 per cent respectively (Table 43.2).

In the present investigation, phanerophytes showed maximum divergence from the normal spectrum as given by Raunkiear, accordingly the phytoclimate of the area may be termed as phanero-therophytic. Similar phytoclimatic association has also been reported by Rajendraprasad *et al.* (1998) from sacred groves of Kerala, Lakshmanan (1962) for Vihar lake Bombay, Misra *et al.* (1979) for Brahmyoni hill, Gaya, Saxena (1980) for North west catchment of Gola river, Nainital, Saxena *et al.* (1982) for oak forest of Kumaon and Khatri (2000) for Satpura National Park M.P.

According to Meher-Homji (1964) the life forms are reflected by bioclimate of the area. Thus in humid regions the bioclimate should be phanerophytic, in arid regions therophytic and in semiarid regions thero-chamaephytic. In Sagar district, both phanerophytes and therophytes share considerably importance in depicting the phytoclimate of dual character extremes *i.e.* warm-moist and warm-dry climate.

In the present study therophytes stand next to phanerophytes with approximately more than half the phanerophtes at most of sites. The predominance of therophytes due to grazing is a common phenomenon (Yadav and Singh, 1977). It is also an indicator of biotic pressures (Barucha and Dave,

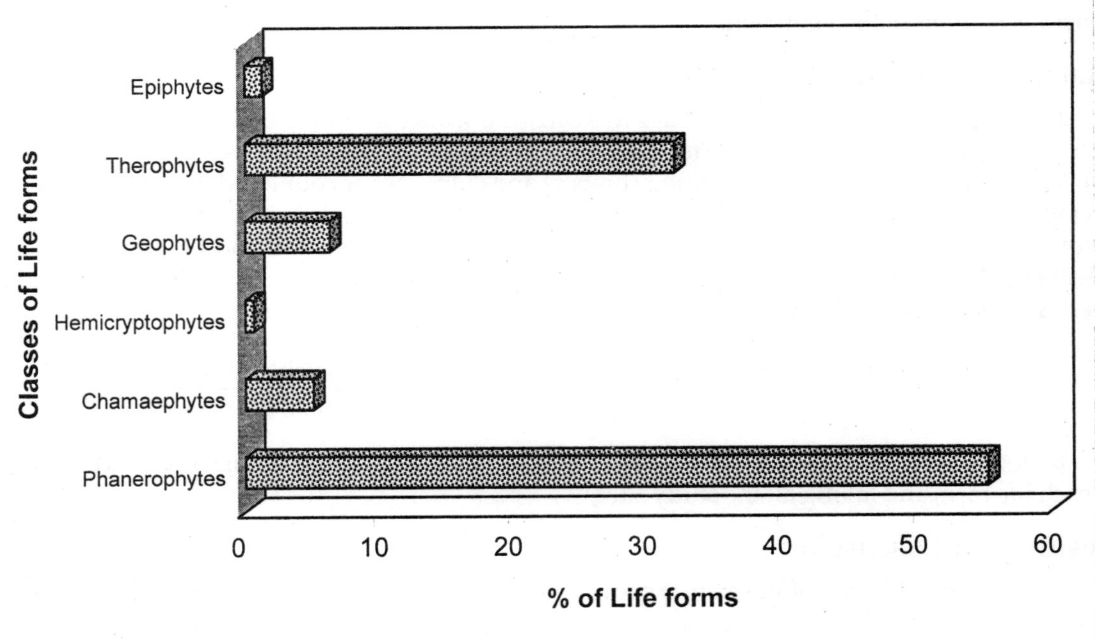

Figure 43.1: Biological Spectrum of Sagar District

1944). Pandeya (1964) observed that the life forms of the flora of different grassland association of Sagar were maintained by intensity of grazing. The high percentage of therophytes in grassland is due to overgrazing resulting in the introduction and spread of weedy grasses (Cain, 1950). Down (1973) also recorded higher number of therophyte in bare and early successional stands. According to Dansereau (1957) the predominance of therophytes indicates warm climate.

The growth of therophyte was much favoured in disturbed areas (Keeley and Albert, 1977; Vora and George, 1987). The dominance of therophytes has also been reported by several workers in grassland and disturbed forests (Srivastava, 1944; Sarup, 1952; Pandeya, 1964; Trivedi and Sharma, 1965; Singh, 1967; Singh and Yadava, 1974; Siddiqui 1972; Singh and Ambasht, 1975; Charan *et al.*1978; Ansari and Singh, 1979; Misra and Misra, 1979; Verma and Das 1980; Ali and Dixit, 1980; Rajwar and Gupta, 1981; Srivastava *et al.*, 1981; Sharma and Dhakre, 1993; Singh, 1995; Kunhikannan, 1999; Baruah, 2003; Kakati and Yadava, 2005 and Subramani *et al.*, 2007).

Percentage composition of chamaephytes varied from 1.66 to 7.84 at different study sites (Table 43.2). They retain their regeneration capacity in favorable season from the above ground and well protected perennating buds and showed hardy nature of the plants for which they can withstand long period of adverse climatic conditions. A number of species such as *Tectona grandis, Diospyros melanoxylon, Terminalia tomentosa, Butea monosperma* and other showed similar behaviour as they sprout after cutting in rainy season. Coppicing is a common character in woody species found in tropical dry deciduous forests.

Table 43.1: Life Forms and Habit Classification of Plants Found in Different Study Sites

Sl.No.	*Family*	*Sl.No.*	*Name of Plant Species*	*Life Form*	*Habit*
			Dicotyledons		
1.	Annonaceae	1.	*Annona squamosa* Linn.	Ph	Tree
		2.	*Miliusa tomentosa* (Roxb.) J.Sinclair	Ph	Tree
2.	Menispermaceae	3.	*Cissampelos pareira* Linn.	Ph	Climber
		4.	*Cocculus hirsutus* (Linn.) Diels	Ph	Climber
3.	Bixaceae	5.	*Casearia tomentosa* Roxb.	Ph	Tree
		6.	*Flacourtia indica* (Burm.F.) Merr.	Ph	Tree/Shrub
4.	Malvaceae	7.	*Hibiscus solandra* L' Herist.	Th	Herb
		8.	*Kydia calycina* Roxb.	Ph	Tree
		9.	*Malvastrum tricuspidatum* A. Grey.	Th	Herb
		10.	*Salmalia malabarica* (DC) Schott and Endl.	Ph	Tree
		11.	*Sida rhombifolia* Linn.	Ch	Herb
		12.	*Sida spinosa* Linn.	Th	Herb
		13.	*Sida veronicaefolia* Lamk.	Ch	Herb
5.	Sterculiaceae	14.	*Helicteres isora* Linn.	Ph	Shurb
		15.	*Sterculia urens* Roxb.	Ph	Tree
6.	Tiliaceae	16.	*Corchorus actangulus* Lam.	Th	Herb
		17.	*Triumfetta neglecta* W. and A.	Th	Herb
		18.	*Triumfetta rhomboidea* Jacq.	Th	Herb
7.	Euphorbiaceae	19.	*Acalypha indica* Linn.	Th	Herb
		20.	*Bridelia retusa* Spreng.	Ph	Tree
		21.	*Emblica officinalis* Gaerth.	Ph	Tree
		22.	*Euphorbia geniculata* Orteg.	Th	Herb
		23.	*E. hypericifolia* Linn.	Th	Herb
		24.	*E. hirta* Linn.	Th	Herb
		25.	*Flueggea microcarpa* Baill.	Ph	Tree
		26.	*Phyllanthus deblis* Ham.	Th	Herb
		27.	*P. simplex* Retz.	Th	Herb
		28.	*P. urinaria* Linn.	Th	Herb
8.	Geraniaceae	29.	*Biophytum sensitivum* DC.	Th	Herb
9.	Rutaceae	30	*Aegle marmelos* Correa.	Ph	Tree
		31.	*Feronia elephantum* Correa.	Ph	Tree
10.	Simarubaceae	32.	*Ailanthus excelsa* Roxb.	Ph	Tree
		33.	*Balanites roxburghi* Planch.	Ph	Shrub
11.	Burseraceae	34.	*Boswellia serrata* Roxb.	Ph	Tree
		35.	*Garuga pinnata* Roxb	Ph	Tree
12.	Meliaceae	36.	*Azadirachta indica* Juss.	Ph	Tree

Contd...

Table 43.1–Contd...

Sl.No.	*Family*	*Sl.No.*	*Name of Plant Species*	*Life Form*	*Habit*
13.	Celastraceae	37.	*Gymnosporia spinosa* Forsk.	Ph	Shrub
		38.	*Elaeodendron glancum* Pers.	Ph	Tree
14.	Rhamnaceae	39.	*Ventilago maderaspatana* Gaerth.	Ph	Climber
		40.	*Zizyphus oenoplia* Mill.	Ph	Shrub
		41.	*Zizyphus jujuba* Lamk.	Ph	Tree
		42.	*Zizyphus rotudifolia* Lamk.	Ph	Shrub
		43.	*Zizyphus xylopyrus* Willd.	Ph	Tree/Shrub
15.	Vitaceae	44.	*Vitis trifolia* Linn.	G	Climber
	(Amplidaceae)	45.	*Leea aspera* Edgw.	G	Climber
16.	Sapindaceae	46.	*Sapindus laurifolius* Vahl.	Ph	Tree
		47.	*Schleichera oleosa* (Lour.)	Ph	Tree
17.	Anacardiaceae	48.	*Buchanania lanzan* Spreng.	Ph	Tree
		49.	*Lannea coromandelica* (Houth.)	Ph	Tree
		50.	*Semecarpus anacardium* Linn.	Ph	Tree
18.	Papilionaceae	51.	*Abrus precatorius* Linn.	Ph	Climber
		52.	*Alysicarpus monilifer* DC.	Th	Herb(legume)
		53.	*Alysicarpus tetragonolobus* Edgew.	Th	Herb(legume)
		54.	*Butea monosperma* (Lamk) Taub.	Ph	Tree
		55.	*Crotalaria prostrata* Roxb.	Th	Herb
		56.	*Dalbergia lanceolaria* L.F.	Ph	Tree
		57.	*Dalbergia paniculata* Roxb.	Ph	Tree
		58.	*Desmodium diffusum* D.C.	Th	Herb(legume)
		59.	*Desmodium gangeticum* D.C.	Ch	Herb(legume)
		60.	*Desmodium triflorum* D.C.	Th	Herb(legume)
		61.	*Erythrina indica* Lamk.	Ph	Tree
		62.	*Indigofera cordifolia* Heyne.	Th	Herb(legume)
		63.	*Indigofera glandulosa* Willd.	Th	Herb(legume)
		64.	*Indigofera trifoliata* Linn.	Th	Herb(legume)
		65.	*Ougeinia dalbergioides* Benth.	Ph	Tree
		66.	*Pongamia pinnata* (Linn.) Pierre.	Ph	Tree
		67.	*Pterocarpus marsupium* Roxb.	Ph	Tree
		68.	*Tephrosia purpurea* Pers.	Ch	Herb(legume)
		69.	*Tephrosia villosa* Pers.	Ch	Herb(legume)
		70.	*Teramnus labialis* (Linn.F.) Spreng.	Th	
		71.	*Xylia xylocarpa* (Roxb.) Tanb.	Ph	Tree
		72.	*Zornia diphylla* (Linn.) Pers.	Th	Herb (legume)

Contd...

Table 43.1–Contd...

Sl.No.	Family	Sl.No.	Name of Plant Species	Life Form	Habit
19.	Caesalpiniaceae	73.	*Bauhinia retusa*	Ph	Tree
		74.	*Cassia fistula* Linn.	Ph	Tree
		75.	*Cassia pumila* Lamk.	Th	Herb(legume)
		76.	*Cassia tora* Linn.	Th	Herb(legume)
		77.	*Delonix regia* Raf.	Ph	Tree
		78.	*Tamarindus indica* Linn.	Ph	Tree
20.	Mimosaceae	79.	*Acacia catechu* Willd.	Ph	Tree
		80.	*Acacia leucophloea* Willd.	Ph	Tree
		81.	*Acacia nilotica* (Linn.) Del.	Ph	Tree
		82.	*Albizzia lebbek* Benth.	Ph	Tree
		83.	*Albizzia odoratissima* Benth.	Ph	Tree
21.	Combretaceae	84.	*Anogeissus latifolia* Wall.	Ph	Tree
		85.	*Anogeissus pendula* Edgew.	Ph	Tree/Shrub
		86.	*Terminalia arjuna* W. and A.	Ph	Tree
		87.	*Terminalia belerica* (Gaearth) Roxb.	Ph	Tree
		88.	*Terminalia tomentosa* W. and A.	Ph	Tree
22.	Myrtaceae	89.	*Eugenia heyneana* Wall.	Ph	Tree
23.	Lecythidaceae	90.	*Careya arborea* Roxb.	Ph	Tree
24.	Lythraceae	91.	*Lagerstroemia parviflora* Roxb.	Ph	Tree
		92.	*Woodfordia fruticosa* Kurg.	Ph	Shrub
25.	Onagraceae	93.	*Ludwigia parviflora* Roxb.	Th	Herb
26.	Cucurbitaceae	94.	*Bryonopsis laciniosa.*	Th	Herb
27.	Rubiaceae	95.	*Adina cordifolia* Hook.F.	Ph	Tree
		96.	*Borreria stricta* Linn. F.	Th	Herb
		97.	*Gardenia latifolia* Aiton.	Ph	Tree
		98.	*Ixora parviflora* Vahl.	Ph	Tree
		99.	*Mitragyna parvifolia* Korth.	Ph	Tree
		100.	*Morinda tinctoria* Roxb.	Ph	Tree
		101.	*Randia spinosa* (Thumb.) Keay.	Ph	Tree/Shrub
		102.	*Wendlandia puberula* D.C.	Ph	Tree
28.	Asteraceae	103.	*Ageratum conyzoides* Linn.	Th	Herb
		104.	*Bidens biternata* (Lour.) Merr. and Sherff	Ch	Herb
		105.	*Elephantous scaber* Linn.	G	Herb
		106.	*Lagascea mollis* Cav.	Th	Herb
		107.	*Pulicaria angustifolia* DC.	Th	Herb
		108.	*Sphaeranthus indicus* Linn.	Th	Herb
		109.	*Tridax procumbens* Linn.	Th	Herb

Contd...

Table 43.1–Contd...

Sl.No.	Family	Sl.No.	Name of Plant Species	Life Form	Habit
		110.	*Xanthium strumarium* Linn.	Th	Herb
		111.	*Vernonia cinerea* Linn.	Th	Herb
29.	Sapotaceae	112.	*Madhuca indica* Gmel.	Ph	Tree
30.	Ebenaceae	113.	*Diospyros melanoxylon* Roxb.	Ph	Tree
31.	Oleaceae	114.	*Nyctanthes arbortristis* Linn.	Ph	Tree
		115.	*Schrebera swietenoides* Roxb.	Ph	Tree
32.	Apocynaceae	116.	*Carissa spinarum* Linn.	Ph	Shrub
		117.	*Holarrhena antidysentrica* Wall.	Ph	Tree/Shrub
		118.	*Wrightia tinctoria* Linn.	Ph	Tree
33	Asclepiadaceae	119.	*Gymnema sylvestre* (Retz) R.Br.	Ph	Climber
		120.	*Hemidesmus indicus* (Linn.) Schultz	Ph	Climber
34.	Gentianaceae	121.	*Canscora diffusa*	Th	Herb
35.	Boraginaceae	122.	*Cordia vestita*	Ph	Tree
		123.	*Ehretia laevis* Roxb.	Ph	Tree
36.	Convolvulaceae	124.	*Convolvulus pluricaulis* Chois.	G	Herb
		125.	*Evolvulus alsinoides* Linn.	G	Herb
		126.	*Ipomaea coccinea* Linn.	G	Climber
		127.	*Merremia emarginata* (Burm.F.) Hau.F.	Th	Herb
37.	Bignoniaceae	128.	*Stereospermum suaveolens* DC.	Ph	Tree
38.	Acanthaceae	129.	*Barleria prionitis* Linn.	Ch	Herb
		130.	*Blepharis boerhaavifolia* Pers.	Ch	Herb
		131.	*Justicia diffusa* Willd.	Th	Herb
		132.	*Justicia simplex* Don.	Th	Herb.
39.	Verbenaceae	133.	*Gmelina arborea* Roxb.	Ph	Tree
		134.	*Lantana camara* Linn.	Ph.	Shrub
		135.	*Tectona grandis* Linn.	Ph.	Tree
		136.	*Vitex negundo* Linn.	Ph	Shrub
40.	Labiatae	137.	*Leucas aspera* Spreng.	Th	Herb
41.	Nyctaginaceae	138.	*Boerhaavia diffusa* Linn.	G	Herb
42.	Amarantaceae	139.	*Achyranthes aspera* Linn.	Th.	Herb
		140.	*Celosia argentea* Linn.	Th	Herb
43.	Proteaceae	141.	*Loranthus longiflorus* Desr.	E	Epiphyte
44.	Ulmaceae	142.	*Holoptelea integrifolia* Planch.	Ph	Tree
45.	Santalaceae	143.	*Santalum album* Linn.	Ph	Tree
46.	Moraceae	144.	*Ficus bengalensis* Linn.	Ph	Tree
		145.	*Ficus glomerata* Roxb.	Ph	Tree
		146.	*Ficus infectoria* Roxb.	Ph	Tree
47.	Loganiaceae	147.	*Mitreola oldenlandioidea* Wall.	Th	Herb

Contd...

Table 43.1–Contd...

Sl.No.	*Family*	*Sl.No.*	*Name of Plant Species*	*Life Form*	*Habit*
			Monocotyledons		
48.	Orchidaceae	148.	*Vanda roxburghii* R.Br.	E	Epiphyte (orchid)
49.	Dioscoreaceae	149.	*Dioscorea bulbifera* Linn.	G	Climber
50.	Commelinaceae	150.	*Murdannia nudiflorum* (Linn.) Brenon.	G	Herb
51.	Palmaceae	151.	*Phoenix sylvestris* Roxb.	Ph	Tree
52.	Cyperaceae	152.	*Cyperus aristatus* Rottb.	Th	Sedge
53.	Zinziberaceae	153.	*Curcuma amada* Roxb.	G	Herb
54.	Gramineae	154.	*Eragrostis interrupta*	Th	Grass
		155.	*Eragrostis pilosa* (Linn.) P. Beauv.	Th	Grass
		156.	*Eragrostis tenella* Linn.	Th	Grass
		157.	*Iseilema anthephoroides* Hack.	H	Grass
		158.	*Ophlismemus burmannii* (Retz. P. Beauv.)	Th	Grass
		159.	*Setaria glauca* (Linn.) P. Beauv.	Th	Grsss
		160.	*Sporobolus diander* (Retz.) P. Beauv.	Th	Grass

Table 43.2: Biological Spectra of All the Study Sites

Sl.No.	*Name of the Sites*	*Life Forms*					
		Ph (%)	*Ch (%)*	*H (%)*	*G (%)*	*Th (%)*	*E (%)*
1.	Patharia	59.59	4.04	1.01	2.02	33.33	-
2.	Mainpani	59.09	4.54	-	6.06	30.30	-
3.	Jaruwakheda	54.54	6.81	-	2.27	36.36	-
4.	Rahatgarh	47.05	7.84	1.96	5.88	37.25	-
5.	Bahadurpur	52.45	6.55	-	6.55	34.42	-
6.	Ramna	58.33	1.66	-	5.00	35.00	-
7.	Ranipura	52.23	7.46	1.49	4.47	34.32	-
8.	Gopalpura	48.43	4.68	1.56	3.12	42.18	-
9.	Baraytha	56.09	6.09	1.21	3.65	31.70	1.21
10.	Nauradehi	57.14	5.71	-	2.85	31.42	2.85
	Total Vegetation of Sagar District	55.00	5.00	0.62	6.25	31.87	1.25

Ph: Phanerophytes; Ch: Chamaephytes; H: Hemicryptophytes; G: Geophytes; Th: Therophytes; E: Epiphytes.

Percentage of geophytes in the present study ranged from 2.02 to 6.55 showing a relatively long period of dryness. More humid areas with fertile upper soil horizon favour the development of perennating organ of geophytes. Agarwal and Paul (1996) confirmed this observation while studying the biological spectrum of flora of Chhotanagpur. Geophytes are good indicators of soil moisture of the regime. This group is first emergents in any vegetation after first rain and adapted to withstand long period of adverse conditions. The storage of food in perennating organs is also important for its survival (Sharma and Singh, 1995).

Hemi-cryptophytes recorded at some of the sites with low percentage value from 1.01 to 1.96 and in total vegetations it was 0.62 per cent (Table 43.2).

Due to alternation of long dry period with moderate rainfall, warm dry and warm moist climate are characteristics of this area. These climatic conditions are responsible for phanero-therophytic phytoclimate. It is experienced that vegetation in a stress of biotic pressure gradually increase the percentage of therophytes. It is pertinent to state that the composition of phanerophytes and therophytes is close in this area, an increase in biotic pressure would change the biological spectrum to therophytic-phanerophytic.

References

Agarwal, V. and S.R. Paul, (1996). Biological spectrum of Chotanagpur flora, *Indian J. Forestry*, 19(1), 35-39.

Ali, S.J. and Dixit, S.N. (1980). Biological spectrum of Lachhmipur forests, *Geobios*, 7(4), 187-188.

Ansari, A.A. and Singh S.K. (1979). Biological spectrum of the Madhaulia forest of Gorakhpur, *Indian J. Forestry*, 2(2), 153-157.

Baruah, P.P. (2003). Biological spectrum of the flora of sand bars (Chapories) of Brahmaputra river, *Indian J. Forestry*, 26(2), 172-176.

Bharucha, F.R. and Dave, R.N. (1944). The biological spectrum of grassland association, *J. Univ. Bombay*, 13, 15-16.

Braun-Blanquet, J. (1951). *Planzensoziologie*. Springer-Verlag, Vienna, 879 pp.

Cain, S.A. (1950). Life-forms and Phytoclimates, *Bot. Rev.*, 16, 1-32.

Champion, H.G. (1936) A preliminary survey of the forest types of India and Burma, *Indian For. Rec.* (N.S.), Vol. 1.

Champion, H.G. and S.K. Seth (1968). A revised survey of forest types of India, Govt. of India Publication, Delhi.

Charan, A.K., Sen, D.N. and Roypurohit, K.S. (1978). Biological spectrum of the vegetation of western Rajasthan Desert India. *Indian J. Forestry*, 1, 313-315.

Dansereau, P. (1957). *Biogeography: An Ecological Perspective*, Ronand Press, New York.

Down, C.G. (1973). Life form succession in plant communities on colliery waste, *Environmental Pollution*, 5, 19-22.

Drude, O. (1890). *Hondbuch der Pflanzengeographie*, Stuttgart J. Engelhorn, 582 pp.

Ellenberg, H. and D. Muller-Dombois (1967). A key to the Raunkiaer plant life-forms with revised subdivision, *Ber. Geobat. Inst. Eidg. Tech. Hochsch. Stift. Rubel.*, 37: 56-73.

Grisebach, A. (1873). Die Vegetation der Erde nach ihrer, klimatischen in del Schweiz, Beiter Geol, *Schweiz. Geotch Ser.*, 17.

Humboldt. A.V. (1806). *De distributione geographica plantanum secundum coeli temperiem et altitudinem montiuna prolegomena* Paris, 28 pp.

Kakati, L.N. and Yadava, P.S. (2005). Floristic composition, Life form and Biological Spectrum of a Grassland Ecosystem at Imphal, Manipur, *Indian Journal of Ecology*, 32(2), 176-179.

Keeley, S.C. and Albert, W.J. (1977). A comparison of pattern of herb, shrub growth in comparable sites of Chili and California, *Am. Hidl. Nat.*, 97, 120-132.

Kerner, M.A. (1890). *Das Pflanzenleben der Donaulander*, 2nd ed. by F. Vierhapper, 1929. University Verlag Wagner, Innsbruck 452 pp.

Khatri, P.K. (2000). Study on biodiversity in tropical forest ecosystem of Satpura National Park, Madhya Pradesh, Ph.D. Thesis Forest Research Institute, Dehra Dun.

Kotiwar, O.S., Pandit, B.R. and Pahurkar, A.J. (1996). Life forms and biological spectrum of the flora of Gir forest, Gujarat, *Geobios New Reports*, 15, 17-20.

Krebs, C.J. (1994). *Ecology: The Experimental Analysis of Distribution and Abundance*, Harper Collins, California, 467 pp.

Kunhikannan, C. (1999). Studies on vegetation ecology of Tadoba National Park, Chandrapur, Maharastra, Ph.D. Thesis Forest Research Institute, Dehra Dun.

Lakshmanan, N.K. (1962). The application of Raunkiaer's life forms, *Journal of Indian Botanical Society*, 41, 585-589.

Lemon, P.C. (1962). *Field and Laboratory Guide for Ecology*, Burgess, Minn, 154 pp.

Malik, S., Bhattacharya, A. and Mukherjee, A. (2006). Biological spectrum of Chandur Forest in Hooghly District, West Bengal, *Indian Journal of Forestry*, 29(2), 145-148.

Meher-Homji, V.M. (1964). Life-forms and biological spectra as epharmonic criteria of aridity and humidity in tropics, *J. Indian Bot. Soc.*, 43(3), 424-430.

Meher-Homji, V.M. (1981). Environmental implications of life form spectra from India, *Journal of Economic Taxonomic Botany*, 2, 23-30.

Milne, L. and Milne, M. (1971). *The Arena of Life. The Dynamics of Ecology.* Double day\Natural History Press, Garden City, New York, 240 pp.

Mishra, M.K. and Mishra, B.N. (1979). Biological spectrum of tropical grassland community of Berhampur, *Indian J. Forestry*, 2, 313-315.

Misra. M.P., Mishra P.N. and Pandey B.N. (1979). An ecological account of the vegetation of Brahmyoni Hills (Gaya), *Proceedings of Indian Science Congress*, 3, 108-109.

Mueller-Dombois, D. and Ellenberg, H. (1974). *Aims and methods of vegetation ecology*, John Wiley and Sons, New York, 525 pp.

Palit, D., Ganguly, G. and Mukherjee, A. (2002). Ecological studies in Ramnabagan Wildlife Sanctuary Burdwan I. Biological spectrum, *Sci. and Cult.*, 68(5-6), 147-149.

Pandeya, S.C. (1964). Ecology of grassland of Sagar M.P. Composition of the fenced grassland association, *J. Indian Bot. Soc.*, 43, 577-605

Rajendraprasad, M., Krishnan, P.N. and Pushpangandan, P. (1998). The life from spectrum of sacred groves-a functional tool to analyse the vegetation, *Tropical Ecology*, 39(2), 211-217.

Rajwar, G.S. and Subodh Gupta, (1981). Flora and biological spectrum of Khoh valley district Pauri (Garhwal), *Indian J. Forestry*, 4(1), 49-55.

Rao, C.C. (1968). Biological spectrum of Karamnasa watershed flora (Varanasi, India). *Proc. Symposium on recent advances in Tropical Ecology*, Part-II (R. Misra and B. Gopal, eds). Banaras Hindu University, Varanasi.

Raunkiaer, C. (1934). *The life form of plants and statistical plant geography*, Being the collected papers of C. Raunkiaer, Oxford, Clarendon Press, 632 pp.

Sarup, S. (1952). The biological spectrum of the flora of Mt. Abu. *Univ. Rajasthan Stub. Biol. Sci.*, 1.

Saxena, A.K., Pandey, P. and Singh, J.S. (1982). Biological spectrum and other structural functional attributes of vegetation of Kumaun Himalaya *Vegetatio.*, 49, 111-119.

Saxena. A.K. (1980). Ecology of vegetation complex of north western catchment of river Gola, Progress report Ecology Research Circle, Dept. of Botany, Kuamaon University, Nainital, pp. 1-4.

Sharma, M. and Singh, H. (1995). *Life forms and biological spectrum of the flora of Champa district (Himachal Pradesh)*, In: Panday, A.K (ed). *Taxonomy and Biodiversity*. CBS Publishers and Distributors, Delhi, pp. 81-86.

Sharma, S.C. and Dhakre, J.S. (1993). Life form classification and biological spectrum of the flora of Shahjahanpur district, Uttar Pradesh (India), *Ind. J. Forestry*, 15(4), 366-371.

Siddiqui, M.O. (1972). Biological spectrum of the forests of Gorakhpur, *Trop. Ecol.*, 3(2), 234-235.

Singh, J.S. (1967). *Seasonal variation in composition, plant biomass and community productivity in the grassland of Varanasi*, Ph.D. thesis, B.H.U., Varanasi.

Singh, J.S. and Yadava, P.S. (1974). Seasonal variation in composition, plant biomass and net primary productivity of a tropical grassland at Kurukhetra, India, *Ecol. Monogr.*, 44, 351-376.

Singh, L.B. (1995). Biological spectrum of the flora of Munger district Bihar, *Taxonomy and Biodiversity*, Ed. A.K. Pandey CBS Publishers and Distributors, Delhi, pp. 105-107.

Singh, V.N. and Ambasht, R.S. (1975). Biotic stress and variability in structure and organic (net primary) production of grass land communities at Varanasi, India, *Trop. Ecol.*, 16, 85-95.

Srivastava, G.D. (1944). The biological spectrum of the Allahabad flora, *J. Ind. Bot. Soc.*, 23, 1-7.

Srivastava, M.M., Srivastava, P.K. and Kukreti, U.D. (1981). Biological spectrum of a marshy grassland at Rajpur, Dehradun (U.P.) India. *Indian J. Forestry*, 4(3), 220-223.

Subramani, S.P., Jishtu V., Verma, R.K. and Kapoor, K.S.(2007). Floristic composition, life-forms and biological spectrum of renuka wildlife sanctuary, Himachal Pradesh, *The Indian Forester*, 133(1), 79-92.

Thakur, A.S. and Khare, P.K. (2006). Species diversity and dominance in tropical dry deciduous forest ecosystem, *J. Environ. Res. Development*, 1, 26-31.

Trivedi, B.S. and Sharma, P.C. (1965). Biological spectrum of Lucknow flora, *Proc. Nat. Acad. Sci. India*, 35B(1), 15-20

Verma, R. and Das R.R. (1980). A new approach towards the use of Raunkiaer's biological spectrum, *Tropical Ecology*, 21(1), 9-15.

Vora, A.B. and George, V.C. (1987). The distribution of various life forms in the ground flora under different canopies of Panchamahal forests: Gujarat, India, *Indian J. Forestry*, 10, 223-225.

Yadav, J.S.P. and Singh, J.S. (1977). *Grassland Vegetation, its structure, function utilization and management*, Today and Tomorrows Printers and Publishers, New Delhi, 132 pp.

Microbial Biotechnology and Ecology (2011) *Pages* **741–765**
Editors: **Deepak Vyas, G.S. Paliwal, P.K.Khare and R.K Gupta**
Published by: **DAYA PUBLISHING HOUSE, NEW DELHI**

Chapter 44

Environmental Impact of Fly Ash on Soil Health, Yield and Nutrient Uptake by Rice

☆ *T. Thomas*[1], *Ram Bharose*[1], *Arun A. David*[1], *H. Thomas*[2]* *and R.K. Tamphasana*[1]

[1]*School of Forestry and Environment, SHIATS-Deemed University, Allahabad*
[2]*Department of Applied Geology, Dr. H.S. Gour University, Sagar – 470 003, M.P.*

ABSTRACT

The research was carried out in the farm of Allahabad Agricultural Institute Deemed University-Allahabad UP. The result generated from the present study show the beneficial effect of fly ash due to essential plant nutrients and fly ash applied @ 40 t ha^{-1} along with $N_{120} P_{60} K_{60}$ was found the most effective. Hence, it is reported that the application of fly ash could be an alternative source of plant nutrients with fertilizers and biofertilizers for sustaining soil fertility status vis-à-vis crop productivity. However, on the basis of one season experimental results, recommendations can not be made; hence further research on this aspect needs to be done for recommendation to the farmers.

Keywords: Fly ash, Nutrients, Soil health.

Introduction

Agriculture is the key to the global agenda on population, environment, poverty reduction, and food security. The world's affluent obtain vital protein through foods such as meat, eggs and dairy

* E-mail: harelthomas@yahoo.com

products, but millions of world poor get most of their protein through rice. It is the foremost cereal crop of the world providing 22 per cent of the world's supply and 17 per cent of protein. About 60 per cent people rely on rice as their staple food.

Rice has 13.7 per cent moisture, 6.8 per cent protein, 0.6 per cent minerals, 0.5 per cent fat, 0.2 per cent fibre, 78.2 per cent carbohydrates and 10mg calcium, 160 mg phosphate, 3.1 mg iron and small amount of vitamin B complex (Bhakra 1996).

Rice is grown in an area of more than 135 million hectares in the world. India has the largest area of about 42 million hectares under rice, with irrigation facilities to cover 43 per cent of the total area. The rice production during 1999-2000 was 88.0, million tones against 84.74 million tones in 1998-99 (71st Annual General Meeting of I.C.A.R. Society, New Delhi, 15 September 2000).

The crop removes the major portion of plant nutrients from soil by crop harvesting. Unless the soils are supplied with nutrients removed by the crop, it will be great threat to sustain crop production. The use of chemical fertilizers is the quickest and surest way of boosting crop production. However, their cost and other constraints frequently deter farmers from using them in recommended quantities and in balanced proportions. As consequence of this and other constraints, there seems to be no option but fully exploit potential alternative sources of plant nutrients. Complementary use of plant nutrients from waste material and biofertilizers along with mineral fertilizers is of great importance for soil producrivity, *i.e.* soil structure, soil bio-activity, cation exchange capacity and water holding capacity (Roy 1994).

Fly ash, grey in colour, abrasive, acidic/alkaline and refractory in nature, is a by-product of thermal power stations where electrical energy is obtained by firing finely powdered coal. Huge amount of fly ash is produced everyday at every thermal power station in the country. As it stands today, about 100 million tones of fly ash are generated per year form the 82 thermal power stations in the country. It has established beyond doubt that fly ash can be advantageously used in agriculture as soil conditioner-improving upon some important physico-chemical properties of soil, such as hydraulic conductivity, bulk density, porosity, water holding capacity, etc. fly ash has also been successfully used as a source of essential plant nutrients like phosphorous, potassium, calcium, magnesium, sulphur, zinc, copper, chlorine, boron, iron, manganese, molybdenum and thus, boosting crop growth and yields (Aitken *et al.*, 1984; Kene *et al.*, 1991).

Fly ash has been successfully applied in different agro-climatic conditions and soil types in different parts of the country using different doses (25 to 500 t/ha). It has been used for the cultivation of different types of crops like paddy, wheat, maize, and mustard, til, sugarcane, cotton, vegetables and fruits. Repeated field trails and residual increase in the crop yield (20 to 50 per cent) with high nutritional value, *i.e.* protein and oil, etc. without any significant carry out of trace/heavy metals and radioactivity in the soil, water bodies and crop produce. Scientists of central fuel research institute have established and successfully demonstrated gainful utilization of fly ash as modifier of agricultural soil and as a source of some plant nutrients. It has the potential to alter the soil texture by increasing the percentage of silt sized particle and thus permanently increasing the soil moisture holding capacity. Fly ash inhibits the infiltration rate of water in sandy type soils and enhances the infiltration rate of clay rich soil due to higher proportion of silt content in fly ash.

Fly ash for its abundant availability and in addition, due to its ameliorating property and a good source of nutrients imparts the demand of an inexpensive product management technology for its fruitful utilization. Its integrated use with chemical fertilizers and biofertilizers would open new avenues to improve soil potential and would boost up the agricultural productivity, simultaneously saving the environment from ill hazards.

Hence, the present investigation entitles "ENVIRONMENTAL IMPACT OF FLY ASH ON SOIL HEALTH, YIELD AND NUTRIENT UPTAKE BY RICE" was undertaken to explore the feasibility of using fly ash as component of integrated plant nutrients system (IPNS) for sustaining soil productivity and crop yield, with the following objectives:

1. To study the effect of various levels of fly ash on yield and nutrient uptake by rice.
2. To study the changes in chemical properties of soil due to fly ash.

Materials and Methods

The details of the materials used and technologies adopted during the course of this investigation with brief description of soil, cropping history of field, planting materials used and climatic conditions prevalent in the locality while this experiment was being conducted is being dealt in this chapter.

Experimental Site

This experiment was conducted during kharif/monsoon season of the year 2001 in the crop research farm of department of agronomy, Allahabad Agricultural Institute- Deemed University, Allahabad and was carried out in plot number 100. The experimental area is very near to the river Yamuna and approximately 5 Km from Allahabad city.

Soil

Soil samples (0 to 15 cm depth) were collected randomly prior to tillage operations, air dried and passed through 2 mm sieve and a composite soil sample was taken for mechanical and chemical analysis. Bouyoucos Hydrometer method were used for the mechanical analysis of soil, to determine sand, silt and clay fraction in the sample. The result of mechanical and chemical analysis is summarized in Table 44.1.

Table 44.1

Analysis	*Particulars*	*Result*	*Method Mechanical and Chemical Analysis of Soil (Pre-sowing)*
Mechanical Analysis	Sand	60.80 per cent	Hydrometer method (Bouyoucos 1952)
	Silt	24.10 per cent	
	Texture of soil	Sandy Loam	
Chemical Analysis	Soil pH (1 : 2)	8.00	Digital pH meter. MK VI
	EC	0.29 dSm^{-1}	Electrical conductivity meter.
	Organic carbon	5.70 g kg^{-1}	Walkley and Black method (1934).
	Available N	270 kg ha^{-1}	Kjeldahl method (Subbiah and Asija 1956).
	Available P	20.40 kg ha^{-1}	OLSEN spectrophotometric method (OLSEN *et al.*, 1954)
	Available K	225.50 kg ha^{-1}	Flame photometric method (Jackson 1973).

Climate

Allahabad has a subtropical and semi-arid climate with temperature reaching the extremes during summer and winter. Rainfall is mostly experienced from July to September. Geographically Allahabad is situated at an altitude of 98 meter sea level at 25.57° North latitude and 81.5° East longitude.

Cropping History

The sequential cropping history of experimental plot is recorded for last years to get an idea about the different species grown. The cropping history summarized in Table 44.2.

Table 44.2: Cropping History

Year	*Cropping History*		
	Kharif	*Rabi*	*Zaid*
1996-97	Maize	Wheat	Fallow
1997-98	Rice	Mustard	Urd
1998-99	Moong	Winter Maize	Fallow
1999-2000	Tile Niger	Wheat	Moong
2000-2001	Maize	Mustard and Maize	Moong

Experimental Details

Plan of Layout

The experiment was laid out in a 3 × 3 factorial design with three levels of fly ash and three levels of fertilizers and their combination. The treatments were replicated three times and were allocated randomly in each replication.

Details of Treatment

The details of the treatments with the notation used under each of them are given in Table 44.3.

Table 44.3

Factors	*Treatments*	*Notation*
Levels of Fly ash	0 t ha^{-1}	F_0
	20 t ha^{-1}	F_1
	40 t ha^{-1}	F_2
Levels of Fertilizers	0 kg ha^{-1}	M_0
	$N_{120} P_{60} K_{60}$ kg ha^{-1}	M_1

Details of Treatment Combinations

Treatments and combination are given in Table 44.4.

Table 44.4

Treatment	*Combination*	*Description*
T_0	F_0M_0	Control
T_1	F_0M_1	$N_{120}\ P_{60}\ K_{60}$ kg ha^{-1}
T_2	F_1M_0	20 t ha^{-1}
T_3	F_1M_1	20 t ha^{-1} + $N_{120}\ P_{60}\ K_{60}$ kg ha^{-1}
T_4	F_2M_0	40 t ha^{-1}
T_5	F_2M_1	40 t ha^{-1} + $N_{120}\ P_{60}\ K_{60}$ kg ha^{-1}

Details of Field Operation

Raising of Nursery

The site of nursery was chosen at Crop Research Farm, Allahabad Agricultural Institute-Deemed University, Allahabad. The nursery was prepared by wet bed method. The field was irrigated, ploughed and puddle. Later the field was demarcated and raised into narrow strips. Needed amount of Urea, DAP and MOP was applied to the strips.

Planting Materials

The rice variety "Pusa Basmati-I" was used in the experiment. It is achieved from a cross between IR- 8 × TKM- 6 at IARI, New Delhi. It is an early maturing rice variety with good plant type responsive to fertilizers management. It possesses good tillering ability with highly synchronous habit. It is resistant to blast and moderately resistant to stem borer but highly susceptible to bacterial leaf blight and tungro virus. Yield potential is about 45 to 50 quintals per hectare of grain yield under optimum conditions of crop management.

Broadcasting of Incubated Seed

After the preparation of nursery the soaked and incubated seeds of the rice were uniformly broadcasted on the standing water in the strips. The nursery was irrigated whenever needed to keep the soil moist to facilitate the germination of rice seeds.

Before sowing of nursery by wet method, seeds were treated with streptocycline + carbendazim @ 0.1 per cent.

Pre-Transplanting Operations of Land

The experimental field was ploughed once with a tractor drawn disc plough followed by harrowing. Stubbles and weeds picked up from the field and puddling was done with the help of tractor drawn puddle. Then the plots were demarcated according to the layout and planking was done. The calendar of operations was given in Table 44.5.

Fly Ash Application

The fly ash used in this experiment was brought from IFFCO, Phulpur. The physical and chemical characteristics of the fly ash are given in Table 44.6.

Table 44.5: Calendar of Pre-transplanting Operations

Operations Done	*Date*	*Remarks*
Ploughing	25.07.2001	By tractor
Harrowing	27.07.2001	By tractor
Puddling	28.07.2001	By tractor
Demarcation and layout	29.07.2001	By manual labour
Fly ash application	31.07.2001	By manual labour
Fertilizer application (Basal dressing)	01.08.2001	By manual labour
Transplanting	02.08.2001	By manual labour

Table 44.6: Physical and Chemical Analysis of Fly Ash to be Observed

Mechanical Analysis	*Unit*	*Results*
Physical characteristics		
Sand	per cent	77.80
Silt	per cent	19.99
Clay	per cent	2.21
Soil texture		Sandy
Porosity	per cent	35.61
Bulk density	g cm^{-3}	0.84
Hydraulic conductivity	m/day	11.04
Chemical characteristics		
pH (1:2)		7.70
EC	dSm^{-1}	0.41
Organic Carbon	per cent	0.64
Total Nitrogen	per cent	0.07
Total Phosphorus	per cent	0.35
Total Potassium	per cent	2.50
Total Sulphur	per cent	2.00
Total Calcium	per cent	0.05
Copper	ppm	33.40
Zinc	ppm	167.00
Manganese	ppm	33.40
Iron	ppm	5.40
Boron	ppm	22.50
Cobalt	ppm	33.40
Molybdenum	ppm	10.24

Fly ash was applied at the rate of 0, 20 and 40 t ha^{-1} to the fly ash treated plots respectively. The fly ash applied was added in surface (0 to 15 cm) soil and mixed thoroughly with the soil within the plots after the demarcation and layout.

Fertilizer Application

Nitrogen, phosphorus and potassium were applied at the rate of 100, 60 and 60 kg per hectare, respectively. Urea and DAP was used as a source of nitrogen and phosphorus. Potassium chloride (MOP) was used as a source of potassium. Half of the nitrogen and total quantity of phosphorus and potassium were applied before the transplanting. The remaining dose of nitrogen was top-dressed in two equal splits before panicle initiating and flowering stage.

Transplanting

Seedlings were uprooted from the nursery and transplanted on the standing water using 2 to 3 seedling per hill at a depth of 2 cm with a spacing of 20 cm between row-to-row and 15 cm between plant-to-plant.

Table 44.7: Post-transplanting operations

Sl.No.	*Operation*	*Date*
1.	1st Irrigation	07.08.2001
2.	Gap filling	09.08.2001
3.	2nd Irrigation	13.08.2001
4.	3rd Irrigation	16.08.2001
5.	4th Irrigation	18.08.2001
6.	5th Irrigation	26.08.2001
7.	Hand weeding	27.08.2001
8.	6th Irrigation	28.08.2001
9.	1st top dressing	30.08.2001
10.	$ZnSO_4$ spraying	07.09.2001
11.	7th Irrigation	17.09.2001
12.	2nd top dressing	24.09.2001
13.	8th Irrigation	29.09.2001
14.	9th Irrigation	11.10.2001
15.	10th Irrigation	23.10.2001
16.	11th Irrigation	01.11.2001
17.	Harvesting	24.11.2001
18.	Threshing and winnowing	27.11.2001

Observation Taken in Crop

Random sampling technique was adopted for recording the observation on various morphological characters of the plant during the course of study. Five plants from each parameter at each stage was computed and recorded. The frequency of plants on which the observations were taken on the plant growth, yield and nutrient uptake are given in Table 44.8.

Table 44.8: Observations Taken in Crop

Sl.No.	*Observation*	*Frequency*
1.	Plant height	5
2.	Tiller count	5
3.	Dry weight	4
4.	Length of panicle (cm)	1
5.	Number of spikelets per panicle	1
6.	Grain yield (q ha^{-1})	1
7.	Straw yield (q ha^{-1})	1
8.	Uptake of Nitrogen by rice grain (kg ha^{-1})	1
9.	Uptake of Phosphorus by rice grain (kg ha^{-1})	1
10.	Uptake of Potassium by rice grain (kg ha^{-1})	1

Pre-Harvest Observation in Crop

Height of Plant

Height was taken from the five tagged plants in each plot. The observations were taken at 20, 40, 60, 80 and 100 DAT (at an interval of 20 days). The height of the main stem or culm (according to IARI) was taken as the height of plants.

Number of Tiller Per Hill

The numbers of tillers per hill were taken from the same tagged plants whenever the plant height was recorded.

Dry Weight

Two hills from each plant were uprooted carefully. These hills were air-dried first and kept in the oven at 70°C for complete drying, to get a constant weight. Mean values of these plants were taken as dry weight per plant at 25, 50, 75 and 100 DAT.

Length of Panicle

Average length of panicle per hill of five samples was recorded from the panicle base to the tip of the same.

Number of Spikelets Per Panicle

From the same plants the number of spikelets per panicle is taken at 100 DAT.

Postharvest Observation

Grain Yield

In order to know the response of different treatments on the grain yield, grain from harvested area (1 square metre from each plot) was dried in the sun, threshed, winnowed and weighed separately.

Straw Yield

After threshing of grain, the straw was dried and weighed individually for individual plots.

Nitrogen, Phosphorous, Potassium Content and its Uptake by Grain

Grain samples were dried in oven and ground in a Wiley Mill, and sieved. These samples were analysed for nitrogen by modified Kjeldahl's method, total phosphorus and potassium was estimated spectrophotometrically and flame photometrically method, respectively after diacid (HNO_3 and $HClO_4$) digestion as described by Jackson (1973).

The Kjeldahl method for total nitrogen content (per cent) essentially involves: digestion of the sample to convert N compounds in the sample to the ammonium (NH_4^+) form. The grain sample is digested with Sulphuric acid and hydrogen peroxide. Hydrogen peroxide destroys organic material material to minimize foaming. Salt/catalyst mixture (K_2SO_4 + $CuSO_4$ + selenium power) is added to each digestion tube to raise the boiling temperature of the digestion mixture and to shorten the digestion time. After the digestion, digest is cooled to room temperature before dilution. Determination of ammonium in digest: (Kjeldahl method). Few ml of digest (10 ml) is distilled with 40 per cent NaOH of the Kjeldahl flask, which gives ammonium. This liberated ammonia is absorbed by the boric acid solution with mixed indicator. After completion of distillation, the boric acid is back titrated against H_2SO_4.

Total phosphorus content (per cent) of the grain sample was carried out using a di-acid 9:4 mixture of HNO_3 : $HClO_4$. Plant phosphorus is converted to orthophosphates during digestion. These orthophosphates react with molybdate and vanadate and give yellow coloured unreduced vanado-molybdo-phosphoric heteropoly complex in acid medium. The intensity of this colour is directly proportional to the concentration of phosphates present in the sample which can be read on colorimeter or spectrophotometer at 430 nm using blue filter. Lastly phosphorus concentration was found out with the help of standard curve.

For total potassium content (per cent) the procedure of plant sample digestion is same as that of phosphorus using diacid mixture. Potassium in the digested is determined using flame photometer.

The nitrogen, phosphorus and potassium uptake in the rice grain was determined by multiplying the N, P, K content (per cent) with the grain yield.

Results and Discussion

The results of the present investigation entitled "ENVIRONMENTAL IMPACT OF FLY ASH ON SOIL HEALTH, YIELD AND NUTRIENT UPTAKE BY RICE" have been presented and discussed accordingly in this chapter along with its confirmation with previous researchers.

Results for all parameters have been taken, summarized and discussed under the following sub-headings:

1 Pre-harvest studies

2. Postharvest studies

The tables of analysis of variance for different parameter have been given in the appendix.

Pre-Harvest Studies

Plant Height

Plant height was recorded at 20, 40, 60, 80 and 100 days after transplanting and the data recorded were analyzed and results were given below:

Effect of Fly Ash Levels on Plant Height

The statistical analysis of data indicate that there was a significant difference in plant height at 20, 40, 60, 80 and 100 DAT, when the plant were supplied with 20 and 40 tonnes fly ash per hectare against the control.

Table 44.9: Effect of Fly Ash Levels on Plant Height

Treatment	*Plant Height (cm)*				
	20 DAT	*40 DAT*	*60 DAT*	*80 DAT*	*100 DAT*
F_0	18.72	24.75	39.73	77.19	77.25
F_1	20.97	27.31	41.29	79.42	79.18
F_2	24.45	30.18	44.02	81.51	82.22
S.E.	0.35	0.43	0.38	0.55	0.45
C.D at 5 per cent	0.78	0.93	0.80	1.16	0.95

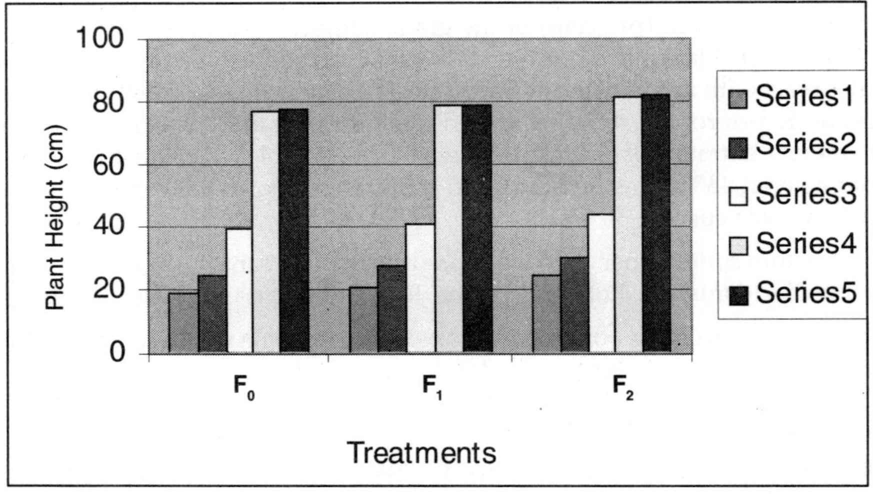

Figure 44.1: Effect of Fly Ash Levels on Plant Height

The effect of fly ash levels on plant height is presented in Table 44.1 and Figure 44.1. The result revealed that the plant height growth was maximum between 60-80 DAT. At 100 DAT, F_2 (Fly ash @ 40 t ha^{-1}) had maximum plant height of 82.22 cm, which was greater than the control (77.25 cm). F_1 (Fly ash @ 20 t ha^{-1}) had also a significant difference over the control. Thus, the plant height showed an increasing trend by increasing levels of fly ash. Increase in plant height with fly ash has also been reported by Dubey *et al.* (1982). Tripathi and Sahu (1997) also reported that 50 per cent fly ash applied to soil increases the plant height.

Number of Tillers Per Hill

The numbers of tillers per hill were recorded at 20, 40, 60, 80 and 100 DAT and results were summarized below:

Effect of Fly Ash Levels on Number of Tillers per Hill

The statistical analysis of number of tillers per hill indicate that there was a significant difference in number of tillers per hill at 20, 40, 60, 80 and 100 DAT when the plot were supplied with 20 and 40 tonnes of fly ash per hectare against the control.

Table 44.10: Effect of Fly Ash Levels on Number of Tillers per Hill

Treatment	*Number of Tillers per Hill*				
	20 DAT	*40 DAT*	*60 DAT*	*80 DAT*	*100 DAT*
F_o	7.23	12.53	12.66	12.05	11.25
F_1	7.65	13.36	13.38	13.13	12.43
F_2	8.25	14.13	14.03	13.74	13.07
S.E.	0.25	0.40	-	0.31	0.43
C.D at 5 per cent	0.54	0.84	NS	0.65	0.91

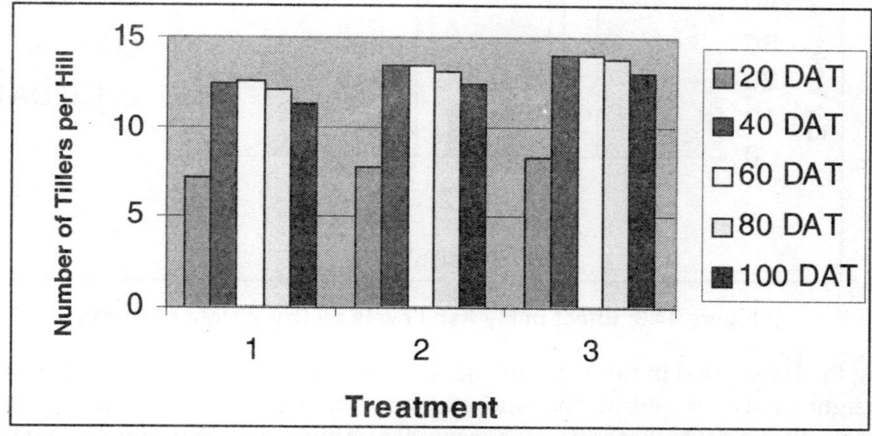

Figure 44.2: Effect of Fly Ash Levels on Number of Tillers per Hill

From the data in Table 44.10 and Figure 44.2. It is revealed that maximum number of tiller (13.07) was recorded with the higher fly ash level (F_2) of 40 t ha^{-1} and minimum (11.25) with the control. The F_1 (Fly ash @ 20 t ha^{1}) had also a significant difference from the control, the number of tiller showed a positive response to the increased fly ash level. This might be due to the fact that fly ash increased the contents of N, P, K in plants at all growth stages. Uptake of these nutrients by the crop also increased with the application of fly ash. These findings are in conformity with the findings of previous workers (Singh *et al.*, 1986 and Kene *et al.*, 1991).

Dry Weight

The dry weight was recorded at 25, 50, 75 and 100 DAT and results are present below:

Effect of Fly Ash Levels on Dry Weight of Plants

The data presented in Table 44.11 and Figure 44.3 shows that all the successive stages of growth in rice shows significant difference in dry weight of plants per hill.

Table 44.11: Effect of Fly Ash Levels on Dry Weight of Plants

Treatment	*Dry Weight (g)*			
	25 DAT	*50 DAT*	*75 DAT*	*100 DAT*
F_o	3.78	11.26	28.91	51.90
F_1	4.30	13.45	32.43	57.56
F_2	7.08	17.03	35.00	60.44
S.E.	0.30	0.17	0.78	0.81
C.D at 5 per cent	0.63	0.36	1.65	1.71

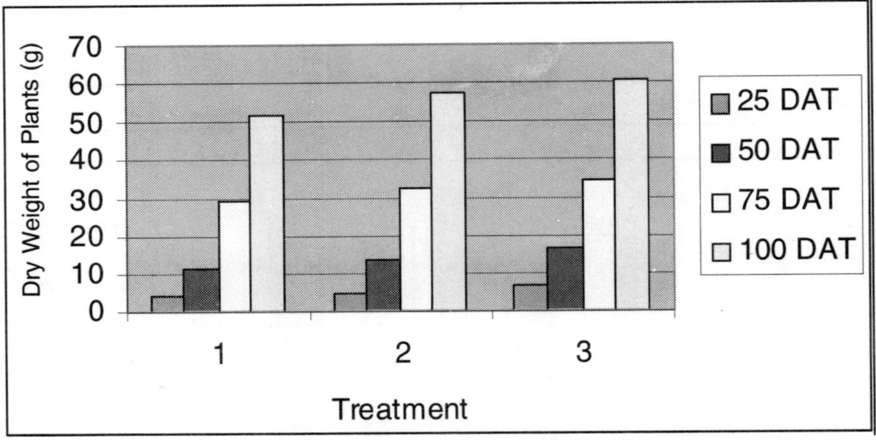

Figure 44.3: Effect of Fly Ash Levels on Dry Weight of Plants

Among the levels tried in this experiment, fly ash @ 40 t ha^{-1} increased the dry weight of plants which was significant over control. The plot supplied with fly ash @ 20 t ha^{-1} was also significant over control. The results revealed that dry weight growth was maximum between 75-100 DAT. In general, F_2 (fly ash @ 40 t ha^{-1}) had maximum plant dry weight than F_1 (fly ash @ 20 t ha^{-1}). The results show that at 100 DAT, the maximum dry weight (60.44 g) was recorded in F_2 (fly ash @ 40 t ha^{-1}) plots and the minimum of 50.90 g with F_0 (control) plots. Rajeev *et al.* (1992) reported that mean dry matter yield increased significantly due to fly ash treatment due to increased inputs of N, S and Fe from fly ash. Sikka and Kansal (1995) also reported that fly ash application had a beneficial effect on the dry matter yield of rice.

Length of Panicle

Effect of Fly Ash Levels on Panicle Length

The data presented in Table 44.12 and Figure 44.4 shows that the effect of different levels of fly ash was statistically significant.

From Table 44.12 is revealed that there was a significant difference in the panicle length between the plots supplied with fly ash @ 20 t ha^{-1} (F_1) and 40 t ha^{1} (F_2) over control. The maximum was found in F_2 (fly ash 40 @ t ha^{-1}) plots with 28.07 cm followed by 27.40 cm in F_1 plots (fly ash 20 @ t ha^{-1}) and minimum in control 26.73 cm panicle length of rice crop was significantly influenced by different

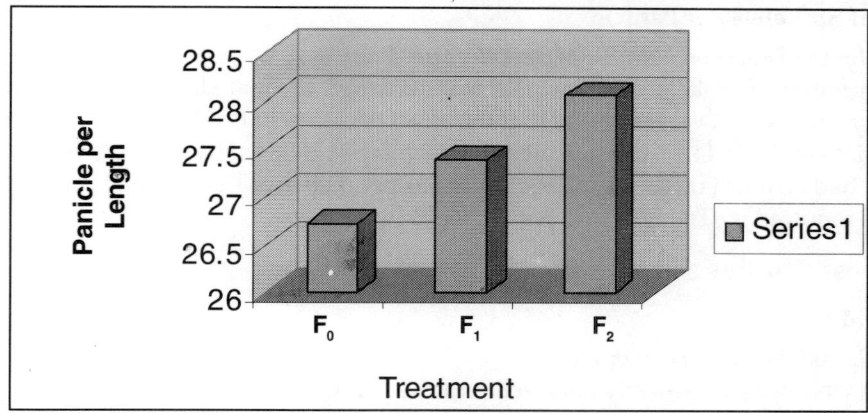

Figure 44.4: Effect of Fly Ash Levels on Panicle Length

levels of fly ash. The maximum length was found with 40 t ha^{-1} fly ash application and minimum in control.

Table 44.12: Effect of Fly Ash Levels on Panicle Length

Treatment	*Panicle Length (cm)*
F_0	26.73
F_1	27.40
F_2	28.07
S.E	0.32
C.D at 5 per cent	0.67

Table 44.13: Effect of Fly Ash Levels on No. of Spikelets per Panicle

Treatment	*No. of Spikelets/Panicle*
F_0	10.27
F_1	10.65
F_2	10.94
S.E	–
C.D at 5 per cent	NS

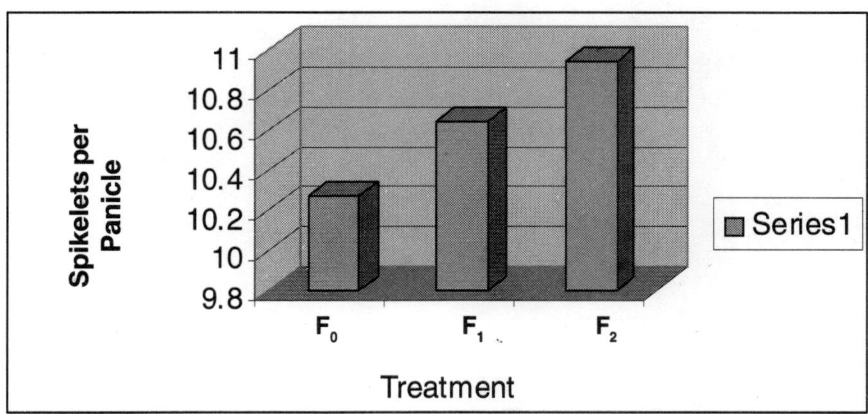

Figure 44.5: Effect of Fly Ash Levels on No. of Spikelets per Panicle

Number of Spikelets Per Panicle

Effect of Fly Ash Levels on Number of Spikelets per Panicle

The number of spikelets per panicle was recorded at final stage of crop growth and it was statistically analysed. It was revealed that the effect of different levels of fly ash was non-significant. From the data in Table 44.13, it is revealed that increasing levels of fly ash from 0-20 t ha^{-1} and from 20 to 40 t ha^{-1} had no effect on the number of spikelets per panicle. These findings are in conformity with the results reported by Tripathy and Sahu (1997).

Postharvest Studies

Grain Yield

Effect of Fly Ash Levels on Grain Yield

Grain yield was statistically analysed and the results are given in Table 44.14.

The grain yield as influenced are presented in Table 44.14 and Figure 44.6. It is clear from the Table that different levels of fly ash influenced the grain yield of rice significantly over the control. The crop showed increasing trend in yield with increasing level of fly ash. The maximum yield (44.53 q ha^{-1}) was recorded when the crop was treated with fly ash @ 40 t ha^{-1} whereas fly ash @ 20 t ha^{-1} produced 41.84 q ha^{-1}. It observed that the treatment received fly ash @ 20 t ha^{-1} and 40 t ha^{-1} recorded a yield increase of 3.64 and 10.30 percent, respectively over the control treatment.

Table 44.14: Effect of Fly Ash Levels on Grain Yield

Treatment	*Grain Yield (q ha^{-1})*
F_0	40.37
F_1	41.84
F_2	44.53
S.E	0.34
C.D at 5 per cent	0.75

Similar results were reported by Matte and Kene (1995). They observed that application of 20 t fly ash per ha gave the best result which increased grain yield by 7 to 30 per cent. Anjali *et al.* (2000) reported that available N P K and micronutrients like Cu, Fe, Zn, Mn and exchangeable Ca and Mg increased

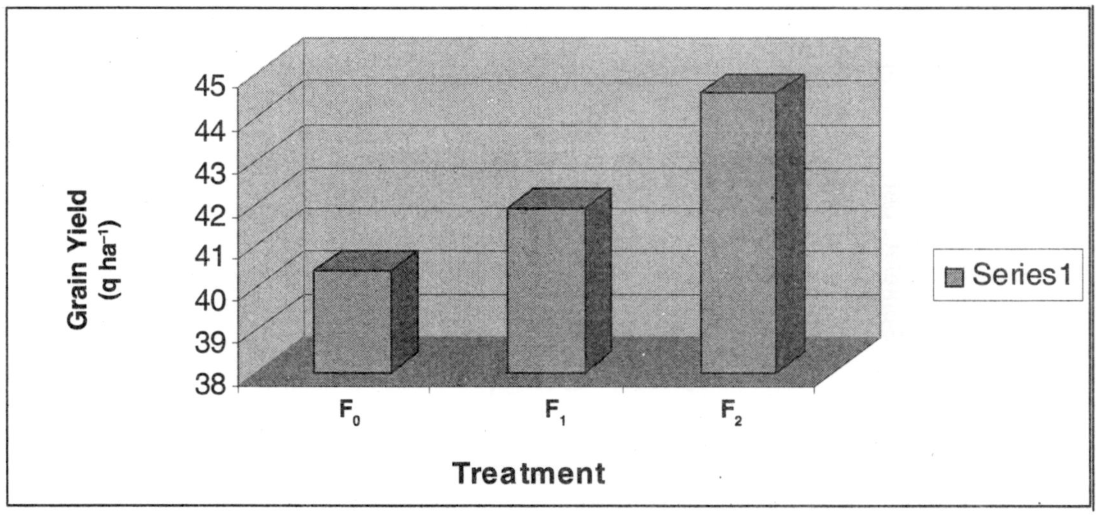

Figure 44.6: Effect of Fly Ash Levels on Grain Yield

with fly ash application which increased the grain yield. Selvakumari *et al.* (2000) also found that treatments which received fly ash at 20 and 40 t ha^{-1} increased the grain yield by 10.3 and 16.3 per cent, respectively over no fly ash application. Also Tiwari *et al.* (1992), Patil *et al.* (1996), Arvind *et al.* (1998), Bharti *et al.* (2001) reported that application of fly ash increased grain yield.

Straw Yield

The effect of different levels of fly ash on straw yield was statistically analysed and the result are given in Table 44.15.

The straw yields are presented in Table 44.15 and Figure 44.7 different levels of fly ash influenced the straw yield of rice significantly over the control. The crop showed increasing trend in yield with each level of fly ash. The maximum straw yield (76.80t ha^{-1}) was recorded with fly ash @ 40 t ha^{-1} whereas fly ash @ 20 t ha^{-1} produced 73.50 q ha^{-1}. There is significant increase in straw yield with both levels of fly ash over control.

Table 44.15: Effect of Fly Ash Levels on Straw Yield

Treatment	*Straw Yield (q ha^{-1})*
F_0	66.35
F_1	73.50
F_2	76.80
S.E	0.45
C.D at 5 per cent	0.95

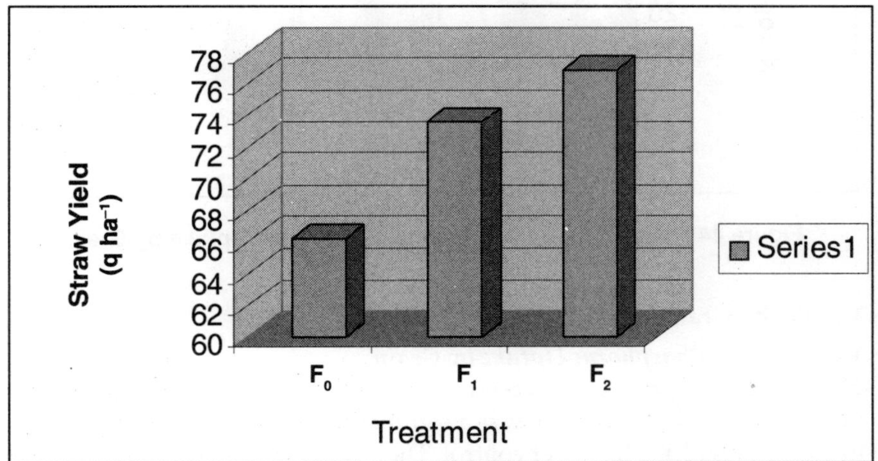

Figure 44.7: Effect of Fly Ash Levels on Straw Yield

Nitrogen, Phosphorus and Potassium Content (per cent) and Uptake by Rice Grain

Nitrogen content in rice grain ranged between 0.98 to 1.59 per cent. Phosphorus content in rice grain ranged between 0.38 to 0.54 per cent. Potassium content in rice grain ranged between 0.22 to 0.41 per cent.

Nitrogen Uptake by Grain

From Table 44.16 and Figure 44.8, the results revealed that different levels of fly ash influenced the N-uptake by rice grain significantly. There was a significant difference in N-uptake between the plot treated with fly ash @ 20 t ha^{-1} and 40 t ha^{-1} over control. The maximum N-uptake (64.33 kg ha^{-1}) was found in plots treated with fly ash @ 40 t ha^{-1} followed by plots treated with fly ash @ 20 t ha^{-1}

(56.82 kg ha^{-1}) and minimum (49.64 kg ha^{-1}) in control. The analysis showed that application of fly ash @ 20 and 40 t ha^{-1} recorded an increase of 7.18 and 14.69 kg ha^{-1} of N-uptake over control. Singh *et al*. (1986) reported that application of fly ash significantly increased the content of N P K at all growth stages. Thus, uptake of nutrients increases both in grains and straw, due to fly ash addition. Sikka and Kansal (1995) also reported that addition of fly ash resulted in a significant increase in the content of N.

Table 44.16: Effect of Fly Ash Levels on Nitrogen Uptake by Grain

Treatment	*N-uptake (kg ha^{-1})*
F_0	49.64
F_1	56.82
F_2	64.33
S.E	0.53
C.D at 5 per cent	1.06

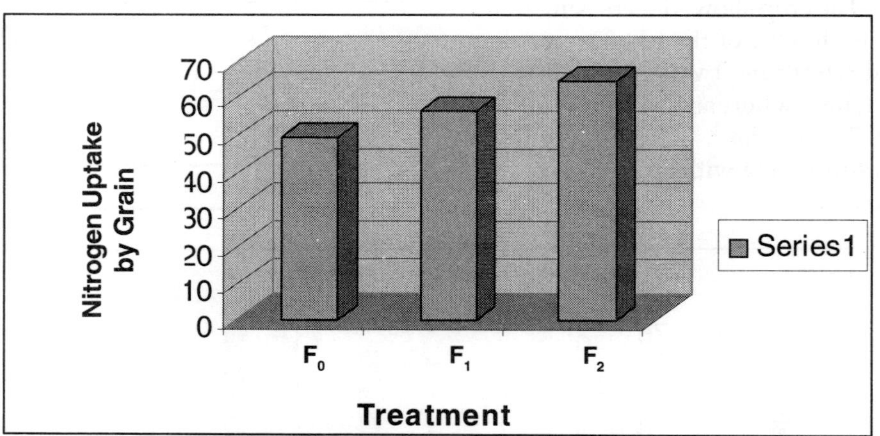

Figure 44.8: Effect of Fly Ash Levels on Nitrogen Uptake by Grain

Phosphorus Uptake by Grain

Effect of Fly Ash Levels on Phosphorus Uptake by Grain

From Table 44.17 and Figure 44.9 the results revealed that different levels of fly ash influence the P-uptake by rice grain significantly. There was a significant difference in P-uptake between the plots treated with fly ash @ 20 and 40 t ha^{-1} over control. The maximum P-take (22.34 kg ha^{-1}) was found in plots treated with fly ash @ 40 t ha^{-1} followed by (20.41 kg ha^{-1}) in plots treated with fly ash @ 20 t ha^{-1} and minimum (18.94 kg ha^{-1}) in control. The analysis showed that the application of fly ash @ 20 and 40 t ha^{-1} recorded an increase of 1.47 and 3.62 kg ha^{-1} of P-uptake over control. Lanjewar (1989), Warambhe *et al*. (1992) and Raghupathy (1993) also reported that increased uptake of P by plant with the application of fly ash.

Table 44.17: Effect of Fly Ash Levels on Phosphorus Uptake by Grain

Treatment	*P-uptake (kg ha^{-1})*
F_0	18.94
F_1	20.41
F_2	22.34
S.E	0.38
C.D at 5 per cent	0.80

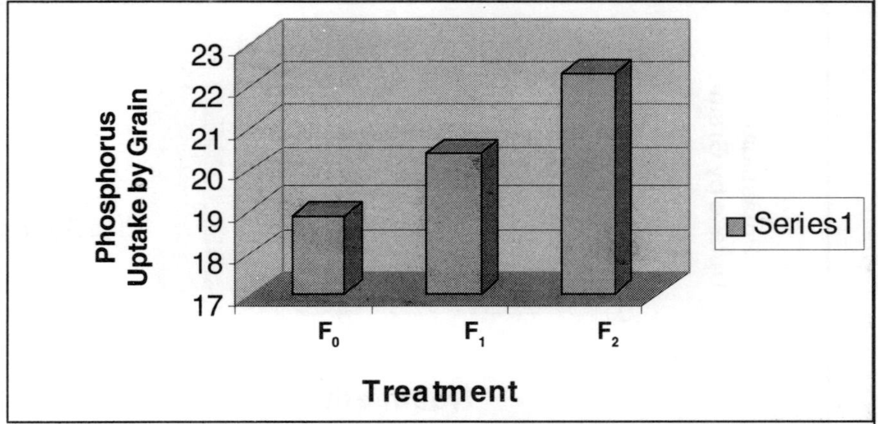

Figure 44.9: Effect of Fly Ash Levels on Phosphorus Uptake by Grain

Potassium Uptake by Grain

Effect of Fly Ash Levels on Potassium Uptake by Grain

From the Table 44.18 and Figure 44.10, the result revealed that different levels of fly ash influenced the K-uptake by rice grain significantly. The plots supplied with fly ash @ 40t ha^{-1} showed a significant increase in K-uptake over control. The maximum K-uptake (16.31 kg ha^{-1}) was found in plots treated with fly ash @ 40 t ha^{-1} and minimum (12.19 kg ha^{-1}) in control. The difference in K-uptake with fly ash @ 20 t ha^{-1} over control was non-significant, but the difference between fly ash @ 20 t ha^{-1} and 40 t ha^{-1} remained significant. The application of fly ash @ 40 t ha^{-1} recorded an increase of 4.12 kg ha^{-1} of K-uptake over control. Grewal *et al.* (2001) reported that application of fly ash increased uptake of N P K both in grain and straw of pearl millet and wheat crops. Increase in K-uptake of corn and bean due to application of fly ash was also reported by Adriano *et al.* (1978).

Table 44.18: Effect of Fly Ash Levels on Potassium Uptake by Grain

Treatment	*K-uptake (kg ha^{-1})*
F_0	12.19
F_1	12.78
F_2	16.31
S.E	0.45
C.D at 5 per cent	0.95

Soil pH

Effect of Fly Ash Levels on pH of the Postharvest Soil

The initial pH of the soil was 8.00. there was decrease in pH of the postharvest soils due to fly ash (pH 7.70) addition as compared to control. The pH decreased from 7.87 to 7.71 due to addition of fly ash @ 20 t ha^{-1}. However, the decrease in pH was not significant. The above findings are in accordance with that reported by Tiwari *et al.* (1992) and Khandar *et al.* (1996). Also Naveen *et al.* (2000) reported that pH of soil decreased with ash content for sandy-loam soils.

Table 44.19: Effect of Fly Ash Levels on pH of the Postharvest Soil

Treatment	*Soil pH*
F_0	7.87
F_1	7.71
F_2	7.81
S.E	-
C.D. at 5 per cent	NS

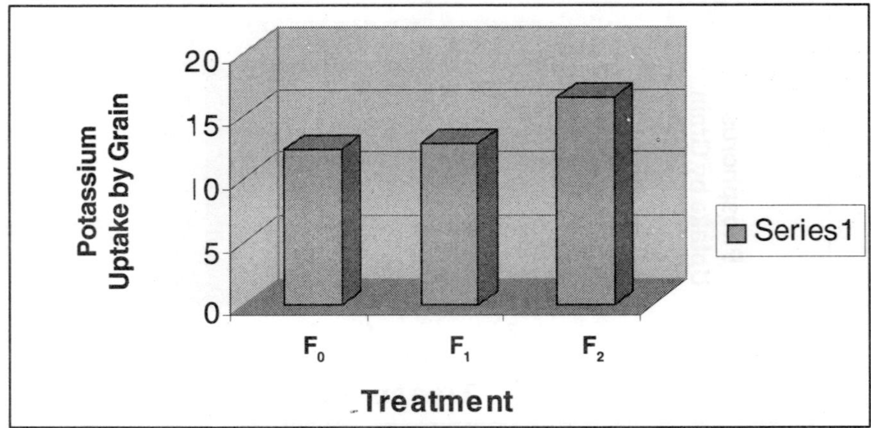

Figure 44.10: Effect of Fly Ash Levels on Potassium Uptake by Grain

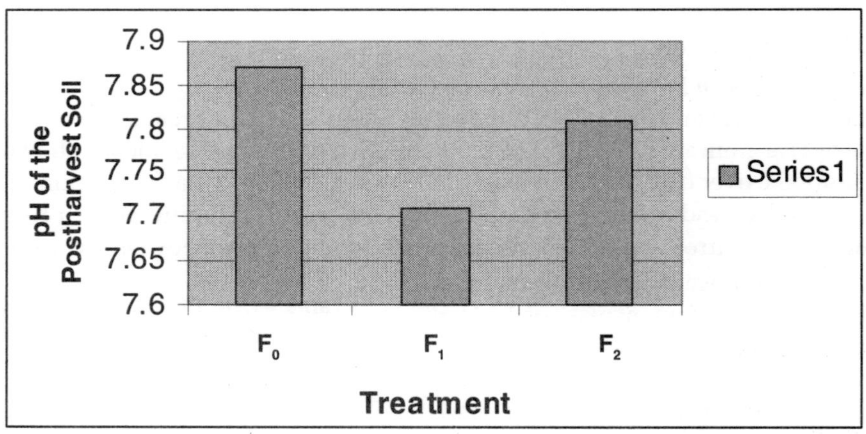

Figure 44.11: Effect of Fly Ash Levels on pH of the Postharvest Soil

Electrical Conductivity (EC)

Effect of Fly Ash Levels on EC of the Postharvest Soil

The initial EC of soil was 0.29 dSm^{-1}. The EC of fly ash was 0.41 dSm^{-1}. The analysis of data indicated non-significant difference in EC for fly ash. The addition of graded levels of fly ash showed no marked influence on EC of the postharvest soil. The EC of plots supplied with fly ash @ 20 t ha^{-1} was 0.20 dSm^{-1} and in control 0.21 dSm^{-1}. This application of fly ash has no marked effect on EC in postharvest soils. These observation corroborate with the earlier work reported by Anjali *et al*. (2000).

Table 44.20: Effect of Fly Ash Levels on EC of the Postharvest Soil

Treatment	*EC (dSm^{-1})*
F_0	0.21
F_1	0.20
F_2	0.21
S.E	-
C.D. at 5 per cent	NS

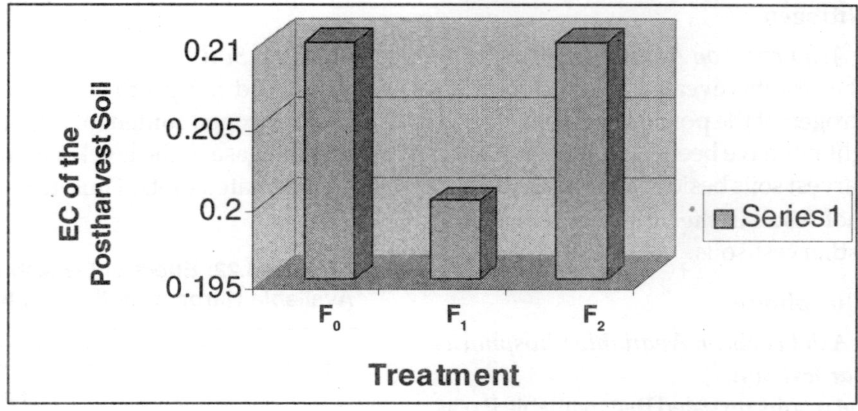

Figure 44.12: Effect of Fly Ash Levels on EC of the Postharvest Soil

Organic Carbon

Effect of Fly Ash Levels on Organic Carbon Content of Postharvest Soil

The analysis of data indicated significant increase in organic carbon content of the postharvest soils due to fly ash addition as compared to control. The organic carbon content in postharvest soil ranged from 5.34 to 5.86 g kg^{-1} with lowest in control and highest in plots treated with fly ash @ 40 t ha^{-1}, as against initial value of 5.70 g kg^{-1} (Pre-sowing). Increasing in organic carbon content in fly ash treated plots over control might be due to higher content of burnt carbon in fly ash. Naveen *et al.* (2000) also reported that organic carbon content of sandy-loam soil increased with the application of fly ash.

Table 44.21: Effect of Fly Ash Levels on Organic Carbon Content of Postharvest Soil

Treatment	*Organic Carbon (g kg^{-1})*
F_0	5.34
F_1	5.74
F_2	5.86
S.E	0.09
C.D. at 5 per cent	0.19

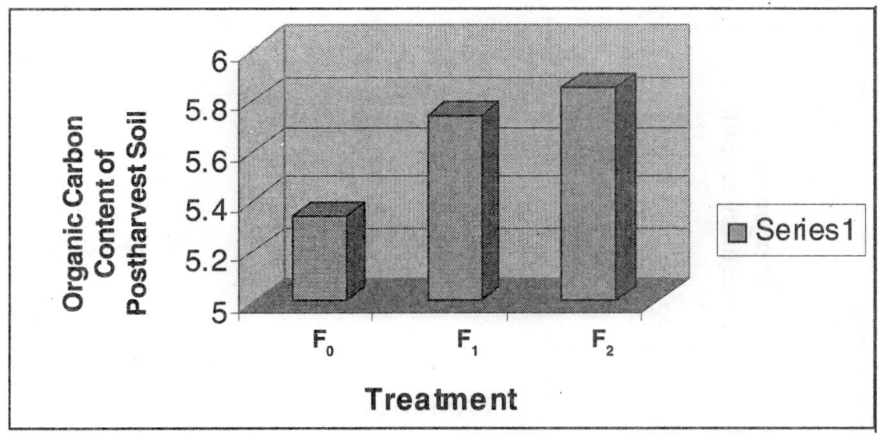

Figure 44.13: Effect of Fly Ash Levels on Organic Carbon Content of Postharvest Soil

Available Nitrogen

Effect of Fly Ash Levels on Available Nitrogen of the Postharvest Soil

From the results revealed that different levels of fly ash did not produce marked variation in available nitrogen of the postharvest soils. The very little total nitrogen content of fly ash (0.07 per cent total N) might not have been sufficient enough to cause any increase in the level of available nitrogen in the postharvest soils besides crop removed more N from the treated plots. Thus, it was revealed that fly ash did not result in the build-up of available N in the postharvest soils.

Table 44.22: Effect of Fly Ash Levels on Available Nitrogen of the Postharvest Soil

Treatment	Available Nitrogen (kg ha^{-1})
F_0	263.20
F_1	265.27
F_2	265.71
S.E	-
C.D. at 5 per cent	NS

Available Phosphorus

Effect of Fly Ash Levels on Available Phosphorus of the Postharvest Soil

From the results revealed that available P was significantly increased by the graded doses of fly ash. The available P content in postharvest range from 20.95 to 22.90 kg ha^{-1} with lowest in control and highest in plots treated with fly ash @ 40 t ha^{-1}(F_2). The application of fly ash @ 20 and 40 t ha^{-1} recorded an increase of 1.77 and 2.50 kg ha^{-1} in postharvest soil, as against initial value of 20.40 kg ha^{-1} (pre-sowing). The favourable effect of fly ash on P availability was ascribed to its effect on biotic activity and the P release via biotic activity. The silicon which is present in fly ash would also have played a major role in releasing insoluble sources in fly ash as well in soil. Anjali *et al*. (2000) reported similar increase in available P content of soil. Koter *et al*. (1984) also observed increase in available P status and they attributed it to the P content of fly ash.

Table 44.23: Effect of Fly Ash Levels on Available Phosphorus of the Postharvest Soil

Treatment	Available Phosphorus (kg ha^{-1})
F_0	20.95
F_1	22.17
F_2	22.90
S.E	0.33
C.D. at 5 per cent	0.69

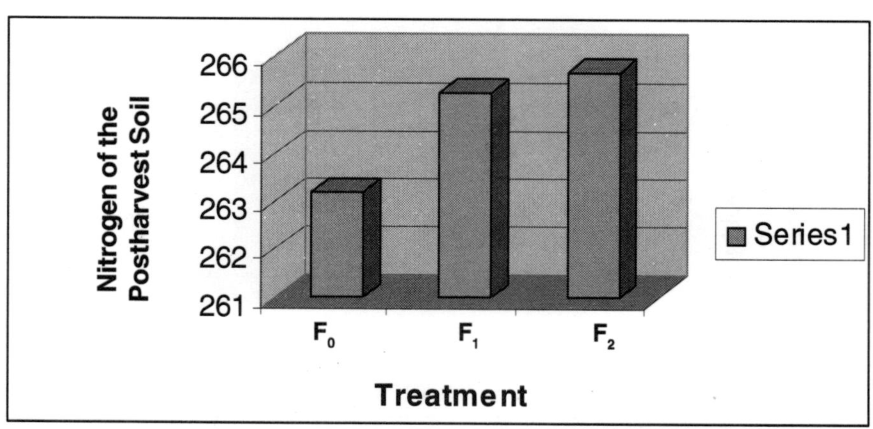

Figure 44.14: Effect of Fly Ash Levels on Available Nitrogen of the Postharvest Soil

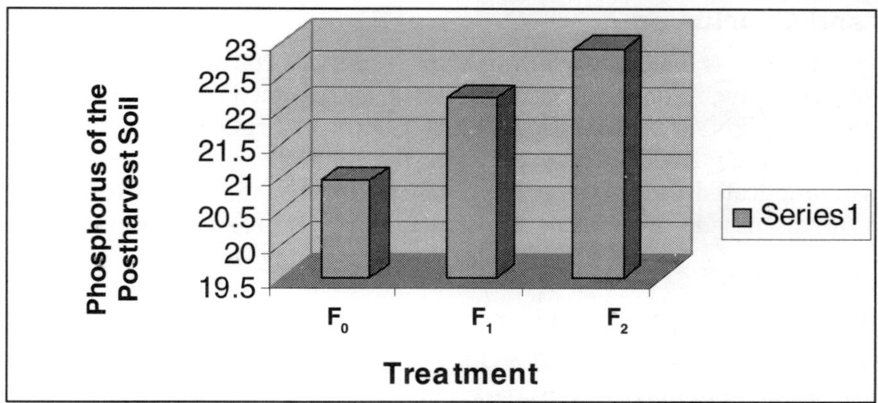

Figure 44.15: Effect of Fly Ash Levels on Available Phosphorus of the Postharvest Soil

Available Potassium

Effect of Fly Ash Levels on Available Potassium of the Postharvest Soil

From the results revealed that available K was significantly increased by the graded doses of fly ash. The increase was 19.16 and 25.50 kg ha^{-1} of the postharvest soil due to addition of fly ash @ 20 and 40 t ha^{-1} as against initial value of 225.50 kg ha^{-1} (pre-sowing). Positive effect of fly ash addition on available K content of soil was also reported by Warambhe *et al.* (1992). Also Anjali *et al.* (2000) and Selvakumari *et al.* (2000) reported that application of fly ash increased K content of soil.

Table 44.24: Effect of Fly Ash Levels on Available Potassium of the Postharvest Soil

Treatment	*Available Potassium (kg ha^{-1})*
F_0	219.33
F_1	244.66
F_2	251.00
S.E	0.76
C.D. at 5 per cent	1.61

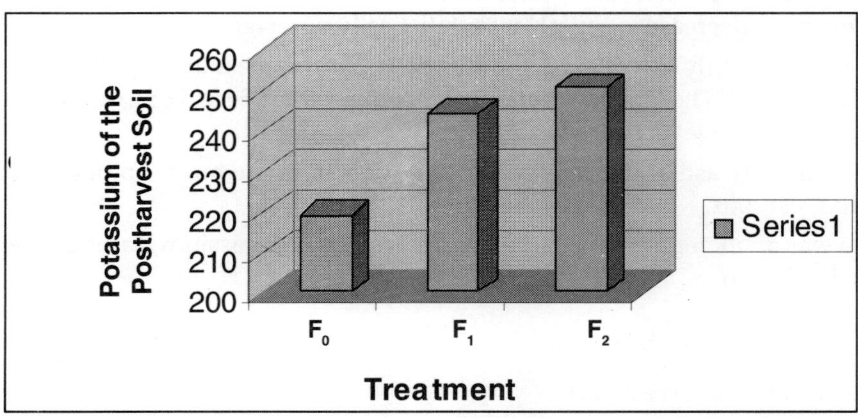

Figure 44.16: Effect of Fly Ash Levels on Available Potassium of the Postharvest Soil

Summary and Conclusion

Field experiment was conducted during kharif season of 2001 at the Crop Research Farm of Department of Agronomy, Allahabad Agricultural Institute- Deemed University, Allahabad, on sandy loam soil, to study the "ENVIRONMENTAL IMPACT OF FLY ASH ON SOIL HEALTH, YIELD AND NUTRIENT UPTAKE BY RICE". The experiment was laid out in 3 × 3 factorial design and the treatments were replicated thrice. The result obtained during the field during the field study are summarized and discussed in previously. The general findings are summarized below:

Pre-Harvest Findings

- ☆ The levels of fly ash significantly increased the plant height.
- ☆ The number of tillers per hill are significantly increased by increasing the levels of fly ash.
- ☆ The dry weight of the plants at successive stages of growth were significantly affected by different levels of fly ash.
- ☆ Panicle length of rice crop was significantly influenced by different levels of fly ash.
- ☆ The number of spikelets per panicle was significantly not influenced by the levels of fly ash.

Postharvest Findings

- ☆ Addition of fly ash at graded doses increased grain yield of rice crop significantly over control. Fly ash applied @ 20 and 40 t/ha increased the grain yield by 3.64 and 10.30 per cent, respectively over the treatment without any addition of fly ash.
- ☆ The straw yield was also significantly increased by the graded doses of fly ash. Apparently, the positive effect of fly ash was found. The maximum grain and straw yield was recorded in the treatment F_2 fly ash @ 40 t/ha.
- ☆ The N P K uptake by rice grain was significantly higher in treatments that received fly ash @ 20 and 40 t/ha than in without fly ash treatment. The maximum N P K uptake by rice grain was observed with the application of fly ash @ 40 t/ha (F_2).
- ☆ There was a decrease in soil pH in the postharvest soil due to fly ash addition as compared to control. The pH decreased from 7.87 to 7.71 due to application of fly ash @ 20 t/ha, however, the decrease in soil pH was statistically non-significant.
- ☆ The addition of fly ash at graded doses did not produce marked influence on EC in the postharvest soil. The organic carbon content range form 5.34 to 5.86 g/kg with highest at (F_2) fly ash @ 40 t/ha level of application.
- ☆ Addition of fly ash at graded levels did not result in the build-up of available N in the postharvest soils.
- ☆ There was an increase in available phosphorous and potassium status of the postharvest soil with fly ash.

Observation Taken in the Soil

Chemical Analysis of Postharvest Soil

Postharvest soil samples were taken to the plough level, *i.e.* upto 0 to 15 cm depth from each plot for determination of important chemical properties of soil, *viz.*, pH, EC, organic carbon, available Nitrogen, Phosphorus and Potassium.

Determination of Soil pH

Digital Electric pH meter MK VI (Systronics) was used for the determination of pH of the 1:2 soil water suspensions. The instrument being a potentiometer requires to be calibrated before use with buffer solution of known pH values of 4.0, 7.0 and 9.2 at 25°C.

Determination of Electrical Conductivity in Soil

Amount of soluble salts in saturated extract or 1:2 soil:water suspension is measured by Direct Reading Conductivity meter-304 (Systronics). The instrument is to be calibrated or checked with 0.01 M standard potassium chloride solution at 25°C.

Determination of Organic Carbon in Soil

For easily oxidizable carbon determination, most widely acceptable method in India is Walkley and Black method (1934). This method is mainly based on the principle of wet oxidation of organic carbon in an acid dichromate solution followed by back titration of the remaining dichromate with ferrous ammonium sulphate.

Determination of Available Nitrogen in Soil (Kjeldahl Method)

Available nitrogen is mainly determined by alkaline permanganate method (Subbiah and Asija 1956). In this method soil is distilled with alkaline potassium permanganate solution (0.32 per cent) and 40 per cent NaOH which gives ammonia. This liberated ammonia is absorbed by boric acid solution with mixed indicator, which is determined volumetrically and serves as an index of available nitrogen status.

Determination of Available Phosphorus by Olsen's Method or Sodium Bicarbonate ($NaHCO_3$) Extractable Phosphorus (Olsen *et al.*, 1954)

Phosphorus determination in soil is a two steps process, *i.e.* extraction of phosphorus from the soil by sodium bicarbonate. After extraction from the soil, phosphate in the extract is measured by the reaction of phosphate with ammonium molybdate in an acid medium to form molybdophosphoric acid. The molybdophosphoric acid is then reduced to a blue coloured complex (reduced phosphomolybdenum blue) through reaction with ascorbic acid. The ascorbic acid method has proved to be reliable and less subjected to interference in colour development than the $SnCl_2$ method. The colour is stable for 24 hours. Absorbance readings are taken at a 730 nm wavelength using a spectrophotometer. A standard curve constructed from absorbance readings standards is used to deduce phosphate concentration of sample.

Determination of Available Potassium (Jackson, 1973)

Potassium is extracted from the soil with the help of suitable extractant neutral normal ammonium acetate (1N CH_3COONH_4) by shaking followed by filtration and is determined in the extract using flame photometer (Mediflame 127-Systronics). The analysis of flame photometer is based on the measurement of the intensity of characteristic wavelength given by the element to be determined. When a solution of a salt is sprayed into a flame, the salt gets separated into its component atoms because of high temperature. The energy provided by flame excites the atom to higher energy levels. When the electrons return back to the ground or unexcited state, they emit radiation of characteristic wave length (Line emission spectrum). The intensity or these radiations is proportional to the concentration of particular element in solution which is measured through a photocell in the flame photometer.

Statistical Analysis

The data recorded during the course of investigation will subjected to statistical analysis as per the method of "analysis of variance technique". The significant and non-significant treatment effects were judge with the help of 'F' table. The significant differences between the means were tested against the critical difference at 5 per cent probability level. For testing the hypothesis the following ANOVA table will used.

The 'F' test will use for judging the significant of treatment means. The significant difference between different means were judge by using least significant difference (C.D) at 5 per cent level of significance, which will calculated by the formula.

Table 44.25: Skeleton of ANOVA Table

Source of Variation	*d.f.*	*S.S*	*M.S.S*	*F(cal)*	*F (tab) at 5 per cent*
Replication	(r-1)	SSR	$\frac{SSR}{d.f}$	$\frac{MSSR}{MESS}$	
Flyash (F)	(f-1)	SSF	$\frac{SSF}{d.f}$	$\frac{MSSF}{MESS}$	
Fertilizer (M)	(m-1)	SSM	$\frac{SSM}{d.f}$	$\frac{MSSM}{MESS}$	
Interaction (F × M)	(f-1)(m-1)	SSFM	$\frac{SSFM}{d.f}$	$\frac{MSSI}{MESS}$	
Error	(r-1)(t-1)	SSE	$\frac{SSE}{d.f}$		
Total	(rfm-1)	TSS			

Sem ± for Flyash levels (F) = $\sqrt{\frac{2 \times MESS}{r \times f}}$

C.D. for Flyash levels = SEm × t_{16} value for error d.f at 5 per cent

SEm ± for Fertilizer levels (M) = $\sqrt{\frac{2 \times MESS}{r \times M}}$

C.D. for Fertilizer levels = SEm × t_{16} value for error d.f at 5 per cent

SEm ± for interaction (F × M) = $\sqrt{\frac{2 \times MESS}{r \times M}}$

C.D. for interaction (F × M) = SEm × t_{16} value for error d.f at 5 per cent

where,

r: Number of replications; t: Number of treatments; d.f: Degree of freedom; S.S: Sum of squares; SSR: Sum of squares due to replication; MSSR: Mean sum of squares due to replication; SSE: Error sum of squares; TSS: Total sum of squares; SE (m): Standard error of means; F (cal): Calculated value of 'F'; F (tab): Value of 'F' from variance table; C.D: Critical difference; SSM: Sum of squares due to fertilizer; SSF: Sum of squares due to fly ash; SSFM: Sum of squares due to interaction (F × M).

References

Anjali, Deshmukh, Matte, D.B., Bhaisare, Bharti, Deshmukh, A. and Bhoisare, B. (2000). Soil properties as influenced by flyash application. *Jour. Soil and Crops* 10 (1) 69-71.

Bharti, B., Matte, D.B., Batole, W.P., Anjali, D., Bhaisare, B. and Deshmukh, A. (2000). Effect of flyash on yield uptake of nutrients and quality of green gram growth on vertisol. *J. Soil and Crops*, 10 (1) 122–124.

Bharti, B., Matte, D.B., Batole, W.P., Anjali, D., Bhaisare, B. and Deshmukh, A. (1999). Effect of fly ash on physico-chemical properties of vertisols and yield of green gram. *J. Soil and Crops*, 9(2): 255-257.

Buck, J.K., Honston, R.J. and Beimborn, W.A. (1990). Direct seedling of anthrotic refuge using coal fly ash a major soil amendment in a process of mining and reclamation conference and exhibition West Virgina University public service.

Deshpande, V.P., Kole, C.K., Godkari, S.K. and Badrinath (1993). Environmental impacts due to fly ash from coal fired thermal power plants. *Paper presented at Nat. sem. Env. Asp. Thermal Power Plants Org.* by R and D center Noida, U.P. from 9-10 Dec.

Dubey, P.S., Pawar, K., Shrigi, S.K. and Trivedi, L. (1982). The effect of flyash deposition on photosynthetic pigments and dry matter production of wheat and grains. *Agro, Ecosystem*, 8(2): 137-140.

Garg, R.N., Singh, G., Kalra, N., Das, D.K. and Singh, A. (1996). Utilization of applied phosphorous by wheat as influenced by fly ash application. *Annals of Biology*, Ludhiana, 12(1): 19-24.

Kuchanwar, T., Matte, D.B. and Kane, D.R. (1997). Effect of fly ash application on physico chemical properties of soil. Nat. Env. Res. Ins. (NEERI) Nehru Marg Nagpur, India.

Kumar, W. and Annanaric, A. (2000). Effect of green manure on growth and yield attributes in pea (*Pisum sativum*). *J. Plant Nutri.*, 24(6): 240-248.

Kene, D.R., Lanjewar, S.A., Ingole, M. and Chaphale, S.P. (1991). Effect of application of fly ash on physico-chemical properties of soil. *J. Soil and Crops*, 1(1): 118.

Microbial Biotechnology and Ecology (2011) *Pages* **766–772**
Editors: **Deepak Vyas, G.S. Paliwal, P.K.Khare and R.K Gupta**
Published by: **DAYA PUBLISHING HOUSE, NEW DELHI**

Chapter 45

Eutrophication: Causes, Consequences and Control Measures

☆ ***Ashu and Mukesh Kumar***

Department of Botany, Sahu Jain P.G. College, Najibabad – 246 763, U.P.

ABSTRACT

Eutrophication is an increase in the concentration of chemical nutrients in an ecosystem to an extent that increases in the primary productivity of the ecosystem. Depending on the degree of eutrophication, subsequent negative environmental effects such as anoxia and severe reductions in water quality, fish, and other animal populations may occur. Eutrophication poses a problem not only to ecosystems, but to humans as well. Reducing eutrophication should be a key concern when considering future policy, and a sustainable solution for everyone, including farmers and ranchers, seems feasible. While eutrophication does pose problems, humans should be aware that natural runoff (which causes algal bloom in the wild) is common in ecosystems and should thus not reverse nutrient concentrations beyond normal levels.

Introduction

Eutrophication is a process whereby water bodies, such as lakes, estuaries, or slow moving streams receive excess nutrients that stimulate excessive plant growth (algae, periphyton attached algae, and nuisance plant weeds). This enhanced plant growth, often called an algal bloom, reduces dissolved oxygen in the water when dead plant material decomposes and can cause other organisms to die. Nutrients can come from many sources, such as fertilizers applied to agricultural fields, golf courses, and suburban lawns; deposition of nitrogen from the atmosphere; erosion of soil containing nutrients; and sewage treatment plant discharges. Water with a low concentration of dissolved oxygen is called hypotoxic.

In Lakes, Eutrophication is frequently a result of nutrient pollution, such as the release of sewage effluent, urban storm water run-off, and run-off carrying excess fertilizers into natural waters. Eutrophication generally promotes excessive plant growth and decay, favors certain weedy species over others, and may cause a severe reduction in water quality. In aquatic environments, Eutrophication enhances growth of problems such as lack of oxygen in the water, needed for fish and shellfish to survive. The water then becomes cloudy, coloured a shade of green, yellow, brown, or red. Human society is impacted as well: Eutrophication decreases the resource value of rivers, lakes, and estuaries such that recreation, fishing, hunting, and aesthetic enjoyment are hindered. Health-related problems can occur where eutrophic conditions interfere with drinking water treatment (Bartram *et al.*, 1999).

Eutrophication was recognized as a pollution problem in European and North America lakes and reservoirs in the mid-20th century (Rodhe 1969), since then, it has become more widespread. Surveys showed that 54 per cent of lakes in Asia are eutrophic; in Europe 53 per cent; in North-America 48 per cent; in South-America 41 per cent; and in Africa 28 per cent. (ILEC/Lake Biwa Research Institute (Eds.) 1988-1993).

Although Eutrophication is commonly caused by human activities, Eutrophication can also be a natural condition for many lakes. Paleolimnologists now recognize that climate change, geology, and other external influences are critical in regulating the natural productivity of lakes. Some lakes also demonstrate the reverse process (meiotrophication), becoming less nutrient rich with time (Walker, 2006; Whiteside, 1983).

Phosphorus is often regarded as the main culprit in case of Eutrophication in lakes. Studies conducted in the Experimental Lakes Area in Ontario have shown a relationship between the addition of phosphorus and the rate of Eutrophication. Humankind has increased the rate of phosphorus cycling on Earth by four times, mainly due to agricultural fertilizer production and application. Between 1950 and 1995; 600,000,000 tonnes of phosphorus were applied to Earth's surface, primarily on croplands (Carpenter and Smith, 1998).

The World Resources Institute has identified 375 hypoxic coastal zones in the world, concentrated in coastal areas in Western Europe, the Eastern and Southern coasts of the US, and East Asia, particularly in Japan (Selman and Mendy, 2007). In addition to runoff from land, atmospheric anthropogenic fixed nitrogen can enter the open ocean. A study in 2008 found that this could account for around one third of the ocean's external nitrogen supply and up to 3 per cent of the annual new marine biological production (Duce, 2008).

Although traditionally thought of as enrichment of aquatic systems by addition of fertilizers into lakes, or other semi-enclosed waters (even slow moving rivers), terrestrial ecosystems are subject to similarly adverse impacts. Increased content of nitrates in soil frequently leads to undesirable changes in vegetation composition and many plant species are endangered as a result of Eutrophication in terrestic ecosystems, *e.g.* majority of orchid species in Europe (Pullin, 2002). Ecosystems (like some meadows, forests and bogs that are characterized by low nutrient content and species-rich, slowly growing vegetation adapted to lower nutrient levels) are overgrown by faster growing and advantage of unnaturally elevated nitrogen level and the area may be changed beyond recognition and vulnerable species may be lost. Example, Species-rich fens are overtaken by reed or reedgrass species, spectacular forest undergrowth affected by run-off from nearby fertilized field is turned into a thick nettle and bramble shrub.

Chemical forms of nitrogen are most often of concern with regard to Eutrophication because plants have nitrogen requirements so that additions of nitrogen compounds stimulate plant growth (primary production). Nitrogen is not readily available in soil because N_2, a gaseous form of nitrogen, is very stable and unavailable directly to higher plants. Terrestrial ecosystems rely on microbial nitrogen fixation to convert N_2 into other physical forms (such as nitrates). However, there is a limit to how much nitrogen can be utilized. Ecosystems receiving more nitrogen than the plants require are called nitrogen-saturated. Saturated terrestrial ecosystems contribute both inorganic and organic nitrogen to freshwater, coastal, and marine Eutrophication, where nitrogen is also typically a limiting nutrient (Hornung *et al.*, 1995). However, in marine environments, phosphorus may be limiting because it is leached from the soil at a much slower rate than nitrogen, which are highly insoluble (Smith *et al.*, 1999).

Causes of Eutrophication

The two major causes of Eutrophication are excess nitrates and excess phosphates in water. It is important to study these nutrients because often times, human activity is responsible for their negative effect on the environment.

Nitrates

Nitrates (NO_3^-) are water-soluble (they dissolve easily in water), and are commonly applied to agricultural fields as fertilizer. Once applied, nitrates may leach into groundwater or erode and end up in surface runoff. Eventually, they may enter in lake, river, or stream and contribute to Eutrophication. Nitrates can also vaporize into the atmosphere, where they become a major source of acid rain. When ingested by organisms in drinking water, nitrates bind to haemoglobin and reduce the oxygen-carrying capacity of the bloodstream. This form of nitrate poisoning seems particularly prevalent among amphibians, and may be contributing to a worldwide decline in the biodiversity of these species.

28 per cent of the annual Nitrogen fixation of the global biosphere is caused by nitrogen fertilizer production, which is energetically expensive and largely based on fossil fuel consumption. A three-fold increase in nitrogen utilization by agriculture in Western Europe and USA has been recorded on agricultural land that actually declines because increased efficiency or over-exploitation. Animal waste from intensive husbandry is of particular significance for nutrient point sources: considerable amounts are directly supplied to freshwater and fields. There are also significant losses by NH_3 emission and denitrification on fields, rivers or shallow estuaries, connecting the agricultural lands directly to the atmosphere. Agricultural run-off has given rise to significant Eutrophication in most estuaries, but also in entire coastal seas such as the southern North Sea, Baltic Sea, Kattegat, northern Adriatic Sea, Chesapeake Bay and Seto Inland Sea in Japan.

Annual global nitrogen fertilizer consumption for 1960-1995 (1 Tg = 10^{12} g; data from FAO 1999). The rate of increase was relatively steady until the late 1980s, when the collapse of the Soviet Union reduced fertilizer use in Russia and former Soviet republics. Fertilizer use is growing again, driven in large part by use in China

Phosphates

Unlike nitrates, phosphates (PO_4^{3-}) are not water-soluble; they do not usually dissolve in water. However, they do adhere to soil particles, and as such often accumulate in soil and erode along with soil into aquatic environments. Phosphates also form a major component of most fertilizers, and in conjunction with nitrates, they have made agriculture the largest source of nonpoint water pollution in the United States.

Effects of Eutrophication

Ecological Effects

Following are the adverse effects of Eutrophication on lakes, reservoirs, rivers and coastal marine waters

1. Increased biomass of phytoplankton
2. Toxic or inedible phytoplankton species
3. Increases in blooms of gelatinous zooplankton
4. Changes in macrophyte species composition and biomass
5. Decreases in water transparency
6. Taste, odour, and water treatment problems
7. Dissolved oxygen depletion
8. Increased incidences of fish kills
9. Loss of desirable fish species
10. Reductions in harvestable fish and shellfish
11. Decreases in perceived aesthetic value of the water body

Many ecological effects can arise from stimulating primary production, but there are three particularly troubling ecological impacts: decreased biodiversity, changes in species composition and dominance, and toxicity effects.

Decreased Biodiversity

When an ecosystem experiences an increase in nutrients, primary producers reap the benefits first. In aquatic ecosystems, species such as algae experience a population increase (called an algal bloom). Algal blooms limit the sunlight available to bottom-dwelling organisms and cause wide swings in the amount of dissolved oxygen in the water.

Oxygen is required by all respiring plants and animals and it is replenished in daylight by photosynthesizing plants and algae. Under eutrophic conditions, dissolved oxygen greatly increases during the day, but is greatly reduced after by the respiring algae and by microorganisms that feed on the increasing mass of dead algae. When dissolved oxygen levels decline to hypoxic levels, fish and other marine animals suffocate. As a result creatures such as fish, shrimp, and especially immobile bottom dwellers die off (Horrigan *et al.*, 2002). In extreme cases, anaerobic conditions ensue, promoting growth of bacteria such as *Clostridium botulinum* that produces toxins deadly to birds and mammals. Zones where this occurs are known as dead zones.

Effect of Fertilizers

Fertilizers containing plant nutrients are sprayed onto fields to make plants grow faster and boost crop yields. When it rains the nutrients may get washed down from the fields and into rivers and lakes (this is called run-off). The result is Eutrophication–which can kill almost everything living in the aquatic environment.

Effect of Pesticides

Pesticides are chemicals used to kill insects, weeds and microorganisms that might damage crops. However, pesticides damage other organisms apart from those they are intended to kill–for example, depriving insect-eating birds of food. Pesticides can also enter local food chains. Organisms that ingest them cannot break them down, so they persist in their bodies. The pesticides may then build up at ever-higher levels until they become toxic to much larger organisms.

New Species Invasion

Eutrophication may cause competitive release by making abundant a normally limiting nutrient. This process causes shifts in the species composition of ecosystems. For instance, an increase in nitrogen might allow new, competitive species to invade and out-compete original inhabitant species. This has been shown to occur in New England salt marshes.

Toxicity

Many algae produce potent toxins. Toxic compounds they produce can make their way up the food chain, resulting in animal mortality (Anderson, 1994). When the algae die or are eaten, neuro and hepatotoxins are released which can kill animals and may pose a threat to humans (Lawton and Codd, 1994; Shumway, 1990). Toxigenics blue green algae like Anabaena, Microcystis and Nostoc have been noted whose toxins can kill fish. The toxin may also contaminate the drinking water supplies.

Sources of High Nutrient Runoff

Point Sources

Point sources are directly attributable to one influence. In point sources the nutrient waste travels directly from source to water. Point sources are relatively easy to regulate.

Nonpoint Sources

Nonpoint source pollution (also known as diffuse or runoff pollution) is that which comes from ill-defined and diffuse sources. Nonpoint sources are difficult to regulate and usually vary spatially and temporally (with season, precipitation, and other irregular events).

It has been shown that nitrogen transport is correlated with various indices of human activity in watersheds, (Cole *et al.*, 1993; Howarth *et al.*, 1996) including the amount of development. There are three reasons that nonpoint sources are especially troublesome:

Soil Retention

Nutrients from human activities tend to accumulate in soils and remain there for years. It has been shown that the amount of phosphorus lost to surface waters increases linearly with the amount of phosphorus in the soil (Raimammake *et al.*, 2003). Thus much of the nutrient loading in soil eventually makes its way to water. Nitrogen, similarly, has a turnover time of decades or more.

Run Off to Surface Water and Leaching to Groundwater

Nutrients from human activities tend to travel from land to either surface or groundwater. Nitrogen in particular is removed through storm drains, sewage pipes, and other forms of surface runoff. Nutrient losses in runoff and leachate are often associated with agriculture. Modern agriculture often involves the application of nutrients onto fields in order to maximise production. However, farmers frequently apply more nutrients than are taken up by crops or pastures (Buol, 1995).

Atmospheric Deposition

Nitrogen is released into the air because of ammonia volatilization and nitrous oxide production. The combustion of fossil fuels is a large human- initiated contributor to atmospheric nitrogen pollution. Atmospheric deposition (*e.g.*, in the form of acid rain) can also affect nutrient concentration in water, (Paerl, 1997) especially in highly industrialized regions.

Controlling Eutrophication

Eutrophication can be controlled by adopting the following methods:

1. Planting vegetation along streambeds to slow erosion and absorb nutrients
2. Controlling application amount and timing of fertilizer
3. Controlling runoff from feedlots
4. Researching use of biological controls; for example, the process of denitrification uses specialized bacteria that convert nitrates to harmless molecular nitrogen
5. Laws regulating the discharge and treatment of sewage have led to dramatic nutrient reductions to surrounding ecosystems, but it is generally agreed that a policy regulating agricultural use of fertilizer and animal waste must be imposed. In Japan the amount of nitrogen produced by livestock is adequate to serve the fertilizer needs for the agriculture industry (Kumuzawa, 2002).
6. Soil Nitrogen Testing (N-Testing) is a technique that helps farmers optimize the amount of fertilizer applied to crops. By testing fields with this method, farmers saw a decrease in fertilizer application costs, a decrease in nitrogen lost to surrounding sources, or both (Haung, Lu and Uri, 2001). By testing the soil and modelling the bare minimum amount of fertilizer needed, farmers reap economic benefits while the environment remains clean and pure.
7. Reseachers at the National Academy of Sciences found that organically fertilizing fields "significantly reduce harmful nitrate leaching" over conventionally fertilized fields.

Acknowledgements

The authors are thankful to the Principal, Sahu Jain P. G. College, Najibabad for providing necessary facilities.

References

Anderson, D.M. (1994). Red tides. *Scientific American*, 27: 62–68.

Bartram, J., Wayne, Carmichael, Ingrid Chorus, Gary Jones, and Olav Skulberg, (1999). Chapter 1 Introduction. In: *Toxic Cyanobacteria in Water: A guide to their public health consequences, monitoring and management*. World Health Organization. URL: WHO document.

Buol, S.W. (1995). Sustainability of Soil Use. *Annual Review of Ecology and Systematics*, 26: 25–44.

Carpenter, S.R., Caraco, N.F. and Smith, V.H. (1998). Nonpoint pollution of surface waters with phosphorus and nitrogen. *Ecological Applications*, 8: 559-568.

Cole, J.J., Peierls, B.L., Caraco, N.F. and Pace, M.L. (1993). Nitrogen loading of rivers as a human-driven process. In: McDonnell, M.J. and Pickett, S.T.A. (Eds) *Humans as Components of Ecosystems*. Springer Verlag, New York, USA, pp. 141-157.

Duce, R.A. *et al.* (2008). Impacts of atmospheric anthropogenic nitrogen on the open ocean. *Science*, 320: 893–897.

Hornung, M., Sutton, M.A. and Wilson, R.B. (Eds.) (1995). Mapping and modelling of critical loads for nitrogen a workshop report. Grange over Sands, Cumbria, UK. UNECE.

Horrigan, L., Lawrence, R.S. and Walker, P. (2002). How sustainable agriculture can address the environmental and human health harms of industrial agriculture. *Environmental Health Perspectives*, 110: 445–456.

Howarth, R.W., Billen, G., Swaney, D., Townsend, A., Jaworski, N., Lajtha, K., Downing, J.A., Elmgren, R., Caraco, N., Jordan, T., Berendse, F., Freney, J., Kudeyarov, V., Murdoch, P. and Zhu Zhaoliang (1996). Regional nitrogen budgets and riverine inputs of N and P for the drainages to the North Atlantic Ocean: natural and human influences. *Biogeochemistry* 35: 75–139.

LEC/Lake Biwa Research Institute (Eds) (1988-1993). Survey of the State of the World's Lakes. Volumes IV. International Lake Environment Committee, Otsu and United Nations Environment Programme, Nairobi.

Lawton, L.A. and Codd, G.A. (1991). Cyanobacterial (bluegreenalgae) toxins and their significance in UK and European waters. *Journal of Soil and Water Conservation*, 40: 87–97.

Paerl, H.W. (1997). Coastal eutrophication and harmful algal blooms: Importance of atmospheric deposition and groundwater as "New" nitrogen and other nutrient sources. *Limnology and Oceanography*, 42:1154-1165.

Pullin, Andrew S. (2002). *Conservation Biology*. Cambridge University Press.

Raimammake, A., Pietilainen, O.P., Rekolainen, S., Kauppila, P., Pitkanen, H., Niemi, J., Raateland, A. and Vuorenmaa, J. (2003). Trends of phosphorus, nitrogen, and chlorophyll *a* concentrations in Finnish rivers and lakes in 1975-2000. *The Science of the Total Environment*, 310: 47–59.

Rodhe, W. (1969). Crystallization of eutrophication concepts in North Europe. In: *Eutrophication: Causes, Consequences, Correctives*. National Academy of Sciences, Washington D.C.

Selman Mindy, (2007). *Eutrophication: An Overview of Status, Trends, Policies, and Strategies*. World Resources Institute.

Shumway, S.E. (1990). A review of the effects of algal blooms on shellfish and aquaculture. *Journal of the World Aquaculture Society*, 21: 65–104.

Smith, V.H., Tilman, G.D. and Nekola, J.C. (1999). Eutrophication: impacts of excess nutrient inputs on freshwater, marine, and terrestrial ecosystems. *Environmental Pollution*, 100: 179–196.

Walker, I.R. (2006). Chironomid overview. In: S.A. Elias (ed.) *Encyclopedia of Quaternary Science*. Elsevier, Amsterdam, 1: 360-366.

Whiteside, M.C. (1983). The mythical concept of Eutrophication. *Hydrobiologia*, 103: 107-111.

Microbial Biotechnology and Ecology (2011) Pages 773–779
Editors: **Deepak Vyas, G.S. Paliwal, P.K.Khare and R.K Gupta**
Published by: DAYA PUBLISHING HOUSE, NEW DELHI

Chapter 46

Aquatic Biodiversity Assessment should Trigger Freshwater Body Monitoring and Conservation

☆ *S.D. Guru[1] and H.K. Goswami[2]**

[1]Department of Botany, Ranchi Women's College, Ranchi, Jharkhand
[2]24, Kaushalnagar, P.O. Misrod, Bhopal – 462 047, M.P.

ABSTRACT

Extensive studies are being carried out under the umbrella of Biodiversity which principally constitute enumeration and listing of species from a particular area and or water body but negligible attempts point out to real interplay of biodiversity which is inherent among related and unrelated species within the ecosystems. Mollusks, fish, sponges and many species of insects invite birds to rest and even nest in the nearby bushes which in turn release their faeces to change pH of the water. Growth of algae is directly related to available chemical and pH factors with in the soil and water. A freshwater lake is bound to be protected because aquatic biodiversity- ecosystems can not be dug and enriched soon; we have enormous wealth in a lake more so when that lake supplies drinking water. Briefly, this is suggested that botanists, zoologists, geochemists and physiologists will be needed to recover a sick lake and only comprehensive and multidisciplinary study, as documented in the past two decades, at Bhojwetland Bhopal, will be needed. The most important follow up step often ignored, is repetition of deweeding programmes. Lake or a waterbody need to be taken care of on regular basis by multidisciplinary teams.

Keywords: *Wetland conservation, Biodiversity assessments and drinking water, Biological monitoring of freshwater lakes, Conservation and management of freshwater.*

---

* E-mail: hkgbhopal@hotmail.com

Introduction

Water has become synonym to life. Life arose in water and more than 90 per cent contents of each functional and dividing cell is water. Since the time immemorial man has been settling around rivers and lakes and in later period, migrating human populations have had dug water bodies to nurture all life forms. Needless to mention, forests, water resources and ever increasing human populations are inseparably interdependent on each other. A greater part of the world has one major biological threat; we will need more water than food to survive for a few more hundred years because rise in human populations is currently inversely proportional to depleting water resources.

Therefore conservation of water bodies with basic biological out put is the major challenge before biologists, environmentalists and planners world over, more so in most Asian countries. In most townships in many Asian countries big lakes are one of the major sources of drinking water supply to millions of inhabitants of that area. Such a situation is most common in Indian subcontinent. Based on International parameters we designate such huge lakes and water bodies as wetlands which have water flooded land mass as well. One of the major wetlands in India was identified in Bhopal (Madhya Pradesh) as bhojwetland. This short communication intends only to emphasize that what we need is to conserve each and every lake and we can not continue to describe floristic composition in the form of biodiversity and end our endeavour before a noble beginning. There have been hundreds of papers and dozens of conferences focusing on need of this exhaustive work but not a single multidisciplinary and real collaborative effort to save and enrich a lake with quality and quantity of water has come to beginning in Central India. Our published monographic treatise on Bhojwetland (Agarker *et al.*, 1994) has been based on comprehensive studies for which seeds were sown in 1984 and major results could be seen after a decade. Further studies have been slowly in progress on this wetland, and also, simultaneously, one of us (HK) has been conducting field work in various states to impress upon teachers in particular, who have a good background of limnological and floristic studies, to share their expertise with chemists, geologists and administrative officials. Academic excellence in at all places has to be brought to safety and security of water availability for our generations.

Background

The bhoj wetland has an area of more than 40 sq kms and supplies drinking water to more than a million people in Bhopal township. The multidisciplinary efforts on conservation of this wetland for more than a decade have had made this as a model for biological conservation and such an exhaustive treatise by any research group have been never documented as was presented by Agarker *et al.* (1994). To begin with, this was estimated that the original upperlake has lost about its 30 per cent area within past 40 years on account of silting, increasing human encroachments, water loss, prolific growth of weeds and erstwhile dragging water for small ponds. The density gradient of weeds (excessive growth of weeds) was found to be biologically supported by in flow of pouring sewage fed water pipes from different nearby localities including wastewater discharge from nearby hospitals and local colonies. Our primary studies had revealed that the lake was biologically very sick and exhibited totally disrupted complex ecosystems. Subsequent follow up studies were carried out to expose the major problems and find out possible remedial efforts. We worked on all possible parameters like enumeration of phytoplankton, zooplankton, a large number of algal forms and aquatic insects, angiospermous, weeds including aquatic ferns, sponges, mollusks, fish and birds (Total about 900 species: very rich biodiversity excluding birds) and distribution with their possible correlation, of metals in water and soil samples from around the lake.

Well planned remedial, both physical (deweeding programmes; removal of top soils and weed assemblages on dry land areas formed due to silting etc in side the lake) as well as biological (strategic conservation of many mollusks, reptiles, amphibians and even bird fauna in adjoining grassland) was undertaken and plantations to check silting was carried out at a large scale. The results were alarmingly fruitful leaving a caution that lakes will continuously need care; leaving at people's mercy would again bring discredit to the water. Condemning deweeding operations will be harmful.

The above background has been emphatically mentioned for a purpose to emphasize the importance of such a massive attempt to be made on every water body which feeds drinking water to a fraction of a population. This will be a matter of only going to the water body for assessments; remedial efforts have to be then urgently planned and executed with the automatic consent of enlightened masses.

Present Reference

Recently, we have initiated collaborative study on conservation and monitoring Kanke reservoir at Ranchi (Jharkhand) which supplies drinking water on multidisciplinary approach involving physico-chemical parameters and their comparative assessments on the same and different water bodies as well as on exhaustive coverage of phytoplankton, zooplankton, higher algal forms. Enumeration of macrophytic vegetation, is being carried out with a reference to explaining utility of each species in the water body. In other words, does these plants offer specific shelter or support in completing life cycles of mollusks/insects/or act as hangers for algal mass? Why are some plants more common in some and not in other parts? Additionally, can we account by metallic separation from different ash samples of these plants and also from soil samples as to why and what severely dangerous microelements are slowly poisoning drinking water resource? We can detect what are the undeclared sewage or other drains pouring effluent are discharged without notice? We know very well from meticulous studies of a large number workers that pollution status and metallic status is reliably demonstrated by selective presence of plant forms.

Our Approach

The exploratory module of research on conservation and wetland management as has been documented by Agarker *et al.* (1994) is by far the best approach applicable in principle to all water bodies in tropics seeking conservation after repair. Hereunder, we mention those major steps on which we are proceeding with a battery of information of publications on limnological and algal biodiversity by various authors in that area.

These steps are:

Zonal Cassification of the Water Body

The lake should be divided in to minimum of two or may be in four zones and identified/marked for further demarcations of sampling spots. For example, North zone, Nzone in to N1/N2– etc depending upon the area of the lake.

Decision of Parameters

There are certain essential parameters which must be investigated on every water body. Physicochemical characteristics of water and soil from different sampling zones are absolutely essential with a reference to seasonal variation.

Depending upon the manpower and finances available for field and equipments' expenses, we plan and also place demand for future repetition. Sampling tools can be designed as per the needs along with standard ones. In order to take out smaller and larger weeds we had designed (Agarker *et al.*, 1994) various shapes with dentate margins from thin iron rods which could catch even floating threads and filaments. Small boats carrying 2 or 3 persons are the best moving agents on the water. Incumbents must know swimming.

Biodiversity Assessments

Sampling and sorting of collection requires a real test of patience. Preparing slides and examining phytoplankton-zooplankton and other forms on the same day before fixation gives more precise information than examining on fixation; whenever this was not actually possible, we preferred to repeat. In order to assess total biodiversity (which is actually needed now) we must share taxonomic expertise of many experts; it is bound to be a collaborative study demanding unshakable faith among workers. Every water body, in and around, has wealth of medicinal plants (Agarker, 1994; Bajpai *et al.*, 1996; Bajpai, 2000) which can be taken up for a proper plantations.

Experimental Trials

In order to prove or rather suggest with confidence that particular macrophyte is positively correlated with the excessive presence of a heavy metal or in other words a species is better adapted to water containing specific chemical has to be ascertained by experimental studies. Bajpai and Goswami (2000) have conducted on metallic tolerance of strontium and chromium (trivalent) on *Polygonum glabrum* under tissue culture. Results indicate the reason why *Polygonum glabrum* is more found at those sites where soil does contain strontium-chromium complexes. Mere presence is not important but it is the absorption and utilization of metallic ions, a problem which would further need well planned physiological study.

Algal samples or any samples collected are being examined and attempts are designed to grow them in sterilized Knop's solution under identical temperature and light source. Hasty description of new species or strains due to abnormal features is not called for; we should see if these were ecophenes?. We guess that even ecotypes of certain alga (example, *Scenendesmus, Chlorella, Cosmarium* etc) may be validated by experimental trials. Attributing abnormal features to pollution should be needed to be taken up by a different experimental approach.

Now a days algal population is rightly being used as pollution indicator during bio-assessment of the water resources (Phillips and Rainbow, 1993; Cairns *et al.*, 1994; De Lang, 1994). Structural abnormalities (Misra *et al.*, 2003) in genera *Oocystis, Oedogonium, Euastrum* and *Cosmarium* and many other algae as well as diversity in distribution in the same and different areas need a careful follow up (Guru and Sahu, 2006; 2007 a,b, c,d,e,f; Guru, 2008 a,b). Among these, the genus *Scenendesmus* alone (An *et al.*, 1999) is taking up a position of water purifier seeking a support for its inoculation studies in different (Guru, 2008) polluted waters.

Shore Line Conservation by Medicinal Plants

Many herbaceous medicinal plants are also hyper accumulators of lead, cadmium and mercury (pteridophytes: *Ceratopteris, Marsilea, Pteris* spp etc.). The Classical medicinal plants are also found in some lake side areas; angiosperms:- *Bacopa, Centella* spp; there is a good list, which can be cultivated around the catchment area or in the marginal fringes of the water body or may even be a small multiplication garden for local medicinal plants can be erected. Initial attempts have already been made by us.

A Practical Suggestion

There are many very large lakes and water bodies in many remote areas, which need biological assessments. Teachers in the Universities should pose very sound and meaningful proposals and convince administrators and related local politicians to realize basic needs of water bodies. Fortunate are those who have lakes and unfortunate are those who can not maintain them?

Lakes are open treasures for survival of every species; plants, mollusks, fish, rodents, arboreal animals and birds all feed on lake water. Must not we save them?

Acknowledgements

We are grateful to Dr Jawed Ahmed, the Principal and other faculty members at Marwari College, Ranchi for accepting our joint endeavour in presenting a two day workshop organized at their institution. In this semiscientific presentation emphasis is laid on seriously taking up such studies on those water bodies which supply drinking water. We acknowledge that our present write up has been mainly guided by following publications mentioned hereunder.

References

Agarker, M.S., Goswami H.K., Kaushik, S., Mishra, S. M., Bajpai, A.K. and Sharma, U.S. (1994). Biology, Conservation and Management of Bhojwetland. I. Upper Lake Ecosystems in Bhopal. *(Bionature) Monograph*, pp. 1-119.

An S. S., Friedel T. and Hegewald E. (1999). Phylogenetic relationships of *Scenedesmus* and *Scenedesmus*–like coccoid green algae as inferred from ITC-2 rDNA sequence comparisons. *Plant Biology* 1: 418-428.

Bajpai, A.K (2000). *In vitro* multiplication of *Bacopa monnieri* and *Centella asiatica*. *Bionature*. 20: 75-79.

Bajpai, A.K. and Agarker, M.S. and Goswami, H.K. (1996). Biology, Conservation and Management of Bhojwetland III. Floristic composition in and around upperlake ecosystem in Bhopal. *Bionature*, 16: 53-64.

Bajpai, A.K. and Goswami, H.K. (2000). Assessment of metallic tolerance in *Polygonum glabrum*. *Physiol. Mol. Biol. Plants*, 6: 149-152.

Becker E. W. (1994). *Microalgae, Biotechnology and Microbiology*. Cambridge Univ. press. Cambridge, U.K.

Bohra C. and Kumar A.(2004). Plankton diversity in the wetlands of Jharkhand. In: *Biodiversity and Environment* (Ed. A. kumar) ABD Pub. New Delhi. pp. 91.

Cairns J. Jr. Mc Cormic P. V. and Nitherlehner B. R. (1994). Bioassay and field assessment of pollution effects. In: *Algae and water pollution*. (*Eds*. Rai L. C, Gaur J. P. and Soider C. J.) Schweizerbort'sch Verlagsbuchhanlung. Stuggert. pp. 267.

Chapman V. J. and Chapman D. J.(1973). *The Algae*. ELBS Publication, Macmillan Press. London. pp. 54.

Das R. N. and Sahu R. (1989). Chloroccocales from freshwater habitats of Ranchi. *Vegetos* (2) 2: 223-229.

De Lang E.(1994). *Mannual of simple water quality analysis.* International Water Tribunal (IWT) Foundation, Amesterdam.

Guru, S.D. and Sahu Radha (2006). Morphological variations in Stigeoclonium (Chlorophyceae) in polluted water in water. *Bionature,* 26 (2): 55-59.

Guru, S. D. (2007a). Effect of Xenobiotic pollution on the algal (Chlorophyceae) population of some freshwater lakes of Jharkhand. *Biospectra,* 2 (1): 143-147.

Guru,S. D.(2007b). A comparative study of the species richness and diversity of chlorophycean assemblage of two city based polluted tanks of Ranchi. *Biospectra,* 2 (2): 343-345.

Guru, S. D. (2007c). Survival Strategies for Medicinal Plants. *Recent Advances in Biological science* (in press).

Guru, S.D. (2007d). Limnological studies of freshwater bodies of Ranchi. *Trans. Zool. Soc. East India,* (in press).

Guru,S. D. (2007e). Prospect of Biomonitoring of Pollution in aquatic system by Algal (Chlorophyceae) Assessment. *Indian J. Environ. and Ecoplan.* 14 (3): 651-654.

Guru, S.D. (2007f). Distribution and biodiversity of desmids in a freshwater lake of Ranchi. *Vegetos,* 20 (2): 81-85.

Guru, S. D. (2008a). Distribution and Biodiversity of Chlorococclean Flora in the Phytoseston of a Freshwater lake. *Journal of Phytological Research,* 21(1).

Guru, S. D. Sushma (2008). Species Richness of *Scenedesmus* (Chlorophyceae) in some sewage fed water bodies of Ranchi. *Bionature,* 28 (1): 1-4.

Hegewald E. and Silva P. (1998). Annotated catalogue of *Scenedesmus* and nomenclaturally related genera including original descriptions and figures. *Bibliotheca phycologica* 80. J. Cramer, Berlin-Stuttgart. Pp. 587.

Johnson J. L., Fawley M. W. and Fawley K. P.(2007). The diversity of *Scenedesmus* and *desmodesmus* (Chlorophyceae) in Itasca-State Park, Minnesota, USA. *Phycologia* 46: 214-229.

Kumar, N., Singh, N., and Agarker, M.S. (1986) Some rare and interesting chlorococcales from Jabalpur, M.P. Bionature, 6: 35-36.

Lewis L. A. and Flechtner V. R. (2004). Criptic species of *Scenedesmus* (Chlorophyta) from desert soil communities of western North America. *Journal of Phycology* 40: 1127-1137.

Misra P. K., Mehrotra R. K., Jai Prakash, Srivastava A. K. and Kishore S. (2002). Freshwater Planktonic algae from Basti. Uttar Pradesh. *Geophytology.* 30(1 and 2): 61-73.

Misra P.K., Srivastava,A.K. and Prakash, J (2003-2004). Structural abnormalities in some green algae from north-eastern part of Uttar Pradesh. *Geophytology* 33 (1 and 2):17-20.

Phillips D. J. H. and Rainbow P. S. (1993). *Biomonitoring of Trace Aquatic contaminants.* Elsevier Applied Science. New York.

Prescott G. W. (1962). *Algae of the Western Grate Lakes Area.* Koenigstein, West Germany. Pp. 977.

Shon Yun-Hee, Nam Kyung-Soo, Kim mi-kyung (2004). Cancer chemopreventive potential of *Scenedesmus* spp. Cultured in medium containing Gioreacted swine urine. *J. microbiol. Giotechnol.* 14: 158-161.

Suseela M. R. and Dwivedi S. (2005). Species diversity of Tola Lake, Uttar Pradesh. In "*Glimpses of Indian phycology*. (Eds. Keshri J. P and Kargupta A. N.) B.S.M.P.S. Publication. Dehra Dun. P. 333-340.

Trainor F. R. (1998). Biological aspects of *Scenedesmus* (Chlorophyceae)–phenotypic plasticity. *Nova Hedwigia* Beiheft 117, J. Cramer, Berlin. Pp. 367.

Voltolina D. Gomez-villa H, Correa G. (2004). Biomass production and nutrient removal in semicontinous culture of *Scenedesmus* sp. (chlorophyceae) in artificial wastewater under stimulated day night cycle. *VIE MILIEU*. 54: 21-25.

Microbial Biotechnology and Ecology (2011) *Pages* **780–826**
Editors: **Deepak Vyas, G.S. Paliwal, P.K.Khare and R.K Gupta**
Published by: **DAYA PUBLISHING HOUSE, NEW DELHI**

Chapter 47

Eco-Physiological Effects of Red Mud Waste of an Aluminium Industry on the Seed Biology of a Crop Plant

☆ *Alka Sahu, Anita R. Patnaik, R.K. Behera and A.K. Panigrahi*

Department of Botany, Berhampur University, Berhampur – 760 007, Orissa

Introduction

Pollution sources can be classified in various ways depending on the origin of pollutants, their main component, property and the effects etc. Very often the classification based on the origin of the pollutants is generally used, which categorizes the pollution sources into domestic, agricultural, industrial and mining. Domestic sewages mostly contain metabolic wastes, various detergent formulations, consumer products and significant amounts of trace elements, making them rich in organic matters and nutrients. The organic matters increase the BOD load of the receiving water bodies and render them unsuitable for the survival of the aquatic animals. The organic matters in the domestic sewages are mostly biodegradable and cause problem only when the rate of input into the environment exceeds the rate of degradation or dispersion. The addition of nutrients by the way of domestic sewage into the water bodies lead to eutrophication, which brings change in the community and the biological composition of inhabiting communities and populations.

Modern agriculture with its rapid mechanization and spreading of fertilizers, besides the use of protective treatments such as herbicides, insecticides, and fungicides exerts an increasing pressure on the natural environment. Some of these chemicals are non-biodegradable, and hence, persist in the ecosystem. These chemicals can be absorbed and concentrated by the living organisms via any mechanism or pathway. This phenomenon is known as bioaccumulation and creates various problems, especially when the pollutants are of high toxic nature with high biological half-life time. This is because the level of pollutants in an organism increases with the increase in its distance from the primary producer in the food chain, *i.e.* with increase in the trophic level. Thus, as a result of biomagnifications, the organisms placed at higher trophic level usually accumulate a persistent pollutant in its tissues to a concentration much greater than those present in the surrounding habitat. Industry is the third and the most important source of pollution. Over 75,000 chemicals are in common use today and several thousands of new compounds are being added to this figure each year (Cairns, 1980 and Miller, 1984). These chemicals are now, an inevitable part of the process of industrialization and mostly they are produced and used by the industry to deliver finished goods. Some of these chemicals, the by-products and the waste discharges of the industry are released inadvertently or accidentally into the environment to such an extent that they really threaten the ecosystem in global scale. The mining operations also contribute significantly to the cause of pollution. The exploitation of ore deposits invariably exposes fresh rock surfaces and large quantities of waste rock or soil to accelerate weathering. In addition, ore processing, smelting and refining operations caused dispersion and deposition of large quantity of chemicals into the water, air and soil of the surrounding environment.

Ramade (1977) has pointed out three principal causes of contamination of the environment. These are: (*i*) the production of energy from combustible fossils or from atom, currently this forms the basis of almost all human activity in industrialized countries and leads to many types of pollution, (*ii*) the chemical industry and its extraordinary expansion over the last few decades, more than half of million chemicals are currently in use, all over the world. (*iii*) Modern agriculture releases substantial quantities of chemicals into the environment by the use of fertilizers, herbicides, fungicides and mechanization. Entries of chemicals into the environment can be classified into three categories (Harris, 1976): point spills, chronic local releases and wide spread releases. By point spill it is meant that a significant amount of chemical has entered an ecosystem at a point in both space and time and the effects of contamination are expected in a well defined more or less local area. Generally this happens when a substance stored in large quantity is released suddenly into the environment. The Bhopal gas tragedy can be an example of this category, wherein 2500 people died and thousands were seriously affected by the accidental release of methyl iso-cyanate, a deadly poisonous gas, from a pesticide industry. Chronic local releases are cases in which discharges have taken place over such periods of time, and in such quantities, that a large region (for example, a river system, a catchments basin or the landscape downwind of a source) has been contaminated. Such a situation is in association with a large industrial or municipal source (Holdgate, 1979). There can be no better example than the Minamata Bay and the Niigata tragedy of mercury poisoning, for this kind of release. Wide spread releases are the release of substances in sufficient quantity and over a wide area. Such releases could result in a noticeable pollution of a significant part of the entire earth's surface. Though this type of release is yet to happen, there are examples of manufacture of a thousand substances in such quantities as to be capable of polluting the entire globe (Butler, 1978). One such situation of this type has arisen due to the increased release of Chlorofluorocarbons (CFCs) and Fluro-bromo-carbons into the atmosphere. This has resulted in progressive destruction of the ozone layer in the last decade, posting a serious threat to result global warming and greenhouse effect. This threat has been responded well in time by the world in the Montreal Protocol, an international treaty which will eliminates CFC use by the year 2000 AD (Hoffman, 1990). Another situation, very close to this, has occurred in the recent Gulf war, where several oil wells in Kuwait caught fire emitting huge quantities of smoke and shoot. These were carried by the wind to the neighboring states of Iraq and Iran covering most of their sky. Even shoot and carbon particles were found in the snowfall on the Himalayas of the Indian sub-continent.

The emission of pollutants into the environment is a complex phenomenon and cannot be limited to the fixed image of waste pipe spilling out its effluents into a lake or river. In almost all cases, substances discharged into the environment are going to be carried a long way from their source. Atmospheric and hydrologic circulation systems then disperse them progressively throughout the biosphere. The pollutants act in many ways on the living systems. Acute and/or long-term actions are the most obvious eco-toxicological impacts of a given pollutant. It results demo ecological effects at population levels, which are displayed through immediate or premature death, reduced reproductive success, reduced growth, and/or increased loss at the juvenile stages. These are ultimately reflected in the lower abundance and perturbed distribution of the exposed populations of sensitive species. The effect of the sub-lethal concentrations of some pollutants is by far the most frequent eco-toxicological problem and it can be far more noxious in the long run for the exposed species resulting in chronic deterioration of the ecosystem. The persistent non-biodegradable pollutants are absorbed by living organisms and are concentrated many times more than the concentration of the surrounding medium. Further, these bio-accumulated pollutants are passed from one trophic level to another and exhibit increasing concentration in organisms related to their trophic status resulting in bio-magnification.

Industrial Pollution and India

Industry is responsible for creating a fantastic array of new chemicals every year all of which eventually find their way into the environment. For most of these chemicals, not even the chemical formula is known and much less is known about their acute, chronic or genetic effect on the living organisms. At present, the industry is the focus of attention, the world-over, as the most important source of pollution of the environment. Chemical industry in India has grown up phenomenally since independence. There are today about 4000 chemical factories in India. They release large quantities of chemicals in the form of gas, liquid and solid wastes, into the environment. Many of these chemicals are toxic and create pollution problem. The problem of toxic hazard has already reached alarming proportions in this country and is bound to grow with increasing industrialization. India is the largest manufacturer of pesticides in the whole of South Asia and Africa. As many as 139 organic chemicals, heavy metals like zinc, lead, chromium, copper, mercury and various other compounds are used in the manufacture of dyes only. Sundaresan *et al.* (1983) have given the growth of industries dealing with toxic chemicals and generating toxic and hazardous wastes during 1950s, 1970s and 1980s, in India.

Industries are known to produce potentially toxic and hazardous wastes are the pesticides, dyes and pigments, organo-chemicals, fertilizers, non-ferrous metals, steel and chloro-alkali plants. The major foci of such industries in India are Bombay, Calcutta, Kanpur, Delhi, Chandigarh, Jamshedpur, Bokaro, Hyderabad, Vishakhapatnam, Madras, Baroda, Cochin etc. The wastes from the industry are generally disposed by land filling or released into water bodies. Generally the toxic effluents from industry are neutralized before their discharge, but still they contain substantial amount of toxic substances that can cause pollution. At present it is believed that rivers are most severely polluted by industries followed by estuaries, lakes and ocean in declining order. Extensive literature on the pollution of surrounding biota through the discharge of effluents and sludge from chlor-alkali industries is available (Weiss *et al.*, 1971; Suckcharoen, 1979 and 1980; Lodenius, 1980; Suckcharoen and Nourteva, 1982; and Lodenius and Tulisalo, 1984). Studies on loss of mercury into the environment from the chlor-alkali industry were carried-out by, Bouveng (1968 and 1972), and Ross (1974). Turney (1970) reported contamination of river Detrait by mercury discharges from a chlor-alkali plant, similar studies were also conducted by Matida and Kumada (1969) on the river Agano of Japan, by Suobodova and Hejtmanek (1976) on the Ohre river and Carlos (1979) on the Jab river of Papua, Newguinea. Hattula *et al.* (1978) indicated a severe pollution of the lake Paijane, which had received in past, the waste discharge from a caustic soda factory.

The purpose of acute toxicity test is to assess various abnormalities caused due to administration of a chemical to live systems on one occasion or other and to determine the order of lethality of the chemical. Many of the schemes are available at present, to test for adverse effects that may result when chemicals enter into the environment. In aquatic toxicology, acute lethal toxicity tests with the fish, seed germination of crop plants and invertebrates are usually intended to assess the numerical value of toxicity, to compare potentials of toxicants, to assess the effects of environmental variables on toxicity. Besides, statistical analysis of toxicity is essentially a tool in all these studies. The rapid increase in contamination of aquatic environments with industrial pollutants in recent years has resulted in an escalation of scientific interests in the biological effects of pollution. Because of the importance of crop in the aquatic environment, any deleterious effect of the toxicant on this is likely to be reflected on the entire ecosystem. Little information is available pertaining to the toxicity studies on crop plants due to the waste of industries. Metallic cations are highly essential for many enzymes to achieve their catalytic activity. These cations maintain the acid base balance; and are also highly essential for the ionic composition of the body fluids. Disturbance in electrolyte concentration are quite common in toxicity. Different studies on electrolyte change resulting from toxic status have produced a variety of diverse effects, because of differential size of toxic actions in the body. The reaction of mercury compounds with sulfahydryl groups has been well established. Bruin (1976) reported that cation movements within tissue cells originate from toxic effects on cellular membranes. Fungicides of diverse chemical structure are capable of changing mitochondria function, thereby making the membrane permeable to cation. Such cations are the mobile co-factors which either firmly bound to metal are called metaloenzymes or metal activated enzymes. Mercurials have long been recognised as agents interact with the poison proteins in general and enzymes in particular (Fox *et al.*, 1975). The DNA molecule is a target site of most, if not all, carcinogenic and mutagenic agents. Additionally, a number of agents are acutely cytotoxic to cells because, they damage the DNA. Numerous chemical agents damage DNA in vivo (Ahmad *et al.*, 1977; Ahuja and Subrahamanyam, 1978). Geener and Jeener (1952) reported the reduced RNA synthesis due to methyl mercury intoxication. Reports are available pertaining to the effects of pesticides on rat; pesticides induced DNA damage in cultured human cells (Ahmad *et al.*, 1977), reappraisal of lead on cell proliferation and influence of lead on nucleic acid metabolism in rat, effect of inorganic mercury on different biochemical parameters of freshwater fish (Panigrahi, 1980). Different aspects concerning the biochemical assessment of functional impairment in vital organs were explored in toxicological studies. Untoward effects can usually be traced back in the functional incompetence of organs. Whenever dysfunction occurs in a tissue it has its origin in biochemical abnormality may become apparent before the onset of morphological changes and precedes the development of chronic degenerative disease. Explanation of biochemical tests facilitates diagnosis of pre-toxic condition in man and it may be valuable in the routine screening of chemicals in animal experimentation. Biochemical studies are the useful tools in aiding diagnostic pathology, which covers a wide range embracing various organs and systems. Pesticides act either as a selective toxicant or may display rather a broad spectrum of adverse biological activities. Toxicant effects on growth may be studied by examining macromolecules involved in growth, such as DNA, RNA, amino acid and protein. Life depends on a complex network of chemical reactions brought about by a specific enzyme. The enzymes are the primary instruments for the expression of gene action. Enzymes are of biological importance in metabolic functions, which have the most highly specialized class of proteins. The change in metabolism can well be correlated with the disturbance in behavior and action of the enzymes (Panigrahi, 1984). The reduction in active metabolism has been correlated with the toxic effective different types of toxicants. The disturbance in enzymatic action can be related to the specific action of certain toxicants by inhibiting the enzymes to act, bind the active sites of the enzyme and enzymes become non functional due to disintegration. Inhibition of enzymes by chemical agents may be reversible or irreversible, competitive or noncompetitive. There are many different mechanisms through which thiol groups of enzymes can be acted upon by heavy metals. The importance of enzymatic studies in the system lies in the functional interpretation of the pollutant causing different types of disorders. Membranes play a role in the structure and function of the cell and its organelles. One of the way by which membranes can affect cellular metabolism is by interacting with enzymes. Some membrane function as the organizing matrix for enzyme systems, the micro environment in all these cases at or near the membrane surface may modulate the activities of the enzymes located in the region.

No information is available on the effects of Red Mud wastes of Aluminium industry on biota. Few preliminary reports and news publications are only available on pollution problems of NALCO plant. Unfortunately, NALCO plant has received the best award for pollution control and management.

The Industry Under Study

The products of his own activities have always burdened man. Hence, the present situation that exists is different from the historic one, in several important ways. Amongst which, the most important remarkable difference is the way at which man has contributed to the environment, both good and bad. This difference is mostly due to inter related phenomena *i.e.* growth of population, increasing urbanization and rapid industrialization. Every underdeveloped or developing country aiming to be highly developed, explore nature and tried to find out methods and adopted industrial revolution, leaving behind the consequence of such trend. When the problems of environmental status and quality was taken into consideration it became apparent that, it was not enough to alleviate undesirable consequences of man's activities by technological means or to prevent them forbidding certain practices of the are of certain chemicals.

Rapid industrialization and exploitation of natural resources on massive scale, accumulated undesirable substances in huge quantity thus, pollute the environment. Pollution is caused due to deliberate or unavoidable discharge of industrially produced wastes. These pollutants causing health hazards and definite and undesirable problems to flora and fauna, apart from influencing the ecological balance and brings significant climatic changes. The field under study refers to the Allumina industry specifically to Mining and Refinery complex, NALCO, Damanjodi in the district of Koraput, Orissa, India. For analysis of various factors of pollution in Allumina industry it becomes imperative for us to discuss the manufacturing process from ore mining to refining in brief with reference to NALCO. The allumina is extracted in two main stages *i.e.* Mining operation and Ore refinery. The ore of Alluminium *i.e.* Bauxite mine is situated at Panchaputamali in the district of Koraput, Orissa. It is at the height of 400ft from sea level. NALCO has marked 17sq. Kilometers of its area for getting deposited Bauxite. 370 million tones deposit in estimated. The mining capacity of NALCO is 24,00,000 tpa and being expanded to 48,00,000 tpa. The method used to mine Bauxite includes exploration and mine planning, removal of topsoil and over burdened and excavation of ore blasting operation. The hard cap rock at the surface is blasted to allow it to be mined together with the ore beneath. Heavy earth moving equipment's like dozer, back-end hoe, front-end loader and dampers etc. are used for mining and transporting operations. Then the ore is crushed by single state double roll tooth crusher of 900 tpa for each transportation and dispatched by various means to the refinery complex, which is done by a long cable conveyer belt systems of 14.6 Km long at single figat multy curve with 900tph capacity at M and

R complex. Damanjodi. It is the longest conveyer belt of the world. The entire distance from the mining site to refinery complex, the air of the area looks cloudy due to heavy dust loading from operation and open transportation by conveyer belt. In the course of mining exploration and transportation, minute dust particles looked like the labourers working in that area as well as the inhabitants residing nearby inhaled few particles. This air heavily loaded with dust or suspended particles cause lung cancer and tuberculosis. A health report indicated that high percentage of the inhabitants suffer from these two diseases and also respiratory distress and bronchitis: Not only the human beings are affected but also this pollution spoils very valuable flora of the environment due to heavy deposition of red coloured dust. The dust are deposited on the green leaves of the plants, reducing the incidence and trapping of sunlight, coming from sun, the only and ultimate sources of energy. Thus reducing the photosynthetic efficiency of plants. It is also noted that during the transportation by conveyer belt, huge amount of crushed Bauxite powders are dispersed, mixed with air, thus, the inhabitants are suffering a lot. Many news items appeared on this issue in different Newspaper and public reacted very badly opposing the way the area is being polluted.

Due to the set up of the industry, not only 17 Km^2 of PANCHAPUTAMALI hills will be deforested but also 1742acres of acquired land were subjected to deforestation, disappearance of valuable flora and disappearance of wild life. The NALCO project-plantation program in barren lands thus reclaimed by back filling and on the two sides of the newly constructed roads. But yet this did not fulfill the purpose of reappearance of the forest species and lead to degradation of biodiversity. The noise and vibration due to continuous blasting and heavy machinery equipment caused noise pollution in the mining area. 'Environment Management Plan' At Allumina Refinery Complex. NALCO has taken all possible measures during construction and also taking all possible measures for monitoring the pollution control parameters so that no pollutant is allowed to be discharged from plant as process effluent or township effluent to the water body without treatment, conforming the IS norms.

Tree Plantation for Ecological Balance

Extensive tree plantation program has been started around for reforestation of the same area. It is very important as trees and forest moderate the climate. Micro- climate in the forested area is distinctly different from the adjoining non-forested area. This occurs mainly through their influence on wind, temperature and humidity. Evapo-transpiration process increased humidity and also lowered atmospheric temperature in the area. Trees not only assimilate CO_2 and release O_2 but also play an important role in trapping some toxic gases and particulate matter in the air. Hence forests function both as filters and sinks for air contaminants. It also reduced noise pollution and enrich aesthetic beauty of the area. For soil conservation and soil stabilisation work, small diversion dams and cross bounds are planned in down flow hills. As well as Lemon grass turfing, Mulberry plantation and cashew-nut plantation are planned. Yet after 14 years, no good forest has been developed. The Alumina plant is surrounded by hills in three sides. Under its "Green belt program" plantation was planned in three concentric rings. First ring of plantation was done in the surrounding hills. Second ring of plantation was carry out in the valley lands and third ring of plantation was done beyond the township area. In this program, first of all soil stabilization work by the sides of newly constructed road, crusher house pump and near conveyer were under taken. Over these dumps and hills sloped so far 1.5 lakhs of plants of different species were planted. Till so far the above green belt plantation is a dream and remained in a planning stage. Land scaping was take-up by planting flowering species like *Jacaranda* and *Cassia siama* of 50mts. width near bauxite storage area and in the township.

Proper program was made for heavy plantation of the hills surrounding the red mud pond and ash pond to keep the ecological balance of the area. The following steps were taken for afforestation of these hills after expansion of Red Mud Pond. (*i*) The D.F.O. Rayagada division under took the afforestation program in central hills. The species selected were mostly of every green in nature and a mixture of monocultures of cashew-nut, mango and jack fruit etc. were planned. (*ii*) With regard to the surrounding hill near Sundhipara and Kantagada afforestation will be taken up by planting:

1. *Accacia auriculiformis*
2. *Hybrid Eucalipatus* sp.
3. *Pongamia pinata* and
4. *Anacardium occidentale*

(*iii*) For stabilisation of the slopes by the sides of the guard land drains in RMP, Lemon grass and Palm rose oil grass will be planted Hills. But in these areas, the dry mud of the industry is being dumped in huge quantities. In future small hillocks of dry red mud will be formed. In rainy season, the leachates of those wastes might enter into the RMP pond. Hills surrounding RM Pond, Dumuriguda and Dengajanigada villages are also planned for afforestation program. The workers NALCO, Damanjodi as well as the tribal inhabitants are affected by the poisonous gases and ash emitted from the chimney. This also affects the natural life in that area. It is also seen that micro particles of allumina and ash emitted during the process are deposited on the leaves of the herb and trees and cause chlorosis. The physicians suspect the increasing number of patients suffering from asthma and lung cancer may also be due to inhalation of powdered allumina and ash from the plant along with the ore dust spread over the area.

Ore Refinery

The capacity of Allumina plant at NALCO, Damonjodi is 8,00,000 tpa and being expanded to capacity of 15,75,000 tpa. The ore refining is done by a classical process called BAYER's Process, in which the aluminum in the Bauxite is digested in caustic at 105°C and ultimately recovered by precipitation with the removal of impurities. After successive operation of digestion, desilication, setting and washing the precipitated hydrate *i.e.* $NaAl(OH)_4$ is filtered and calcined at 1000°C. There are two production stream of 4,00,000tpa capacity each atmospheric pressure digestion process is carried out at 107°C with energy efficient fluidised bed calciners of 1400tph (3 × 18.5MW) power is co-generated by use of back pressure turbine in steam generation plant. The residual mud is separated and pumped to the red mud pond.

Red Mud Pond

In the process of bauxite refining the red mud, which is generated after digestion is the major waste product. For 8 lakhs MT allumina production 10 lakhs MT of red mud is generated and is being discharged in red mud pond by 2nd stage pump in slurry form at the rate of $370m^3/hr$ with 150gps solid consistency and 2.3 gpl Na_2O the dry red mud flow in the RMP is 110MT/hr. To store such a huge quantity of red mud slurry, the Red Mud Pond has been constructed towards the west of refinery complex. Three earthen dams called Orissa Dam-1, 2 and 3, flank the Red mud pond. Fortunately or unfortunately natural hill ridges with high elevation surround the red mud pond. These three earthen dams connect the natural ridges. The Orissa Dam-1 is towards east *i.e.* towards the refinery complex, the Orissa Dam-2 towards north, the Orissa Dam-3 is towards west *i.e.* opposite to dam-1 to dam1 this dam separated RMP from ash pond area. Hill ridges with high elevation covered South of the pond.

Orissa dam-2 has a natural hill ridge with 930 meters elevation. No spill way is provided in the dams to avoid spillage contamination to natural nalaha. Elevation of dams during the first phase is 930 meters the anticipated life is for 3.5 years. It is planned to expand the elevation up to 945 mts and 957 meters during second and 3rd phase operation. The anticipated life of the pond is 7 and 11 years respectively.

The initial elevation of RMP was 905 mts at different increased elevations the catchment area and the capacity of RMP are given below. At 920 mt elevation catchment area is 16.544 hectares with total capacity of 301×10^4 m^3 at present elevation *i.e.* system which needs very less area for the disposal and stacking of 930 meters the area is raised up to 108.6 Hectares and 1016.17×10^4 m^3 capacity. After second phase expansion up to 945 meters; the area will be raised to 187 Hectares with capacity of 3305.87×10^4 m^3. At final phase of expansion up to 957 meters elevation the total catchments area of the pond will be 212.40 hectares with total capacity of 5728.82×10^4 m^3 with 2mts free board. After the life of the red mud pond is over, one area has been already ear marked during the feasibility study for the construction of second pond. Horizontal expansion of red mud pond is feasible to certain extent. During last 3 years it is noted that the pond level is rising abnormally due to more precipitation than evaporation at Damanjodi. In order to check the pond water level the alkaline water is returned back from the pond and is recycled for use in plant various process mainly to carry fresh generation of red mud slurry as a result alkalinity of the pond water is increasing day by day. The shore of this pond is extremely affected. The water of the pond is toxic to the plants. Although the life of the dam in phase-I is over, yet the second phase expansion work has not started, rather in order to explore the long-term solution to the wet tailing system, Dry mud disposal system, which needs very less area for the disposal and stacking of dry mud. It does not call for construction of large earthen dams. The system multiplies alkalinity of the area of dispersal. The run-off leachates of red mud stacked near RMP are entering into the pond with rainwater. This is also an addition to the alkali strength to the RMP water instead of diluting it.

Table 47.1: Analysis of Mud of RMP

Parameter (per cent)	*Sample–I*	*Sample–II*	*Sample–III*
Al_2O_3	19.11	16.60	18.56
Fe_2O_3	56.88	57.93	58.77
TiO_2	4.56	4.03	4.15
SiO_2	5.97	6.67	6.94
Na_2O	3.86	4.40	4.10
pH	9.90	10.02	10.06
Return water pH	14	–	–
NaOH	30-35 per cent	–	–
Na_2CO_3	65-70 per cent	–	–

NALCO the Industry

National Aluminium Co. Limited (NALCO) is considered to be a turning point in the 50 years old history of Indian Aluminium Industry. In a major leap forward NALCO has addressed itself to the country's need for self sufficiency in aluminium as well given the country a technology edge in making this strategic metal on the best of world standard. NALCO was set up in 1981, in the public

Table 47.2: Physical Properties of Alumina

	Typical	*Guaranteed Range*
LOI (300-1000° C) per cent	0.6–0.8	0.5–1.0
BET surface area (M^2/gm)	60–70	60–80
Alpha Aluminium content per cent	–	10 Max.
Granulometry		
+125 Micron (per cent)	–	15 Max.
–45 Micron (per cent)	10	12 Max.

Chemical Properties

	Typical	*Limit*
Al_2O_3(per cent)	98.7	98.5 Min.
Na_2O (per cent)	0.38	0.5 Min.
Fe_2O_3 (per cent)	0.01	0.015 Max.
SiO_2 (per cent)	0.012	0.02 Max.
CaO (per cent)	0.042	0.050 Max.

Alumina Hydrate: Physical Properties

	Typical	*Maximum*
LOI (110–1000°C) per cent	34–36	36
Moisture	3–6	8

Granulometry

	Typical	*Maximum*
–45 Micron (per cent)	3–6	7

Chemical Properties

	Typical	*Max/Min*
Al_2O_3 (per cent)	65+0.5	64 Min.
Na_2O (per cent) Total	0.23–0.30	0.33 Max.
Na_2O (per cent) Soluble	0.015–0.025	0.30 Max.
SiO_2 (per cent)	0.007–0.010	0.016 Max.
Fe_2O_3 (per cent)	0.006–0.008	0.016 Min.
Hydrate Content (per cent)	99.0	98.5 Min.

sector, following a major investment decision of government of India in 1980,to exploit a part of large deposit of Bauxite, discovered in the east coast in 1975. Aluminium Pechiny of France provided the technology and basic engineering for Bauxite refinery, smelter and mine. The project cost of Rs.2408 crore was partly financed by Rs.1119 crore equivalent of Euro- dollar lone extended by a consortium of international banks. The project was most expeditiously implemented, different, segments of NALCO want into production in a phased manner from November 1985 sale of Aluminium was commercial on May 1987 and export was started on September 1988. Initially 1987-88 the Aluminum production was 160,000 tones the production rate remarkably increased to 807000 tones in 1995-96, in 1996-97, 840,000 MT and in 1997-98 it was 883,000 MT and has chartered a course of international confidence in India's industrial capability. To day NALCO has emerged as the largest integrated Bauxite Alumina -Aluminium complex in Asia, enabling India to witness a quantum jump in Alumina and Aluminium production. NALCO produces calcined allumina at refinery complex, Damanjodi with following specifications.

Topology and Location

The mines and refinery complex of NALCO, Damonjodi is situated Similiguda block, under Potangi tahasil in the district of Koraput, Orissa state, India. From the district head quarter Koraput, it is 38 kilometers towards southeast on road, *i.e.* 27 kms towards south in NH-43 up to Similigude junction and further 11kms towards east on project road. It is 60 kms from Jeypore, the oldest city of Koraput district. It is 560 Kms away from Bhubaneswar the state capital city of Orissa and 172 kms from Visakhapatnam (A.P), nearest air port. Damonjodi is at a highest of about 1300 mts from sea level, located at latitude 18°-6′–18°-58′ towards North and longitude 82°.57′-83°.04′ East. The area enjoys an annual rainfall of 1723 mm in 1998. The relative humidity of area ranges from a minimum of 47 per cent in April and maximum of 85 per cent in July 1998. The temperature of the area varied from a minimum of 15°C to maximum 35°C in 1997-98 and from a minimum of 9°C to maximum of 42°C in 1998-99. Southeast side is covered by Deomali hill range. The slope of the area is towards the northwest. A small river Karandia is flowing near by the Refinery complex and the Damanjodi township. It carries almost all the emissions of the plant and township. At its down stream mixed with the Kolab River at its catchment area of Upper Kolab project near Sunabeda.

Affected Area

As we know the Red Mud pond is situated in such a place that the pond water is restricted by high hill ridges at south, ash pond at west separated Orissa dam-3. But at its north seepage is marked as a natural nalaha at its down stream about 100mts away from Orissa Dam-2 of RMP. This seepage might be due to the storage of huge quantity of effluent at a high level from the original point of leaching. The leachates gradually flow downwards mixed with natural nalaha and ultimately enter into the crop field. These leachates from RMP gone down in its slope towards the river Karandi in the north west direction and finally mixes with the river Kolab near Sunabeda. As a result, cultivators of villages, Sukuriguda, Janigada, Dengajaniguda, Kharaguda, Khajuriguda, Kalapadar and other village in the vallery, depending on the water source for their agricultural purpose are being harassed. The contaminated water in the catchment area of upper kolab project is being lifted for Sunabeda as well as Damanjodi town-ship for all domestic use and human consumption. Ultimately this polluted water flows down along the river and being used by the inhabitants of Jeypore town as well as the village at the riverbank.

Toxic Effects

The leachates at its initial point is highly alkaline in nature with Fe, Al, Ti, Na ions the pH of it ranging from 9 to 10 even more. Gradually when the leachates entered into the rice crop field, it influenced the rice plants very badly. The cultivators generally use the medium high yield and resistant variety (Lalat). Due to the effects of toxic chemicals rice plants do not grow well. It is found that the soil colour of the crop field changed to violet red with high caustic smell. On the stem, and leaf lamina radish colouration is developed ultimately resulting chlorosis. Straw-yellow long slender grains of lalat variety of rice do not reproduce; the size became smaller with development of reddish brown colour on the seed grains as well as on the panicle. The peduncle was weak to bear the load of the inflorescence. At the alternate year the seedlings could not be established due to less rainfall during month of the crop (May-June), the concentration of the leached chemicals became very high with pH more than 8.

Year Wise Study

In 1995, it is studied that the rice plant become very short, reddish colour spots developed on leaf lamina and on the stem. Roots became thickened and curled and number of lateral roots is relatively less. The grain size is remarkably reduced and the colour of the grain was brick red instead of straw yellow. The husk production is relatively more. In 1996, from the study in the field it is observed that- maximum seedlings after germination attained an height of 6" to maximum 1ft (at low density of pollution area), the rottening of roots started the seedling could not be established within a period of 25 to 30 days. These effects ultimately resulted nil production that year. This happened due to increased alkalinity on the crop field (pH –<10) for less rail fall during first month (April-May). The colour of the soil in the crop fill was violet red with high caustic smell.

In the year 1997, the rainfall during the period of seed germination was better then the last year. Hence alkalinity of the leachate contaminated crop field was also relatively low (pH–7.68). It also found that the typical effects due to the toxic leachate were lesser as we go far from the RMP. In that year the typical symptoms reappeared as on the 1995. Through personal interview with the cultivators of the nearby village Sukriguda, it was reported that-

1. In general the production rate is decreasing every year.
2. Before the construction of RMP, the production of Lony baele was good.
3. Rice grain size became smaller.
4. Seed colour turned reddish.
5. Red colouration developed on the leaf lamina and the stem.
6. Root was not well developed, no lateral roots are less and those are thickened and curled.
7. Most of the rice plants are affected by chlorosis.
8. Peduncles were so week that, they do not bear the load of the inflorescence.

Other Effects

The general public opinion flashed several times in local dailies and weekly news papers that the undesirable waste emissions of NALCO mixing with water bodies, pollute the river and the reservoir, which man used. It was reported in one of the newspaper that, there is every possibility of loosing the memory power as well as reproduction ability by animals including man, if the polluted water is used for consumption. It is published in a newspaper that by using the contaminated water for drinking purpose, many people suspected their deafness and some have lost their reproductive ability. Now users report different types of skin diseases caused by polluted water is to be because of the contamination. On the present issue/problem many physicians have expressed their fear and also apprehension that in future, this industry causing pollution may create wide spread health hazards. Not only the human community is facing hazards but also animals, aquatic flora and fauna are also affected. It is expected that the toxic pollutants might be accumulated in the body of the contaminated fishes, which can be observed from the symptoms like the scale souring. Some time heavy emission lead to fatal condition of fish and aquatic organism. The abnormal deposit of red mud in the red mud pond and increasing in alkalinity of red mud pond water may become a future threat for the people near by locality in Koraput district, because of heavy leaching from the red mud pond.

Keeping in view; the leaching of chemicals from the Red mud pond of the industry (Damonjodi) and entry of these chemicals into paddy fields of the locality and runoff water of the dumps during rainy seasons and its entry into paddy fields and their possible effect on the crop plant in the crop fields, this project was undertaken to evaluate the eco-toxicological effects of the leached wastes on the germination, seedling growth and establishment of the rice plant, *Oryza sativa*, L.

Materials and Methods

Study Material

The seeds of *Oryza sativa* L. (Cult: LALAT, OR 26.2014-14) [Parentage-OBS 677/IR 2071/VIKRAM/W1268, Released by Orissa] was selected as test material for this study. The pure line seeds were collected from O.U.A.T. Rice Research Center, Jeypore Branch, Koraput. Before conducting any investigation, the seeds were further sampled by hand sieving and sorting, to obtain healthy and uniform seeds.

Choice of the Test Material

1. A popular early and high yielding variety of rice, found to be suitable for cultivation in medium and high lands.
2. Grains of this variety show high percentage of germination both in the field and in laboratory conditions.
3. It is cultivated in all seasons and in various agro-climatic conditions because of its special type of physiological adaptations such as: Weak photosensitivity and minimal variation in physiological processes in response to climatic changes.
4. Seed disinfections is recommended for this variety as seeds and seedlings/plants are very much susceptible to fungal, bacterial and viral pathogens rather than insects and pests. This variety is resistant to Gall fly, BPH, sheath rot and medium resistant to stem borer.
5. Adopted to direct seed sowing and also by transplantation methods.

Some important information about Cult: Lalat of *Oryza sativa* L. as relevant to this piece of work is detailed as follows:

Important Technical Information About the Seed Material (Rice)

A) Cultivation Manual

1. Name of the cultivar: Lalat
2. Type: Medium high yielding resistance variety (Irrigated type). This can also be used in non-irrigated land, widely cultivated by the cultivators of Koraput.
3. Suitability: For both high and medium land

4. Duration: 125-130 days
5. Sensitivity: Weakly photoperiod sensitive can be grown in various agro-climatic conditions.
6. Tillering ability: 299/25 plants or 10-12/plant
7. Average plant height: 85-90 cm (80.7cm (av.)
8. Plantation practice: 15 × 15 cm. Distance to be maintained between plants during plantation.
9. Seed quantity/acre: 30 Kg.
10. Leaf sheath colour: Yellowish green; Spikelet colour: Straw yellow; Kernel colour: White
11. Panicle length: 22.2cm
12. Yield: 45 quintal/hectre (Average)

B) About Grain Character

1 Average no. of grains/panicle: 124 ± 08
2. Grain type: Long and slender
3. Length/breadth of the grain: 8.5/2.5
4. Number of grains/Kg.: 45000

Test Chemical

The leached chemicals of the red mud pond of the NALCO plant prepared in the laboratory have been used as the test chemical for the experimental study. The red mud collected from RM pond is air dried, powdered and sieved. A known (2kg.) quantity of dried powder is mixed with known amount (2lit.) of distilled water and stirred for 15 days. The mixture was allowed to stand for one day and the supernatant was decanted and again passed through a multisieve soaking and filtering system and the obtained extract is the leached chemical of the waste, which is stored for future experiments. This is the red mud extract and known as the test toxicant.

Study of Seed Viability

The seeds were soaked with different concentrations of test solution from 12h to 96h. After scheduled period of exposure, the grains were washed with tap water, followed by distilled water and their viability were tested according to the procedure of Moore (1969). The result was expressed as percentage of mortality.

Germination Study

Before the utilization of seeds in the field, the germination studies must be conducted under controlled and standardized laboratory conditions, because:

1. Results of germination test should be known before sowing.
2. Care can be taken to reproduce the results of laboratory conditions in the field condition.
3. The maximum germination potential of the seed lot can be known easily.
4. Undesirable factors can be eliminated, so that influence/effect of test extract can be sorted and without any interference.

But all these above conditions are neither possible nor practicable in field conditions (Annonymous, 1989). Hence for germination, the sterilized petridishes with sterilized absorbent cotton and blotting paper were utilized. Always twenty-five seeds were kept in each petridish and each treatment including control. For germination and growth studies mainly two types of treatments were carried out:

1. Short-term treatment in recommended concentrations of toxicant in petriplates both in racks and seed germinator.
2. Long term treatment in experimental concentrations of the toxicant in pot culture.

Short-term experiments were conducted in petriplates. A selected concentration of the extract was applied and the constancy of the medium was maintained both in open rack culture condition and in Seed Germinators. Long-term experiments were conducted in pot cultures. Where exact amount of dried red mud powder was mixed with soil: biological fertilizer mixture and water was added daily to maintain constancy.

In short term experiments readings were noted after 144hrs of exposure. In long term experiments, the parameters were studied after 15, 30, 45 and 60 days of exposure. In the third type of investigation, the seeds were treated with different concentrations of RM leached chemical for 24 hours and then kept for germination in those concentration media, as the seeds were soaked previously. For this experiment, a graded series of concentrations of the toxicant was prepared for this pilot test considering the actual amount of the test chemical present and the amount of this test chemical available in the affected areas at Damonjodi, Koraput. On the next day, 2nd dose was given *i.e.* petridishes were supplied with same quantity of freshly prepared solutions of different concentrations. On the next day, 3rd dose was given to compensate the possibility of biological detoxification, oxidation or loss of the toxicant in the process of evaporation. Then after the set was regularly supplied with distilled water at an interval of 12 hour. In all sets, the seeds were allowed to germinate in normal photo inductive cycles, normal humid atmosphere and at a temperature of $30 \pm 2^{\circ}$ C for 48 hours. After 48 hours of normal soaking and incubation, all seedlings were transferred to growth chamber (Culture rack and Seed Germinator [Remi].

To calculate the percentage of germinations, periodical observations were made at an interval of 24 hours from 48 hours to 144 hours. First emergence of coleorhiza (Referred as Root) about 2 mm. in length was considered as normal germination, so also appearance of coleoptile (Referred as Shoot) before emergence of coleorhiza was considered as abnormal germination. From this pilot test, a range was selected by visual screening and percentage of germination and percentage of seedling establishment was noted. The seeds were allowed to grow in petridishes in growth chamber. Visual screening was carried out basing on the growth and the percentage of seed germination and percentage of seedling establishment was also calculated. A test was run within the expected range to select the concentrations for the study.

Study of Seedling Growth (Petriplate Culture)

In petriplate culture, first the petriplates are cleaned with tap water then with chromic acid and then tap water and finally with double distilled water, and dried in an oven. Twenty-five soaked seeds were sown in petriplates at uniform distance in all the sets. All petriplates were kept at room temperature and normal photo-inductive cycle was maintained by providing light from fluorescent tubes in daytime. For all other studies, seeds were grown up to seedling establishment stage (up to 7th day of exposure to the toxicant), inside petriplates in different concentrations of the toxicant including control set, as it was done in germination studies. On each 7th day of exposure, seedlings were harvested for respective experimental analysis. From the above-recorded parameters, three concentrations were selected. Future experiments were conducted at LC_0 (MAC value–Maximum Allowable Concentration) LC_{10}, LC_{50} and

LC_{90} values, to find out the effects of the toxicant on the growth performance of crop plant, *Oryza sativa* L. Same concentrations were selected for pot culture experiments and three doses of the toxicant was applied.

Table 47.3

Lethal Concentration	*Concentration of the RM Leachate*
LC_0 (A)	0.21 per cent
LC_{50} (B)	1.25 per cent
LC_{90} (C)	2.02 per cent

Values were selected from the toxicity test.

In future experiments always ten seeds were kept in each petridish and each treatment including control instead of twenty five seeds as was done in pilot tests.

Study of Morphological Parameters

Shoot and Root Length

From each replicate shoot and root lengths were measured, with the help of a scale.

Shoot and Root Weight

Seedlings from each replicate were taken. The shoots were separated from the roots. These were washed thoroughly, surface dried with the help of blotting paper. Then fresh weight of roots and shoots was taken separately by a single pan electric balance.

Pigment Studies

The amount of total chlorophyll and total phaeophytin was calculated by using the formula given by Vernon (1960). The amount of carotene was calculated by using the formula given by Davies (1976).

$$\text{Total chlorophyll (mg g}^{-1}) = (6.45 \times \text{OD at 665 nm}) + (17.22 \times \text{OD at 649 nm})$$

$$\text{Total phaeophytin (mg g}^{-1}) = (6.75 \times \text{OD at 666 nm}) + (26.03 \times \text{OD at 655 nm})$$

$$\text{Carotene content (mg)} = \frac{\text{D V K}}{2500 \times 100}$$

where,

D = Optical density at 475 nm, V = Volume of the extract, K = Dilution factor, 2500 = Specific extinction coefficient at 475 nm

Oxygen Evolution and Consumption Measurements

The evolution of oxygen due to photosynthesis and consumption of O_2 in respiration were measured manometrically with the help of a Photo-warburg's apparatus (New Paul, India) following the procedure of Hannan and Patouillet (1972) and Oser (1965). Rate of photosynthesis was expressed in ml of O_2 evolved hr/1 g of the plant and respiration rate was expressed in ml of oxygen consumed hr^{-1} g^{-1} of leaf of the plant. The GPP (Gross Primary Production) and NPP (Net Primary Production) values were calculated from the values obtained from both the oxygen evolution and oxygen consumption studies.

ATPase activity studies: The enzyme activity was studied following the method described by Sahu (1987). Estimation of inorganic phosphate by molybdenum blue method (Martineck, 1970) was followed.

Estimation of Nitrogen: Nitrogen was estimated by Nesslerization method (Herbert *et al.*, 1971).

Estimation of Glucose: The glucose was estimated following Herbert's method (Herbert, 1971).

Results

Healthy selected seeds were exposed to graded series of concentrations of leached chemicals of the red mud waste in sterilized petriplates, to find out the lethal concentration and percent survival values for the present set of experiments. Series of pilot tests were conducted and the experiments were repeated at least thrice to determine the lethal concentration values. The Table 47.4 indicate the percent survival (PS) and lethal concentration (LC) values for the leached chemicals of the red mud waste.

Table 47.4: Per cent Survival and Lethal Concentration values, when Rice Seeds were Exposed to Leached Chemicals of the Red Mud Waste

Percent (PS) Survival Value	*Concentration of the Toxicant (per cent, v/v)*	*Lethal Concentration (LC) Value*
PS_{100}	0.075	LC_0
PS_{90}	0.2	LC_{10}
PS_{50}	1.25	LC_{50}
PS_{10}	2.0	LC_{90}
PS_{00}	2.2	LC_{100}

During lethal concentration studies, seeds and seedlings were carefully watched to find out the abnormalities during seed germination and seed establishment. No significant morphometric changes were observed. Blackening of the shoot at the base of the exposed seedlings was marked. The entire root became black after few days of exposure. Some of the plants became pure white, the green colour of the plant totally disappeared. Control seedlings remained clinically healthy. After prolonged exposure, the exposed seedlings became brown and dry. At very high concentrations, roots became small and less in number.

Cent percent germination after 144hrs of exposure was recorded in the control and at 0.1 and 0.2 per cent RM extract. The percentage of seed germination decreased with the increase in RM extract concentration. No germination was recorded beyond 2.6 per cent RM extract. Cent percent seedling establishment was recorded in control and 0.1 and 0.2 per cent RM extract. Seedling establishment decreased with the increase in the RM extract. No seedling establishment was recorded beyond 2.2 per cent RM extract (Table 47.5). Basing on the data, 0.2 per cent RM extract concentration was considered as 'A', where cent percent seed germination and seedling establishment was recorded, as maximum allowable concentration for the toxicant under study. Concentration 'B' and concentration 'C' were selected basing on the same data, where approximately 50 per cent and 10 per cent germination and seedling establishment were recorded. The correlation coefficient analysis indicated the existence of highly significant ($P \leq 0.001$) correlation between percentage of seed germination and toxicant concentration in petriplate culture. But in case of pot culture, non-significant negative correlation existed at 24 and 48 hrs of germination. At 72 hrs of exposure, significant ($P \leq 0.05$) correlation existed and beyond this period higher significant level ($P \leq 0.01$) was observed.

Table 47.5: Changes in Seed Germination, Seedling Establishment, Shoot and Root Length, Ratio Value and Per cent Change Value, when Compared to Control, of 144 hrs Old Rice Seedlings, Grown in Different Concentrations of the Toxicant in Petriplate Culture. Data calculated from the mean of the samples ± standard deviation.

Concentration of the Toxicant	*Percentage of Seed Germination*	*Percentage of Seedling Establishment*	*Shoot Length, in cms*	*Root Length, in cms*	*Root/ Shoot Length Ratio*	*Percent Change in Shoot Length*	*Percent Change in Root Length*
Control	100	100	8.12±0.31	8.96±0.22	0.91	--	--
0.2 per cent (A)	100	100	8.16±0.42	7.11±0.08	1.15	+0.9	-20.64
1.25 per cent (B)	48	32	3.14±0.14	2.42±0.04	1.29	-61.33	-72.99
2.0 per cent (C)	20	12	1.14±0.32	0.84±0.06	1.36	-85.96	-90.62

In the control set, 100 per cent seed germination and 100 per cent seedling establishment was observed. In concentration A (0.2 per cent), all the seeds germinated and 100 per cent seedlings established. To conduct experiments in the seed germinator the selected concentrations were: A–0.2 per cent, B–1.25 per cent, C–2.0 per cent. In concentration B, 48 per cent seeds germinated, out of which only 32 per cent germinated seedlings established. The rest died because of the toxicant. In concentration C, seeds swelled and the seeds started germinating but 72 per cent seeds could not reach to 2mm size to be counted as germinated. At this stage, no further germination or prolongation of plumule was marked. In case of 'C' only 14 per cent seedlings established with stunted growth. No germination was marked beyond 2.2 per cent of the toxicant. The rest 14 per cent seeds though germinated but these germinated seeds could not establish altogether (Tables 47.5 and 47.6). The percentage of germination decreased showing negative significant correlation at all exposure periods except 24h and 144h, where non-significant correlation was marked. The two-way analysis of variance ratio test indicated that there was no significant difference between rows and columns.

Table 47.6: Changes in Seed Germination, Seedling Establishment, Shoot and Root Length, Ratio Value and Per cent Change Value when Compared to Control, of 144 hrs Old Rice Seedlings, Grown in Different Concentrations of the Toxicant in Pot Culture. Data calculated from the mean of the samples ± standard deviation.

Concentration of the Toxicant	*Percentage of Seed Germination*	*Percentage of Seedling Establishment*	*Shoot Length, in cms*	*Root Length, in cms*	*Root/ Shoot Length Ratio*	*Percent Change in Shoot Length*	*Percent Change in Root Length*
Control	100	100	9.6±0.4	9.1±0.3	1.05	--	--
0.2 per cent (A)	100	100	10.2±0.8	8.2±0.7	1.24	+6.25	-9.89
1.25 per cent (B)	48	32	5.4±0.2	3.2±0.4	1.69	-43.75	-64.83
2.0 per cent (C)	28	14	2.1±0.3	1.1±0.4	1.91	-48.12	-87.91

The shoot length declined from 8.12 ± 0.31 cm to 1.14 ± 0.32 cm at 0.2 per cent of the toxicant. No shoot was present in concentration beyond 2.2 per cent of the toxicant. A maximum of 85.96 per cent decrease in shoot length was marked at concentration C, when compared to the control value. The root length of the control seedling was 8.96 ± 0.22 cm and the root length declined 7.11 ± 0.88 cm at conc. A and 2.42 ± 0.04 cm at conc. B and the length further decline to 0.84 ± 0.06 cm conc. C. In concentration A, 20.64 per cent, in conc. B., 72.99 per cent and in conc. C. 90.62 per cent decrease in root length was noted, when compared to the control value (Tables 47.5 and 47.6). The root/shoot length ratio increased from 0.91 to 1.15 in conc. A and to 1.29 in conc. B and 1.356 in conc. C. A maximum of 49.45 per cent increase in R/S ratio value was observed at conc. C of leached chemicals of the red mud waste. The shoot fresh weight increased from 32.91 ± 3.14 mg to 34.22 ± 5.82 mg at concentration A, where a maximum increase by 3.98 per cent was recorded. Where as, at higher concentration of the toxicant, the shoot weight decreased showing a maximum decrease by 74.63 per cent at concentration C. The changes in physiological variables in control and toxicant exposed rice seedlings in petriplate cultures. All the experiments were conducted in a seed germinator under controlled conditions, to evaluate the toxicity of the toxicant, excluding the effect of environmental variables. The shoot fresh weight declined from 32.91± 3.14 cm declined to 12.81±4.02 mg in conc. B and further depleted to 9.35 ± 2.14 mg in conc. C, where a maximum of 74.63 per cent decrease was recorded in conc. C. The root fresh weight decreased significantly from 18.5 ± 3.1 mg to 1.2 ± 0.4 mg at concentration C, where a maximum of 93.5 per cent decrease in root fresh weight was marked (Table 47.7). With the increase in toxicant concentration, the root weight significantly declined. Beyond 2.2 per cent toxicant concentration of the red mud waste, no root was seen. The root/shoot fresh weight ratio showed significant increase, when compared to the control value. The ratio value increased at all the three selected concentrations and the ratio value increased from 1.78 to 6.96 at concentration C. The shoot dry weight increased from 6.9 ± 0.2 mg to 7.10.4 mg at conc. A. With the increase in toxicant concentration, the shoot dry weight gradually decreased, when compared to control. A maximum of 88.4 per cent decrease at conc. C was recorded, when compared to control (Table 47.8).

Table 47.7: Changes in Shoot and Root Fresh Wt., Ratio Value, and Shoot and Root Dry Weight and Per cent Change when Compared to Control, of 144 hrs Old Rice Seedlings, Grown in Different Concentrations of the Toxicant in Petriplate Culture. Data calculated from the mean of the samples ± standard deviation.

Concentration of the Toxicant	*Shoot Fresh Wt., in gms*	*Root Fresh Wt., in gms*	*Root/Shoot Weight Ratio*	*Shoot Dry Wt., in gms*	*Root Dry Wt., in gms*	*Per cent Change in Shoot Weight*	*Per cent Change in Root Weight*
Control	32.9±3.14	18.5±3.1	1.78	6.9±0.2	3.6±0.4	---	---
0.2 per cent (A)	34.2±5.82	13.6±2.8	2.52	7.1±0.4	3.1±0.3	+3.98	-26.49
1.25 per cent (B)	12.8±4.02	4.9±1.4	2.61	2.1±0.3	1.2±0.1	-61.07	-73.51
2.0 per cent (C)	8.35±2.14	1.2±0.4	6.96	0.8±0.1	0.3±0.08	-74.63	-93.51

Table 47.8: Changes in Shoot and Root Fresh Wt., Ratio Value, and Shoot and Root Dry Weight and Per cent Change when Compared to Control, of 144 hrs Old Rice Seedlings, Grown in Different Concentrations of the Toxicant in Pot Culture. Data calculated from the mean of the samples ± standard deviation.

Concentration of the Toxicant	*Shoot Fresh Wt., in gms*	*Root Fresh Wt., in gms*	*Root/Shoot Weight Ratio*	*Shoot Dry Wt., in gms*	*Root Dry Wt., in gms*	*Per cent Change in Shoot Weight*	*Per cent Change in Root Weight*
Control	36.8±1.8	26.4±2.8	1.39	8.6±0.8	6.2±0.6	---	---
0.2 per cent (A)	41.6±2.8	14.9±4.2	2.79	9.2±0.4	4.1±0.3	+13.4	-43.56
1.25 per cent (B)	16.4±1.9	5.2±1.8	2.15	4.4±0.7	1.9±0.4	-55.43	-80.03
2.0 per cent (C)	9.2±0.8	1.8±0.6	5.11	1.6±0.3	0.7±0.2	-75.0	-93.18

The root dry weight also decreased with the increase in toxicant concentration. The root dry weight decreased from 3.6 ± 0.4 to 0.3 ± 0.08 mg at concentration C, when compared to control. The root/shoot dry weight ratio increased from 1.92 to 2.67 at conc. C. The increase in ratio value was not linear with the increase in toxicant concentration. A maximum 39.06 per cent increase in the dry weight of the root was recorded at concentration C (Tables 47.7 and 47.8). Only 8.85 per cent decrease in the root/shoot dry weight was recorded at conc. B, when compared to the control value. A careful examination of the percent values revealed that the variables studied showed lesser values in the exposed seedlings, when compared to the control value. The correlation co-efficient analysis revealed the existence of negative correlation between variables with the toxicant concentration and the percent decrease showed the existence of a positive correlation with the toxicant concentration. All the values were statistically significant. Another set of experiment was conducted to study the effect of the toxicant in pot culture. The obtained data can be compared with the data obtained in the seed germinator, when the environmental parameters were controlled. The shoot length declined from 9.6 ± 0.4 to 2.1 ± 0.3 cm at conc. C, where, a maximum of 78.12 per cent decrease was recorded. In petriplate culture, the decrease was 85.96 per cent and in pot culture the decrease was 78.12 per cent in shoot length. So here, 7.84 per cent benefit in shoot length was available in pot culture (Table 47.7). The benefit might be due to the interaction of environmental parameters and most important was the availability of nutrients in the soil. And in addition, the advantage of toxicant natural detoxification or binding of the toxicant with the soil might have played a crucial role in giving such advantage in the pot culture. The root length in pot culture declined from 9.1 ± 0.3 cm to 1.1 ± 0.4 cm at concentration C. The decrease was linear and steady with the increase in toxicant concentration, where a maximum of 87.91 per cent decrease was recorded. In petriplate culture, a maximum 90.62 per cent decrease was recorded. A difference of 2.71 per cent decrease, when compared to petriplate culture was marked at conc. C. In pot culture, this is not significant. The non-significant difference observed in the pot culture indicates significantly the adverse effect of the toxicant. The root/shoot length ratio increased showing a maximum increase by 81.90 per cent at concentration C. The shoot fresh weight increased from 36.8 ± 1.8 to 41.6 ± 2.8 mg at concentration A and than the fresh weight value decreased to 16.4 ± 1.9 mg at conc. B. The shoot fresh weight declined at concentration C, showing a maximum decline by 75 per cent, when compared to control. The decrease in shoot fresh weight was again linear, with the increase in toxicant concentration except at conc. A (Table 47.8). The shoot weight in exposed seedling declined indicating decrease in growth induced by the toxicant. The root fresh weight declined at concentration C, where a maximum of 98.18 per cent decrease was recorded, when compared to the control value, in pot culture. The root/shoot weight ratio increased from 1.39 to 5.11 at concentration C, where a maximum of 267.62 per cent increased was recorded. The shoot dry weight decreased from 8.6 ± 0.8 mg to 1.6 ± 0.3 mg at concentration C. A maximum of 81.39 per cent decrease when compared to control was recorded. The root dry weight declined from 6.2 ± 0.6 to 0.7 ± 0.2 mg at conc. C. Here, a maximum of 88.71 per cent decrease in root dry weight was recorded at concentration C, when compared to control value. A maximum of 66.19 per cent and 64.03 per cent increase in the ratio value was recorded at conc. B and conc. C, respectively (Table 47.8). All the exposed parameters were found to be less than the control values except at few cases, where an increase was recorded. Higher toxicity values were recorded in petriplate cultures and less toxicity values were recorded in pot culture. The difference in both was the environmental influence and the common factor in both the experiment was the application of the toxicant at the same concentration.

The changes in pigments content of control and leached chemicals of the red mud waste exposed seedlings of a rice plant at different concentrations of the toxicant, after 144 hour of exposure in petriplate culture. The chlorophyll-a content increased from 0.566 ± 0.08 to 0.58 ± 0.11 $mg.g^{-1}$ fresh weight at concentration A, decreased from 0.56 ± 0.08 to 0.22 ± 0.04 $mg.g^{-1}$ fresh weight at concentration B, and from 0.56 ± 0.08 to 0.06 ± 0.02 $mg.g^{-1}$ fresh weight at conc. C (Table 47.9). The decrease was steady and linear. A maximum of 89.28 per cent decrease (Table 47.10) was recorded at con. C. The chlorophyll-b increased from 0.54 ± 0.11 to 0.59 ± 0.06 at conc. A decrease from 0.54 ± 0.11 to 0.19 ± 0.22 at conc. B and from 0.54 ± 0.11 to 0.22 ± 0.01$mg.g^{-1}$ fresh weight at concentration C. Where a maximum of 96.29 per cent decrease was recorded at conc. C of the toxicant. The total chlorophyll content increased from 1.19 ± 0.22 to 1.24 ± 0.31 $mg.g^{-1}$ fresh weight at conc. A; decrease from 1.14 ± 0.3 to 0.48 ± 0.2 $mg.g^{-1}$ fresh weight at conc. B and from 1.19 ± 0.22 to 0.09 ± 0.2 $mg.g^{-1}$ fresh weight at concentration C after 144 hours of exposure (Tables 47.9 and 47.10). A maximum of 92.44 per cent decrease in total chlorophyll content was recorded at concentration C, when compared to the control value. The total phaeophytin content decreased from 0.96 ± 0.06 to 0.91 ± 0.04 $mg.g^{-1}$ fresh weight at concentration A; from 0.96 ± 0.06 to 0.21 ± 0.05 $mg.g^{-1}$ fresh weight at concentration B and from 0.96 ± 0.66 to 0.08 ± 0.01 $mg.g^{-1}$ fresh weight at concentration C. A maximum of 91.67 per cent decrease was recorded at concentration C when compared to the control value. The carotene decreased from 0.0146 ± 0.0014 to 0.0141 ± 0.0008 $mg.g^{-1}$ fresh weights at concentration B and from 0.0146 ± 0.0014 to 0.0008 ± 0.0001 $mg.g^{-1}$ fresh weights at concentration C. A maximum of 94.52 per cent decrease over the control value was recorded at concentration C (Table 47.9). The chlorophyll a/b ratio increased with the increase in toxicant concentration from 1.04 to 3.0. The total chlorophyll/phaeophytin ratio decreased from 1.24 to 1.12 at conc. C and the total chlorophyll/total carotene ratio increased from

Table 47.9: Changes in Chlorophyll-a and b; Total Chlorophyll, Phaeophytin and Carotene Content of Control and Exposed 144 hrs Old Rice Seedlings, Grown in Different Concentrations of the Toxicant in Petriplate Culture. Data calculated from the mean of the samples ± standard deviation.

Concentration of the Toxicant	*Chlorophyll-a $mg.g^{-1}$ Fresh Weight*	*Chlorophyll-b $mg.g^{-1}$ Fresh Weight*	*Total Chlorophyll $mg.g^{-1}$ Fresh Weight*	*Phaeophytin $mg.g^{-1}$ Fresh Weight*	*Carotene $mg.g^{-1}$ Fresh Weight*
Control	0.56±0.08	0.54±0.11	1.19±0.22	0.96±0.06	0.0146±0.0014
0.2 per cent (A)	0.58±0.11	0.59±0.06	1.24±0.31	0.91±0.04	0.0141±0.0008
1.25 per cent (B)	0.22±0.04	0.19±0.02	0.42±0.03	0.21±0.05	0.0032±0.0004
2.0 per cent (C)	0.06±0.02	0.02±0.01	0.09±0.02	0.08±0.01	0.0008±0.0001

Table 47.10: Percent Changes in Chlorophyll-a and b; Total Chlorophyll, Phaeophytin and Carotene Content of Exposed Rice Seedlings, when Compared to the Control Value, Grown in Different Concentrations of the Toxicant in Petriplate Culture. Data calculated from the mean of the samples.+- increase;– decrease.

Concentration of the Toxicant	*Per cent Change in Chlorophyll-a Content*	*Per cent Change in Chlorophyll-b Content*	*Per cent Change in Total Chlorophyll Content*	*Per cent Change in Phaeophytin Content*	*Per cent Change in Carotene Content*
Control	--	--	--	--	--
(A)	+3.57	+9.26	+4.20	-5.21	-3.42
(B)	-60.71	-64.81	-64.70	-78.12	-78.08
(C)	-89.28	-96.29	-92.44	-91.67	-94.52

81.51 to 112.5 at conc. C, where a maximum increase of 38.02 was recorded at conc. C. The correlation coefficient values of pigment content of the 144-hour-old seedlings in petriplate culture, where significant negative correlations were marked between toxicant concentrations and pigments like chl-a, chl-b, total chlorophyll, phaeophytin and carotene content. The analysis of variance ratio test conducted basing on the data indicated the existence of significant difference between columns and non-significant difference between rows. The changes in total chlorophyll in control and leached chemicals of the red mud waste exposed rice plant leaves at different period of exposure in pot culture (Table 47.11). The total chlorophyll content was 2.28 ± 0.16 $mg.g^{-1}$ fresh weight on 15th day of exposure in the control rice plant. The total chlorophyll content increased from 2.28 ± 0.16 to 2.44 ± 0.24 $mg.g^{-1}$ fresh weight at concentration A of the toxicant and on 15th day of exposure in pot culture, where a maximum 7.02 per cent increase was recorded. With the increase in toxicant concentration, the percent decrease of total chlorophyll increased showing a significant correlation on 30th day of exposure, the total chlorophyll content decreased steadily from 3.14 ± 0.62 to 0.41 ± 0.02 $mg.g^{-1}$ fresh weight at concentration C and where, a maximum of 86.94 per cent decrease was recorded. On 45th day of exposure, the total chlorophyll content declined from 3.08 ± 0.44 to 0.08 ± 0.02 $mg.g^{-1}$ fresh weight at concentration C. On 45th day of exposure, a maximum of 97.4 per cent decrease, when compared to control value was recorded at concentration C. The decrease in values with the increase in toxicant concentration and the increase in percent decrease with the increase in toxicant concentration indicated stress. On 60th day of exposure, the total chlorophyll content decreased from 1.01 ± 0.11 to 0.01 ± 0.005 $mg.g^{-1}$ fresh weight at concentration C, where, a maximum 99.02 per cent decrease was recorded (Table 47.11).

Table 47.11: Changes in Total Chlorophyll Content ($mg. g^{-1}$ fresh weight) of Leaves of Rice Plant at Different Concentrations of the Toxicant at Different Days of Exposure in Pot Culture. Values in parentheses indicate percent change values when compared to control values. Data calculated from the mean of samples ± standard deviation.

Concentration of Toxicant	*Exposure in Days*			
	15	*30*	*45*	*60*
Control	2.28±0.16	3.14±0.62	3.08±0.44	1.02±0.11
0.2 per cent (A)	2.44±0.24 (+7.02)	3.26±0.18 (+3.82)	2.84±0.22 (–7.79)	0.88±0.24 (–13.72)
1.25 per cent (B)	1.26±0.08 (–44.74)	1.36±0.29 (–56.69)	1.65±0.14 (–46.43)	0.28±0.08 (–72.54)
2.0 per cent (C)	0.38±0.04 (–83.33)	0.41±0.02 (–86.94)	0.08±0.02 (–97.40)	0.01±0.005 (–99.02)

The changes in total phaeophytin content in control and leached chemicals of the red mud waste exposed rice plant leaves at different days of exposure and at different concentrations of the toxicant. The same table and figure indicate the percent change in phaeophytin content in the exposed seedlings in pot culture. The total phaeophytin content declined from 1.82 ± 0.27 to 1.74 ± 0.38 $mg.g^{-1}$ at concentration A, from 1.82 ± 0.27 to 0.91 ± 0.29 $mg.g^{-1}$ at concentration B, and from 1.82 ± 0.27 to 0.52 ±0.18 $mg.g^{-1}$ at concentration C on 15th day of exposure (Table 47.12). With the increase in toxicant concentration, the phaeophytin content decreased and the percent decrease increased with the increase in toxicant concentration and 95.95 per cent maximum decrease was recorded at concentration C. After 30 days of exposure the total phaeophytin content decreased from 1.86 ± 0.28 to 1.31 ± 0.47 $mg.g^{-1}$ at concentration A, from 1.86 ± 0.28 to 0.76 ± 0.38 $mg.g^{-1}$ at concentration B, and from 1.86 ± 0.28 to

0.43 ± 0.28 mg.g^{-1} at concentration C. A maximum of 76.88 per cent decrease in phaeophytin content was recorded at concentration C, on 30th day of exposure (Table 47.12). The total phaeophytin content decreased from 2.12 ± 0.54 to 1.42 ± 0.51 mg.g^{-1} at concentration A, from 2.12 ± 0.54 to 0.54 ± 0.28 mg.g^{-1} at concentration B and from 2.12 ± 0.54 to 0.28 ± 0.08 mg.g^{-1} at concentration C on 45th day of exposure. A maximum of 86.79 per cent decrease was recorded at conc. C and on 45th day of exposure. The total phaeophytin content decreased from 2.72 ± 0.82 to 1.14 ± 0.22 mg.g^{-1} at concentration A, from 2.72 ± 0.82 to 0.31 ± 0.07 mg.g^{-1} at conc. B (Table 47.12) and from 2.72 ± 0.82 to 0.11 ± 0.02 mg.g^{-1} at conc. C and was recorded on 60th day of exposure in pot culture. A maximum of 95.95 per cent decrease was recorded at concentration C and on 60th day of exposure. With the increase in toxicant concentration and day of exposure, the phaeophytin content decreased showing a negative and significant correlation. With the increase in exposure period and toxicant concentration, the percent decrease in phaeophytin content showing the existence of positive correlation. Both the assessments indicated the toxicant stress.

Table 47.12: Changes in Total Phaeophytin Content (mg. g^{-1} fresh weight) of Leaves of Rice Plant at Different Concentrations of the Toxicant at Different Days of Exposure in Pot Culture. Values in parentheses indicate percent change values when compared to control values. Data calculated from the mean of samples ± standard deviation.

Concentration of Toxicant	*Exposure in Days*			
	15	*30*	*45*	*60*
Control	1.82±0.27	1.86±0.28	2.12±0.54	2.72±0.82
0.2 per cent (A)	1.74±0.38 (–4.39)	1.31±0.47 (–29.57)	1.42±0.51 (–33.02)	1.14±0.22 (–58.09)
1.25 per cent (B)	0.91±0.29 (–50.0)	0.76±0.38 (–59.14)	0.54±0.28 (–74.53)	0.31±0.07 (–88.6)
2.0 per cent (C)	0.52±0.18 (–71.43)	0.43±0.28 (–76.88)	0.28±0.08 (–86.79)	0.11±0.02 (–95.95)

The changes in carotene content in control and leached chemicals of the red mud waste exposed rice plant leaves at different exposure periods and at different toxicant concentrations. The carotene content declined from 0.0148 ± 0.0016 to 0.0088 ± 0.0016 mg.g^{-1} fresh weights at 15th day of exposure, where 40.54 per cent decrease, when compared to control was recorded. On 30th day of exposure, 1.78 per cent increase in carotene content over the control value was recorded at concentration A and 45.83 per cent decrease was recorded at concentration C (Table 47.13). On 45th day of exposure, 5.75 per cent increase in carotene content over control value was recorded in concentration A. However, 59.16 per cent decrease was recorded in concentration C, in contrast to concentration a. On 60th day of exposure in concentration A, 6.08 per cent increase in carotene content was recorded over the control value and in contrast, 58.01 per cent and 82.32 per cent decrease in carotene content over the control value was recorded on concentration B and concentration C, respectively. At lower concentration of the toxicant, increase in carotene level and at higher concentrations decrease in carotene level was marked at all exposure periods. Significant negative correlation was marked at all exposure periods for total chlorophyll. For total phaeophytin non-significant correlation at 15th day exposure and significant negative correlation at higher exposure period was marked. Non-significant negative correlation was marked at all exposure periods for carotene content change. The chlorophyll/carotene ratio value declined at all exposure periods and highest depletion was recorded at concentration-C. Lowest value was recorded at concentration C and on 60th day of exposure in pot culture (Table 47.13). The carotene/phaeophytin ratio indicated that the ratio values increased with the increase in exposure periods and with the increase in toxicant concentration in all exposed plants. No trend was recorded in the control set of the pot culture experiments. The chlorophyll/phaeophytin ratio decreased with the increase in toxicant concentration at all exposure periods. No definite trend was recorded with the exposure period. The phaeophytin/carotene ratio indicated significant depletion of the ratio value at higher exposure period and at higher concentration of the toxicant (Table 47.13).

Table 47.13: Changes in Carotene Content (mg. g^{-1} fresh weight) of Leaves of Rice Plant at Different Concentrations of the Toxicant at Different Days of Exposure in Pot Culture. Data in parentheses indicate percent change values, when compared to control values. Data calculated from the mean of samples ± standard deviation.

Concentration of Toxicant	*Exposure in Days*			
	15	*30*	*45*	*60*
Control	0.0148±0.0016	0.0168±0.0024	0.0174±0.0031	0.0181±0.0014
0.2 per cent (A)	0.0151±0.0008 (+2.03)	0.0171±0.0020 (+1.78)	0.0184±0.0051 (+5.75)	0.0192±0.0022 (+6.08)
1.25 per cent (B)	0.0092±0.0012 (–37.84)	0.0099±0.0012 (–41.07)	0.0096±0.0026 (–44.83)	0.0076±0.0012 (–58.01)
2.0 per cent (C)	0.0088±0.0016 (–40.54)	0.0091±0.0008 (–45.83)	0.0071±0.0004 (–59.19)	0.0032±0.0002 (–82.32)

Table 47.14: Changes in the Respiration Rate (ml of CO_2 evolved g^{-1} hr^{-1}), Rate of Photosynthesis (ml of O_2 evolved g^{-1} hr^{-1}) and Gross Production (ml of O_2 evolved g^{-1} hr^{-1}) of Control and Exposed Rice Seedlings After 144hrs of Germination in Petriplate Culture. Data calculated from the mean of samples ± standard deviation

	After 144 hrs of Germination (ml of CO_2/O_2 evolved g^{-1} hr^{-1})		
Concentration of Toxicant	*Rate of Respiration*	*Rate of Photosynthesis (Net Primary Production, NPP)*	*Gross Primary Productivity (GPP)*
Control	236.5±18.4	224.8±16.4	461.3
0.2 per cent (A)	208.4±19.6	246.2±28.5	454.6
1.25 per cent (B)	102.6±28.8	126.4±18.5	229.0
2.0 per cent (C)	64.5±12.6	74.6±8.5	131.1

Interesting changes in rate of respiration, rate of photosynthesis (NPP) and Gross Primary Productivity (GPP) in control and toxicant exposed 144-hour-old seedlings in petriplate culture, grown in a seed germinator, under controlled conditions, were observed (Table 47.14). The rate of respiration decreased from 236.5 ± 18.4 to 208.4 ± 19.6ml of CO_2 evolved hr^{-1} g^{-1} dry weight of the seedling at concentration A, from 236.5 ± 18.4 to 102.6 ±28.8ml of CO_2 evolved hr^{-1} g^{-1} at concentration B and from 236.5 ± 18.4 to 64.5 ± 12.6ml of CO_2 evolved hr^{-1} g^{-1} at conc. C in 144 hour old rice seedlings. The rate of photosynthesis increased from 224.8 ± 16.4 to 246.2 ± 28.5 ml of O_2 evolved hr^{-1} g^{-1} dry weight of the seedlings in conc. A; the rate of photosynthesis decreased from 224.8 ±16.4 to 126.4 ± 18.8 ml of O_2 evolved hr^{-1} g^{-1} dry weight of the seedlings in conc. B and from 224.8 ± 16.4 to 74.6 ± 8.5 ml of O_2

evolved $hr^{-1} g^{-1}$ dry weight of the 144 hour old seedlings in petriplate cultures (Table 47.14). The gross primary productivity decreased in exposed seedlings, when compared to control seedlings. The GPP value decreased from 461.3 to 454.6 at concentration A, from 461.3 to 229.0 and from 461.3 to 139.1ml of O_2 evolved $hr^{-1} g^{-1}$ dry weight of the 144-hour-old seedlings in petriplate culture (Table 47.14).

Change in photosynthetic rate, respiration rate and GPP values at different concentrations of the toxicant and at different days of exposure in pot culture indicated interesting features. The photosynthetic rate (NPP) decreased from 184.6 to 91.2ml of O_2 evolved $hr^{-1} g^{-1}$ dry weight on 15th day of exposure, where a maximum of 50.59 per cent decrease in NPP value was recorded. On 30th day of exposure, the NPP value depleted from 191.2 to 82.4ml of O_2 evolved $hr^{-1} g^{-1}$ dry weight at concentration C, where a maximum of 56.9 per cent decrease was recorded (Table 47.15). On 45th day of exposure, the NPP value depleted from 202.4 to 71.6 ml of O_2 evolved $hr^{-1} g^{-1}$ dry weight of the seedlings at concentration C, where a maximum of 64.62 per cent decrease was recorded. On 60th day of exposure, the NPP value depleted from 212.6 to 48.5 ml of O_2 evolved $hr^{-1} g^{-1}$ dry weight of the seedling at concentration C, where a maximum of 77.19 per cent decrease in NPP value was recorded (Table 47.15). With the increase in exposure period and toxicant concentration, the NPP value declined indicating a negative correlation. With the increase in exposure period and toxicant concentration,

Table 47.15: Changes in the respiration rate (ml of CO_2 evolved $g^{-1} hr^{-1}$), rate of photosynthesis (ml of O_2 evolved $g^{-1} hr^{-1}$) and gross production (ml of O_2 evolved $g^{-1} hr^{-1}$) of control and exposed rice seedlings at different days of exposure in pot culture. Data calculated from the mean of samples ± standard deviation. Data in parentheses indicate percent increase (+)/percent decrease (–) in the values, when compared to control.

Concentration of Toxicant	*Exposure Period in Days (Respiration rate–ml of CO_2 evolved $g^{-1} hr^{-1}$)*			
	15	*30*	*45*	*60*
Control	142.3	151.4	158.6	161.2
0.2 per cent (A)	144.6(+1.62)	136.2(–10.04)	101.4(–36.06)	88.9(–44.85)
1.25 per cent (B)	114.2(–19.75)	91.6(–39.63)	74.8(–52.84)	36.6(–77.29)
2.0 per cent (C)	82.4(–42.09)	42.7(–71.79)	21.6(–86.38)	8.4(–94.79)
Concentration of Toxicant	*Exposure Period in Days (Photosynthetic rate–ml of O_2 evolved $g^{-1} hr^{-1}$)*			
	15	*30*	*45*	*60*
Control	184.6	191.2	202.4	212.6
0.2 per cent (A)	188.4(+2.06)	198.7(+3.92)	218.2(+7.81)	260.4(+22.48)
1.25 per cent (B)	128.6 (–30.33)	171.4(–10.35)	145.8(–27.96)	126.2(–40.6)
2.0 per cent (C)	91.2(–50.59)	82.4(–56.90)	71.6(–64.62)	48.5(–77.19)
Concentration of Toxicant	*Exposure Period in Days (GPP–ml of O_2 evolved $g^{-1} hr^{-1}$)*			
	15	*30*	*45*	*60*
Control	326.9	342.6	361.0	373.8
0.2 per cent (A)	333.0(+1.87)	334.9(–5.02)	319.6(–11.47)	349.3(–6.39)
1.25 per cent (B)	242.8(–25.73)	262.8(–25.47)	220.6(–38.89)	162.8(–56.37)
2.0 per cent (C)	173.6(–46.89)	125.1(–64.52)	93.2(–74.18)	56.9(–84.75)

the percent decrease in NPP value increased showing a positive and significant correlation in pot culture. The respiration rate increased from 142.3 to 144.6ml of CO_2 evolved $hr^{-1}g^{-1}$ dry weight in conc. A; from 142.3 to 114.2ml of CO_2 evolved $hr^{-1}g^{-1}$ dry weight conc. B and from 142.3 to 82.4 ml of CO_2 evolved $hr^{-1}g^{-1}$ dry weight at conc. C, on 15th day of exposure, where a maximum of 42.09 per cent decrease was recorded in conc. C. The respiration rate on 30th day of exposure declined from 151.4 to 42.7 ml of CO_2 evolved $hr^{-1}g^{-1}$ dry weight at conc. C, where a maximum of 71.79 per cent decrease was recorded at conc. C and on 30th day of exposure. On 45th day of exposure, the respiration rate of the exposed seedlings depleted from 158.6 to 21.6ml of CO_2 evolved $hr^{-1}g^{-1}$ dry weight at conc. C, showing a maximum depletion by 86.38 per cent in pot culture experiment. On 60th day of exposure, the respiration rate significantly declined from 161.2 to 8.4 ml of CO_2 evolved $hr^{-1}g^{-1}$ dry weight at conc. C in pot culture, where a maximum of 94.79 per cent decrease was recorded (Table 47.15). The gross primary productivity of the exposed seedlings drastically reduced, when compared to the control value. The GPP value decreased from 326.9 to 173.6 ml of O_2 evolved $hr^{-1}g^{-1}$ dry weight at conc. C and on 15th day of exposure; the GPP value depleted from 342.6 to 125.1ml of O_2 evolved $hr^{-1}g^{-1}$ dry weight at conc. C and on 30th day of exposure; the GPP value depleted from 361.0 to 93.2 ml of O_2 evolved $hr^{-1}g^{-1}$ dry weight at conc. C and on 45th day of exposure and the GPP value depleted from 373.8 to 56.9 ml of O_2 evolved $hr^{-1}g^{-1}$ dry weight at conc. C and on 60th day of exposure in pot cultures (Table 47.15). With the increase in toxicant concentration and exposure period, the GPP value significantly declined at all exposure periods. Highest depletion in GPP value was recorded in concentration C. With the increase in exposure period, the GPP value declined significantly on 15th day 46.89 per cent; on 30th day 64.52 per cent; on 45th day 74.18 per cent and on 60th day 84.75 per cent decrease was recorded, when compared to the control value. On 15th day the percent decrease was 25.73 per cent and 46.89 per cent in conc. B and C, respectively. On 30th day, the percent decrease was 5.02 per cent, 25.47 per cent and 64.52 per cent in conc. A, B and C, respectively. On 45th day, the percent decrease was 11.47 per cent, 38.89 per cent and 74.18 per cent in conc. A, B and C, respectively. On 60th day, the percent decrease was 6.39 per cent, 56.37 per cent and 84.75 per cent in conc. A, B and C, respectively. Maximum depletion in GPP value was recorded on 60th day of exposure and in concentration C (Table 47.15). The data indicated the existence of significant ($p< 0.05$) negative correlation between toxicant concentration and NPP, GPP, rate of respiration values in 144-hour-old seedlings in petriplate culture. The analysis of variance ratio test related to rate or respiration, NPP value and GPP value in 144 hour old seedlings and rice plants in pot culture at different exposure periods indicated the existence of non significant difference between rows and columns was quite clear from the analysis of variance ratio test. The NPP value showed non-significant correlation at 15 and 30 days of exposure and significant correlation at 45 and 60 days exposure. The respiration rate showed all significant negative correlation values at all exposure periods. The GPP values showed significant ($p<0.05$) negative correlation values at all exposure periods. Changes in glucose content of both control and exposed leaves of rice plants at different exposure periods and at different selected concentrations of the toxicant, in pot culture showed the effects caused by the toxicant.

The glucose content declined from 17.4 ± 2.8 to 6.2 ± 0.8 mg/g fresh weight after 15th day of exposure; from 18.9 ± 3.5 to 5.1 ±1.2 mg/g fresh weight after 30th days of exposure; from 20.4 ± 5.5 to 3.6 ± 0.9 mg/g fresh weight after 45 days of exposure and from 22.2 ± 1.4 to 1.8 ±0.4 mg/g fresh weight after 60 days exposure. Highest depletion was recorded at conc. C (2.0 per cent of the toxicant) at all exposure periods. Drastic depletion in glucose level was recorded at all concentrations and at all exposure periods, except 45th and 60th day of exposure in conc. A, when compared to control values (Table 47.16). Significant ($p<0.001$) negative correlation existed between the parameter with exposure period and between the parameter and toxicant concentration. Steady and linear increase in percent decrease in glucose content with the increase in toxicant concentration and exposure period was marked. Maximum of 54.37 per cent, 73.01 per cent, 82.35 per cent and 91.89 per cent decrease was observed at 15, 30, 45 and 60 days of exposure at concentration C. All the values were statistically significant. Positive significant ($p<0.001$) correlation exists between the percent decrease and toxicant concentration and exposure period. Changes in nitrogen content in shoot and root of both control and toxicant exposed rice plants grown in pots, at different exposure period and at different toxicant concentrations revealed interesting sequences (Table 47.16). Highest depletion in nitrogen content of the shoot of the exposed plant was recorded at conc. C and at 60th day of exposure, when compared to the rest of the values. The nitrogen contents depleted from 3.8 ± 0.8 to 1.4 ± 0.7 from 4.1 ± 1.1 to 1.4 ± 0.6; from 4.4 ± 1.4 to 1.2 ±0.6 and from 5.1 ± 0.9 to 1.1 ± 0.5 mg/g fresh weight was recorded at 15, 35, 45 and 60 days of exposure in shoot of the exposed seedlings. Drastic depletion in nitrogen content was marked in the exposed roots. The nitrogen content decreased from 4.1 ± 0.4 to 1.3 ± 0.9 mg/g dry weight at 15 days of exposure; from 4.5 ± 0.6 to 1.4 ± 0.3 mg/g dry weight after 30 days of exposure; from 5.1 ±0.6 to 0.8 ± 0.2 mg/g dry weight after 45 days of exposure and from 5.6 + 0.8 to 0.2 + 01 mg/g dry weight after 60 days of exposure (Table 47.16). Highest depletion in nitrogen content was recorded at concentration C in root and shoot of the exposed seedlings, when compared to control, conc. A and conc. B rice plants. At all exposure periods and toxicant concentration, the nitrogen content significantly declined. Highest depletion was marked at conc. C both in shoot and root. Maximum depletion by 63.16 per cent, 65.85 per cent, 72.72 per cent and 78.43 per cent was recorded at 15, 30, 45 and 60 days exposure period at conc. C. Drastic depletion in nitrogen content in the root of the exposed plants when compared to control plants was marked. Maximum decrease by 68.29 per cent, 68.89 per cent, 84.31 per cent and 96.43 per cent was noted at noted at 15, 30, 45 and 60 day exposure period at conc. C (Table 47.16). The values of shoot did show significant trend and significant correlation was marked. In case of root, significant positive ($p<0.01$) correlation was marked between the percent decrease in nitrogen content with the exposure period and with the toxicant concentration.

Table 47.16: Changes in Glucose Content and Nitrogen Content in Control and Exposed Rice Leaves at Different Concentrations of the Toxicant and at Different Days of Exposure. Data calculated from the mean of the samples ± standard deviation. Data in parentheses indicate percent decrease(–) and percent increase(+) in the parameters, when compared to control values.

Concentration of Toxicant	*Exposure Period in Days (Glucose content, mg. g^{-1})*			
	15	*30*	*45*	*60*
Control	17.4±2.8	18.9±3.5	20.4±5.5	22.2±1.4
0.2 per cent (A)	16.2±4.9(–6.89)	18.1±4.2(–4.23)	21.6±3.2(+5.88)	23.6±3.6(+6.31)
1.25 per cent (B)	11.5±2.2(–33.91)	12.4±3.9(–34.39)	11.2±1.8(–45.09)	9.1±1.2(–59.01)
2.0 per cent (C)	6.2±0.8(–64.37)	5.1±1.2(–73.01)	3.6±0.9(–82.35)	1.8±0.4(–91.89)
Concentration of Toxicant	*Exposure Period in Days (Nitrogen content, mg. g^{-1})*			
	15	*30*	*45*	*60*
Control	3.8±0.8	4.1±1.1	4.4±1.4	5.1±0.9
0.2 per cent (A)	3.6±0.3(–5.26)	4.0±0.8(–2.44)	3.9±2.6(–11.36)	3.7±1.1(–27.45)
1.25 per cent (B)	2.6±1.1 (–31.58)	2.8±1.4(–31.71)	2.4±1.1(–45.45)	1.8±0.2(–64.70)
2.0 per cent (C)	1.4±0.7(–63.16)	1.4±0.6(–65.85)	1.2±0.6(–72.72)	1.1±0.5(–78.43)

The root was more affected than the shoot of the exposed rice plants. Control plants remained throughout the experimental period and served as standard for comparison. The data of petriplate culture was more prominent than the pot culture. As the pot culture experiments were subjected to environmental influence. The changes in ATPase activity of 144-hour-old rice seedlings in different concentrations of the toxicant in petriplate culture, grown in a seed germinator under controlled conditions showed features related to toxicity. The ATPase activity of the 144-hour-old seedlings, decreased with the increase in toxicant concentration, when compared to the control value. The ATPase activity decreased from 3.4 + 0.3 to 2.6 + 0.6 at conc. A; from 3.4 + 0.3 to 1.4 + 0.5 at conc. B and from 3.4 + 0.3 to 0.3 + 0.2 mg i.p liberated/hr/100 mg dry weight in concentration C. A significant ($r = -0.993, p<0.01$) negative correlation between the parameter with the toxicant concentration was marked. The ATPase activity decreased by 23.53 per cent in conc. A, 58.82 per cent in conc. B and 91.18 per cent decrease in conc. C, when compared to the control value. All the obtained values were statistically significant. ATPase activity of the 144-hour-old seedlings showed the existence of significant ($p<0.01$) negative correlation with the toxicant concentration.

When all the data were considered along with the statistical data it can be inferred that the toxicant was more effective in petriplate culture, when compared to pot culture experiment. Higher percent of inhibition was recorded in petriplate culture experiments. Petriplate experiments were conducted in side a seed germinator, where all environmental factors were controlled. But in pot culture experiments, the environmental factors played a crucial role and reduced the effect of the toxicant on the crop plant. In both the cases the root was more affected than the shoot, in all the variable parameters. The residual accumulation of the toxicants in the exposed rice plants could have provided much better information. But due to lack of facilities and equipments, residual analysis part was not carried out. In presence of residual accumulation of toxic ant data, the obtained data can be analyzed, correlated and interpreted properly. However, in absence of residual accumulation data, concrete conclusion may not be drawn but to a greater degree of accuracy, the data was presented and interpreted. All the obtained data were statistically significant. Further, higher-level work is necessary to assess the toxic nature and site of the action studies. Further work is needed to find out possible ways of detoxification of the leached chemicals of the red mud. No doubt, leaching will be there, in addition groundwater contamination cannot be avoided, as there is no bottom lining. At least, care could be taken to stop surface leaching leading to run off water, entering into water bodies.

Discussion

The eco-toxicological assessments of toxic chemicals depend on two basic items of information. First, the environmental available concentrations of the chemical which occur as a result of discharge and distribution in the natural environment and secondly, the toxicological properties of the chemical at that concentration and its possible impact on the biota including humans. Environmental concentrations and toxicological properties also include the concentrations of by-products or transformation products as well. Different methods and procedures are used to draw all the available eco-toxicological information's together to arrive at an assessment. The basic requirements for such procedures are the pattern of use of chemicals; their disposal and release; physico-chemical characteristics; degradation and bioaccumulation; and biological factors such as growth inhibition, toxicity testing etc. Thus, the eco-toxicology of chemicals is an important aspect of environmental management and the management of pollution.

High percentage of seed germination and seedling establishment, disease free seedling and healthy growth of the plant are considered to be some of the reliable indications about high yield potential of any crop plant. However, in nature, crop plants experience extensive damage due to insect pests, fungi, and mainly because of different type of industrial effluents and wastes etc. The infected seeds spread the disease when grown in fields. Thus, to avoid decline in food grain productions, killer chemicals are applied to crop plants (Butler, 1978). It is essential to understand the amount of toxicant present, its movement and biological magnification along the critical pathways finally reaching to man. Compared to other chemicals, specially, the unrestricted use of pesticides in agriculture towards the last past of the 18th century has increased substantial amount of pesticides in the aquatic and terrestrial environment, and has created a serious threat to biotic components of the earth (Fiskesjo, 1979). Now it stands as a global problem. It is highly essential to understand the amount of toxic pesticides present, its movement and biological magnification along the critical path to man. It was realized that from pesticide-contaminated environment, the entry and accumulation into the biological system, occurs at a very slower rate and also it takes a longer time period for its dreadful expressions. But, the pesticide, which enters into, the agricultural soil in the form of seed dresser, or by mass spray finds its way into the living system through direct consumption of food grain.

The industrial wastes once thrown into the environment, these wastes spread all over and affect the flora and fauna. For example, the red mud waste discharged from the NALCO plant was stored in a natural pond surrounded by hills from all sides except one side, where the industry people have constructed three dams. Unfortunately, they have never visualized probably that the leached chemicals from the red mud pond, will create future problems. The data obtained in this piece of investigation revealed that the extract of the red mud is deadly toxic and can seriously affect the crop plants. We have selected a resistant variety, still then, the extract effected the crop plant seriously, particularly to the production/yield of the crop plant. The morphological changes were clearly visible and effects were more pronounced. Hence, care should be taken to check leaching of the chemicals from the red mud pond or they must find out ways and means for safe disposal of the waste. We are not conservative enough to request/direct the closure of the industry but some safe disposal methods are ought to be adopted to safe guard the interest of the public in general and environment in particular. According to Baicu and Diaconu (1972), smaller seeds abosorb/retain more amount of the treated chemicals due to exposure of more surface area, resulting in high transfer/entry of mercury/pesticide/toxicant to the agricultural soil through smaller seeds. Hence, the agricultural soil increases substantial amount of toxicant within a notable period of time making it dangerous for human health, when red mud wastes enter nutritional cycle through dressed seeds or other treated parts of plants intentionally or due to carelessness (Koronowski,1973). However, literature explaining the following aspects in details is lacking.

1. Toxicant dynamics in different seeds and seed types disinfected with different types of insecticides formulations and leached chemicals of red mud wastes.
2. Red mud waste dynamics in seeds in relation to seed biology.
3. Amount of red mud leached chemical transfer to agricultural soil in relation to seed type, seed size, seed quantity etc.
4. Leached chemicals of the red mud transfer from seed to soil and again from soil to seed in crop rotation is a usual practice in modern agriculture.
5. Interferences of the toxicant in seed physiology during germination and establishment and its biochemistry.

In the present investigation, the red mud waste dynamics in seed and seed biology during germination and seedling establishment was studied in RM waste treated seedlings. The decrease in root and shoot length of the treated seedlings at higher concentration was in agreement with Lipsey (1978) and Pradhan (1998) who observed inhibition in growth of maize seedlings grown in methyl mercury hydroxide (MMH) and rice seedlings in pesticide exposure. Retardation in growth of crop plants treated with organo-mercurial formulation was reported by Sorteberg (1974), Weaver *et al.* (1984) and Semu *et al.* (1985). At low concentrations of PMA and ethyl-mercuric chloride the winter wheat showed changes in the seedling vigour (Bateman, 1975). The seedlings of tomato, corn and bean grown in a complete nutrient solution containing MMH (Haney and Richard, 1973), showed the tomato seedlings were killed within 4-8 days at concentration of 0.05 mg/l. The growth was inhibited at concentration of 0.01 mg/l for corn and beans. In this study, growth of the seedlings was inhibited beyond 2.2 per cent of red mud leached chemicals in only petriplate culture. At 1.2 per cent, root growth significantly declilned when compared to shoot growth. Although the seeds germination was inhibited beyond 2.6 per cent of red mud waste but seedling establishment was inhibited at lower doses (beyond 2.0 per cent) of RM leached chemicals. It seems that these rice seeds were more effective, when compared to mustard grains (Padhi, 1990) in respect of seed germination. Padhi (1990) reported significant variation or no germination at all, when rice grains were exposed to MEMC (an organo-mercurial compound), such an observation was marked here. When sugar beet seeds were treated with ethyl mercuric phosphate, phytotoxic effects were observed (Byford, 1971). The same author reported that methyl mercury- dicyano-diamide was found to be more phyto-toxic than the less volatile ethyl and phenyl mercury compounds. Toubey (1972) reported that the emergence of summit wheat seeds was reduced significantly when the seed was stored for a long period after being treated with normal doses of PMA, a fungicide. Here also, with higher concentrations of red mud leached chemicals and longer period of exposure reduced the percent germination and seedling establishment. Hasset *et al.* (1976) stated that inhibition of root elongation is one of the sensitive parameters to assess the toxicity of toxicants. Further they stated that compared to the growth rate, pesticide was found to be more toxic than mercury, cadmium and zinc. Godbold and Huttermann (1985) observed that the root elongation was severely inhibited by 0.1 to 0.5 m mole of mercury after 24 hours. At 5 and 15 m mole the root elongation was ceased completely and radial shrinkage was observed in 1.5 mm from behind the root tip. Application of $HgCl_2$ to primary root tip of *Zea mays* in the form of droplets, showed reduction of root growth and also inhibited their gravy response (Pilet and Jean, 1981). Treatment of various concentrations of metallic compounds (both inorganic and organic); Mercury (Mukherji and Ganguly, 1974) on different varieties of rice have shown that, towards lower concentration the inhibition of germination was not at all marked rather stimulation was noticed (Padhi, 1990).

Siegel *et al.* (1984) studied the seed germination and early growth of the seedling of 15 species treated with mercury vapour and observed that, more than 50 per cent plants did not show inhibition of root and shoot length, but occasional stimulation was noticed. Sai (1998) reported an initial decrease by 11.3 per cent in shoot length and 22.3 per cent decrease in root length at 100 ppm of pesticide in petriplate culture. It was the indication of no stimulation. No stimulation was observed in the present investigation with red mud extract. The length of ratio shoot and root calculated for all types of treatments, showed positive trend in relation to concentration, which indicated that root length was much affected than the shoot system (Sai,1998 and Pradhan,1998). This might be due to the fact that the root being the primary absorbing organ, was in direct contact with a toxic medium and hence resulted higher reduction in different parameters of root. The distribution of red mud leached chemical in plant was asymmetrical with greater amount of elements in the roots than the shoots. Although the level of red mud leached chemical gradually increases in plant tissues, with increasing amount in external levels, the proportion retained in the roots to that of shoots was almost constant (*i.e.* approximately 95 per cent). The initial blackening followed by browning and the observed chlorosis was only due to the red mud extract chemical waste. Similar observations were not found in pesticide poisoning or mercury poisoning. The type of deposition should be identified and characterised to reach to a logistic conclusion. As the apical meristem of *Elodia densa* showed deposition of more methyl mercury, so also the deposition of more mercury in the region of the root might have caused inhibition. When mercuric chloride was applied in droplets to the cap of primary roots of the maize, it reduced their elongation (Pilet and Jean, 1981). Sharma (1982) reported that seeds of different varieties *Phaseolus aureus* treatment with mercuric acetate solution showed inhibition of seedling growth. Sharma (1983 and 1985) also reported that the seeds of *Pisum sativum* C. V. Bonneville, when treated with mercuric acetate solution shown promotion of radicle and epicotyle length at lower concentration (10 mg/l) but in higher concentration at 50 mg/l, a significant reduction in seedling growth was observed. The decrease in shoot, root length and seedling establishment with the increase in the concentration of the stress probably suggests and supports the idea that (1) the toxicant increases the osmotic pressure of the medium by reducing or preventing the availability of water required for germination, (2) the toxicity of the chemical and (3) presence of higher concentrations of ions and active ingredients, help jointly for the reduction of the seedling growth and establishment (Donovan and Dey, 1969; Panigrahi and Misra, 1978 and Pradhan, 1998). Experiments were conducted to study the toxic effect of various mercury compounds such as inorganic monovalent mercurous chloride, divalent mercuric chloride, mercuric acetate and organic compound of mercury as phenyl mercuric acetate on seed germination, pigment content, root and shoot lengths, fresh and dry weights of barley. It was observed that phenyl mercuric acetate was more toxic, followed by mercuric acetate and mercuric chloride (Mukhiya *et al.*, 1983). In case of red mud leached chemicals poisoning, drastic depletion in the parameters were marked but the extent of pollution was far less when compared to above mentioned compounds. Interestingly in case of insecticide poisoning no stimulation was marked at low concentrations and also at low exposure periods but Patra (1993) reported that at low exposure period, inhibition was not marked rather stimulation was observed. The stimulation might be due to change in certain biochemical parameters caused due to mercury toxicity. Inhibition of root growth was considered to be important and an indication of metal toxicity (Godbold *et al.*, 1984; Godbold and Hutterman, 1985), the promotion of the shoot might be the secondary effect reflected due to root inhibition. The differential effect of PMA on root and shoot, might be due to the asymmetrical distribution of mercury (Baeuford *et al.*, 1977), which might be imparting a differential toxicity to the seedling parts. Our interpretation agrees fully with Padhi (1990) and partly with Baeuford *et al.* (1977). It is very difficult at this stage to infer the toxic effects of red mud leached chemical on the seedling establishment of the rice seed. The pigment analysis, physiological change studies of the seedling, might throw light on detailed aspects of RM waste toxicity. Photosynthetic pigments of the plant system play a vital role in trapping solar energy and CO_2 fixation (Kashyap and Gupta, 1981). The chlorophylls have long been recognized as the primary light acceptors in plants and they are invariably present in every organism, which carries out photosynthesis with absorption of CO_2 and evolution of molecular oxygen. Zingmark and Miller (1975), De Filippis and Pallaghy (1976 a), Rai and Khatonair (1980), and Rai *et al.* (1981 b) reported that heavy metals reduce chlorophyll content and inhibit photosynthesis. De *et al.* (1985) suggested that at 20 ppm the Hg (II) lowered the chlorophyll by decreasing the synthesis of chlorophyll as well as possibly by increasing chlorophyllase activity in *Pistia*. De Filippis and Pallaghy (1976 b) reported that among the heavy metal solution PMA and $ZnCl_2$ caused the greatest and least inhibition respectively. These levels were reflected in the levels of phaeophytin (De Filippis and Pallaghy, 1976 c), a degradation product of chlorophyll (Wolken *et al.*, 1955). The above authors added that the chlorophyll and phaeophytin a/b ratios were similarly affected. Cultures treated with heavy metal solutions increased their carotenoid/chlorophyll ratios. Rai *et al.* (1981 a) in their review article mentioned the acute toxicity of cadmium to green algae, which inhibited photosynthesis [$^{14}CO_2$ uptake] (Stratton and Carke, 1979). Conway (1978) found a significant lowering of pigment content in *Asterionella formosa* after addition of cadmium. Excessive concentrations of copper cause loss of photosynthetic pigments in *Chlorella* and in a natural phytoplankton community dominated by *Aphonizmenon flos-aque* (Whittakar *et al.*, 1978).

Sai (1998) reported significant variations in chlorophyll content in the exposed plants indicated the presence of stress. Chlorosis was marked in the exposed plants. Similar type of chlorosis was observed by Padhi (1990) and Sai (1998) in exposed rice seedlings. Hence, it can be indicated that the observed chlorosis in exposed seedlings might be due to breakdown of chlorophyll pigments by the toxicant. The growth rate depleted significantly, even at very low concentration of the red mud leached chemicals. It indicated that red mud leached chemicals at lower concentrations acts as a growth inhibitor by way of affecting the biochemical mechanism during seed germination and at higher concentrations acts as a growth inhibitor due to the red mud leached chemicals toxicant. As red mud leached chemicals at lower concentrations, it reduced transpiration, thus decreasing growth of the plant. However, with increase in concentration of red mud leached chemical, the amount of pigment content decreased significantly, with slight increase in the initial concentration applied over the control values (Sai, 1998). An initial increase in pigment content might be due to the stimulatory effect of the pesticide (Sai, 1998). Pesticide, Monocrotophos showed dichotomous behaviour in the investigation carried out by Sai (1998), we could not notice such a change in behaviour in the present investigation. The pigment change in exposed seedlings was due to only red mud leached chemical. Harris *et al.* (1970) and Overneil (1975) reported the reduction of chlorophyll pigment as a result of reduction in growth and suggested that the chlorophyll estimation can be considered as a parameter of measuring growth of the system. The phaeophytin content in the leaf of plant has an important role for the fact that any unfavourable change in the environment inhabited by the plant is reflected through a change in phaeophytin level. Chlorophylls are known to be converted to phaeophytins as a consequence of exposure to weak acids, by replacement of Mg^{2+} with two atoms of hydrogen and thereby changing the spectral properties (Rao and Le Blanc, 1966 and Singh and Singh, 1984 a). Degradation to phaeophytins might be the first step towards the breakdown of chlorophyll, which was evident from the increased level of phaeophytin in the initial concentration in the treated culture. In high concentration of red mud leached chemical, the amount of carotenoid content also decreased significantly as the case of chlorophyll content. It clearly indicates that red mud leached chemical in lower concentration degrades chlorophyll pigments to phaeophytin, but in higher concentration it also destroys phaeophytin pigments alongwith chlorophyll pigments. That means red mud leached chemical is highly toxic in higher concentrations and also at lower concentrations. Carotenoids play a vital role as a protector of photosynthetic tissues against photosensitized oxidation. The decrease in carotenoid content in the leaves exposed to red mud waste stress lead to a decrease in protection from the stress to the photosynthetic tissue. Here, in our experiment also there was decrease in chlorophyll and phaeophytin content with the decrease in carotenoid content. So clearly the decrease in carotenoid content in shoot exposed to red mud leached chemicals stress lead to a decrease in protection from the stress to the photosynthetic tissue. The ratio of chlorophyll to carotenoid has long been cosidered as a valuable parameter for defining environmental conditions unfavourable for growth of the plant. The variation in the ratio value with the increase in the concentration of the toxicant indicated stress. When the nutrients in the medium are exhausted or a toxicant was introduced into the medium the ratio increased due to decrease in the chlorophyll content (Rai *et al.*, 1981 b). The same result was found in higher concentration (2.0 per cent) when compared to that of control. Increased ratio indicated inhibition of chlorophyll biosynthesis, inactivation of enzyme system and disruption of many physiological and biochemical processes (Leland *et al.*, 1979; Sorentino, 1979). The insecticide at relatively low concentrations also effect the energy transfer by selectively affecting the phycocyanin and phycobilisomes of intact cells of *Spirulina*, which was reported by Murthy and Mohanty (1991). It is a common observation that toxicity of metals showed great variation under laboratory and field conditions (Whitton, 1970). The phaeophytin/carotenoid ratio increased at lower concentrations and also at higher concentrations of red mud leached chemical. A significant increase at higher concentration might be either due to the interaction of environmental parameters or due to the increase in red mud leached chemical toxicity. According to Pradhan (1998) the seedlings grown under field condition showed significant growth than those grown under laboratory-controlled conditions. Hence it becomes explicit that laboratory based information cannot solely be used to stimulate field conditions, because many environmental and nutritional factors operate to bring about metal/pesticide/industrial waste toxicity in field conditions (Harding and Whitton, 1977; Gadd and Griffiths, 1978). Pure petriplate culture in open racks, provide some sort of environmental influences. In the present investigation, petriplates culture experiments were conducted in a seed germinator, under total controlled conditions. The obtained data will vary strongly to open rack culture experiments. Field experiments were conducted in pots and the culture will have restricted environmental influence. Pot was selected to restrict the leaching and drainage of the red mud waste after application, which generally happens in field conditions.

Almost all the cellular chlorophyll and carotenoid pigments are localized in the photosynthetic lamellae of the cells, the thylakoids (Wolk, 1973). The lamellae are proteinaceous (Schmitz, 1967) and increase in thylakoid surface area with metal exposure may indicate an increase in photosynthetic potential by active synthesis of thylakoidal protein and associated pigments or it may reflect an uncoupling of the bonds in protein causing the lamellae to stretch (Rachlin *et al.*, 1982). The metals cause a reduction in the volume of the intra-thylakoidal spaces. The significance of such reduction is not understood but the result is to bring the thylakoids into closer approximation. This may have some value in facilitating photosynthetic activity in the metal stresses cell so that the necessary ATP is manufactured to drive the metabolic machinery required to effect detoxification (Rachlin *et al.*, 1982). Rothstein (1959) has demonstrated that metals interact with sulphyhydryl groups in cell membranes to produce–S–metal–S–bridges, and Simkis (1979) has discussed the importance of proteins and lipoproteins in binding with metal as means of inactivating them within the cell. Lipsey (1978) also tested under *in vitro* conditions, MMH inhibited photosynthesis of chloroplast and phosphate uptake by mitochondria. The same author also opined that MMH showed stunted growth and respiration of isolated mitochondria were inhibited. Haumann (1987) showed that mercury affects the chloroplast by causing considerable increase of the grana stacks in *Chara vulgaris*. In addition, mercury caused dilation of the endoplasmic reticulum and of the mitochondrial tubuli. Many of the above results and interpretations tally with our findings and ideas. Hence, it might be a common man's observation that red mud leached chemicals significantly affects the pigments and cause great physiological changes evinced from the observation of NPP, GPP and respiration studies.

The observed toxic changes in both the sets of experiments might be due to red mud leached chemicals only. Considering the reports that PMA inhibits electron transport and photo-phosphorylations, its effectiveness as an anti-transparirant may depend primarily on its restriction to the epidermal layer of the leaf. The disturbances in growth and growth substances are always related with metabolic changes inside the plant body. Biochemical changes proceed any change in growth because growth is the outcome of many biochemical processes; and physiological and biochemical effects, are the underlying cause of measurable whole organism effects. Complexes between Hg^{2+} and certain purine and pyrimidines especially thymine, are quite stable (Katz, 1962) and complexes with phosphates are probably formed readily; thus one would expect nulceotides and nucleic acids also to bind Hg^{2+} rather well. Inogaki (1940) found various nucleotides, such as AMP, GMP and IMP to be precipitated by mercuric compounds. Hg^{2+} has been found to produce complex with nucleic acids from thymus, plants (Trim, 1959), Pneumococci (Dove and Yamane, 1960), and TMV (Katz and Santilli, 1962 b). Interference with cellular functions via interaction with various nucleic acid components is undoubtedly in large part responsible (Ramel, 1969; Mulvihilli, 1972) for the mutagenecity of mercurials. The excessive discharge of red mud leached chemicals in recent years tends to contaminate the environment. Controversy has centered around both the mode of action of red mud leached chemical in effecting plant metabolism and the extent of its toxicity resulting from penetration into the mesophyll. The literature on residual accumulation of red mud leached chemical and its effects on crop like rice is scanty. Vascular plants accumulate red mud leached chemicals by three routes of uptake: through the root from the soil (ionic), through the stomata from the leaf surface deposition and by the retentions of particulate dust, atmospheric uptake predominating in the above ground (mostly leaves) parts of herbaceous plants. As the Hg concentrations prevailing in soils, plants retain Hg almost exclusively within the root, where it seem to be relatively tightly bound to acidic groups of cell walls only at exceptionally high soil mercury contents, there occurred significant translocation to shoot (Lorenz, 1979). Higher concentrations of red mud leached chemical in leaves than in other tissues of the plants, as well as in grasses, draw the attention of ecologists because, grazers mostly depend on grasses and leaves of the plants. Thus the grazers of the area (cows, sheep, goat) must be accumulating red mud leached chemicals in their tissues via food chain since they are totally dependent on the live flora of the area. Hamilton and Ruthvein (1967) analyzed potato seeds, which had been treated with organo-mercurial disinfectants, for export purposes. The potatoes grown from the seed contained very small amount of mercury and were indistinguishable from those grown from untreated seeds. Plants treated with red mud leached chemical compounds may have high red mud leached chemical concentrations in certain parts but it is not known whether the chemical was absorbed and translocated by plant tissues to these parts, or only occurred as a superficial deposit. Plants are capable of absorbing red mud leached chemical and translocating it through their tissues. Thus, red mud leached chemicals deposited/transported to leaves might be translocated to the fruit and other parts. Red mud leached chemical concentrations in water, due to the ultimate discharge of Red Mud from the NALCO plant; cause a considerable reduction in the photosynthetic capability of phytoplankton. High percentage of seed germination and seedling establishment, disease free seedling and healthy growth of the plant are considered to be some of the trustworthy indications about high yield potential of any crop plant. In nature, as the plants are very much exposed to different environmental changes, wastes, insects and pests, they suffer from variety of diseases at different stages of their life cycle. So, the crop plants cannot maintain a perfect toxicant/disease free life, unless proper care is being taken. The seeds produced from the affected plants cannot be utilized in agriculture or for food purposes, because these lack germination vigor and nutritional value. Rather these seeds contain a lot of toxicants that also gets distributed throughout the plant and finally the seeds of this plant again accumulate a lot of toxicants. Really, the cultivation of this crop is a challenging task for a cultivator, because, the cultivation needs a lot of experience and much care. All phases of its life cycle (*i*) Germination phase, (*ii*) Seedling phase, (*iii*) Growth and tillering phase, (*iv*) Flowering phase, (*v*) Fruiting phase and (*vi*) Harvesting phase are very much sensitive to toxicant stress, industrial wastes, pest infection and also minor changes in the climate and environment. Out of all the phases, the germinating phase needs more attention, because it is the basic and most sensitive phase from which the life cycle of the plant starts. If seed and soil borne pathogens, will be eradicated before or at this stage, the future seedling becomes healthy and can resist/tolerate up and downs of natural changes by application of specific insecticides/pesticides. On the other hand, compared to other chemicals, specially, the unrestricted use of organo-mercurial compounds/formulations in industry and agriculture towards the last part of the nineteenth century has increased substantial amount of mercury in the aquatic and terrestrial environment, and has created a serious threat to biotic component of the earth (Fiskesjo, 1979). Now it stands as a global problem. According to Sahu (1987) the toxic hazards of red mud leached chemicals and mercury has now gained sociological and political importance. Hence, it is highly essential to understand the amount of toxic red mud leached chemical present, it's movement and biological magnification along the critical path to the man. Though the process of bio-accumulation, bio-magnification of the heavy metal, mercury, and red mud leached chemical was recently understood, but it was realized that, from the red mud leached chemical contaminated the entry and accumulation into the biological system, occurs at a very slower rate and also it takes a longer time period for its dreadful expressions. But, the pesticide, which enters into the agricultural soil by leaching and through irrigation, finds its way into the living system through direct consumption of food grain. Hence the pesticide burden of the biological system had increased in an astounding rate in a short time. Recently it has been reported that, besides the seeds, the largest in-put of pesticide into U.K. agricultural soil arise from atmospheric deposition after mass fumigation. The cultivators of the area reported several times, the reporters, the NGO's reported and protested several times regarding the effects of the leached chemicals of the red mud pond and also demonstrated several times regarding the destruction of crop plant and crop production many a times, but neither the government nor the industry people show any interest on the issue. Rather NALCO plant gets the award as the best non-polluting industry obeying all the norms for the protection of the environment and the surrounding.

The prediction of Koronowski (1973) become a reality and opined that the agricultural mercury becomes dangerous for human health, when mercury containing fungicides enter into nutritional cycle through dressed seeds or other treated parts by mistake, ignorance and carelessness. Similar predictions can also be attributable for the red mud leached chemical and mercury present in the irrigated water or the leached chemicals of the red mud waste. Siegel *et al.* (1977) have shown that he use of mercurial seed dresser, year after year has not only increased the mercury burden or the agricultural soil but also contaminated the abiotic and biotic components of the ecosystem. Mercury based pesticides treated seed grains, which is flooded after planting (*e.g.* rice) can directly contribute this toxic metal to water and soil. Including above statements, further seed dressing can introduce approximately 10g/ha of mercury into the soil. As all most all the components of the environment are polluted with pesticide and mercury, the entry of it into the living system through food chain is a must and cannot be avoided (Jernelov and Lann, 1971). Hence, the idea of mistake, ignorance and carelessness as quoted by Koronowski (1973) at this stage are found to have no meaning. In Poland, it has been first realized that the mercury content of water (River and Stream) draining the agricultural soils was found to be increasing during sowing time of cereal crops. In future, Damonjodi area and its surrounding will face the consequences of the leached chemicals of the red mud pond. A big poison lake is under preparation for the destruction of the future of Damonjodi, Koraput area. Towards last part of the present century the agricultural contamination of red mud leached chemical and its entry through food chain, have not only drawn the attention of the scientists of all over the world, but also a lot of research work in this line have already been undertaken. Many countries have enacted their legislation to restrict the use of pesticide and mercury both in industry and in agricultural sectors. Some developed countries like Japan, Sweden, USA, Canada, and France etc. have totally banned the use of mercurial compounds in agriculture. Here it is interesting to note that in Sweden, the mercury content of freshwater (arising from leaching and non-off of fungicide etc.) is still increasing even though the use of mercury compound was banned some ten years ago. The restriction and also the ban on the use of mercurial compounds and pesticides by advanced/developed countries have indirectly compelled the industrial entrepreneurs of those countries to shift their market and dump those in developing and underdeveloped countries of the world. Many compounds banned by those countries due to their hazardous effect are dumped in the third world countries in the form of charity or in liberal soft business terms/loans. So the people of developing countries usually suffer from various types of dreadful diseases. To have better, non-toxic, potent and bio-degradable pesticide chemical, the desire and unending search of man through decades no doubt have produced/introduced various chemical formulations from time to time, but no chemical was found to be satisfactory to man till to-day. The banning of one, and introduction of new chemical has become the common practice. Hence, it is a general feeling in developing countries that all chemicals introduced till to-today are/were in the experimental phase only. The same condition has also happened for mercurial compounds as these were proved to be hazardous both to the nature and also to the biotic component of the ecosphere. Therefore, at present, it is logical to predict that the seed dressing chemicals which are introduced in recent past (non-mercurials) after some more years again these will be obsolete and may be banned by assigning some other negative reasons. In future, a similar step might be taken by the government to ban the industry but by the time sufficient harm might have occurred in the affected area. Here it can be stressed that, before introduction of any chemical proper scientific scrutiny, from all possible aspects is essential, so the reckless handling of the chemical, cannot cause any residual toxicity problem in future. Secondly, sound knowledge on chemical behavior and toxicity will be very much essential prior to introduction of the chemicals either through irrigation or natural entry through leaching. Literature explaining the following aspects in details is lacking:

1. Leached chemicals of the red mud waste dynamics in seeds in relation to seed biology. 2. Amount of leached chemical transfer to agricultural soil and its transfer to seedlings. 3. Leached chemical of the red mud pond transfer from soil to seed from seed to seedling and from seedling to plant and from the plant again to the seeds. 4. Interferences of leached chemical of red mud in seed physiology during germination and establishment and its biochemistry. 5. Comparative study of RM leached chemical toxicity in petriplate culture, pot culture and field culture. The agricultural contaminated waste poses to be a threat to the present generation. The study of the above aspects, certainly add additional information pertaining to the contribution of man for enriching the agricultural soil. Further, it can be said that, the degree and the process of bioaccumulation of such added chemicals through various crop plant could be identified and investigated. Hence, the present piece of work was designed to study the effects of Red mud leached chemical on a rice seed, seedling and the plant. Usually the protrusion of the radical through seed coat though considered as germination, but this simple process comprises of four phases: (*i*) Imbibition phase, (*ii*) Activation phase, (*iii*) Phase of mitosis and (*iv*)The radical protrusion phase. Each distinct phase can be influenced by an external or internal factor. During germination, the seeds not only imbibe water, but also absorb inorganic and organic substances present in the imbibing medium other physiological processes of the seedling. But actually the nature of the chemical substance entered and also nature of the seed, both combined determine the degree of response and direction of the effect. During normal course of germination, according to Young (1938), the emergence of primary root to the external environment precedes to that of coleoptile. But in the investigation conducted by Padhi (1990), a reverse process was observed in the long term treated seeds or seeds treated with high concentration of MEMC. The coleoptile was observed not only to emerge prior to radical but also there was a considerable delay in radical emergence. This type of germination reported by Padhi (1990) was designated as abnormal germination. This finding was similar to the findings of Taylor (1942 a and b). Delayed germination as observed in the present

investigation was also reported in case of beans, cabbage, carrot, millet, onions, tomato (Bache *et al.*, 1973), Oats (Sorteberg, 1974), Maize (Bache *et al.*, 1973 and Lipsey, 1975) and Bermuda grass (Bache *et al.*, 1973 and Weaver *et al.*, 1984). High MEMC content in the soil (50 mg Kg^{-1}, Aretan) also delayed the germination of wheat for 5 days, but at this concentration the seedlings of $HgCl_2$ treatment, did not show delay in germination (Semu *et al.*, 1985). The delay and reduction in germination might be due to accumulation of more amounts of toxic ions in the seed or toxic effect of the chemical. It was claimed that the reduced percentage of germination was directly proportional to the osmotic pressure it produces and thus reducing/preventing the availability of water needed for imbibition or toxic effect of specific ions in the medium where the seeds were exposed. We agree with the findings of the above authors. At still higher concentrations, the seed germination was totally stopped. According to Semu *et al.* (1985), the germination in bean failed completely, when the soil contained 50 mg of Hg Kg^{-1}. Even after repeated sowing no germination was recorded in that contaminated soil. Similar cases were reported in pesticide and waste contaminated agricultural fields.

The characteristic malformations of seedlings of cereals were produced from organic mercury exposure (ethyl mercury phosphate) when applied at high doses. The maize seedling grown in methyl mercury hydroxide showed severe decrease in growth (Lipsey, 1975). At 50 mg of Hg Kg^{-1} Aretan (MEMC) in the soil, the wheat plant not only showed stunted growth of the seedling but also remained shorter throughout the life period. The wheat plants grown in soil containing similar concentrations of Hg treated with $HgCl_2$, showed stunted growth up to flowering but the plants could recover to its normal size at the time of maturity (Semu *et al.*, 1985). Growth retardation of crop plants were also reported by Sorteberg (1974), Lipsey (1975) and Weaver *et al.* (1984) as the seeds were treated with different types of organo-mercurial formulations. At low concentrations of PMA and ethyl mercuric chloride the winter wheat showed changes in the seedling vigor (Bateman, 1975). The seedlings of tomato, corn and bean grown in complete nutrient solution containing MMH (Haney and Richard, 1973) showed that tomato seedlings were killed within 4-8 days at concentrations of 0.05 ppm. The growth was inhibited at concentration of 0.01 ppm for tomatoes and 0.05 ppm for corn and beans. Hassett *et al.* (1976) and Godbold *et al.* (1984) stated that inhibition of root elongation is one of the sensitive parameters to assess the toxicity of the heavy metals and pesticides. Godbold and Huttermann (1985) observed that the root elongation was severely inhibited by 0.1 to 0.5 mM of mercury after 24 hours. At 5 and 15 mm the root elongation was ceased completely and radial shrinkage was observed in 1.5 mm from behind the root tip. The treatment of PMA to the root tip Secale cereal (Sokolowska *et al.*, 1975) and treatment of Methoxy-beta ethyl mercuric chloride to *Allium cepa* (Venot and Glachhero, 1971) showed irregularity in cell division in root and also showed growth inhibition. The cytological study revealed that the treated seeds of Apel-*pine* (*Pinus halepensis*) showed precocious mitosis, accelerated lipolysis, proteolysis and inhibition of synthesis of organelles, especially in radical portion of the seedling. According to Ganesan and Monoharan (1983) the effect of cadmium and mercury on root length, stem length, leaf area and dry matter production *of A. esculantus* is inversely proportional to their concentration. When mercuric chloride applied in droplets to the cap of primary roots of the maize it reduced their elongation (Pillet and Jean, 1981). Sharma (1982) also reported that seeds of different varieties *Phaseolus aureus* treated with mercuric acetate solution showed inhibition of seedling growth. The same author, Sharma (1983 and 1985), reported that the seeds of *Pisum sativum* C.V. Boneville when treated with mercuric acetate solution shown promotion of radical and epicotyle length at lower concentration (10 mg l^{-1}), but in higher concentration at 50 mg l^{-1}, a significant reduction in seedling growth was observed. Inhibition of seedling growth was also observed by Mukherji and Ganguly (1974) in rice. The root inhibition was much more pronounced than the shoot inhibition, which was recorded in lettuce seedling (Mukherji and Das Gupta, 1972) in rice (Das Gupta and

Mukherji, (1977) treated with copper and rice (Banerjee and Mukherji, (1980) treated with Nickel. Increase in duration of pretreatment, increased the inhibition of rice seedlings in case of Barium exposure. Further, depending on the root elongation of ryegrass, the toxicity of various heavy metals was compared (Wong and Bradshaw, 1982). The length ratio of shoot and root calculated for all types of treatments, showed the negative trend in relation to concentration and period of treatment. This indicated that root length was much affected than the shoot system. This might be due to the fact that, the root being the primary absorbing organ, was in direct contact with a toxic medium and hence resulted higher reduction in different parameters of root. No doubt it is a confirmatory test which depicts the nature of growth of the root and shoot. According to Baeuford *et al.* (1977), the uptake of mercury in plants growth in hydroponic solutions was a function of external concentration. Over the concentration range considered, the accumulation of mercury in root was linear on a log-log basis although the uptake of elements in shoots appeared to be biphasic. The distribution of mercury in plant was asymmetrical with greater amounts of element in the roots than the shoots. As the apical meristem of *Elodi densa* showed deposition of more methyl mercury (Czuba and Mortimer, 1982), so also the deposition of more mercury in the apical region/meristematic region of the root might have caused inhibition. The observation made in the present investigation agrees with the findings of all the workers reported here except Siegel *et al.* (1984) and Padhy (1990). But in the present observation, water content of the seedling decreased in shoot and root portion of the seedling, the toxicity of the chemical might be the real reason of growth inhibition. Hence at this stage it will be premature to infer but it can be predicted that if growth studies of seedlings are undertaken at very low doses of leached chemicals of the red mud waste, at low exposure periods and also in case of very young seedlings, significant and notable inhibition of shoot system could be marked. The stimulation observed might be due to change in certain bio-chemical parameters caused due to mercury toxicity. So far, most of the research efforts were concentrated after 144 h of seed germination in normal and toxic mediums. References pertaining to the physiology and biochemical changes during germination and seedling establishment before 144 h of germination is scanty and the only report of Padhy (1990) and Pradhan (1998) is interesting. In absence of sufficient literature pertaining to the early phases of germination, satisfactory explanations and logical conclusions might face strong criticism. However, Padhy (1990) made an effort to illustrate the probable mechanism in a simpler way and the work indicated a separate line of thinking and suggested the real mechanism during early phases of germination and seedling growth.

In this study, inhibition of root was more pronounced than the shoot, which is probably the characteristic of toxicity as root is the first site to absorb the toxicants. Hassete *et al.* (1976); and Godbold *et al.* (1984) indicated with positive confirmation of the idea and support of findings presented in this piece of investigation. On seedling basis, it become clear that the decrease in fresh weight was only due to decrease in water content, as the dry weight of the seedling decreased significantly. Increase in shoot/root dry weight ratio confirmed the above explanation. Hence, in the treated seedling water stress condition was created. Inhibition of root growth was considered to be an indication of pesticide toxicity (Godbold *et al.*, 1984), depletion of the shoot might be the secondary effect reflected due to root inhibition. Hence, at this stage it was difficult to infer, whether stimulation of shoot was due to toxicity of the leached chemical or this chemical had no effect on the shoot system in lower concentrations and also in very young seedlings (Patra, 1993). According to present investigation, acquisition of more amounts of toxic ions by the root from the leached chemical contaminated soil might be imparting high toxic effect on root cells. On the other hand the low amount of leached chemical probably deposited in shoot might have shown inhibitory action. Very low concentrations of pesticide induce stimulation in growth and here in case of red mud waste such a trend was not marked. The above finding was confirmed by Sahu (1987), Shaw (1987) and Padhy (1990). As in lower concentration, the stimulation in seed germination and shoot growth was not observed, so also, the chlorophyll content of the seedling decreased with the dose. It can be said that inhibition of shoot growth might have inhibited the chlorophyll biosynthesis which in turn showed decrease in total chlorophyll content of the seedling. No doubt the inhibition of root growth and the stimulation of shoot growth are the consequences of mercury toxicity at lower concentrations, so also the increase in chlorophyll was the consequence of toxic behavior of mercury in sub-acute concentrations (Padhi, 1990). The effect of $HgCl_2$, MMC, MEMC, PMA on this species also have shown striking decrease in chlorophyll, and dry matter content. Lee and Young (1972) also reported that when compared to cadmium and zinc, mercury depressed the growth rate and chlorophyll content of *Chlorella ellipsoidea*. Rai *et al.* (1981) had suggested that specific growth rate and final yield of *Chlorella* treated with zinc, mercury and methyl mercury, showed decrease in total chlorophyll content and increase in carotenoid/ chlorophyll ratio with increase in heavy metal concentration. Lipsey (1975) also stated that *in vitro* conditions, MMH inhibited photosynthesis of chloroplast and phosphate uptake by mitochondria. The same author reported that when maize seedlings were treated with MMH, showed stunted growth and respiration of isolated mitochondria were inhibited. In addition, the mercury caused dilation of the endoplasmic reticulum and of the mitochondrial tubuli. Lee *et al.* (1973) demonstrated that binding of Hg to chloroplast depend on concentrations and nature of the compound. The binding of Hg governs the blockage of electron flow by altering the Hills reaction. Mercury abolishes the communication between photosystems and associated redox pool. But according to Kimimura and Sakae (1972)–the $HgCl_2$ completely inhibits methyl viologen Hill reaction as well as methyl viologen photo-reduction with reduced DCPIP as electron donor. The extent of inhibition of Hill activity was much higher under high intensity of light. Here it can be added that in activation of photosynthesis and loss of leaf protein are both related to total mass of leaf chloroplast during senescence of rice seedling. Both actinomycin–A and $HgCl_2$ inhibited the development of ATP producing system, linked with most part with the development of non-cyclic photo-phosphorylation, which may be due to participation of ATP, synthesized in cyclic electron transport in the formation of chloroplast during greening. According to Huising and Kline (1972) it has been reported in Barley that the absorption and translocation of mercury from treated seeds to seedling leaves and roots showed a definite dosage–concentration dependence. Further, the same authors have stated that, the anionic moiety to which mercury is attached, influence absorption and translocation. Mercury levels in plants decreased with time. The level in leaves decreased more rapidly than that in roots. Actually the entry of mercury in relation to seed behaviour during germination could not be explained in a better way (Radha, 1993). The residual mercury was found to be located in the rice bran (specially in protein components of the bran) portion of the grain as the plants were sprayed with inorganic mercury during vegetative and flowering stages of growth. From the observations and available literature, it clearly indicated that the organo-mercurial fungicide–MEMC induced significant alternation in germination and in normal morphology of the seedling. Simultaneously the entry of mercury into the endosperm was also realized. Hence the findings of the present investigation have not only induced to study the bio-chemical changes of the germinating seedling but also their behaviour in the growth and productivity of the crop plant. Significant changes in respiration rate of the different aged seedlings, when exposed to different concentrations of the red mud waste leachates indicated clearly the effect of the test chemical. At lower exposure periods, the low aged seedlings, the effect seems to be more drastic than the higher aged seedlings. The effect of the toxicant at higher doses (2 per cent) was much more drastic when compared to low doses of the test chemical. Debnath and Mukherji (1982), reported identical observations under $BaCl_2$ stress in different types of aged seedlings. The decrease in respiration rate in young germinating seedlings might be due to the stress, the red mud waste. Because, at this stage, the body burden of Red mud leached chemical might be the maximum, which gets diluted with the aging of the seedling. But the significant variation observed at 144 h old seedling was interesting. At lower concentrations of the toxicant, decrease in rate was observed. Sahu (1987), Shaw (1987), Padhy (1990), and Pradhan (1998) reported an initial increase followed by a decrease in respiration rate both in inorganic and organic mercurial compound exposure. This result did not support the biphasic or dual behavior of the toxicant in different biosystems. After a decrease, again an increase in respiration rate can be correlated with the dilution of the toxicant in the seedlings and also at higher exposure period. This supports the idea that low stress causes depression and high stress induces inhibition.The germination of seeds was subjected to activity changes, which are regulated by exogenous and endogenous factors. In the moment of soaking, the complex reaction began in dormant embryo and also in its nutritive tissue. RNA, Protein and DNA conversions are set in a predetermined way of germination and seedling development. All these processes are bio-chemically reflected in alteration of enzyme status. Investigation on changes in enzyme activities and pattern, in germinating seeds, suggest not only the information's about the course of germination process but also they may contribute to a deeper understanding of gene activators. Since all cellular processes are essentially enzyme catalyzed, the intersection of a toxicant agent with living matter generally causes disturbance in the enzymatic reactions. Further such interference at the enzymatic level provides clue to the mode of action of the toxic substance (Bruin, 1976). Hence in view of the above fact the effect of an exogenous toxic chemical the Red mud leached chemical on bio-chemical and enzymatic changes of young rice seedling in different cultures needs proper investigation.

At very high concentrations of the toxicant significant bimolecular changes can be marked. But at very low concentrations of the toxicant, the observed insignificant inhibition might be a transitional short stayed phase. Pradhan (1998) and Sahu (1987) stressed the dichotomous behaviour of the mercurial toxicant. Both the authors emphasized stimulation at very low concentrations of the toxicant and shorter periods of exposure and inhibition both at higher concentrations of the toxicant and longer period of exposure. When we overview the works of Rath (1984), Sahu (1987), Shaw (1987) and Panigrahi (1990) which gives clear indication of dichotomous behaviour of the mercury compounds on different plant systems. It becomes rather too difficult here to explain the dual behavior in germinating seedlings, where as, we have only observed one type of effect *i.e.* inhibition. The only probable note, we can leave here just to escape from the present situation might be due to the following reasons: (*i*) the real detailed bio-chemical and physiological mechanisms in germinating seedlings are yet to be ascertained, (*ii*) non-existence of a dynamic sequence of events occurring in germinating seedlings, (*iii*) insufficient amount of bio-macromolecule production, (*iv*) phasic changes in the rates of metabolism in germinating seedlings, (*v*) role of water and its highest absorption disturbing the osmotic resistance and mechanical fragility of the cells of the germinating seedlings, (*vi*) fast and unstable macromolecular conversions in a very limited time. Here it can be stressed that, the inhibited amount of RNA produced, certainly takes part in the protein synthesis, so that low amount of protein formation occurs in the root and shoot portion. But in the shoot, only a significant decrease in protein content was noticed. Hence, it is suggested that the low amount of protein synthesized might have been derived towards the formation of more hydrolysing enzymes, such as proteases abundantly seen in rice seeds. It is known that protease is related to dynamic state or << turnover >> of protein in the cell than to the absolute protein level at any one time (Das Gupta and Mukherji, 1977). In copper treated lettuce seedlings, a considerable rise in the level of soluble protein was marked (Mukherji and Das Gupta, 1972). The same authors opined that, this type of behavior of soluble protein formation probably synchronizes with the similar increase in enzyme activity. In addition, they suggested that the increase in enzyme activity. In addition, they suggested that the increase in the activity of the enzymes studied (Mukherji and Das Gupta, 1972) was due to enhanced protein synthesis and the entire happenings were probably due to copper (a heavy metal) toxicity. However, the present investigation did not agree 100 per cent with the above findings. But at this stage, it will be premature to reach to a firm conclusion. Mukherji and Das Gupta (1972) and Das Gupta and Mukherji (1977) conducted the experiments in old seedlings of rice. Secondly, the type of toxicant was different, which shows differential activity based on their site of action and site of stimulation or inhibition. Further detailed work on enzymes explained late, might suggest again a total different picture and even the story may take a different turn. On this basis, protein levels may rise even though the protease shows increasing activity. To put it in the other way, enzymatic degradation by protease may be rapid but the coincident rate of protein synthesis may also be rapid (Das Gupta and Mukherji, 1977). Our findings agree with the above-mentioned workers. Hence accumulation of free amino acids in the system is facilitated and DNA/protein ratio is almost maintained at a steady state. However, this phase is a purely temporary one and in later phase (increase in exposure period to toxic chemical) all above parameters will show differential trends, because stimulation of RNA and synthesis of protein will be ceased and degradation of the bio-macromolecules will set in. Salt sensitive cultivars (TKM 9) of rice showed accumulation of excess soluble protein in shoots and roots. Lead toxicity on growth and metabolism of germinating rice (Mukherji and Maitra, 1977), mercury toxicity in rice seedling (Mukherji and Nag, 1977 a) are available. They have reported that the oxidising enzymes *viz.*, catalase, peroxidase, IAA oxidase and ascorbic acid oxidase, all showed constant enhancement and have been envisaged as general biochemical symptoms of metal toxicity. Consequently, a close correlation between reduced growths and increased activity of these enzymes has been established (Debnath and Mukherji, 1982). Mukherji and Das Gupta, (1972) showed in lettuce seedlings, that, respective of age of the seedling, the catalase activity showed about 2 fold increase at the highest copper dose. Enzyme level decreased both in control and copper with aging, which was presumed to be result of an impaired metabolic status of the older seedlings. Steeman and Wium-Anderson (1969), Steeman and Kamp-Nelson (1970) recorded that excess copper in the growing medium caused drastic reduction in the growth of an alga and attributed this phenomenon to a permanent injury to the photosynthetic mechanism. The same authors opined that product change might be due to the imbalance of the enzyme systems responsible for growth. They have suggested that Ni, Hg, Co, Cd application brought changes in quantity of citric, malic and aconitic acids. The amphiphilic nature of Me-Hg favoured the interactions of lipophilic cell structure, above all with the membranes, which may represent the primary target of organo-metallic attack. Further, both $HgCl_2$ and CH_3HgCl_2 (MMC) crossed the bio-molecular lipid membranes and entered into the cell and consequently act on different substrates and enzymes of the cell. Most of the results obtained in the present investigation do not tally with the results as reported by earlier workers as pointed out during discussion. Most of the references cited here were related to either heavy metal toxicity or pesticide toxicity. We do not find sufficient literature on this type of poisoning related to leached chemicals of red mud waste coming from the Alluminium industry, which might contain several other metals and might be heavy metals. The peculiar behavior shown by this toxicant (Red mud waste) might be due to synergistic effect of all types of chemicals available in the red mud waste.

Most of the results of different parameter were found to be statistically significant; it does mean that, the trend or changes observed in the present piece of work are to be taken into confidence. In this connection, here it can be stressed that as the study was undertaken during transition phase of growth or at active growth phase or the phase, in between emergence (embryo) and establishment (seedling), hence most of the parameters did confirm to the statistical 'significance' test, as observed by other workers. From the above observations and interpretations, erecting a model becomes a difficult task in absence of residual level data. However, many interferences and predictions raised during discussion, provides gaps or fields unexplored yet. In this piece of investigation, though we felt to a link a gap but after completion of this piece, we find many questions remain unanswered. In this piece of investigation, we tried to find out the effects of Red mud leached chemical, on seed germination and seeding establishment of rice crop, *Oryza sativa*, L. From the results obtained in present study, it is clearly evident that, Red mud leached chemical, which is now well known for its interference in biochemical metabolism, becomes phyto-toxic when used in lower and moderate concentrations. Thus, we can conclude that even though many advantages have been derived from the industry but we must not neglect the environment by way of constructing poison ponds like RED MUD PONDS near NALCO. Many similarities exist in biological process among all forms of life, and investigative effects of this nature are not only important to plants, fish and wildlife, but to all life forms, including man. However, as long as these chemicals are thrown into the environment without proper check, this type of leaching will always be there. These leached chemicals will always enter into crop fields; contaminate the groundwater and water bodies. There is always the possibility in future that unexpected and undesirable complication may arise even though minimum immediate hazards are occurring at present. Safe disposal of these wastes and proper care to avoid leaching of these chemicals can protect the non-target organisms, the blue-green algae. These tiny particles perform a fantastic job of atmospheric nitrogen fixation, increasing the fertility of paddy fields, maintaining the balance, used as biofertilizer. Due to careless handling of chemicals, unplanned disposal of wastes, future and fate of the waste chemicals in the environment, non adoption of safety measures, non-maintenance of ecological balance, improper adoption of plantation, non-selection of pollution reducing plantation, will significantly harm the man made agricultural ecosystem in particular and the ECOSYSTEM in general. Hence, protection of non-target systems is equally essential like protection of the crop plants. Due to heavy and constant discharge of these waste chemicals without following the directions given by Center and State Pollution Control Boards, Department of Environment, many a times, failure of the crop was marked. This failure was always attributed and pointed towards the seed banks. They are always accused of supplying bad seeds or non-viable seeds. But the fact lies at the site, where the seeds are sown to grow a crop. Hence, proper care and proper and safe disposal of these killer chemicals is essential to protect the agricultural ecosystem, hence, protecting the main users of these agricultural produce, *i.e.* M A N.

Summary

In petriplate culture, with the increase in toxicant concentration in the soil, the percentage of germination significantly declined and above 2.0 per cent leached Red mud waste chemical, germination of the seeds was not marked. The percentage of germination increased with the increase in exposure period and the same parameter decreased with the increase in toxicant concentration. The control set showed normal germination and a maximum of 100 per cent germination of seeds was marked after 144 hrs of exposure. Out of which, 100 per cent seedlings established. With the increase in toxicant concentration, the percent of seed germination reduced significantly. The difference between control and exposed sets was significant at higher exposure periods. Higher percentage of seed germination was marked in the pot, when compared to petriplate culture experiments. At higher conc. of the toxicant, the percentage of seedling establishment showed significant decline in pot culture experiments and the decrease showed the existence of negative correlation between the percentage of seedling establishment and toxicant concentration. A maximum of 85.96 per cent decease in shoot length was marked at 2.0 per cent of the toxicant exposed seedlings when compared to control seedlings, with the increase in the toxicant the shoot length decreased significantly. The length of the roots was more than the length of the shoots in the control set. The length of the root decreased from 8.96 ± 0.22cms in the control set to 0.84±0.06 cm in conc. C (2.0 per cent). In petriplate culture experiments, the changes observed in shoot, root length and fresh weight, root and shoot dry weight were highly significant, where the correlation coefficient values were all negative and significant. The gradual decrease in shoot fresh wt with the increase toxicant concentration dose was probably due to the toxicant in laboratory controlled petriplate culture. A maximum of 88.4 per cent and 82.35 per cent decrease was marked in shoot and root dry weight respectively in exposed seedlings exposed to toxicant. In pot culture, with the increase in toxicant concentrations, the shoot length decreased significantly, showing a maximum of 47.22 per cent decrease, when compared to the control value. The root and shoot fresh weight ratio did show significant variation and the exposed values were less than the control value. Significant variation was observed in pot culture, when compared to the petriplate culture. Significant differences were marked between petriplate culture and pot culture data. A maximum of 89.28 per cent decrease in chlorophyll 'a' content was marked in seedlings exposed to conc. C, when compared to the control value in petriplate culture. At 2.0 per cent of red mud leached waste, 92.44 per cent depletion in total chlorophyll content was marked. Interestingly the total phaeophytin content declined significantly with the increase in toxicant concentration in exposed rice seedlings and 91.67 per cent decrease in phaeophytin content when compared to control value was marked in 144 hr old seedlings in petriplate culture, at conc. C. The total carotene content decreased with the increase in toxicant concentration significantly, when compared to the control value. In pot culture, in each exposure period, the total chlorophyll content of the leaves, decreased from the control value and maximum decrease was marked at conc. C. In conc. A on 15th and 30th day of exposure, increase in chlorophyll content by 7.02 per cent and 3.82 per cent was recorded. In pot culture, in each exposure period and at all the three concentrations of the toxicant, the phaeophytin content depleted significantly and a maximum of 58.09 per cent, 88.6 per cent and 95.95 per cent decrease was marked at concentration A, B and C, respectively indicated highly toxic nature of the toxicant, leached chemicals of the red mud. Changes in carotenoid content followed, almost the same trend indicating the toxic nature of the toxicant, red mud waste.

The respiration rate decreased with the increase in the conc. of the toxicant. Significantly, the net primary productivity decreased in conc. C of the toxicant. Similarly the gross primary productivity decreased with the increase in concentration of the toxicant in 144 hr old rice seedlings. Maximum depletion in net primary productivity was marked at conc. C of the toxicant on 60th day of exposure. The changes in gross primary productivity in control and exposed seedlings in pot culture followed an identical trend. At lower exposure periods and lower doses of the toxicant, stimulation in the net primary productivity values were marked when compared to the control values. Significant negative correlation coefficient values were marked between the respiration rates of the rice plant leaves at different concentrations of the toxicant. Under field conditions in pot culture, the respiration rate of exposed plants declined with the increase in time period and concentration of the toxicant. Highest decrease in NPP value was recorded at conc. C and 60th day of exposure. The NPP value decreased significantly. The effects were more in pot culture in prolonged period of experiment. In petriplate culture, probably less amount of the toxicant was absorbed. But in prolonged period of experiment, higher amount of toxicant was absorbed and accumulated in the exposed plant. The body burden might have increased significantly showing the effects. The gross primary productivity was the calculated value of NPP and RR. Hence GPP values showed an identical trend like that of NPP and RR. Highest depletion was recorded at conc. C and on 60th day of exposure. Glucose content decreased significantly by 88.36 per cent at conc. C, when compared to the control value. Approximately 90.32 per cent decrease in nitrogen content was marked in seedlings exposed to the toxicant, when compared to control seedlings. With increase in the toxicant, the glucose content of the exposed leaves, declined significantly except in conc. A. The decrease in glucose content in the leaves of control plant at 60th day of exposure might be due to the collaborative effort of the toxicant and aging and senescence of the exposed rice plants. A maximum of 78.43 per cent and 96.43 per cent decrease in nitrogen content was marked at conc. C after 60th day of exposure in shoot and root, respectively. The ATPase activity of the exposed seedlings showed significant depletion and 91.18 per cent decrease was recorded in conc. C in petriplate culture.

From the above observations, it can be concluded that the toxicant, leached chemicals of the red mud pond is deadly toxic. The variation in toxicity was only due to the concentration of the toxicant. Every year during the rainy season, these toxicants leach heavily and leaching was continuous in all seasons and in all days, enters into the paddy fields, thereby increasing the toxicant concentration. It was observed that toxicants enter into the plant and there might be a gradual build up of toxicant level in the rice plant. From the plants, toxicant might be getting deposited in the rice grains. Toxicant build up in the plants and than in the grains, and consequent build up in grazers may lead to availability of toxicant in milk and meat of herbivores or grazers. From milk, meat and rice grain, toxicant(s) may enter into human body. This build up of toxicant in the human system may lead to another significant incident, like many other incidents related to pollution.

References

Ahmad, F. E., R. W. Hart and N. J. Lewis (1977). *Mut. Res.*, 42: 161.

Ahmad, M. R., P. N. Saxena, D. V. Amla and R. Shyam (1978). *Beitr. Biol. Pflanzen*, 54: 33.

Ahuja, A. K. and D. Subrahmaniyam (1978). *Proc. Ind. Acad. Sci.*, 87: 189.

Annonymous (1989). Special short Course Training on Seed Testing. Seed testing Laboratory, Directorate of Agrl. and Food Production, Bhubaneswar.

Bache, C.A., W.H. Gutenmann and D.J.Hisk (1971). *Science*, 172: 951.

Baicu, T. and T. Diaconu (1972). *An Inst. Cercet. Prot. Plant.*, 10: 381.

Banerjee, A. and A.S. Mukherji (1980). *Indian Journal of Exp.Biol.*18: 438.

Barron, M.G and Adelman, I.R. (1984). Nucleic acid. Protein content, and growth of larval fish sub-lethally exposed to various toxicants. *Can. J. Fish. Aquat. Sci.*, 41: 141.

Barrineau, P., P. Gillbert, W.J.Jackson, C.S.Jones, A.O. Summers and S. Wisdom (1984). *Mol. Appl. Genet.*, 2: 601.

Beauford, W. J. Barber and A.R.Barringer (1977). *Physiol. Plant.*, 39: 261.

Bouveng, H.O.(1968). The chlorine industry and mercury problem. *Modern. Kemi.*, 3: 45.

Bruin, A. De. (1976). Nucleic acid metabolism. In: *Biochemical Toxicity of Environmental Agents*. Ed. Bruin. A. De. pp. 605-655. Elsevier/North Holland Biomedical Press, The Netherlands.

Butler, G.C. (1978). *Principles of Ecotoxicology*. John Wiley and Sons, Chisester, New York, Brisbane, pp. 350.

Byford, W.J. (1971). *Ann. Appl.* 79(3). 221.

Cairns, J. (1980). *Bioscience*, 30: 101.

Cairns, J. Jr., D. Gruber, K. L. Dickson, A. C. Hendrick and S. W. H. Van Deer (1977). Developing an on site continuous biological monitoring system for chemical industry. In : *Proc. 5th Annual Industrial Pollution Conf. 1.* Delpino and Krigman (eds.), 285.

Cairns, J. Jr., D. K. L. Dickson and G. F. Wastelake (1976). Biological monitoring of water and effluent quality. Philadelphia, American Society for Testing of Materials, STP, 607.

Cairns, J. Jr., G. R. Lanza and B. C. Parker (1972). *Proc. Acad. Nat. Sc.*, Philadelphia, 124: 79.

Cairns, J. Jr., K. L. Dickson and A. W. Maki (eds.) (1978). Estimating the hazard of chemical substances to aquatic life. *ASTM*, Philadelphia.

Czuba, M. And D.C.Mortimer (1982). *Can J. Bot.*, 60(5). 657.

Das Gupta, B. And S. Mukherji (1982). *Z. Pflanzen Physiol.*, 82: 95.

De Filippis, L. F. (1979). *Zietschrift fur Pflanzen Physiologie*, 92: 39.

De Filippis, L. F. and C. K. Pallaghy (1976 a). *Z. Pflanzen-physiol. Bd.*, 78: 197.

De Filippis, L. F. and C. K. Pallaghy (1976 b). *Z. Pflanzen-physiol. Bd.*, 78: 323.

De Filippis, L. F., R. Hamp and H. Zeigler (1981). *Z. Pflanzen Physiol. Bd.*, 101: 37.

De, A.K., A.K. Sen, D.P. Modak and S. Jana (1985). Studies of toxic effects of Hg(II) on *Pistia stratioles. Water, Air and Soil Pollution*, 24: 351.

Debnath, R. and S. Mukherji (1982). *Biologia Plantarum (PRAHA)*, 24(6). 423.

Desiah, D., L.K.Cutkomp, R.B.Koch and G. A. Garvinean (1975). *Arch. of Environ. Contam. Toxicol.*, 3(2). 132.

Dove, W.F. and T. Yamane (1960) : *Biochem. Biophys. Res. Commun.*, 3: 608.

Donovan, T.J. and A.D.Day (1969). Some effects of high salinity on germination and emergence of barley (Hordeum vulgare, L. and Lati) *Agron. J.*, 61: 236.

Dove, W.F. and T.Yamane (1960). *Biochem. Biochem. Biophys. Res. Commun.*, 3: 608.

Filip, D. S. and R. T. Lynn (1972). *Chemosphere*, 6: 251.

Fox, J.H.K. Patel-Mandlik and M.M. Cohen (1975). Comparative effects of organic and inorganic mercury on brain slice respiration and metabolism. *J. Neuro-chemistry*, 24: 757.

Frenkel, G.D. and K. Randles (1982). Specific stimulation of a-amanitin sensitive RNA synthesis in isolated HeLa Nuclie by methyl mercury. *J. Biol. Chem.* 257-6275.

Frenkel, G.D., R.Cain and E.S-E. Chao (1985). Exposure of DNA to methyl mercury results in an increase in the rate of its transpiration by RNA polymerase-II. *Biochemical and Biophysical Research Communications*, 127: 849.

Furukawa, K., T. Suzuki and K. Tonomura (1969). *Agric. Biol. Chem.*, 33: 128.

Gadd, G.M. and A.J. Griffith (1978). *Microbial Ecol.*, 4: 303.

Geener, H. and J.R.Jeener (1952). *Exptl. Cell Res.*, 3: 675.

Gill, T.S., J.C. Pant and H.Tewari (1988). *Bull. Environ. Contam. Toxicol.*, 41: 241.

Godbold, D.L., and A.Hutterman (1985). Environmental Pollution (Ser.A.). *Ecological and Biological*, 38: 375.

Gross, R. E., P. Pungo and W. M. Dugger (1970). *Plant Physiology*, 46: 183.

Hamilton, G. and A. Ruthvein (1967). *Journal of Science of Food and Agriculture*, 18 (12) : 558.

Hannan, P.J. and C. Patouillet (1972). Effects of Pollutants on growth of algae, *Reports of Naval Res. Lab. Progress*, p.1-8.

Hannan, P. J., P. E. Wilkniss, C. Patouillet and R. A. Carr (1973). Measurement of mercury sorption by algae, *NRL Report*, 7623.

Hanumann, H.G. (1987). *Potoplasma*, 136 (1). 37.

Harris, R.C., D.B. White and R.B. Mac Farlane (1970). Mercury compounds reduce photosynthesis of plankton. *Science*, 170: 736.

Hattula, M.L., J. Sarkka, J.Janatuinen, J. Passivirta and A.Roos (1978). *Env. Pollut.*, 17: 19.

Holdgate, M.W. (1979). *A perspective of environmental pollution*. Cambridge University Press, Cambridge, London, New York, Melbourne, p.278.

Huckabee, J. W., J. W. Elwood and S. G. Hildebrand (1979). In: *Biogeochemistry of Mercury in the Environment*, Nriagu, J. O. (Ed.) Elsevier, Holland, 277-302.

Huckabee, J.W., S.D.Francisco, S.A. Janzen and J.Solmon (1983). *Environ. Pollut. Ser.* A. 30: 211.

Jernelov, A. and H. Lann (1971). *Oikos*, 22: 403.

Joy, C. M. (1990). *Bull. Environ. Contam. Toxicol.*, 45: 915.

Kar, S. and P. K. Singh (1978). *Bull. Environ. Contam. Toxicol.*, 20: 707.

Kashyap, A.K. and S.L. Gupta (1981). *Acta Botanica Indica*, 9: 265.

Katz, S. (1962). *Nature*, 194: 569.

Katz, S and V. Santilli (1962). *Biochem. Biophys. Acta.*, 55: 621.

Kimamura. M. and S. Kotoh (1972). *Biochem. Biophys. Acta.*, 283: 178.

Koronowski, K. (1973). *Mitt. Biol. Bundesanst.* Land Forstwirtsch Berling-Dahlem. 153: 1-21.

Kumar, K. B. (1984). Studies on physiology of senescence in crop plants. II. Effect of growth regulators and photo period on leaf senescence in *Eleusine coracana,* Gaertn. *Ph. D. Thesis*, Berhampur University, India.

Leland, H. V., S. N. Luoma and J. M. Fielden (1979). *J. Wat. Pollut. Contr.Fed.*, 51: 1592.

Levitt, J.(1972). *Response of plants to environmental stresses*. Academic Press, Inc. N. Y.

Lodenius, M. (1980). *Ann. Bot. Fenn.*, 17: 336.

Lodenius, M. and E. Tulisalo (1984). Environmental mercury contamination around a Chlor-alkali plant. *Bull. Environ. Contam. Toxicol.*, 32: 439.

Misra, S.R. (1984). Analysis of the effects of solid waste extracts of a caustic-chlorine factory on growth and physiology of rice seedlings. *Ph.D. thesis*. Berhampur University, Orissa, India.

Mukherji, S. and G. Ganguly (1974). *Indian J. Exp. Biol.*, 12: 432.

Mukherji, S. and P. Nag (1977). *Biochem. Physiol. Pflanzen.*, 171: 227.

Mukherji, S. and P. Maitra (1977). *Z. Pflanzen. Physiol.*, 81: 26.

Murthy, S. D. S. and P. Mohanty (1991). *Plant Cell Physiol.*, 32(2). 231.

Odum, E.P. (1971). *Fundamentals of Ecology*, 3rd Edition. W.B.Saunders Co., Philadelphia, London.

Oser, B. L. (1965). *Hawks Physiological Chemistry*, 14th edn., Edited by B. L.Oser, TMH Publishers, New Delhi, reprinted 1979, p. 179, 224 and 444.

Padhi, N. P. (1990). Eco-physiological response of germinating rice seedlings to an organo-mercurial fungicide, MEMC., *Ph.D. Thesis*, Berhampur University, India.

Panigrahi, A.K. and B.N .Misra (1978). *Comp. Physiol. Ecol.*, 8: 253.

Patra, R.R. (1993). Eco-physiological effects of an organomercury based pesticide on a crop plant. *Ph.D. Thesis*. Berhampur University. Orissa. India.

Phillip, J.R. (1958). *Plant Physiol.*, 33, 23.

Poljakoff-Mayber, A. and J. Gale (1975). *Plants in Saline Environments (Ecological studies–15)*. Springer-Verlag. Berlin.

Pradhan, P. (1998). Eco-toxicological effects of a pesticide on a crop plant. *Ph.D. Thesis*. Berhampur University. Orissa. India.

Rai, L. C. and N. Khatoniar (1980). *Indian J. Environ. Hlth.*, 22: 113.

Rai, L. C., J. P. Gaur and H. D. Kumar (1981, a). *Biol. Rev.* 56: 99.

Rai, L. C., J. P. Gaur and H. D. Kumar (1981, b). *Environmental Research*, 25: 250.

Sai Babu, T. (1998). Eco-physiological effects of a pesticide on a crop plant. *M.Phil. Thesis*, Berhampur University. Orissa, India.

Sax, I.N. (1974). *Industrial pollution*. Van Nostrand Reinhold Company, New York.

Semu, E., B.R. Singh, A.R. Selmen-Olsen and K. Steenberg (1985). *Plant and Soil.*, 87: 347.

Sharma, B.K. and H. Kaur (1993). *Environmental Chemistry*. Goel Publishing House, Krishna Prakashan Media (P) Ltd., Meerut.

Shaw, B.P. (1987). Eco-physiological studies of industrial effluent of a cholr-alkali factory on biosystems. *Ph.D. Thesis*. Berhampur University, Orissa. India.

Siegel, B.Z., M. Lasconta, E.Yaeger and S.M. Siegel (1984). *Water Air Soil Pollut.*, 23(1). 15.

Siegenthaler, P.A. and L. Packer (1965). Light dependent volume changes and reactions in chloroplasts.I. action of alkenylsuccinic acids and phenyl mercuric acetate and possible relation to mechanism of stomatal control. *Pl. Physiol. Lancaster*, 40: 785.

Smith, L. and M.Baltscheffsky (1959). Respiration and light induced phosphorylation in extracts of *Rhodospirillum rubrum*. *J. Biol. Chem.*, 234: 1575.

Srivastava, A.K., V.K.Sharma and Ahuja, K.L. (1972). Effect of salt stress on seed germination and survival of soyabean seedlings. *Trop. Ecol.*, 18: 27.

Suckcharoen, S. (1979). *Ann. Bot. Fenici.*, 16: 173.

Sunderesan, B.B., P.V.R. Subrahmanyam and A.D. Bhinde (1983). An overview of toxic and hazardous waste in Indian Industry and Environment. Special issue (1983). In: The State of India's Environment 1984-85. *The Second Citizen's Report*, p. 196.

Toubey, C.L. (1972). *Aust. J. Exp. Agric. Anim. Husk.*, 12(55). 176.

Weaver, R.W., J.R. Melton, D.Wang and R.L.Dable (1984). *Environmetal Pollution*. Series-A. *Ecol. Biol.*, 33(2). 133.

Whitton, B.A. (1970). Toxicity of heavy metal to freshwater algae. A review. Phykos, 9: 116.

Wolk, C. P. (1973). *Bacteriol. Rev.*, 37: 32.

Wong, M.H. and A.D.Bradshaw (1982). *New Phytol.*, 91(2). 255.

Yung, Chi-Tung (1938). Development anatomy of the seedling of rice plant. *Bot. Gaz.*, 99: 786.

Zingmark, R.C. and T.G. Miller (1975). *Belle W. Baruch Libr. Marine Science*, 3: 45.

Microbial Biotechnology and Ecology (2011) *Pages* **827–836**
Editors: **Deepak Vyas, G.S. Paliwal, P.K.Khare and R.K Gupta**
Published by: **DAYA PUBLISHING HOUSE, NEW DELHI**

Chapter 48

Effect of Pollution in Groundwater Quality and Soil Health of Naini Area at Allahabad City

☆ ***Saurabh Upadhyay*[1], *Arun A. David*[1], *T. Thomas*[1], *H. Thomas*[2]*, *R.K. Tamphasana*[2] *and Ram Bharose*[1]**

[1]*School of Forestry and Environment, SHIATS-Deemed University, Allahabad*
[2]*Department of Applied Geology, Dr. H.S. Gour University, Sagar – 470 003, M.P.*

ABSTRACT

The experiment was conducted to assess the quality of soil and groundwater in Naini area of Allahabad, U.P. India. The 4 sampling sites were selected S_1–AAI-DU research farm of Soil Science and Agricultural Chemistry Farm as center, S_2–Arail, S_3–Cotton mill, and S_4–Kharkauni (village) and observation were taken in pre–monsoon and post–monsoon seasons for groundwater and soil properties respectively. pH 7.1-7.82, Turbidity 0.02-0.20 NTU, EC 0.47-0.88 dS m^{-1}, Hardness 430.6-490.4 mg l^{-1}, DO 2.8-4.5 mg l^{-1}, BOD 0.31-0.67 mg l^{-1}, Alkalinity 37-84 mg l^{-1}, Chloride 25.48-69.9 mg l^{-1} and for soil pH 7.65-7.26, EC 0.46-0.43 dS m^{-1} Bulk density 1.62-1.83 g cm^{-3}, Particle density 2.6-3.6 g cm^{-3}, per cent OC 0.27-0.8, Available Nitrogen 239-271 $kgha^{-1}$, Available Phosphorus 27.4-31.6 $kgha^{-1}$, Potasium 256-306 $kgha^{-1}$, Cu 0.32-0.95 $mgkg^{-1}$ were recorded respectively. These values were analyzed by appropriate statistical desined *viz.*, two way analysis of variance and determination and analysis were done with the standard methods. According to the results obtained by analyzing various physico-chemical parameters of groundwater and soil quality the sites S_1–AAI- DU and S_2–Arail was safe as compared to other locations *viz.* S_3–Cotton mill and S_4–Kharkauni (village).

---

* E-mail: harelthomas@yahoo.com

Introduction

Soil quality is the key to agricultural productivity, soil organic matter and nutrient levels, prime indicators of soil quality, readily decline when soils are taken under cultivation (Lobe *et al.*, 2001). Fertilizer use will improve the nutrient status of soils, but rarely over comes the soil organic matter and few ideas are around to remedy this crucial step in soil degradation (Marticus *et al.*, 2001). It is widely recognized that water and soil degradation problem is man made problem. It has been taking place since the down of agriculture (Barrow 1991; Hillel 1991). What is now the intensity of degradation in recent times where is the soil of the world, on average, lost 25.3 million tonnes (Mt) of Humus per year since agriculture began some 10,000 years ago, these loses were, on average, 300 Mt yr^{-1} in the last 300 years and 760 Mt in the past 50years (Rozauov *et al., 1990*). Thus the growth of population, expansion of crop lands, and destruction of vegetation, global warming emergence of yield-enhancing technologies all seem to have played a role. In essence, the last 50 years have been a saga of economic growth and ecological losses.

There is an urgent need to develop indicators, threshold limits or symptoms, potential indicators should be quantitative, change, widely applicable, able to asses the present status and trend, able to distinguish change due to natural cycles as apposed to anthropogenic interventions, and relevant to ecologically significant phenomena (Rubio and Bichet 1998). The assessment of degradation on the basis of yield trend is however difficult due to the use of improved varieties and fertilizer masking ongoing degradation (Oldewau 1994; Swaling and Braun 1998). May elaborate methods such as classical soil testing or modern technologies such as soil genomics may eventually after new means of assessing the health of our soil (Torsvik and Oureas 2002).

Keeping in view of the problem stated above mentioned about may be a suitable solution for the Allahabad region. The problem was taken during the period 2007-2008 on topic entitled "Effect of pollution in groundwater quality and soil health of Naini area at Allahabad city", were studied with the following objectives:

To check the quality of groundwater and soil in Naini area of Allahabad City. To compares groundwater quality with Indian standards. To compare soil quality with standards of Soil testing Laboratory, State Agricultural Department (U.P.).

Materials and Methods

Study Area

The area selected for the present study was Naini town located in Allahabad city. Which is located at 25.57° N latitude, 81.56°E longitude and 98 m elevation above the mean sea level. Naini is an industrial town of Allahabad lodging various types of industries manufacturing products. It comes under sub tropical climate receiving the mean annual rainfall of about 807.4 mm, major rains are received from July to end of September. However, occasional precipitation is also not uncommon during winter. The winter months are cold while summer months are very hot and dry. The minimum temperature during the crop season was 7.3°C and maximum was 31.4°C. The maximum humidity was 93 per cent and minimum was 21 per cent during study period.

***Source*: Metrological data of College of forestry AAI-DU (Allahabad)**

Water and Soil sampling were done in pre–monsoon (March, April, and May) and post-monsoon (October, November and December) period 2007–2008, with the standard methods, groundwater samples were collected from the different sites/points of Naini area Soil sampling were done with help of soil auger from the upper soil layer having depth of (0–15cm) from different Sites *viz.* S_1-AAI–DU Allahabad, S_2- Arail, S_3–Cotton mill and S_4–Kharkauni village, Naini Allahabad.

Table 48.1: General Information about Allahabad District- 2008

Area	2,261 sq.km
Population	49,21,313 (census 2001)
STD Code	0532
Best Season	November–March
State	Uttar Pradesh
Language	Hindi, Urdu, English
Altitude	98 meters above sea level
Temperature	Minimum 4 degree Celsius to max 48 degree Celsius
Local Transport	Taxi, Bus, Tempo, Auto-rickshaw, Cycle rickshaw
Accessibility	Air, Rail, Road

Source: ADA Allahabad (2008).

Table 48.2: Experimental Sites/Locations and their Distance from AAI-DU

Sl.No.	*Site Symbol*	*Site: Name*	*Distance from AAI–DU (Km)*
1	S_1	AAI–DU, Alld.	0
2	S_2	Arail	2
3	S_3	Cotton mill	4
4	S_4	Kharkauni village	3

Table 48.3: Different Biochemical Parameters Taken for Groundwater Study their Respective Methods Used for Analysis

Parameters	*Methods*
pH	Jackson (1958)
Turbidity (NTU)	APHA (1985)
EC (dS m^{-1})	APHA (1995)
Hardness (mg l^{-1})	APHA (1985)
Alkalinity (mg l^{-1})	APHA (1985)
Chloride (mg l^{-1})	APHA (1985)
Dissolved oxygen (mg l^{-1})	APHA (1985)
Biochemical oxygen demand (mg l^{-1})	APHA (1985)

Table 48.4: Different Soil Parameters and their Respective Methods Used for Analysis

pH 1:2 (w/v)	Jackson (1958)
EC (dS m^{-1})	Digital Electrical Conductivity Meter
Bulk density (g cm^{-3})	Black (1965)
Particle density (g cm^{-3})	Black (1965)
Percentage Organic Carbon (per cent)	Walkley (1947)
Available Nitrogen (kg ha^{-1})	Walkley (1947)
Available Phosphate (kg ha^{-1})	Olsen *et al.* (1954)
Available Potash (kg ha^{-1})	Toth and Prince (1949)
Copper (mg kg^{-1})	Cheng and Bray (1953)

Results and Discussion

Groundwater

In the pre-monsoon pH of investigated sites varied from 7.1-7.82 given in Table 48.5, pH value of groundwater to be was recorded at four different sites was found to be maximum in Cotton mill 7.82 followed by Kharkauni 7.30, Arail 7.21 and the lowest in AAI-DU, Alld. 7.10. As represented in the Table 48.5 the Turbidity value of groundwater to be was recorded at four different locations was found to be maximum in Cotton mill 0.18 followed by Arail 0.13, Kharkauni 0.07 and the lowest in AAI.–DU 0.01 NTU respectively. Electrical Conductivity concentration of groundwater was recorded at four different sites were found to be maximum in Kharkauni 0.87 followed by Arail 0.84, Cotton mill 0.82 and the lowest in AAI–DU 0.46 dS m^{-1}. This may be found due to leachate infiltration from the refuse dumps. Hardness value of groundwater to be were recorded at four different sites was found to be maximum in Kharkauni 483.20, followed by Arail 451.00, Cotton mill 438.10 and the lowest in AAI.–DU 423.00 mg l^{-1} respectively. Alkalinity concentration of groundwater were recorded at four different sites was found to be maximum in Kharkauni 82.00 followed by Cotton mill 81.30, Arail 64.00 and the lowest in AAI–DU 35.60 mg l^{-1} respectively, this alkalinity values having lower concentration as compared to BIS standards recommendations. Chloride value of groundwater were recorded at four different sites were found to be maximum in Cotton mill 68.70 followed by Kharkauni 56.50, Arail 43.90, and the lowest in AAI.–DU 22.20 mg l^{-1} respectively. DO concentration of groundwater were recorded at four different sites was found to be maximum in AAI.–DU 5.20 followed by Cotton mill 4.40, Kharkauni 3.60 and the lowest in Arail 2.70 mg l^{-1} respectively. BOD concentration of groundwater were recorded at four different sites was found to be maximum in Kharkauni 0.63 followed by Cotton mill 0.51, Arail 0.38 and the lowest in AAI–DU 0.28 mg l^{-1} respectively.

In the post-monsoon pH of investigated sites varied from 7.31-7.95 given in Table 48.6, pH concentration of groundwater to be was recorded at four different sites were found to be maximum in Cotton mill 7.95 followed by Kharkauni 7.65, Arail 7.31 and the lowest in AAI-DU, Alld. 7.40. The neutral to alkaline pH may be attributed to the reaction of applied fertilizer material with soil colloids which resulted in the reaction of basic cations on the exchangeable complex of the water. The pH concentration values were found under the permissible limits of the standards. As represented in the Table 48.6 the Turbidity value of groundwater to be was recorded at four different sites were found to be maximum in Kharkauni 0.98 Cotton mill 0:50 followed by Arail 0.18, and the lowest in AAI.–DU 0.02 NTU respectively. This turbidity indicating presence of suspended and colloidal matterial such

Table 48.5: Effect of Groundwater on Physico-chemical Properties of Water in Pre-monsoon Period at Different Sites

Sl.No.	*Parameters*	*Sites*				*Permissible Limit (WHO)*
		AAI-DU	*Arail*	*Cotton mill*	*Kharkauni*	
1.	pH	7.1	7.21	7.82	7.3	6.5-8.5
2.	Turbidity (NTU)	0.01	0.13	0.18	0.07	5NTU
3.	E.C. (dS m^{-1})	0.46	0.84	0.82	0.87	
4.	Hardness (mg l^{-1})	423	451	438.1	483.2	500
5.	Alkalinity (mg l^{-1})	35.6	64	81.3	82	
6.	Chloride (mg l^{-1})	22.2	43.9	68.7	56.5	250
7.	Dissolved oxygen (mg l^{-1})	5.2	2.7	4.4	3.6	
8.	Biochemical oxygen demand (mg l^{-1})	0.28	0.38	0.51	0.63	

Table 48.6: Effect of Groundwater on Physico-chemical Properties of Water in Post-monsoon Period at Different Sites

Sl.No.	*Parameters*	*Sites*				*Permissible Limit (WHO)*
		AAI-DU	*Arail*	*Cotton mill*	*Kharkauni*	
1.	pH	7.4	7.31	7.95	7.65	6.5-8.5
2.	Turbidity (NTU)	0.02	0.18	0.50	0.98	5NTU
3.	EC (dS m^{-1})	0.52	0.92	0.95	0.98	
4.	Hardness (mg l^{-1})	426.00	456.00	445.40	490.60	500
5.	Alkalinity (mg l^{-1})	36.40	66.50	85.40	87.80	
6.	Chloride (mg l^{-1})	28.70	55.20	75.60	65.80	250
7.	Dissolved oxygen (mg l^{-1})	4.90	2.30	3.90	3.20	
8.	Biochemical oxygen demand (mg l^{-1})	0.31	0.42	0.58	0.82	

as clay, silt and fibrous particle such as asbestos minerals. Electrical Conductivity, concentration of groundwater was recorded at four different sites were found to be maximum in Kharkauni 0.98, followed by Cotton mill 0.95, Arail 0.92, and the lowest in AAI.–DU 0.52 dS m^{-1} respectively. This may be found due to leachate infiltration from the refuse dumps. Hardness value of groundwater to be were recorded at four different sites was found to be maximum in Kharkauni 490.60, followed by Arail 456.00, Cotton mill 445.40 and the lowest in AAI.–DU 426.00 mg l^{-1} respectively. Alkalinity concentration of groundwater were recorded at four different sites were found to be maximum in Kharkauni 87.80 followed by Cotton mill 85.40, Arail 66.50 and the lowest in AAI.–DU 36.40 mg l^{-1} respectively, this alkalinity values having lower concentration as compared to BIS standards recommendations. Chloride value of groundwater were recorded at four different sites were found to be maximum in Cotton mill 75.60, followed by Kharkauni 65.80, Arail 55.20, and the lowest in AAI.–DU 28.70 mg l^{-1} respectively. A direct correlation between the chloride content and EC was recorded in the present study high level of chloride can also be contributed by mineral deposits, and industrial wastes. DO concentration of groundwater were recorded at four different sites was found to be maximum in AAI.–DU 4.90 followed by Cotton mill 3.90, Kharkauni 3.20, and the lowest in Arail 2.30 mg l^{-1} respectively. BOD concentration of groundwater were recorded at four different sites was found to be maximum in Kharkauni 0.82, followed by Cotton mill 0.58, Arail 0.42 and the lowest in AAI.–DU 0.31 mg l^{-1} respectively. This BOD values having lower concentration as compared to WHO/BIS standards recommendations.

Soil

As represented in the Table 48.7, the pH concentration of soil was recorded in pre-monsoon period, at four different sites was found to be maximum in Cotton mill 7.62 followed by Kharkauni 7.58, Arail 7.57 and the lowest in AAI–DU 7.23. Alkaline range of pH in most of the soil sample may be due to the general alkaline nature of the effluents being released into sampling sites/locations. EC concentration of soil to be were recorded at four different sites was found to be maximum in Cotton mill 0.44 followed by AAI.–DU 0.42 and the lowest were in Kharkauni 0.41, and Arail 0.41dS m^{-1} respectively. Particle density values of soil were recorded at four different sites was found to be maximum in Kharkauni 2.80, followed by Cotton mill 2.70, Arail 2.70 and the lowest in AAI.–DU 2.40g cm^{-1} respectively. Bulk density values of soil were recorded at four different sites was found to be maximum in Cotton mill 1.80, followed by Kharkauni 1.73, Arail 1.72 and the lowest in AAI.–DU 1.57g cm^{-1} respectively. Per cent Organic Carbon value of soil were recorded at four different sites was found to be maximum in Kharkauni 0.81 followed by Cotton mill 0.76, Arail 0.27 and the lowest in AAI.–DU 0.25 per cent respectively. Available Nitrogen concentration of soil to be were recorded at four different sites was found to be maximum in Kharkauni 271.00 followed by Cotton mill 263.00,

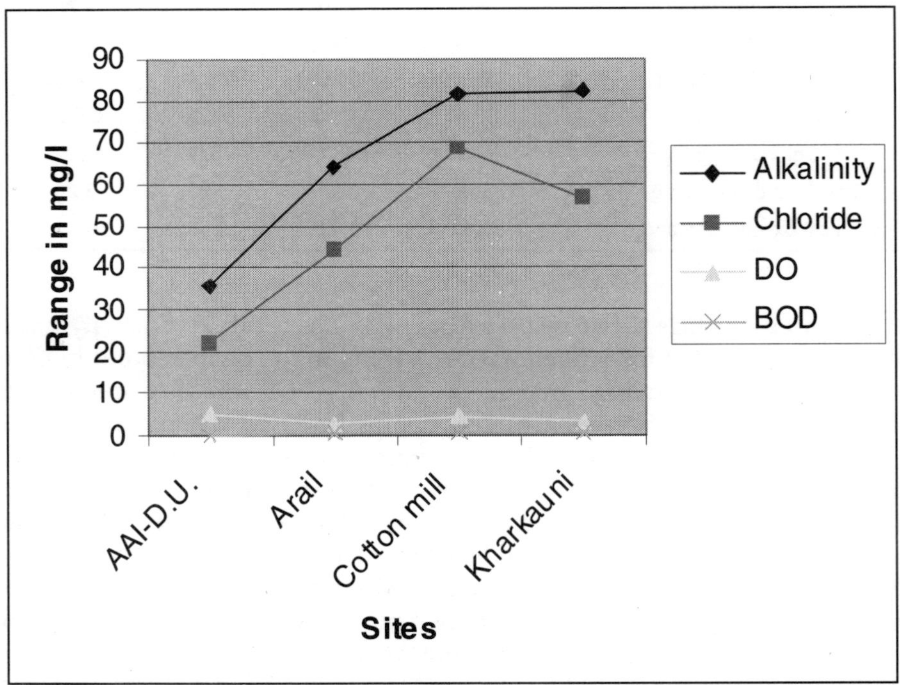

Figure 48.1: Response of Alkalinity, Chloride, DO and BOD on Water at Different Sites of Naini Area in Pre-monsoon Period

Arail 252.00 and the lowest in AAI–DU 241.00kg ha^{-1} respectively. Available Phosphorus concentration of soil were recorded at four different sites was found to be maximum in Kharkauni 31.60 followed by Cotton mill 35.00, Arail 29.40 and the lowest in AAI–DU 28.20kg ha^{-1}kg ha^{-1} respectively. Available Potassium concentration of soil were recorded at four different sites was found to be maximum in Khaekauni 280.30 followed by Cotton mill 303.30, Arail 313.00 and the lowest in AAI.–DU 256.00kg ha^{-1} respectively Cu concentration of soil were recorded at four different sites was found to be maximum in Kharkauni 0.93 followed by Cotton mill 0.83, Arail 0.72 and the lowest in AAI–DU 0.30mg kg^{-1} respectively.

Table 48.7: Effect on Soil on Physico-chemical Properties of Soil in Pre-monsoon Period at Different Sites, Naini Allahabad

Sl.No.	*Parameters*	*Sites*				*Permissible Limit (Agricultural Deptt. U.P. 2008)*
		AAI-DU	*Arail*	*Cotton mill*	*Kharkauni*	
1	pH 1:2 (w/v)	7.23	7.57	7.62	7.58	7.0-8.5
2	EC (dS m^{-1})	0.42	0.41	0.44	0.41	1.40-1.50
3	Particle density (g cm^{-3})	2.40	2.70	2.70	2.80	2.60-2.70
4	Bulk density (g cm^{-3})	1.57	1.72	1.80	1.73	1.40-1.50
5	Percentage Organic Carbon (per cent)	0.25	0.27	0.76	0.81	0.6-0.80
6	Available Nitrogen (kg ha^{-1})	241.00	252.00	263.00	271.00	240-320
7	Available Phosphorus (kg ha^{-1})	28.20	29.40	30.50	31.60	28-34
8	Available Potassium (kg ha^{-1})	256.00	313.00	303.30	280.30	240-320
9	Copper (mg kg^{-1})	0.30	0.72	0.83	0.93	0.4-1.0

As represented in the Table 48.8, the pH concentration of soil were recorded in post-monsoon period, at four different sites was found to be maximum in Kharkauni 7.89 followed by Cotton mill 7.73, Arail 7.62 and the lowest in AAI–DU 7.28. Alkaline range of pH in most of the soil sample may be due to the general alkaline nature of the effluents being released into sampling sites/locations. EC concentration of soil to be were recorded at four different sites was found to be maximum in Kharkauni 0.52 followed by Cotton mill 0.49, Arail 0.48 and the lowest in AAI.–DU 0.43dS m^{-1} respectively. This E.C may be due to mineralization by soil organism and conductivity increase is due to leachate infiltration from the refuse dump. Particle density values of soil were recorded at four different sites was found to be maximum in Kharkauni 2.90, followed by Arail 2.80, Cotton mill 2.70 and the lowest in AAI.–DU 2.50g cm^{-1} respectively. Bulk density value of soil to be were recorded at four different sites was found to be maximum in Cotton mill 2.10 followed by Arail 1.78, Kharkauni 1.73 and the lowest in AAI.–DU 1.59g cm^{-1} respectively. Per cent OC concentrations of soil were recorded at four different sites was found to be maximum in Kharkauni 0.83 followed by Cotton mill 0.78, Arail 0.29 and the lowest in AAI.–DU 0.27 respectively. Available Nitrogen concentation of soil to be were recorded at four different sites was found maximum in Kharkauni 273.00 followed by Cotton mill 264.00, Arail 253.00 and the lowest in AAI–DU 242.00kg ha^{-1} respectively. Available Phosphorus concentration of soil were recorded at four different locations was found to be maximum in Kharkauni 32.10 followed by Cotton mill 31.20, Arail 29.80 and the lowest in AAI–DU 28.40kg ha^{-1} respectively. Available Potassium concentration of soil were recorded at four different sites was found to be maximum in

Arail 314.00 followed by Cotton mill 304.00, Kharkauni 281.00 and the lowest in AAI.–DU 257.00kg ha^{-1} respectively. Cu concentration of soil to be were recorded at four different sites was found to be maximum in Kharkauni 0.97 followed by Cotton mill 0.85, Arail 0.74 and the lowest in AAI–DU 0.32mg kg^{-1} respectively.

According to the result obtained by analyzing various physico-chemical parameters groundwater and soil quality in AAI.–DU. and Arail were safe as compared to other locations *viz.* Cotton mill and Kharkauni.

Table 48.8: Effect of Soil on Physico-chemical Properties of Soil in Post-monsoon Period at Different Sites

Sl.No.	*Parameters*	*Sites*				*Permissible Limit (Agricultural Deptt. U.P. 2008)*
		AAI-DU	*Arail*	*Cotton mill*	*Kharkauni*	
1	pH1:2 (w/v)	7.28	7.62	7.73	7.89	8.0–8.5
2	EC (dS m^{-1})	0.46	0.48	0.49	0.52	1.40–1.50
3	Particle density (g cm^{-3})	2.50	2.80	2.70	2.90	2.60–2.70
4	Bulk density (g cm^{-3})	1.59	1.78	2.10	1.73	1.40–1.50
5	Percentage Organic Carbon (per cent)	0.27	0.29	0.78	0.83	0.6–0.80
6	Available Nitrogen (kg ha^{-1})	242.00	253.00	264.00	273.00	240–320
7	Available Phosphorus (kg ha^{-1})	28.40	29.80	31.20	32.10	28–34
8	Available Potassium (kg ha^{-1})	257.00	314.00	304.00	281	240–320
9	Copper (mg kg^{-1})	0.36	0.74	0.85	0.97	0.4 -1.0

Summary and Conclusion

Monitoring the health of our soil is urgently needed and will require a long term commitment, a dense network of monitoring sites and well functioning laboratory facilities. It will require the development of indicators, threshold limits or symptoms that can predict the on set of land degradation. Combined with the use of satellite imagery as discussed in this paper; such a system may be made cost effective.

Human needs of change the natural system of new one that is stable and virtually closed to one that is degrading and more or less open, dependent on the severity of the human interferences. The rapid decline in water and productivity of land following conservation to agriculture has been demonstrated again and again. The present study represents an in-depth investigation of the current status of Groundwater and Soil quality of Naini area of Allahabad city (U.P.). The findings of the research have resulted in environmental degradation with regarding to water and soil. As such the present environmental status of Naini area is not so alarming. The Industrial Complex and its surroundings have been growing fast due to rapid urbanization and industrialization in the last four decades. However, if proper environmental management is not followed, then the situation may degrade further. The groundwater in some localities are found to be polluted due to various industrial activities as well as domestic activities. Some water quality parameters have already exceeded the permissible limits and some parameters are approaching towards the permissible limits because of leaching, percolating and other such phenomenon for groundwater. There are various measures which can be made to control the water and soil pollution; however the following measures are important depending on the topographic and metrological consideration of the area under study.

Municipal and sewage water should be treated before it is released to the water bodies and irrigation use in the farmer's field. For industrial houses, provision of zero according to the guideline of the pollution control board/bodies/departments/Govt. (Central and State) emission or minimum emission should be enforced. Proper planning should be implemented before allowing any body to draw the water from under ground. Groundwater used for infant feed must be pretreated and reanalyzed so as to ensure the safety for live-stock and human mankind.

Acknowledgements

Authors sincerely acknowledge and express thanks to Prof. (Dr.) S.B.Lal, Director Research/ Dean College of Forestry, SHIATS-DU Allahabad for providing guidance and facilities for conducting research work and preparing manuscript.

References

Adekunlel, M., *et al.* (2007). "Assessment of Groundwater Quality in a Typical Rural Settlement in Southwest Nigeria". *Int. J. Environ. Res. Public Health* 4(4), 307-318.

Bharambe, P.R. *et al.* (2005). Water table fluctuations, quality of groundwater and soil health in Jayakwadi command". *Environment and Ecology*,. 34(4): 431 521.

Black, C.A (ed). (1965). *Methods of Soil Analysis Vol. 1.* Am. Soc Agron.Madison, Wisconsin, U.S.A.

Brady, N. C. (1980). *The Nature and Properties of Soils.* Eurasia Publishing House Private Limited, Ram Nagar, New Delhi-110 055.

Cheng, K.L., and R.H. Bray (1953). Two specific methods of determining Cu in soil and plant material. *Anal. Chem.* 25: 655-659.

Chaudhary, S. *et al.* (2004). Studied that "Soil and groundwater pollution in Faridabad." Environment and Ecology, 2004. 22(3): 636-641.

Hillel, D.J. (1991). *Out of the earth: civilization and the life of the soil.* The free press, New York, NY, USA.

Hutson, J.L. (1997). The Soil Quality Indices Literature Compiler's Report; Appendix D-"W and Listings *Journal of Environmental Quality* 26: 41–48.

Jackson, M. L. (1958). *Soil Chemical Analysis.* Prentice Hall of India. Private Ltd. New Delhi.

Lobe, I., Amelung, W. and Dee Preez, C.C. (2001). Losses of carbon and nitrogen with prolonged arable cropping from sandy soil of the South African Highveld. *E uropean Journal of Soil Science* 52 pp. 93-101.

Mayan Kutty, P.C. *et al.* (1995). examined that "Monitoring of trace metals in desalinated Drinking water and their permissible levels". Paper presented at the IDA conference, Abu Dhabi, held during 18–24 Nov., 1995.

Marticus, C., Tiessen, H. (2001). The management of organic matter in tropical soils; What are the priorities ? *Nutrient Cycling in Agroecosystems* 61, 1-6.

Moti R. Sharma (2004). Assessment of Groundwater quality of Hamirpur area in Himachal Pradesh. 23(1): 131-134, *Enviromedia.*

Muhr, G.R. N.P. Datta, H. Sankarasubramoney, V.K. Leley, and R.P. Donahue (1965). *Soil Testing in India.* U.S.Agency for Intern. Development Mission to India, New Delhi.

Oldman L. R. (1994). The global extent of soil degradation. In: *Soil Resistance and Sustainable Land Use.* (D. J. Greenland and I, Szaboles, Eds.) pp. 99-118 CAB International, Wallingford, U. K.

Olsen, S.R., Cole, Cv., Watnahe,F.S. and Dean, L.A. (1954). Estimation of available phosphorus in soils by extraction with sodium bicarbonate *U.S. Deptt.Agr. Circ.* 939.

Palanisamy, P. N., Geetha, A., Sujatha, M., Sivakumar, P. and Karunakaran, K. studied that Groundwater samples collected from different localities in and around Gobichettipalayam town, Erode District, Tamil Nadu. Journal of environmental biology USEPA.

Rozanov, B. G., Targulian V., Orlov D. S. (1990). Soils in the Earth as transformed by human action (B. L. Turner, W. C. Clark, J.f. Richards, J. T. Mathews and W. B. Meyer, Eds.). Cambridge University Press, Cambridge, U. K.

Rubio J. L. and Bichet, E. (1998). Desertification indicators as diagnostic criteria for desertification in Europe. *Journal of Arid Environments.* 39: 113-120.

Torsvik, V. and Ovreas, L. (2002). Microbial diversity and function in soil: from genes to ecosystems. *Current Opinion in Microbiology,* 5: 240-245.

Toth, S.J. and A.L. Prince (1949). Estimination of cation exchange capacity and exchangeable Ca, K and Na content of soil by flame photometer technique. *Soil Sci.* 67: 439-445.

Walkley, A. (1947). Critical examination of rapid method for determining organic carbon in soils. Effect of variation in digestion conditions and of inorganic soil constituents. *Soil Sci.* 632: 251.

Wick, B., R. F. Kuhne, K. Vielhauer, and P. L. G. Vlek. (2002). Temporal variability of selected soil microbiological and biochemical indicators under different soil quality conditions in south-western Nigeria. *Biology and Fertility of Soils* 35, No. 3: 155-167.

Wilcox L.V (1950). Electrical conductivity. *Amer. Water Works Assoc.* J. 42: 775-776.

Microbial Biotechnology and Ecology (2011) *Pages* **837–845**
Editors: **Deepak Vyas, G.S. Paliwal, P.K.Khare and R.K Gupta**
Published by: **DAYA PUBLISHING HOUSE, NEW DELHI**

Chapter 49

Modifying Influence of Woody Perennials on Atmospheric Deposition of Nutrient Ions in a Dry Tropical Region of India

☆ *J. Pandey*

Department of Botany, Banaras Hindu University, Varanasi – 221 005, U.P.

ABSTRACT

Atmospheric depositions of SO_4^{2-}, NO_3^-, PO_4^{3-}, NH_4^+, Na^+, K^+, Ca^{2+} and Mg^{2+}, both as clearfall and throughfall were measured in a seasonally dry tropical region of India. Significant spatial variations in the deposition of these cations and anions were observed. In general, depositions of these ions were high at source oriented sites (industrial and traffic oriented locations), and lower at comparatively remote forested sites. The pH of bulk deposition was alkaline at sites influenced by local sources of basic cations. Among the anions, maximum deposition was observed for SO_4^{2-} followed by NO_3^- and minimum of PO_4^{3-}. For cations, the deposition of Ca^{2+} appeared maximum followed by NH_4^+, Na^+, K^+ and Mg^{2+}. The pH as well as the deposition of cations and anions were higher in throughfall received under woody perennials than in clearfall samples. This modifying influence of woody perennials on atmospheric deposition may leads to long-run consequences on nutrient cycling and on soil characteristics even for areas void of direct human interference and has relevance in adopting practices towards forest management.

Introduction

Increased atmospheric deposition of nutrient elements as a result of anthropogenic activities such as fossil fuel combustion in urban–industrial areas and fertilizer application in agriculture has become a common phenomenon in many parts of the world. Atmospheric emission coupled with wind action is adding pollutants and nutrients even in areas far away from source oriented sites (Pandey and Pandey, 2005). Although developed countries, such as United States, have made considerable progress during past few decades reducing the amount of pollutants discharged from point sources, the control of pollutants generated by dispersed or non–point sources is still a big challenge. The problem is more acute in developing countries where, due to new establishing industries and extensive urban growth, atmospheric loading and deposition of pollutant aerosols is continued to rise.

India is a rapidly developing country where air pollution levels are steadily rising in urban industrial areas (Pandey and Agrawal, 1994a; 1994b; Pandey, 2005). Our country has been rapidly increasing its food and energy needs to sustain exponentially growing population and industrial development. For instance, due to continued population pressure, increase in fertilizer use has become unavoidable to achieve maximum agricultural harvest. This has led to rapid growth of fertilizer factories in India. Furthermore, at present, coal based electric generation accounts for about 64 per cent of the total installed capacity. These activities coupled with massive number of automobiles continue to increase the atmospheric emission in metropolitan cities and in the industrial areas.

Chemicals from atmosphere can stimulate, inhibit or have variable effects on growth and productivity of agricultural crops and on forest vegetation. Studies have shown stronger dependence of forest maintenance of nutrients derived from atmosphere and even in some ecosystems, atmospheric input of nutrients provide an important mechanism for replacing hydrologic losses as well as losses due to timber extraction (Friedland and Miller, 1999). However, the relative importance of such deposition often depends upon specific nutrient and site. For instance, N in bulk deposition is equivalent to about 70 per cent of nitrogen incorporated annually in above ground woody tissues in some temperate hardwood forests (Swank, 1984). The contribution of atmospheric deposition in many part of our country has been shown to be significantly high to modify the accumulation pattern in vegetation and soil (Singh and Agrawal, 2005; Pandey and Pandey, 2009) and productivity in aquatic ecosystems (Pandey and Pandey, 2005). This has particular relevance for dry tropical regions where removal of nutrients by leaching remains very slow. Under such condition, atmospheric deposition could shorten the time of nutrient saturation. In agroecosystem, excessive atmospheric nutrient input may lead nutrient cycle to remain open and unsustainable. Relatively less information however, are available on atmospheric inputs of nutrient elements with modifying influences of woody perennials in dry regions of India. The main objectives of this study were to characterize source and non–source oriented variations in deposition of nutrient elements and the role of vegetation in modifying the deposition in a dry tropical region of India.

Materials and Methods

Study area: This study site lies between 24°35' N lat and 73°42' E long and 510 to 580 m above msl in Udaipur district of Rajasthan. The climate of the region is tropical with three distinct seasons, a hot and dry summer (March–June), a short rainy season (July–September) and a cold and dry winter season (November–February). Mean monthly maximum temperature ranges between 23°C in January and 42°C in May and mean monthly minimum temperature ranges between 5°C in January and 25°C in May. Mean annual rainfall remains below 650 mm, about 90 per cent of which occurs during rainy season. Wind direction shifts from predominantly south–westerly during November through March and south–westerly to southerly for most of the remaining months.

Ten sites were selected in and around urban settlement of Udaipur considering the source of emission, relief features and vegetation. Three of the sampling sites were located adjacent to three different lakes, two under partial influence of road emission (Fateh Sagar and Udai Sagar) and third situated in the midst of a deciduous forest with least human influence. Two of the sites, Sukher and Madri, receive emission from industries. Rest of the sites represents traffic oriented urban and sub-urban locations. The details of study sites, emission characteristics, vegetation types etc are presented in Table 49.1. The sampling period consisted of November 15, 2003 to October 14, 2005.

Table 49.1: Characterization of Study Sites

Site No.	*Site*	*Location/source*	*Vegetation*
1.	Delhi Gate	City center, high frequency of petrol driven vehicles	Few avenue trees
2.	Sukher	Sub-urb, marble industry and heavy duty vehicles	Avenue trees and shrubs
3.	Fateh Sagar	Lake site, NW margin of city, petrol driven vehicles	Deciduous trees and shrubs on uplands
4.	Shilpgram	3 km NW from the city, Low frequency of petrol driven vehicles	deciduous forest with ground vegetation
5.	New Campus	3 km NE from the city, residential, low frequency of petrol driven vehicles	Plantation of avenue trees, agricultural field
6.	Sector 5	5 km from the city, sub-urb, low frequency of petrol driven and heavy duty vehicles	Avenue trees and shrubs
7.	Savina	3 km S from the city, sub-urb, heavy duty vehicles	Avenue trees and shrubs
8.	Madri	8 km SE from the city, industrial area	Plantation of avenue trees
9.	Udai Sagar	Lake site, 14 km E from the city, highway, agricultural field	Avenue trees, agricultural land and grasses
10.	Baghdara	Lake site, 20 km SE from the city, remote but partial industrial influence	Deciduous forest, shrubs and grasses

Dust Deposition

The settleable particulates were collected using dry polyethylene collectors having 30 cm height and 15 cm diameter. Collectors were placed at heights of 5 m for known period of time at all sites in open locations for collection of clearfall and under the canopy of *Cassia fistula* for throughfall measurements. *Cassia fistula*, selected as a representative of tropical woody perennials for this study, is an ornamental tree found uniformly at all sites including traffic–orientated urban locations.

$$\text{Dust deposition rate } (g\ \text{m}^{-2}\ \text{d}^{-1}) = \frac{g \text{ particulates}}{a \times d}$$

where,

a is the cross–sectional area (πr^2) of the mouth of the particulate collector and d is the number of days for which the collector was exposed to atmospheric deposition.

Deposition of Nutrient Ions

Bulk atmospheric depositions were collected by using properly washed and dried five liter polyethylene bulk collectors mounted with stainless steel funnel of 30 cm diameter. These collectors were exposed to atmosphere for a period of 30 days to collect bulk deposition as clearfall in open locations and throughfall under the canopy of *Cassia fistula*. A protective guard ring was fitted around each funnel to avoid materials from birds, insects etc. A nylon membrane (240 μm) was placed between the collector and funnel. At each site, triplicate sampling collectors were placed. At the end of each sampling period (30 d), atmospheric deposits were quantitatively transferred from the collectors to properly washed polythene containers. The wall of the funnel and nylon membrane was carefully rinsed with deionized water to incorporate the deposits adsorbed on these surface. The final volume was made 100 ml and after proper stirring, these were left for overnight to extract the maximum water soluble ions. During the rain events, the wet samples were preserved with chloroform. These were filtered through Whattman filter paper and kept under refrigerated condition until the completion of chemical analysis.

Chemical Analysis

The pH was measured with the help of a digital photovolt pH meter (EI, model 101E) using a glass electrode standardized with pH 4.7 and 9.2 reference buffers. Conductivity was measured using a conductivity meter (Electronic India). All the atmospheric depositions were analyzed for SO_4^{2-}, NO_3^-, NH_4^+, PO_4^{3-}, Na^+, K^+, Ca^{2+} a nd Mg^{2+}. Sulphate–S content was determined by turbiditimetric method (Rossum and Villaruz, 1961). $NO_3^-$and NH_4^+ contents were determined by using nitrate and ammonium electrodes attached to an ion analyzer. Concentrations of Na^+, K^+ and Ca^{2+} were measured using a flame photometer (ELICO, India). Magnesium concentration was determined by Atomic Absorption Spectrophotometer (Perkin Elmer, USA).

Quality Assurance and Statistical Analysis

For quality assurance, data comparisons were made between calculated vs measured conductivity and cation *vs* anion balance of individual samples. The data were treated as reliable when the differences were below 10 per cent. Blank analyses were performed for about 10 per cent of all samples according to standard operating procedures. The analytical precision expressed as relative standard deviation was below 10 per cent in all the cases.

Effects of sites were tested using analysis of variance (ANOVA). Means were separated by using Duncan's multiple range tests. Correlation coefficients were calculated between the atmospheric deposition parameters and pollutant concentrations.

Results and Discussion

The dust deposition rates, both as clearfall as well as throughfall, were maximum at site 8 and minimum at site 10 (Figure 49.1). Site–wise variation in dust deposition rates was significant ($P < 0.01$; ANOVA). Throughfall dust deposition rates appeared uniformly higher than the clearfall. Sitewise variations in atmospheric dust depositions clearly indicated the influence of local sources including urban and industrial activities as well as the partial influence of local soil sources.

The pH of the clearfall varied between 6.00 at site 10 to 7.80 at site 2 (Figure 49.2). Site–wise variation in pH of bulk deposition was significant ($p < 0.01$). The pH of the clearfall remained lower than that of the throughfall deposition. The pH of the deposition was comparatively lower in forested areas (site 4 and 10). The low pH at site 1 may be ascribed to be due to relatively higher SO_4^{2-}- S and comparatively lower proportion of base cations. At site 2 on the other hand, high proportion of base cations could neutralize the acidity of depositions even at higher SO_4^{2-}- S. Jain *et al.* (2000) have reported atmospheric bulk deposition pH between 6.3 to 6.5 at urban sites, 6.6 to 6.7 at urban industrial sites and 7.1 at certain rural areas in India.

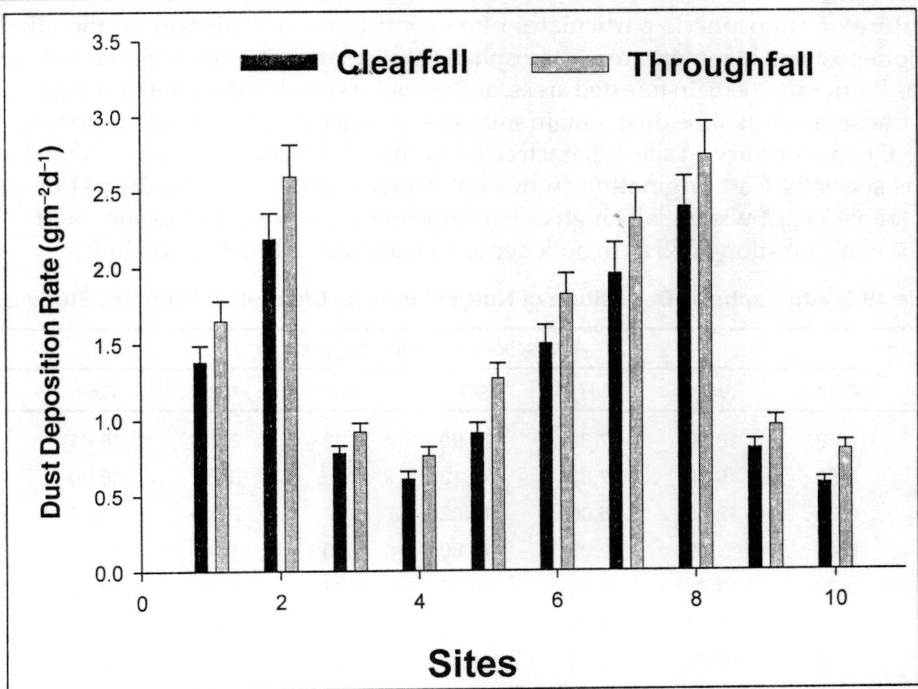

Figure 49.1: Dust Deposition Rates Measured as Clearfall and Throughfall at Different Study Sites. Bars represent mean of three replicates ± 1SE.

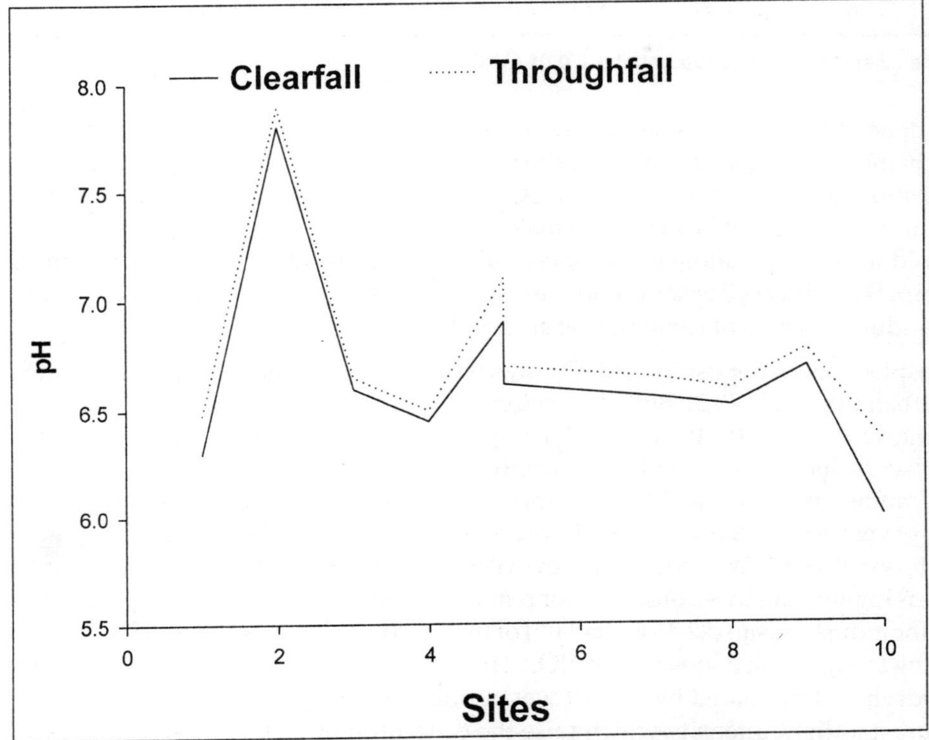

Figure 49.2: pH of Clearfall and Throughfall at Different Study Sites

The nature of atmospheric particulates often contributes in maintaining the alkaline pH of atmospheric deposition. In remote areas, atmospheric particulates are often enriched with soil oriented basic cations (Jain *et al.*, 2000). In forested areas, as the case of sites 4 and 10, with no local dust sources, long range transport of alkaline dust remain smaller and hence the pH of the atmospheric deposition remain low. On the contrary, at site 2 characterized by marble based industries, potential influence of base cations specially Ca^{2+} originating from local sources can be seen on the pH of atmospheric deposition (Table 49.2). Substantially high Ca^{2+} in atmospheric deposits of this site could make the pH alkaline. The concentration of NH_4^+ in bulk deposition also contributes to alkalinity.

Table 49.2: Atmospheric Deposition of Nutrient Ions as Clearfall at Different Study Sites

Site	Atmospheric Deposition (kg ha^{-1} yr^{-1})*							
	PO_4^{3-}	NO_3^-	NH_4^+	SO_4^{2-}	Na^+	K^+	Ca^{2+}	Mg^{2+}
1.	0.48	18.92	7.32	23.90	3.90	2.24	18.61	4.20
2.	0.59	19.80	7.80	25.12	11.25	5.19	48.90	10.66
3.	0.75	12.85	5.06	16.02	2.87	2.08	14.26	3.72
4.	0.46	7.92	2.90	11.80	2.00	1.05	10.15	2.66
5.	0.78	13.74	5.76	18.05	4.98	4.00	18.20	3.96
6.	0.70	14.28	5.10	17.15	4.95	3.05	14.51	4.85
7.	0.78	16.63	5.90	20.38	6.01	3.14	18.95	6.80
8.	1.08	22.45	8.78	26.95	9.65	5.36	26.86	10.25
9.	1.12	14.50	4.91	17.64	4.18	5.80	20.98	5.18
10.	0.98	5.83	2.01	7.25	3.02	1.12	7.35	2.15

*Between site differences were significant at $p < 0.01$ (ANOVA).

Bulk deposition of SO_4^{2-} as clearfall was maximum at site 8 and minimum at site 10 (Table 49.2). Variation in this anion was significant due to site and showed significantly positive correlations with dust deposition rate ($r = 0.71; p < 0.01$) and SO_2 concentration ($r = 0.79; p < 0.01$). Sulphur dioxide (36 to 167 μg m^{-3}) was found to be one of the major air pollutants in the area (Pandey and Chasta, 2006). As observed for site 2, alkaline particulates could favour the adsorption of SO_2. Atmospheric bulk deposition of SO_4^{2-}observed at source oriented sites in this study was higher than the values measured in urban–industrial areas of Delhi (Jain *et al.*, 2000).

Atmospheric bulk deposition of NO_3^- was typically high at industrial sites (2 and 8) and traffic oriented urban site (Table 49.2). Bulk deposition of NO_3^- showed significant positive correlations with dust fall rate ($r = 0.82; p < 0.01$) and NO_2 concentration in the ambient air ($r = 0.72; p < 0.01$). This indicates that the industrial activities are mainly responsible for high atmospheric NO_3^- deposition in the area (Pandey and Chasta, 2006). Further, high NO_3^- deposition at site 1 may be due to high frequency of vehicles. Miller *et al.* (1993) have reported atmospheric N input of 16.7 kg ha^{-1} y^{-1} at a high elevation forest of Whiteface mourtain, New York receiving regional transport of pollutant aerosols. This value is higher than those observed for remote forested site (5.83 kg ha^{-1} y^{-1}) but lower than those recorded for industrial site (22.45 kg ha^{-1} y^{-1}) of this study. Dry deposition of HNO_3 could be a factor contributing to high bulk deposition of NO_3^-. The climate of this region is characterized by extended period of dryness terminated by a short wet period. Formation of HNO_3 is favoured by high day temperature and light intensity which raise the concentration of OH^- radicals. The NO_3^- particles formed by the reaction of atmospheric HNO_3 with particulates could lead to high deposition of NO_3^- at site 1, 2 and 8 (Table 49.2).

Atmospheric deposition of PO_4^{3-} varied from 0.46 kg ha^{-1} y^{-1} at site 4 to 1.12 kg ha^{-1} y^{-1} at site 9. The bulk deposition of orthophosphate observed in this study remained lower in comparison to all other nutrient ions (Table 49.2). Pandey and Pandey (2005) reported relatively lower deposition of P in some remote areas of dry tropics. These observations indicate that the forested remote sites of this study are also under strong industrial influence. In particular, sites 9 and 10, although away from direct anthropogenic activity, receive atmospheric loading of P from phosphate factories by temporal flushing of north–westerly winds. Furthermore, site 9 is also under the influence of vast stretch of agricultural land as far as nutrient loading is concern.

Atmospheric deposition of Ca^{2+} was observed maximum at site 2 (48.90 kg ha^{-1} y^{-1}) and minimum at site 10 (7.35 kg ha^{-1} y^{-1}). A similar trend appeared for bulk atmospheric deposition of Na^+ and Mg^{2+}. The deposition of K^+ was maximum at site 8 (Table 49.2). Atmospheric deposition of Ca^{2+} showed significant positive correlation with Na^+ ($r = 0.86; p < 0.01$), Mg^{2+} ($r = 0.89; p < 0.01$) and K^+ ($r = 0.79; p < 0.01$). Correlation coefficients between cations indicate their common source of origin. Values of correlation coefficient between Ca^{2+} and SO_4^{2-} ($r = 0.75; p < 0.01$) and between Ca^{2+} and NO_3^- ($r = 0.80; p < 0.01$) were also significant.

Table 49.3: Atmospheric Deposition of Nutrient Ions as Throughfall at Different Study Sites

Site	*Atmospheric Deposition (kg ha^{-1} yr^{-1})**							
	PO_4^{3-}	*NO_3^-*	*NH_4^+*	*SO_4^{2-}*	*Na^+*	*K^+*	*Ca^{2+}*	*Mg^{2+}*
1.	0.54	21.26	8.20	26.18	4.16	2.51	20.69	4.80
2.	0.67	23.05	8.71	28.01	13.00	5.71	56.18	11.19
3.	0.84	14.01	6.80	18.10	3.70	2.39	15.90	4.09
4.	0.52	8.50	3.25	12.51	2.65	1.26	11.05	3.10
5.	0.88	14.80	5.98	19.19	5.60	4.88	20.10	4.18
6.	0.85	15.90	6.11	20.00	5.19	3.62	16.02	5.60
7.	0.90	18.05	6.78	22.01	6.70	3.76	20.18	7.56
8.	1.17	25.01	9.60	30.15	10.80	5.94	29.50	11.80
9.	1.30	16.15	5.75	20.18	4.78	6.61	23.15	6.20
10.	1.09	6.74	2.69	8.00	3.48	1.33	8.76	2.40

*Between site differences were significant at $p < 0.01$ (ANOVA).

Bulk atmospheric deposition as measured in terms of throughfall (under the influence of woody perennial) also showed significant between site variations in pH as well as in anions and cations (Figure 49.2 and Table 49.3). Higher pH of throughfall than that of the clearfall may be ascribed to continued deposition and neutralizing effects of basic cations on leaf surfaces. Furthermore, according to Liu *et al.* (2002), the hydrogen ion exchange with other cations at canopy exchange site increases the cations on leaf surfaces. Higher pH of throughfall has also been reported in earlier studies (Singh and Agrawal, 2005). Throughfall deposition of anions and cations were also higher than the clearfall at all sites. Such enrichment effects of plant leaves have also been reported in other studies including the Silent Valley forest in south India (Rao *et al.*, 1995) and subtropical montane moist forest on Ailao

Mountains, China (Liu *et al.*, 2002). Chemical enrichment observed in throughfall can be attributed to impaction, leaching of substances from plant tissues and the influence of foliar microflora. Throughfall enrichment can be major pathway in nutrient cycling in natural ecosystems especially for those areas where direct anthropogenic flushing of nutrient is almost negligible.

In the present study, N deposition at industrial site 8 (31.23 kg ha^{-1} y^{-1}) was about 4 times higher than the distantly situated forested site 10 (7.84 kg ha^{-1} y^{-1}). The former value is more than 10 times higher than that reported for non-source oriented northern forested ecosystems (Aber *et al.*, 1989). This suggests that, site 10 in this study, although situated away from direct human influence, is under the strong influence of atmospheric loading through airshed. Miller *et al.* (1993) reported annual N and S input at the rate of 16.7 kg ha^{-1} y^{-1} and 17.5 kg ha^{-1} y^{-1} respectively, at high elevation forest site at Whiteface mountain of New York receiving regional transport of pollutants.

The SO_4^{2-}- S deposition as clearfall was 26.95 kg ha^{-1} y^{-1} at heavily polluted site and 7.25 kg ha^{-1} y^{-1} at distantly situated forested site (Table 49.2). Singer *et al.* (1996) have reported atmospheric bulk deposition of SO_4^{2-}- S to be 14.3 kg ha^{-1} y^{-1} at a forest site on Mt. Carmel. These values appear close to SO_4^{2-}- S deposition measured at suburban sites of this study. For cations with few exceptions, bulk deposition was maximum for Ca^{2+} followed by Mg^{2+}, Na^+ and K^+ (Table 49.2). The depositions of all the nutrient elements were uniformly higher in throughfall than in clearfall depositions (Tables 49.2 and 49.3). In a study, conducted in a deciduous forest on the Walker branch watershed, Lindberg and Harriss (1981) recorded 75 per cent of dryfall input when hard woods were in leaf, indicating the importance of aerosol impaction on foliage. Liu *et al.* (2002) have also reported enrichment of throughfall bulk deposition of Ca^{2+}, Na^+, Mg^{2+}, K^+ and SO_4^{2-}- S.

Conclusions

The present study indicates that the bulk atmospheric deposition, both the clearfall and throughfall as observed at different sites are greatly influenced by anthropogenic sources including urban-industrial activities and agricultural practices and by regional wind patterns. Among anions, the deposition was recorded maximum for SO_4^{2-}- S followed by NO_3^- and PO_4^{3-}, whereas among cations, the deposition was maximum for Ca^{2+} followed by NH_4^+ and then Na^+, Mg^{2+} and K^+. The pH of deposition was greatly influenced by the atmospheric loading of anions and base cations. Source oriented loading of base cations showed strong neutralizing effect on the pH of the deposition. Both, pH and nutrient elements remained significantly higher in throughfall than in clearfall. This strong modifying influence of vegetation on atmospheric deposition may leads to long–run consequences on biogeochemical cycling of nutrients with consequent ecosystem level implications even for those areas situated far away from direct human interference. Continuous atmospheric deposition of nutrient aerosols will alter tree leaf microflora, composition of herbaceous vegetation, microbial biomass and activity and mineralization and release of nutrients with long–term effects on structure and composition of terrestrial ecosystems. In addition, direct atmospheric input of nutrient aerosols will change the trophic status of aquatic ecosystems with subsequent change in phytoplankton composition, species diversity and water use. Thus, quantification of air–driven nutrient input need serious attention for forest management as well as for restoration of aquatic ecosystems.

References

Aber, J. D., Nadelhoffer, K. J., Steudler, P. and Melillo, J. M. (1989). Nitrogen saturation in northern forest ecosystems. *Bioscience* (39): 378–386.

Friedland, A. J. and Miller, E. K. (1999). Major elemental cycling in a high elevation Adirondack forest: patterns and changes. 1986–1996. *Ecological Applications* (9): 958–967.

Jain, M., Kulshrestha, U. C., Sarkar, A. K. and Parashar, D. C. (2000). Influence of crustal aerosols on wet deposition at urban and rural sites in India. *Atmospheric Environment* (34): 5129–5137.

Lindberg, S. E. and Harriss, R. C. (1981). The role of atmospheric deposition in an eastern United States deciduous forest. *Water, Air and Soil Pollution* (16): 13–31.

Liu, W., Fox, J. E. D. and Xu, Z. (2002). Nutrient fluxes in bulk precipitation, through fall and stream flow in montane subtropical moist forest on Ailao Mountains in Yunnan, south–west China. *Journal of Tropical Ecology* (18): 527–548.

Miller, E. K., Panek, J. A., Friedlnd, A. J., Kadlecek, J. and Mohnen, V. A. (1993). *Atmospheric deposition to a high elevation forest at Whiteface mountain*, New York, USA. Tellus (45): 209–227.

Pandey, J. and M. Agrawal (1994a). Evaluation of air pollution phytotoxicity in a seasonally dry tropical urban environment using three woody perennials. *The New Phyologist* (126): 53–61.

Pandey, J. and M. Agrawal (1994b). Diurnal and seasonal variations in air pollutant concentrations in a seasonally dry tropical urban environment. *Current Science* (66): 293–303.

Pandey, J. (2005). Evaluation of air pollution phytotoxicity downwind of a phosphate fertilizer factory in India. *Environmental Monitoring and Assessment* (100): 249-266.

Pandey, U. and J. Pandey (2005). The influence of catchment modifications on two freshwater lakes of Udaipur. In: *Urban Lakes in India: Conservation, Management and Rejuvenation* (Part-I). K.K.S.Bhatia and S.D. Khobragade (Eds.) National Institute of Hydrology, Roorkee. pp. 256-262.

Pandey, J. and A. Chasta (2006) Evaluation of air pollution phytotoxicity in urban environment of Udaipur, Rajasthan. *Plant Archives* 6 (1): 93-96.

Pandey, J. and U. Pandey (2009). Accumulation of heavy metals in dietary vegetables and cultivated soil horizon in organic farming system in relation to atmospheric deposition in a seasonally dry tropical region of India. *Environmental Monitoring and Assessment* 148 (1): 61–74.

Rao, P. P. S., Momin, G. A., Safai, P. D., Pillai, A. G. and Khemani, L. T. (1995). Rain water and throughfall chemistry in the Silent Valley forest in South India. *Atmospheric Environment* (29): 2025–2027.

Rossum, J. R. and Villarruz, P. (1961). Suggested methods for turbidimetric determination of sulphate in water. *Journal of American Water Works Association* (53): 873.

Singer, A., Ganor, E., Fried, M. and Shamay, Y. (1996). Throughfall deposition of sulfur to a mixed Oak and Pine forest in Israel. *Atmospheric Environment* (30): 3881–3889.

Singh, R. K. and Agrawal, M. (2005). Atmospheric depositions around a heavily industrialized area in a seasonally dry tropical environment of India. *Environmental Pollution* (138): 142–152.

Swank, W. T. (1984). Atmospheric contributions to forest nutrient cycling. *Water Resources Bulletin* (20): 313–321.

Microbial Biotechnology and Ecology (2011) *Pages* **846–858**
Editors: **Deepak Vyas, G.S. Paliwal, P.K.Khare and R.K Gupta**
Published by: **DAYA PUBLISHING HOUSE, NEW DELHI**

Chapter 50

Trends and Determinants of Health Practices Profile Among the Baigas

☆ ***Arun K. Jain[1] and A.N. Sharma[2]***

[1]*Department of Anthropology and Tribal Development, G.G. University, Bilaspur, C.G.*
[2]*Department of Anthropology, Dr. H.S. Gour University, Sagar – 470 003*

ABSTRACT

The Baigas of Mandla district has a good account of indigenous medicines and they know the medicine for the cure of most each and every type of disease. There are folk healers called guniya who cure disease of village people by giving medicines or performing magico-religious acts. The objective of the present chapter is to study health practices profile among the Baigas of Mandla district (M.P.), India. The present investigation is based on interviews of 400 Baiga households from five different blocks of Mandla district. A sizable medicinal plant wealth exists in Mandla district, which still awaits scientific exploration. The indiscriminate deforestation should be checked, so that rare plants could not become extinct. Promoting the indigenous medicines system of Baigas, can fulfill the World Health Organization's important issue, *i.e.*, people must be involved as partners in the decision making and management process for health at all levels.

Keywords*: Health practices, Indigenous medicines, Baiga, Mandla district.*

Introduction

The history of evolution of medicine is a long story stretching from prehistoric to modern times. The 'art of healing' began thousands of years ago with the primitive man trying to provide relief with his limited knowledge, to the kind in sickness and suffering. In the absence of explanation, disease

* E-mail: arun_raj_jain@yahoo.com

and calamites were attributed to wrath of gods, the invasion of the body of evil spirits or malevolent influence of stars and planets (Park and Park, 1997).

Anthropologist's interest in the study of disease and cure is as old as their interest in the study of tribal culture. Rivers (1924) stated that art of medicine of the people was in some respect more rational than our own, in that its mode of diagnosis and treatment follow more directly from the ideas concerning the causation of disease, even though there are wrong ideas from the civilized point of view (Dwivedi, 2003).

Since long tribal and forests are intertwined related to each other. Forests are not only the source of major and minor forest produces, but they depend much on forest for their day-to-day needs. From the very beginning of human civilization, men depend on nature for his food, shelter and medicine.

It is true that use of medicinal plants for curing disease in human society is as old as existence itself. The earliest mention of use of medicinal plants is found in 'Rigveda', which happens to be the oldest scripture. In 'Rigveda' and 'Charak Samhita', 2000 names of medicinal plants have been listed. Out of which, 1600 species of medicinal plants have so for been established.

Indigenous medicine is to be studied, as medicine in a primarily spoken not written tradition. The importance of tribal medicine and like could draw the attention of Mittal (1979), Mathur (1982), Tiwari (1984), Banerjee and Jalota (1988), Rizvi (1991), Sharma and Sharma (2000), Jain and Sharma (2006), Jain and Sharma (2006), Shukla, Chakravarty and Gautam (2008).

The Baigas of Mandla district has a good account of indigenous medicines and they know the medicine for the cure of most each and every type of disease. There are folk healers called *guniya* who cure disease of village people by giving medicines or performing magico-religious acts. The local people depend for medical cure on indigenous methods. They initially do not prefer to go to allopathic doctors. In case of such diseases, which are beyond the cure of their indigenous remedies, they consult allopathic practitioners, occasionally.

Materials and Methods

The present investigation is based on interviews of 400 Baiga households from five different blocks of Mandla district. Mandla district is located in the east central part of the Madhya Pradesh. It lies between the latitude 220.2′ and 230.22′ north and longitude 800.18′ and 810.50′ east. The total area of the district is 13,269 Sq. Km. The block and villages were selected randomly as per the concentration of blocks. In this regard 80 samples were selected randomly from the five villages of each block and approximately 16 samples were selected randomly from each village. The data were collected from the households of the Baigas of Mandla district, Madhya Pradesh. One sample was collected randomly from each household of randomly selected villages. The present study has been conducted through interview schedule. Simultaneously, group discussions and informal interview methods has been used. Observations have been conducted through semi-participants methods.

Results and Discussions

Keeping in mind these views, an attempt has been made to investigate the indigenous medicines for the cure of different diseases among the Baigas. The observations and results of the study are presented in the following tables:

Table 50.1 shows information regarding type of treatment received by the family members, who feel sick during last one year, it could be seen from the table that maximum individuals received self treatment (36.00), rather than allopathic treatment (33.00) and other peoples were also noticed who do their indigenous or ethno medicines during sickness (31.00). It could be concluded that, 67.00 per cents Baigas used the indigenous or ethno-medicine and self treatment and 33.00 percents Baigas are received allopathic treatment, but allopathic treatment received secondary. The Baigas are firstly preferred indigenous or ethno-medicines and self treatment and secondary preferred allopathic treatment.

Table 50.1: Information Regarding Type of Treatment Received by the Family Members, during Last One Year

Sl.No.	Type of Treatment	AB.	PC.
1.	Allopathic	132	33.00
2.	Indigenous or ethno-medicines	124	31.00
3.	Self treatment	144	36.00
	Total	400	100.00

Table 50.2 shows indigenous medicine used for the cure of fever. It could be seen from the table that Baigas use the root of Jhilmili to get relief from fever.

Table 50.2: Information Regarding Medicine Used for the Cure of Fever

Sl.No.	Name of Indigenous Medicine or Herb (Local name)	Botanical Name	Part of the Herb Used	Method of Applying	Probable Dosages	Duration of Application
1.	Jhilmili	–	Root	Crush it and boil in water	Two times Two spoon	2 Days

Table 50.3 reveals information regarding indigenous medicine used for the cure of Malaria. It could be seen from the table that the different medicines, which are used for the cure of Malaria, are the leaves of Neem, bark of Jamun, seeds and leaves of Banjeet and an equally made mixture of grinded roots of Mainer and Kadi Kudaiya. The method of application can be seen from the table.

Table 50.3: Information Regarding Medicine Used for the Cure of Malaria

Sl.No.	Name of Indigenous Medicine or Herb (Local name)	Botanical Name	Part of the Herb Used	Method of Applying	Probable Dosages	Duration of Application
1.	Neem	*Azadirachta indica* (Meliaceae)	Leaves	Boil the leaves in water and take it	2-3 Times One spoon	2 Days
2.	Jamun	*Eugenia jambolana* (Myrtaccae)	Bark	Grind well to make powder and take it with Gur (Jaggery)	Once in the morning Two spoon	2 Days
3.	Banjeet	–	Seed or leaves	Grind well or boil in water and take the water	Two Times Two Spoon	2 Days
4.	Mainar+ Kadi Kudaiya	–	Root+ Root	Grind well equally both the roots and dissolve in water take the solution orally	Two Times Two spoon	3 Days

Table 50.4 shows information regarding indigenous medicines used for the cure of Typhoid. It could be observed from the table that root of Khirrari and leaves of Amla are used for the cure of Typhoid. Both these are boiled in water, in a clay pot (Khapra) and the resultant solution is taken as such by the patient.

Table 50.4: Information Regarding Medicine Used for the Cure of Typhoid

Sl.No.	*Name of Indigenous Medicine or Herb (Local name)*	*Botanical Name*	*Part of the Herb Used*	*Method of Applying*	*Probable Dosages*	*Duration of Application*
1.	Khirrari+ Amla	– *Phyllanthus emblica* (Euphorbiaceae)	Root+ Leaves	Take same water in a clay pot (Khapra) and boil the root and leaves in it. Take the solution as Medicine.	Once time Two spoon	2-3 Days

Table 50.5 exhibits information regarding indigenous medicines used for the cure of Cough and Cold. It can be observed from the table that root of Akuvan can be used for the cure of Cough and Cold. The leaves of Harrah are also an effective medicine to cure cough and cold.

Table 50.5: Information Regarding Medicine Used for the Cure of Cough and Cold

Sl.No.	*Name of Indigenous Medicine or Herb (Local name)*	*Botanical Name*	*Part of the Herb Used*	*Method of Applying*	*Probable Dosages*	*Duration of Application*
1.	Akuvan (Akaua)	*Calotropis gigantea* (Asclepiadeceae)	Root	Crush the root and boil in one liter water Add sugar and take it	Once time Two spoon	1 Day
2.	Harrah	*Terminalia-chebula* (Combretaceae)	Leaves	Boil the leaves in water and take the water	Two times Two spoon	2 Days

Table 50.6 shows information regarding indigenous medicines used for the cure of wounds, cuts and burns. It can be observed from the table that the bark of Khamher, leaves of Kubbi and leaves of Chirchitta are all effective medicines for the cure of wounds, cuts and burns. All these are applied externally on the wounds etc. and the use of these medicines varies from individual to individual or folk healer to folk healer.

Table 50.6: Information Regarding Medicine Used for the Cure of Wounds, Cuts and Burns

Sl.No.	*Name of Indigenous Medicine or Herb (Local name)*	*Botanical Name*	*Part of the Herb Used*	*Method of Applying*	*Probable Dosages*	*Duration of Application*
1.	Khamher (Gurja)	*Cimelina arborea*	Bark	Grind it to make its powder and apply it on the wound externally (only on the skin).	Two Times	Applied up to the relief
2.	Kubbi	–	Leaves	Crush it to make paste like, and apply it on the wound	Two times	Applied up to the relief
3.	Chirchitta	*Lyciuin barbatum*	Leaves	Crush and apply it on the wound	Three Times	Applied up to the relief

Table 50.7 exhibits information regarding indigenous medicines used for the cure of toothache or caries. It could be seen from the table that the lactin of papaya is an effective medicine for the cure of toothache or caries.

Table 50.7: Information Regarding Medicine Used for the Cure of Toothache

Sl.No.	*Name of Indigenous Medicine or Herb (Local name)*	*Botanical Name*	*Part of the Herb Used*	*Method of Applying*	*Probable Dosages*	*Duration of Application*
1.	Papita	*Carica papaya*	Lactin of the Papaya	Apply the lactin on teeth and fill it in the Tooth depressions/ carries	Two or Three times	2 Days

Table 50.8 reveals information regarding indigenous medicine used for the cure of stomachache or diarrhea. It can be observed from the table that there are mainly five type of medicines used for the same. These are–root of Tinkapari, root of Padhin, root of using these medicines varies from individual to individual or folk healer. The use of specific type of medicine also depends on the availability of herbs etc.

Table 50.8: Information Regarding Indigenous Medicine Used for the Cure of Stomachache or Diarrhoea

Sl.No.	*Name of Indigenous Medicine or Herb (Local name)*	*Botanical Name*	*Part of the Herb Used*	*Method of Applying*	*Probable Dosages*	*Duration of Application*
1.	Tinkhapari	*Oxalis* sp.	Root	Grind it to make the powder and take with water	One or Two times One spoon	Applied up to relief
2.	Padhin	*Mentha arvensis*	Root	Give the patient to chew it and suck the juice	Two times Two spoon	2 Days
3.	Phulchuhi	–	Root	Crush the root and boil in water. Take the water as medicine	Two times Two spoon	1 Day
4.	Tinpariya	*Oxalis corniculata Holarina*	Root	Chew the root to take the juice Grind it to make	Two times One cm. above Two times	2 Days
5.	Kadi Kudaiya	*Intidisen-erica*	Root	The powder and take with water	One spoon	1 Day

Table 50.9 shows information regarding indigenous medicines used for the cure of head-ach. It could be seen from the table that Baigas use the leaves of Bantulsi for the cure of head-ache. The medicine was reported to be very effective for the cure of head-ache.

Table 50.9: Information Regarding Indigenous Medicines Used for the Cure of Head-ache

Sl.No.	*Name of Indigenous Medicine or Herb (Local name)*	*Botanical Name*	*Part of the Herb Used*	*Method of Applying*	*Probable Dosages*	*Duration of Application*
1.	Bantulsi/ Mahatulsi	*Hypits suaveolens*	Leaves	Crush the leaves to get the juice and apply it on the forehead	2-3 times	Apply up the relief

Table 50.10 shows the information regarding about indigenous medicines used for the cure of earache. It can be seen from the table that powder of dried burnt shrub of Sanpavur is an effective medicine, used by the Baigas for the cure of earache.

Table 50.10: Information Regarding Indigenous Medicines Used for the Cure of Earache

Sl.No.	*Name of Indigenous Medicine or Herb (Local name)*	*Botanical Name*	*Part of the Herb Used*	*Method of Applying*	*Probable Dosages*	*Duration of Application*
1.	Sanpavur	–	Dried Bush	Burn the plant to get the dried bush of ash and mix it in mustard oil Pour it in ear of the patient	Two times and Two drops	3 Days

Table 50.11 exhibits information regarding indigenous medicines used for the cure of Oral ulcer. It can be seen from the table that the three important medicines used by the Baigas for the cure of ulcers are bark or leaf of Khirrari, leaves of Amla and honey. The medicines were reported to be very effective for the cure of mouth ulcers.

Table 50.11: Information Regarding Indigenous Medicines Used for the Cure of Dial Ulcer

Sl.No.	*Name of Indigenous Medicine or Herb (Local name)*	*Botanical Name*	*Part of the Herb Used*	*Method of Applying*	*Probable Dosages*	*Duration of Application*
1.	Khirsari	*Euphorbia titirucalli*	Bark or Leaves	Grind and apply on ulcers	Two times	2-3 Days
2.	Amla	*Phyllanthus emblica* (Euphorbiaceae)	Leaves	Eat the leaves orally to take the juice	2-3 times	2 Days
3.	Honey	–	As such	Eat a spoonful honey and take the juice slowly	2-3 times	One dose

Table 50.12 reveals information regarding indigenous medicines used for the cure of blood dysentery. It could be seen from the table that the lactin of Badh and sugar when mixed in equal amount, proves to be a good medicine for the cure of blood dysentery.

Table 50.12: Information Regarding Indigenous Medicines Used for the Cure of Blood Dysentery

Sl.No.	*Name of Indigenous Medicine or Herb (Local name)*	*Botanical Name*	*Part of the Herb Used*	*Method of Applying*	*Probable Dosages*	*Duration of Application*
1.	Badh+ Sugar	*Bengalensis* (Urticaceae)	Lactin of Badh Sugar grains	Mix equal amount of both and take it with warm water	Once	2 Days

Table 50.13 shows information regarding indigenous medicines used for the cure of Jaundice. It could be seen from the table that root of Jhilmili is an effective medicine for the cure of Jaundice, which is used in different ways.

Table 50.13: Information Regarding Indigenous Medicines Used for the Cure of Jaundice

Sl.No.	*Name of Indigenous Medicine or Herb (Local name)*	*Botanical Name*	*Part of the Herb Used*	*Method of Applying*	*Probable Dosages*	*Duration of Application*
1.	Jhilmili	–	Root	Grind it to make its powder and take with water	Two times Two spoons	2 Days

Table 50.14 shows information regarding indigenous medicines used for the cure of vomiting. The Baigas use the medicine for the cure of vomiting, *i.e.*, root of Dooba.

Table 50.14: Information Regarding Indigenous Medicines Used for the Cure of Vomiting

Sl.No.	*Name of Indigenous Medicine or Herb (Local name)*	*Botanical Name*	*Part of the Herb Used*	*Method of Applying*	*Probable Dosages*	*Duration of Application*
1.	Dooba	*Cynodon dactylon*	Root	Grind it and add in water. Take it as medicine	Once time One spoon	Once day

Table 50.15 reveals information regarding indigenous medicines used for the cure of worms of stomach. It could be seen from the table that the seeds of Chewla are used by the Baigas for the cure of stomach worms. The medicine is reported to be very effective.

Table 50.15: Information Regarding Indigenous Medicines Used for the Cure of Worms of Stomach

Sl.No.	*Name of Indigenous Medicine or Herb (Local name)*	*Botanical Name*	*Part of the Herb Used*	*Method of Applying*	*Probable Dosages*	*Duration of Application*
1.	Chewla	*Butea monosperma*	Seeds	Grind seeds to make the power and take with water	Once time One spoon	2 Days

Table 50.16 exhibits information regarding indigenous medicines used for the cure of weakness or body-ache. It could be seen from the table that there are two medicines, which are used by the Baigas to remove weakness. These are very effective medicines.

Table 50.16: Information Regarding Indigenous Medicines Used for the Cure of Weakness

Sl.No.	Name of Indigenous Medicine or Herb (Local name)	Botanical Name	Part of the Herb Used	Method of Applying	Probable Dosages	Duration of Application
1.	Okhad (Badi Davai)	–	Root or Bark	Boil the root or bark in water and add some gur take the solution as medicine	Two times One spoon	2 days
2.	Bijnauri	–	Root	Chew the root to suck the juice	Two times One cm. above	1 Day

Table 50.17 shows information regarding indigenous medicines used for the cure of skin diseases. It could be seen from the table that fat of Goh animal is an effective medicine for the cure of skin diseases. This medicine is very effective.

Table 50.17: Information Regarding Indigenous Medicines Used for the Cure of Skin Diseases

Sl.No.	Name of Indigenous Medicine or Herb (Local name)	Botanical Name	Part of the Herb Used	Method of Applying	Probable Dosages	Duration of Application
1.	Goh (Varanus)	–	Fat of Goh	Apply the fat on affected part externally	Applied up to the relief	Apply up to the relief

Table 50.18 Shows information regarding indigenous medicines used for the cure of wounds, which due to itching, forms locally known as Biskuti, or Baltodh. It could be seen from the table that leaves and seed of Kharenta are applied by the Baigas as an effective medicine.

Table 50.18: Information Regarding Indigenous Medicines Used for the Cure of Wounds Due to Itching

Sl.No.	Name of Indigenous Medicine or Herb (Local name)	Botanical Name	Part of the Herb Used	Method of Applying	Probable Dosages	Duration of Application
1.	Kharenta	*Dodonoea visocosa* (Sapindaceae)	Seed and leaves	Crush the seeds and leaves and apply juice on the part	Two times	2 Days

Table 50.19 shows information regarding indigenous medicines used for the cure of scorpion sting. It could be seen from the table that leaf of grass and leaves or Ber are used as medicine for the cure of scorpion sting among the Baigas.

Table 50.20 shows information regarding indigenous medicines used for the cure of snake bite. It could be seen from the table that the root of Bariyari, which is uprooted in one attempt, and a combination of three medicines–root of Mua, root of Kansa and root of Tumba, used for the cure of snake bite. These medicines are very effective.

Table 50.19: Information Regarding Indigenous Medicines Used for the Cure of Scorpion Sting

Sl.No.	Name of Indigenous Medicine or Herb (Local name)	Botanical Name	Part of the Herb Used	Method of Applying	Probable Dosages	Duration of Application
1.	Grass	–	Leaves	Rub and crush the grass and apply on the bite	Once time	Once
2.	Ber	*Zizyphus-jujube* (Rhamnaceae)	Leaves	Take 1 grm. leaves of Ber	Once time	Once
3.	Guard (bitter)	*Benincasa-hispida*	Root	Crush the root and apply on the bite	Once time	Once

Table 50.20: Information Regarding Indigenous Medicines Used for the Cure of Snake Bite

Sl.No.	Name of Indigenous Medicine or Herb (Local name)	Botanical Name	Part of the Herb Used	Method of Applying	Probable Dosages	Duration of Application
1.	Bariyari	*Sida spinosa*	Root	Take the root and eat it to get the juice	Once a time Two spoons	One day
2.	Mua+ Kansa+ Tumba	–	Root + Root + Root	Grind all the three roots properly. Mix them well and take it.	Once time Two spoon	One day

Table 50.21 reveals information regarding indigenous medicines used for the cure of dog bite. It could be seen from the table that the seeds of Khutlaiya are used by the Baigas as the medicine of dog bite, which is reported to very effective.

Table 50.21: Information Regarding Indigenous Medicines Used for the Cure of Dog Bite

Sl.No.	Name of Indigenous Medicine or Herb (Local name)	Botanical Name	Part of the Herb Used	Method of Applying	Probable Dosages	Duration of Application
1.	Khutlaiya	–	Seeds	Eat the seeds as the medicine	Once a time One spoon	One day

Table 50.22 shows information regarding indigenous medicines used for the cure of bleeding. It can be observed from the table that bark of Gurja is used as an effective medicine to cure the bleeding, where as Chuna and Kattha is also applied by many people for the same purpose. These medicines are very effective.

Table 50.23 shows information regarding use the medicines for anti fertility purpose. It could be seen from the table that bark of white flowers of Tilya are the effective medicine. This medicine is very effective.

Table 50.22: Information Regarding Indigenous Medicines Used for the Cure of Bleeding

Sl.No.	*Name of Indigenous Medicine or Herb (Local name)*	*Botanical Name*	*Part of the Herb Used*	*Method of Applying*	*Probable Dosages*	*Duration of Application*
1.	Gurja	*Lania coromandilica*	Bark	Rub or Grind the bark and apply on the wound	Once a time	One day
2.	Kattha + Chuna	*Acacia catechu*	Powdered bark As it is	Tie the mixture on the bleeding wound	Once a time	One day

Table 50.23: Information Regarding Use the Medicines for Anti Fertility Purpose

Sl.No.	*Name of Indigenous Medicine or Herb (Local name)*	*Botanical Name*	*Part of the Herb Used*	*Method of Applying*	*Probable Dosages*	*Duration of Application*
1.	Tiliya	–	Bark or the white flower	Bark or crush the flower and make its tablets with gur. Take with water or milk	Two tablets in the evening	2 days

Table 50.24 shows information regarding indigenous medicines used for re-fertility purpose. It could be seen from the table that *talka* fruit are the effective medicine of re-fertility purpose. This medicine is very effective.

Table 50.24: Information Regarding Use the Medicines for Re-fertility Purpose

Sl.No.	*Name of Indigenous Medicine or Herb (Local name)*	*Botanical Name*	*Part of the Herb Used*	*Method of Applying*	*Probable Dosages*	*Duration of Application*
1.	Talka	–	Fruit	Eat the Vega	Two times above 50 gm	1 day

Table 50.25 shows information regarding indigenous medicines used for the cure of swelling of body and stomach, which is locally known as *'Fulni'*. It could be seen from the table that this is the common indigenous medicine, which are used for the cure of 'Fulinf is root of Chittawar'. The medicines are very effective.

Table 50.25: Information Regarding Indigenous Medicines Used for the Cure and Stomach Swelling

Sl.No.	*Name of Indigenous Medicine or Herb (Local name)*	*Botanical Name*	*Part of the Herb Used*	*Method of Applying*	*Probable Dosages*	*Duration of Application*
1.	Chittawar	*Plumbago zelaniya*	Root	Grind the root and make its tablets in gur. Take with water	Time 10 mg.	2 Days

Table 50.26 shows information regarding indigenous medicines used for the cure of fever with unconsciousness and tight teeth, which are locally known as Maura. It could be seen from the table that to cure such fever, Kalihari is tied in the neck of the patient. The medicines are very effective.

Table 50.26: Information Regarding Indigenous Medicines Used for the Cure of Fever with Unconsciousness

Sl.No.	*Name of Indigenous Medicine or Herb (Local name)*	*Botanical Name*	*Part of the Herb Used*	*Method of Applying*	*Probable Dosages*	*Duration of Application*
1.	Kalihari	*Gloriosa suberva*	Dried bark	The kalihari in the neck	Once	One day

Table 50.27 shows information regarding use of indigenous medicine used for the cure of 'heat of winter'. In this disease itching and burning sensation is felt in the urine. It could be observed from the table that the root of Tejraj proves to be a good medicine for the cure of this disease, which is reported to be very effective.

Table 50.27: Information Regarding Use of Indigenous Medicine Used for the Cure of Heat of Winter

Sl.No.	*Name of Indigenous Medicine or Herb (Local name)*	*Botanical Name*	*Part of the Herb Used*	*Method of Applying*	*Probable Dosages*	*Duration of Application*
1.	Tejraj	*Peucedanum dhana*	Root	Eat the root as the medicine	Once a time, one cm-above	2 Days

Table 50.28 shows information regarding use the medicines for the cure of cracks. It could be seen from the table that oil of the *wilma* are the effective medicine of cure of the cracks of the heals. This medicine is very effective.

Table 50.28: Information Regarding Use the Medicines for Cracks of the Heals

Sl.No.	*Name of Indigenous Medicine or Herb (Local name)*	*Botanical Name*	*Part of the Herb Used*	*Method of Applying*	*Probable Dosages*	*Duration of Application*
1.	Wilma	–	Fruit	Cut the Wilma fruit, burn the mud pot and collect in the lower side. Lape the hill	Two time	2 days

It could be concluded from the foregoing brief reporting of indigenous practices that:

1. The 46.07 per cent individuals received indigenous or ethno medicines.
2. There are a large number of herbal medicines and plant wealth which should be explored through modern techniques and pharmaceutical investigations.
3. These herbal resources could generate a good source of income for the Baigas of Mandla district.
4. A socio-psychological and therapeutic investigation should be made to find out the reliability of the usefulness of magi-co-religious acts.

5. A proper and reliable list of indigenous medicines with diseases should be proposed for the awareness of the tribals, so that they can uplift their health status without modern medical facilities.
6. The proper and reliable list of indigenous medicines with diseases should be evolved within same ecological conditions.
7. The reported medicinal plants should be further investigated concerning the availability of various species and botanical identification of the therapeutic values through scientific analysis.
8. The Baigas have a good knowledge about the indigenous medicines for anti-fertility.
9. The medicines are used for fever, malaria, cough and cold, wounds, cuts, burns, toothache, stomachache, diarrhoea, headache, earache, ulcers, blood dysentery, jaundice, vomiting, worms of stomach, weakness, body-ache, skin diseases, wounds due to itching, scorpion bite, snake bite, dog bite, bleeding, anti fertility, reflectivity, body or stomach swelling, fever with unconsciousness and tight teeth, typhoid, crack etc. and need extensive scientific investigations for wider spectrum of human welfare.

In short, a sizable medicinal plant wealth exists in Mandla district, which still awaits scientific exploration. The indiscriminate deforestation should be checked, so that rare plants could not become extinct. Promoting the indigenous medicines system of Baigas, can fulfill the World Health Organization's important issue, *i.e.*, people must be involved as partners in the decision making and management process for health at all levels. In the words of Nakajima (1990), "The time has now come to galvanize our efforts. The knowledge and technology already exist, what we need now is determination, courage and foresight. Health is a product of special action. Active community participation and supportive social policies are necessary for progress in health and here in lies our challenge". So, it may be stated from the foregoing brief reporting of indigenous health practices that there are number of indigenous medicines and plant wealth, which should be explored through modern techniques and pharmaceutical investigation. Such attempts will give new material and direction in the field of pharmaceutical researchers.

References

Banerjee, B.G. and Jalota, R. (1977). *Folk Illness and Ethno-medicine*. Northern Book Centre, New Delhi.

Dwivedi, P. (2003). Demographic Profile and Health Care Practices among the Baigas of Samanpur Block of Dindori District, Madhya Pradesh, *Unpublished Dissertation*, Department of Anthropology, Dr. H.S. Gour University, Sagar (M.P.).

Jain, A.K. and Sharma, A.N. (2006). *The Berias (Rai Dancers), Socio-Demographic and Reproductive Health Care Practices*. Sarup and Sons, New Delhi.

Jain, A.K. and Sharma, A.N. (2006). Indigenous Health Care Practices among the Beria Women of Sagar District, M.P. India. In: *Indigenous Health care and Ethno-Medicine*, Edited By, A.N. Sharma, R.K. Goutam and A.K. Gharami, Sarup and Sons, New Delhi, p. 50-53.

Mathur, P.R.G. (1982). Anthropology of Tribal Medicine: Disease and Curing Techniques among the Tribal of North Wynad (Kerla), *Man in India*, 62: 295-312.

Mittal, K. (1979). *Primitive Medicine Versus Modern Medicine among the Santhal*. Dr. of Social Research, 22: 49-54.

Park, J.E. and Park, K. (1977). *Textbook of Preventive and Social Medicine*, Banarsidas Bahanot, Jabalpur.

Rizvi, S.N.H. (1991). Health practices of the Jounsaris: A socio-cultural analysis. In: *Tribal Health: socio-Cultural Dimensions*, Edited by Budhadev Chouhari. Inter India Publications, New Delhi.

Sharma, A.N. and Sharma, N.M. (2000). Indigenous health practices related to fever among Bharias of Patalkot, M.P. *Tribal Health Bulletin*, 6(1): 6-8.

Shukla, R., Chakravarty, M. and Gautam, M.P. (2008). Indigenous medicine used for treatment of gynecological disorders by tribal of Chhattisgarh, India. *Journal of Medicinal Plants Research*, 2(12): 356–360.

Tiwari, S.C. (1984). Socio-cultural and genetico-environmental determinants of tribal health: Measures for health development. In: *Tribal Health in India*, Edited by Salil Basu. Inter India Publications, New Delhi.

Author Index

Adhikary SP, 3
Agrawal Pooja, 571
Akhtar Nasim, 501
Ashu, 766
Atri DC, 853

Banerjee Meenakshi, 34
Behera RK, 780, 827
Bharose Ram, 741, 827
Bhatt RK, 683
Bhattacharya Abhishek, 439
Biradar DP, 484
Byatanal Mahesh B, 472

Chakravarty Neha, 209
Chauksey P, 268
Chaurasia Bhaskar, 201
Choubey Anjuli, 344, 353, 606, 616
Chouhan AKS, 544

David Arun A, 741, 827
De Car Valho MAAP, 484
Dehariya Poonam, 344, 353, 606, 616
Dikshit Anupam, 393
Dwivedi Om Prakash, 256

Goswami HK, 773
Gupta Pushpa, 577
Gupta Rajan Kumar, 60, 94, 225
Gupta US, 94
Gupta Umesh Dutta, 577
Guru SD, 773,

Hegde Ganesh R, 484

Jadhav SK, 724
Jain Arun K, 846
Jain Devendra, 591
Jamaluddin, 29

Jha Anuradha, 209

Kamran Ahsan, 393
Kamalvanshi M, 209
Kango Naveen, 303
Karwa Alka, 452
Kaushik BD, 525
Khare MN, 275
Khare Pramod Kumar, 201, 729
Kumar Anil, 209
Kumar Mukesh, 150, 766
Kunjam S, 724

Lakshman HC, 168, 472

Maya C, 472
Mehta A, 520
Mehta P, 520
Mishra AK, 41, 683
Mishra Meenakshi, 225, 256

Biotechnological potential, 553
Blue green algae, 579
Breeding, 503
Buffer solution, 632

Carbohydrate, 346
Carbon sequestration, 226, 701
Carbonic anhydrase, 440
Carboxy Methyl Cellulose, 631
Cell division, 545
Cellulase enzyme assay, 631
Cellulases, 624
Cellulose powder, 624
Chamaephytes, 729
Charcoal rot, 276
Chemical control, 157
Chemical method, 594
Chitin, 170
Climate moderation, 708
Communicator, 233
Conservation, 30, 320, 484, 708, 773
Crop improvement, 503
Crude extract, 618
Cryopreservation, 505
Culinary awareness, 453
Cultivation, 354
Culture medium, 71
Cyanobacteria, 41, 158, 162
Cyanobacterial toxins, 151
Cylindrospermopsins, 125
Cytotoxic alkaloids, 105
Cytotoxic compounds, 562

Dalbergia sissoo, 714
Damping off, 276
Denitrification, 163
Dermatotoxic alkaloids, 105
Diazotroph, 162, 526
DNA, 172, 546
Dry deciduous forest, 729
Dry tropical region, 837

Ecophysiological effects, 780
Ecosystem, 29
Endo-glucanase, 303
Enzymatic potential, 303
Enzymes, 561
Epiphytes, 729
Esterase, 174
Eucalyptus, 712
Eurythermal fungi, 305
Eutrophication, 766
Exo Glucanase (FPU) activity (FPase), 634

Fatty acids, 559
Fertilizers, 769
Fluxomics, 237
Fly ash, 741
Folicolous fungi, 268
Foot rot, 276
Forest flora, 268
Fungal diseases, 276
Fungitoxic potential, 393
Fungitoxic, 394

Gallic acid, 606
Ganoderma, 457
Genetic diversity, 31
Genomics and proteomics, 236
Genotypic, 41
Geophytes, 729
Glucoamylase, 303
GM crops, 473
Gram staining, 574
Ground water, 827
Growth promoting effect, 528

Habitat diversity, 31
Health practices, 846
Hemicrytophytic, 729
Hepatoprotection, 521
Hepatoprotective drug, 521
Host specificity, 4
Hydrocarbon, 168
Hydrogen metabolism, 61

Immobilization, 78
Immunodulators, 562
Immunostimulation, 459
Indigenous medicines, 846
Intercropping, 217
Isolation, 322

Jagdal region, 724
Jatropha curcas, 169
Jatropha gossypifolia, 169

Laccase, 309
Leucaena leucocephala, 713
Lichen communities, 669
Lipases, 308
Lipids, 173
Live vaccine, 580
Lytic enzymes, 378

Madhuca indica, 169

Marketing strategy, 371
Mass production, 2, 575
Medicinal plant, 189, 521
Metal sequestration, 229
Metallic silver, 593
Microbial diversity, 31
Microcystis, 293
Microorganism, 29
Minerals, 347
Minimum Bacterial Concentration (MBC), 618
Minimum Inhibitory Concentration (MIC), 618
Moisture, 347
Morchell esculenta, 606, 616
Mushroom, 320, 353, 452
Mycoparasitism, 378
Mycorrhiza induced resistance, 232
Myotoxin, 394

Nanoparticles, 591
Nanosilver synthesis, 593
Nanotechnology, 592
Natural resources, 708
Neurotoxic, 101
Neurotoxic Cyanobacteria, 105
Neutraceuticals, 345, 557
Neutral lipids, 173
Nif genes, 21
Nitrates, 768
Nitrogen fixation, 4
Nitroginase, 61
Nodulation and mechanism, 21, 572
Novel vaccine, 580
Nucleic acid, 546
Nutrient ions, 837
Nutrient sequestration, 228

Ofloxacin, 293
Ore refinery, 786
Organogenesis, 504
Ornamental plants, 201

Pathogen interaction, 378
Pathogenic, 616
Perennials, 837
Peroxidase enzyme, 173
Pertoplant, 169
Pesticides, 769
Petrocrops, 169
Phanero therophytic phytoclimate, 729
Phanerophytes, 729
Pharmaceuticals, 345, 554
Pharmacological potential, 452
Phenol, 608
Phenolic quantification, 606
Phenotypic, 41
Phosphates, 768
Photochemical fuel cell, 76
Photosynthetic pigment, 691
Phycobiliprotien, 557
Physico-chemical properties, 831
Phytopathora parasitica, 297
Phytoprotector, 231
Piper bitle, 293
Plant DNA banking, 484
Plant genetic resources, 486
Pollution, 827
Polyphosphatase, 174
Polysaccharides, 171, 559
Population, 321
Preservation, 322, 574
Productivity, 21
Protease, 308
Pseudomonas, 258

Radioprotection, 563
Red mud pond, 786
Red mud waste, 780
Relative density, 203
Reproductive modulators, 563
Restriction enzymes, 561
Reversible hydroginase, 65
Rhizobium, 575
Rhizobium biofertilizer, 3
Rhizodeposition, 227
Rhizosphere, 192
Ricinus communis, 169
RNA, 172
Root rot, 276

Salinity tolerance, 505
Saxitoxins, 101
Secondary metabolites, 379
Seed biology, 780
Silver, 591
Silvipastoral system, 683
Soil amelioration, 698
Soil health, 741, 827
Soil microflora, 724
Soil organic matter, 529
Soil parameter, 830
Soil retention, 770
Somatic embryogenesis, 504

Species diversity, 31
Starch, 170
Stem rot, 276
Sterothermal fungi, 305
Symbiotic Cyanobacteria, 76

Theophytes, 729
Therapeutic, 364
Thermal environment, 36
Thermophilic fungi, 303
Thermophillic Cyanobacteria, 37
Thermotolerant fungi, 305
Toxic blooms, 109
Toxic Cyanobacteria, 107
Toxicity , 770
Transformation, 530
Transgenic plants, 475
Transition thermophiles, 305
Trichoderma species, 293, 378
Tropical lowlands, 162
Tuberculosis, 577

Vaccine, 577
VAM histology, 214
VAM inoculum, 215
VAM morphology, 214
Viscometric Method, 630
Vitamins, 347, 559

Wetland conservation, 773
Wheat, 256
Wilt rot, 276
Woody species, 686

Xylanase, 303

Zooplankton, 127
Zygomycotina, 726